MEDICINAL PLANTS

Bioprospecting and Pharmacognosy

Holy Basil or Tulsi	Neem
Indian Pennywort	**Turmeric**

Innovations in Horticultural Science

MEDICINAL PLANTS

Bioprospecting and Pharmacognosy

Edited by
Amit Baran Sharangi, PhD
K. V. Peter, PhD

A∧P | APPLE
ACADEMIC
PRESS

First edition published 2023

Apple Academic Press Inc.
1265 Goldenrod Circle, NE,
Palm Bay, FL 32905 USA

4164 Lakeshore Road, Burlington,
ON, L7L 1A4 Canada

CRC Press
6000 Broken Sound Parkway NW,
Suite 300, Boca Raton, FL 33487-2742 USA

2 Park Square, Milton Park,
Abingdon, Oxon, OX14 4RN UK

© 2023 by Apple Academic Press, Inc.

Apple Academic Press exclusively co-publishes with CRC Press, an imprint of Taylor & Francis Group, LLC

Library and Archives Canada Cataloguing in Publication

Title: Medicinal plants : bioprospecting and pharmacognosy / edited by Amit Baran Sharangi, PhD, K.V. Peter, PhD.
Other titles: Medicinal plants (2023)
Names: Sharangi, A. B. (Amit Baran), editor. | Peter, K. V., editor.
Series: Innovations in horticultural science.
Description: First edition. | Series statement: Innovations in horticultural science | Includes bibliographical references and index.
Identifiers: Canadiana (print) 20210394072 | Canadiana (ebook) 20210394137 | ISBN 9781774638453 (hardcover) | ISBN 9781774638460 (softcover) | ISBN 9781003277408 (ebook)
Subjects: LCSH: Medicinal plants. | LCSH: Pharmacognosy.
Classification: LCC RS164 .M45 2022 | DDC 615.3/21—dc23

Library of Congress Cataloging-in-Publication Data

Names: Sharangi, A. B. (Amit Baran), editor. | Peter, K. V., editor.
Title: Medicinal plants : bioprospecting and pharmacognosy / edited by Amit Baran Sharangi, K. V. Peter.
Other titles: Innovations in horticultural science.
Description: First edition. | Palm Bay, FL, USA : Apple Academic Press, 2023. | Series: Innovations in horticultural science | Includes bibliographical references and index. | Summary: "With chapters written by scientists from respected institutes and universities around the world, this book looks at the bioprospecting of medicinal plants for potential health uses and at the pharmacognosy of a selection of medicinal and aromatic plants. The book touches on a diverse selection of topics related to medicinal plants. Chapters look at the use of medicinal plants in healthcare and disease management, such as to treat inflammation, anti-hyperglycemia, and obesity and as immunity boosters. The authors also address the conservation, maintenance, and sustainable utilization of medicinal plants along with postharvest management issues. A chapter discusses the use of synthetic seeds in relation to cryopreservation, and a chapter is devoted to the use of microcomputed tomography and image processing tools in medicinal and aromatic plants. Other topics include consumption, supply chain, marketing, trade, and future directions of research. Some specific plants discussed include fennel, basil, clove, ginger, lavender, turmeric, ginsing, and asparagus in connection with their various therapeutic properties, including anti-rheumatic, anti-asthmatic, anti-diabetic, carminative, diuretic, fever-reducing, and hypotensive. Medicinal Plants: Bioprospecting and Pharmacognosy will prove informative for scientists and researchers in medicinal plants as well as for faculty and students, pharmaceutical researchers, and others"-- Provided by publisher.
Identifiers: LCCN 2021060274 (print) | LCCN 2021060275 (ebook) | ISBN 9781774638453 (hardback) | ISBN 9781774638460 (paperback) | ISBN 9781003277408 (ebook)
Subjects: LCSH: Medicinal plants. | Materia medica, Vegetable. | Pharmacognosy. | Botanical drug industry.
Classification: LCC RS431.M37 M44 2022 (print) | LCC RS431.M37 (ebook) | DDC 615.3/21--dc23/eng/20220111
LC record available at https://lccn.loc.gov/2021060274
LC ebook record available at https://lccn.loc.gov/2021060275

ISBN: 978-1-77463-845-3 (hbk)
ISBN: 978-1-77463-846-0 (pbk)
ISBN: 978-1-00327-740-8 (ebk)

INNOVATIONS IN HORTICULTURAL SCIENCE

Editor-in-Chief:

Dr. Mohammed Wasim Siddiqui, Assistant Professor-cum-Scientist
Bihar Agricultural University | www.bausabour.ac.in
Department of Food Science and Post-Harvest Technology
Sabour | Bhagalpur | Bihar | P. O. Box 813210 | INDIA
Contacts: (91) 9835502897
Email: wasim_serene@yahoo.com | wasim@appleacademicpress.com

The horticulture sector is considered as the most dynamic and sustainable segment of agriculture all over the world. It covers pre- and postharvest management of a wide spectrum of crops, including fruits and nuts, vegetables (including potatoes), flowering and aromatic plants, tuber crops, mushrooms, spices, plantation crops, edible bamboos etc. Shifting food pattern in wake of increasing income and health awareness of the populace has transformed horticulture into a vibrant commercial venture for the farming community all over the world.

It is a well-established fact that horticulture is one of the best options for improving the productivity of land, ensuring nutritional security for mankind and for sustaining the livelihood of the farming community worldwide. The world's populace is projected to be 9 billion by the year 2030, and the largest increase will be confined to the developing countries, where chronic food shortages and malnutrition already persist. This projected increase of population will certainly reduce the per capita availability of natural resources and may hinder the equilibrium and sustainability of agricultural systems due to overexploitation of natural resources, which will ultimately lead to more poverty, starvation, malnutrition, and higher food prices. The judicious utilization of natural resources is thus needed and must be addressed immediately.

Climate change is emerging as a major threat to the agriculture throughout the world as well. Surface temperatures of the earth have risen significantly over the past century, and the impact is most significant on agriculture. The rise in temperature enhances the rate of respiration, reduces cropping periods, advances ripening, and hastens crop maturity, which adversely affects crop productivity. Several climatic extremes such as droughts, floods, tropical cyclones, heavy precipitation events, hot extremes, and heat waves cause a negative impact on agriculture and are mainly caused and triggered by climate change.

In order to optimize the use of resources, hi-tech interventions like precision farming, which comprises temporal and spatial management of resources in horticulture, is essentially required. Infusion of technology for an efficient utilization of resources is intended for deriving higher crop productivity per unit of inputs. This would be possible only through deployment of modern hi-tech applications and precision farming methods. For improvement in crop production and returns to farmers, these technologies have to be widely spread and adopted. Considering the above-mentioned challenges of horticulturist and their expected role in ensuring food and nutritional security to mankind, a compilation of hi-tech cultivation techniques and postharvest management of horticultural crops is needed.

This book series, Innovations in Horticultural Science, is designed to address the need for advance knowledge for horticulture researchers and students. Moreover, the major advancements and developments in this subject area to be covered in this series would be beneficial to mankind.

Topics of interest include:

1. Importance of horticultural crops for livelihood
2. Dynamics in sustainable horticulture production
3. Precision horticulture for sustainability
4. Protected horticulture for sustainability
5. Classification of fruit, vegetables, flowers, and other horticultural crops
6. Nursery and orchard management
7. Propagation of horticultural crops
8. Rootstocks in fruit and vegetable production
9. Growth and development of horticultural crops
10. Horticultural plant physiology
11. Role of plant growth regulator in horticultural production
12. Nutrient and irrigation management
13. Fertigation in fruit and vegetables crops
14. High-density planting of fruit crops
15. Training and pruning of plants
16. Pollination management in horticultural crops
17. Organic crop production
18. Pest management dynamics for sustainable horticulture
19. Physiological disorders and their management
20. Biotic and abiotic stress management of fruit crops
21. Postharvest management of horticultural crops
22. Marketing strategies for horticultural crops
23. Climate change and sustainable horticulture
24. Molecular markers in horticultural science
25. Conventional and modern breeding approaches for quality improvement
26. Mushroom, bamboo, spices, medicinal, and plantation crop production

BOOKS IN THE SERIES

- **Spices: Agrotechniques for Quality Produce**
  Amit Baran Sharangi, PhD, S. Datta, PhD, and Prahlad Deb, PhD

- **Sustainable Horticulture, Volume 1: Diversity, Production, and Crop Improvement**
  Editors: Debashis Mandal, PhD, Amritesh C. Shukla, PhD, and Mohammed Wasim Siddiqui, PhD

- **Sustainable Horticulture, Volume 2: Food, Health, and Nutrition**
  Editors: Debashis Mandal, PhD, Amritesh C. Shukla, PhD, and Mohammed Wasim Siddiqui, PhD

- **Underexploited Spice Crops: Present Status, Agrotechnology, and Future Research Directions**
  Amit Baran Sharangi, PhD, Pemba H. Bhutia, Akkabathula Chandini Raj, and Majjiga Sreenivas

- **The Vegetable Pathosystem: Ecology, Disease Mechanism, and Management**
  Editors: Mohammad Ansar, PhD, and Abhijeet Ghatak, PhD

- **Advances in Pest Management in Commercial Flowers**
  Editors: Suprakash Pal, PhD, and Akshay Kumar Chakravarthy, PhD

- **Diseases of Fruits and Vegetable Crops: Recent Management Approaches**
  Editors: Gireesh Chand, PhD, Md. Nadeem Akhtar, and Santosh Kumar

- **Management of Insect Pests in Vegetable Crops: Concepts and Approaches**
  Editors: Ramanuj Vishwakarma, PhD, and Ranjeet Kumar, PhD

- **Temperate Fruits: Production, Processing, and Marketing**
  Editors: Debashis Mandal, PhD, Ursula Wermund, PhD, Lop Phavaphutanon, PhD, and Regina Cronje

- **Diseases of Horticultural Crops: Diagnosis and Management, Volume 1: Fruit Crops**
  Editors: J. N. Srivastava, PhD, and A. K. Singh, PhD

- **Diseases of Horticultural Crops: Diagnosis and Management, Volume 2: Vegetable Crops**
  Editors: J. N. Srivastava, PhD, and A. K. Singh, PhD

- **Diseases of of Horticultural Crops: Diagnosis and Management, Volume 3: Ornamental Plants and Spice Crops**
  Editors: J. N. Srivastava, PhD, and A. K. Singh, PhD

- **Diseases of Horticultural Crops: Diagnosis and Management, Volume 4: Important Plantation Crops, Medicinal Crops, and Mushrooms**
  Editors: J. N. Srivastava, PhD, and A. K. Singh, PhD

- **Biotic Stress Management in Tomato**
  Editors: Shashank Shekhar Solankey, PhD, and Md. Shamim, PhD

- **Medicinal Plants: Bioprospecting and Pharmacognosy**
  Editors: Amit Baran Sharangi, PhD, and K. V. Peter, PhD

- **Tropical and Subtropical Fruit Crops: Production, Processing, and Marketing**
  Editors: Debashis Mandal, PhD, Ursula Wermund, PhD, Lop Phavaphutanon, PhD, and Regina Cronje

ABOUT THE EDITORS

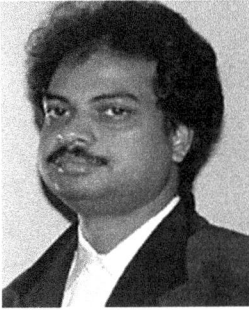

Amit Baran Sharangi, PhD
Professor and former Head,
Department of Plantation, Spices,
Medicinal and Aromatic Crops,
Faculty of Horticulture,
BCKV (Agricultural University),
Nadia, West Bengal, India

Amit Baran Sharangi, PhD, is a Professor in Horticultural Science and former Head of the Department of Plantation, Spices, Medicinal and Aromatic Crops in the Faculty of Horticulture at Bidhan Chandra Krishi Viswavidyalaya (Agricultural University), India. He has been teaching for 23 years and was instrumental in the process of coconut improvement leading to the release of a variety Kalpa Mitra from the Central Plantation Crops Research Institute. He spent time at several laboratories around the world, including the laboratories of Professor Cousen in Melbourne, Australia; Professor Picha in the USA; and Dr. Dobson in the UK. He has published about 85 research papers in peer-reviewed journals, 60 conference papers, and 26 books with reputed publishers including Springer Nature. He has also published chapters in books published from Springer, CRC Press, Nova Science Publishers, and others. One of his papers was ranked among the top 25 articles in ScienceDirect. Presently he is associated with 50 international and national journals in a variety of roles, including editor-in-chief, associate editor, regional editor, technical editor, editorial board member, and reviewer.

Professor Sharangi has visited abroad extensively on academic missions and has received several international awards, such as the Endeavour Post-doctoral Award (Australia), INSA-RSE (Indian National Science Academy) Visiting Scientist Fellowship (UK), Fulbright Visiting Faculty Fellowship (USA), Achiever's Award (Society for Advancement of Human and Nature, Man of the Year—2015 (Cambridge, UK), Outstanding Scientist (Venus International Foundation), Bharat Ratna Mother Teresa Gold Medal Award in 2020, etc. He has delivered invited lectures in the UK, USA, Australia, Thailand, Israel, and Bangladesh on several aspects of herbs and spices. Professor

Sharangi is associated with a number of research projects as Principal and Co-Principal Investigator. He is an elected Fellow of the WB Academy of Science and Technology (WAST) and a Fellow of the International Society for Research and Development (ISRD, UK), the Society for Applied Biotechnology (SAB), International Scientific Research Organisation for Science, Engineering and Technology (ISROSET), Academy of Environment and Life Sciences (AELS), and the Scientific Society of Advanced Research and Social Change (SSARSC). He is an active member of many other science academies and societies, including the New York Academy of Science (NYAS), World Academy of Science, Engineering and Technology (WASET), African Forest Forum (AFF), Association for Tropical Biology & Conservation (ATBC, USA), Society of Pharmacognosy & Phytochemistry (SPP),International Society for Noni Science (ISNS),SAS Eminent Fellow, to name a few.

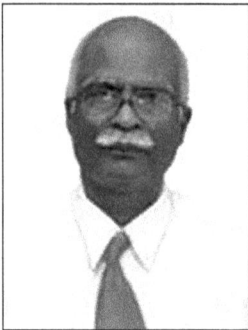

K. V. Peter, PhD

K. V. Peter, PhD, is a former Vice-Chancellor at Kerala Agricultural University (KAU) India; Director of the ICAR–Indian Institute of Spices Research, Calicut; Director of Research at KAU; and Professor of Horticulture since 1979. He is an acknowledged teacher and science manager. A postgraduate from G.B. Pant University of Agriculture and Technology Pantnagar, Uttarakhand (1969–1975), he is associated with the development of biotic stress resistant varieties in chili (Pant-CI, Pant-C2), tomato (Sakthi), and brinjal (Surya) grown throughout the Indian sub-continent.

Dr. Peter is the recipient of several national awards, including the Rafi Ahmad Kidwai Award; Dr. M H Marigowda National Award; HSI-Shiva Sakthi Award for Life Time Contributions to Vegetable Research; recognition award and Dr. K. Ramiah Memorial Award of the National Academy of Agricultural Sciences, New Delhi; PNASF Gold Medal; KRLCC Award–2015 for contributions to Education and Science; Suganda Bharati Award–2015 from the Indian Society of Spices Calicut; gold medal from the Indian Society of Vegetable Science, Varanasi; VEGNET International Award–2018 from PNASF Bengaluru; and Gurupuja Puraskar–2018 from the KCBC Media Commission. He is a fellow of the National Academy of Agricultural Sciences, New Delhi; National Academy of Sciences,

Prayagraj, U.P.; National Academy of Biological Sciences, Chennai; International Society of Noni Science, Chennai; Indian Academy of Horticulture Science, New Delhi; and Confederation of Horticultural Associations of India (CHAI), New Delhi.

National Book Trust (NBT), New Delhi, published his authored book Plantation Crops in three languages (English, Hindi, and Malayalam) and Tuber Crops in English. Woodhead Publishing (Elsevier) published the three-volume series titled Handbook of Herbs and Spices, now revised into two volumes (2012). ICAR New Delhi published the book Genetics and Breeding of Vegetable Crops. New India Publishing Agency, New Delhi, published Dr. Peter's 12-volume series Horticultural Science; five-volume series Underutilized and Underexploited Horticultural Crops, two volumes of Science of Horticulture, much read Climate Resilient Horticultural Crops of Future and Production and Protection of Horticultural Crops. Dr. Peter's co-edited the books Agricultural Bioinformatics, Fruit Breeding, Horticulture Biotechnology-Methods and Applications, and Ornamental Horticulture. Daya Publishing Company (Astral International Pvt. Ltd.) published six volumes of Biodiversity of Horticultural Crops, two volumes of Future Crops and the books Nutri-Horticulture and Horticultural Crops for Nutritional Security. He co-edited the book Handbook of Industrial Crops with late Prof. V. L. Chopra, published by Taylor and Francis, USA. Brillion Publishing, New Delhi, published his edited books Horticultural Crops of High Nutritive Values, Horticultural Sciences: Perspectives and Applications, Phytochemistry of Fruits and Vegetables, Zero Hunger India: Policies and Perspectives, Vegetables for Nutrition Security, and Origin and Biological Diversity of Horticulture Crops. He published monographs on jackfruit and mangoes in two volumes, co-edited by him, and published by Studium Press, LLC, which are informative and widely read. Orient Blackswan UK (Universities Press Hyderabad) published the books Biotechnology: Methods of Gene Transfer and Tissue Culture and Spiders of India, along with renowned scientists in the respec-tive fields. With Prof. G. R. Rout, Dr. Peter co-edited Genetic Engineering in Horticultural Crops, published by Elsevier USA.

Dr. Peter is a trustee of Federal Aswas Trust, Ernakulam, India. He is chairman and member of scientific review committees of several research institutes. He is also President of the Indian Society of Vegetable Science and Editor (Horticulture) of Agricultural Research, published by the National Academy of Agricultural Sciences, New Delhi. He is also President of the Kerala Chapter of the National Academy of Sciences.

CONTENTS

CONTRIBUTORS

Md. Nasim Ali
Department of Agricultural Biotechnology, Faculty of Agriculture, Bidhan Chandra
KrishiViswavidyalaya, Mahanpur, Nadia, West Bengal, India, E-mail: nasimali2007@gmail.com

M. Anitha
Department of Plantation, Spices, Medicinal, and Aromatic Crops, Dr. YSRHU, Venkataramannagudem,
West Godavari, Andhra Pradesh – 534101, India, E-mail: anithamajji01@gmail.com

Meraj Alam Ansari
ICAR Research Complex for NEH Region, Manipur Center, Imphal – 795004, Manipur, India

K. Nirmal Babu
Director, ICAR Indian Institute of Spices Research, Calicut – 673012, Kerala, India

Vikas Bajpai
Sophisticated Analytical Instrument Facility, CSIR-Central Drug Research Institute,
Lucknow – 226001, Uttar Pradesh, India

Dnyaneshwar U. Bawankule
Molecular Bioprospection Department, Central Institute of Medicinal and Aromatic Plants, Near
Kukrail Picnic Spot, P.O. CIMAP, Lucknow – 226015, Uttar Pradesh, India

Navneeta Bhardavaj
Department of Biotechnology, Delhi Technological University, Shahbad Daulatpur Village, Rohini,
New Delhi – 110042, India, E-mail: navneetab@dce.ac.in

Karanpreet Singh Bhatia
Department of Biotechnology, Delhi Technological University, Shahbad Daulatpur Village, Rohini,
New Delhi – 110042, India

Preeti Chandra
Sophisticated Analytical Instrument Facility, CSIR-Central Drug Research Institute,
Lucknow – 226001, Uttar Pradesh, India

Ankan Das
Department of Horticulture, Institute of Agricultural Science, University of Calcutta,
51/2 Hazra Road, Kolkata – 700019, West Bengal, India

Suddhasuchi Das
Department of Plantation, Spices, Medicinal, and Aromatic Crops, Faculty of Horticulture,
Bidhan Chandra Krishi Viswavidyalaya (Agricultural University), Mohanpur – 741252,
West Bengal, India

N. Surmina Devi
College of Horticulture and Forestry, CAU, Pasighat, Arunachal Pradesh – 791102, India

Sunita Singh Dhawan
Biotechnology Division, CSIR-Central Institute of Medicinal and Aromatic, Lucknow, Uttar Pradesh,
India, E-mails: sunsdhawan@gmail.com; sunita.dhawan@cimap.res.in

Minoo Divakaran
Assistant Professor, Providence Women's College, Calicut – 673009, Kerala, India,
E-mail: minoodivakaran@gmail.com

Shalini Dixit
Analytical Chemistry Department, CSIR-Central Institute of Medicinal and Aromatic Plants,
Near Kukrail Picnic Spot, P.O. CIMAP, Lucknow – 226015, Uttar Pradesh, India

Mahomoodally Mohamad Fawzi
Department of Health Sciences, Faculty of Science, University of Mauritius, Réduit – 80837,
Mauritius; Institute of Research and Development, Duy Tan University, Da Nang – 550000, Vietnam,
E-mails: f.mahomoodally@uom.ac.mu; mohamadfawzimahomoodally@duytan.edu.vn

Pankhuri Gupta
Biotechnology Division, CSIR-Central Institute of Medicinal and Aromatic, Lucknow, Uttar Pradesh,
India

Yogini S. Jaiswal
Center for Excellence in Post-Harvest Technologies, North Carolina Agricultural and Technical State
University, The North Carolina Research Campus, 500 Laureate Way, Kannapolis, NC – 28081, USA,
E-mail: yoginijaiswal@gmail.com; ysjaiswa@ncat.edu

A. C. Jnanesha
CSIR-Central Institute of Medicinal and Aromatic Plants, Research Center, Boduppal, Hyderabad,
Telangana – 500092, India, E-mail: jnangowda@gmail.com

Jyotshna
Analytical Chemistry Department, CSIR-Central Institute of Medicinal and Aromatic Plants,
Near Kukrail Picnic Spot, P.O. CIMAP, Lucknow – 226015, Uttar Pradesh, India

Hiroko F. Kasai
Faculty of Pharmaceutical Sciences, Hoshi University, Ebara 2-4-41, Tokyo – 142-8501, Japan,
E-mail: kasai@hoshi.ac.jp

Palakdeep Kaur
Department of Pharmaceutical Sciences and Technology, Maharaja Ranjit Singh Punjab Technical
University (MRSPTU), Bathinda, Punjab – 151001, India

Fahad Khan
Department of Biotechnology, Noida Institute of Engineering Technology, 19, Knowledge Park-II,
Institutional Area, Greater Noida, Uttar Pradesh – 201306, India

Mohammad Mustufa Khan
Department of Basic Medical Sciences, Integral Institute of Allied Health Sciences & Research
(IIAHS&R) and Department of Biochemistry, Integral Institute of Medical Sciences & Research
(IIMS&R), Integral University, Lucknow, Uttar Pradesh – 226026, India

Navneet Kishore
Department of Chemistry, University of Delhi, North Campus, New Delhi – 110007, India

Pintubala Kshetri
ICAR Research Complex for NEH Region, Manipur Center, Imphal – 795004, Manipur, India

Ashish Kumar
CSIR-Central Institute of Medicinal and Aromatic Plants, Research Center, Boduppal, Hyderabad,
Telangana – 500092, India

Brijesh Kumar
Sophisticated Analytical Instrument Facility, CSIR-Central Drug Research Institute, Lucknow – 226001, Uttar Pradesh, India, E-mail: gbrikum@yahoo.com

Raj Kishori Lal
Division of Genetics and Plant Breeding, CSIR-Central Institute of Medicinal and Aromatic, Lucknow, Uttar Pradesh – 226015, India

Debashis Mandal
Department of Horticulture, Aromatic, and Medicinal Plants, Mizoram University, Aizawl – 796004, Mizoram, India, E-mail: debashismandal1982@gmail.com

Uttam Kumar Mandal
Department of Pharmaceutical Sciences and Technology, Maharaja Ranjit Singh Punjab Technical University (MRSPTU), Bathinda, Punjab – 151001, India, E-mail: mandalju2007@gmail.com

Manas Mathur
School of Agriculture, Suresh Gyan Vihar University, Jaipur, Rajasthan – 302017, India

Priyanka Maurya
Analytical Chemistry Department, CSIR-Central Institute of Medicinal and Aromatic Plants, Near Kukrail Picnic Spot, P.O. CIMAP, Lucknow – 226015, Uttar Pradesh, India

Kalkame Ch. Momin
College of Horticulture and Forestry, CAU, Pasighat, Arunachal Pradesh – 791102, India, E-mail: kalkame.momin@gmail.com

Dhiman Mukherjee
Directorate of Research, Bidhan Chandra Krishi Viswavidayalaya, Kalyani – 741235, West Bengal, India, E-mail: dhiman_mukherjee@yahoo.co.in

Sunil Kumar Nagar
School of Agriculture, Suresh Gyan Vihar University, Jaipur, Rajasthan – 302017, India

Pratibha Pandey
Department of Biotechnology, Noida Institute of Engineering Technology, 19, Knowledge Park-II, Institutional Area, Greater Noida, Uttar Pradesh – 201306, India

K. V. Peter
Former Vice-Chancellor, Kerala Agricultural University, and Former Director, ICAR Indian Institute of Spices Research, Calicut; Mullakkara, P O Mannuthy – 680651, Thrissur, Kerala, India

Rakesh Kumar Prajapat
School of Agriculture, Suresh Gyan Vihar University, Jaipur, Rajasthan – 302017, India

M. Chandra Surya Rao
MS Swaminathan School of Agriculture, Centurion University of Technology and Management, Odisha – 761211, India

Syandan Sinha Ray
IRDM Faculty Center, Ramakrishna Mission Vivekananda Educational and Research Institute, Ramakrishna Mission Ashrama, Narendrapur, Kolkata – 700103, West Bengal, India

Arpita Roy
Department of Biotechnology, Delhi Technological University, Shahbad Daulatpur Village, Rohini, New Delhi – 110042, India

Subhra Saikat Roy
ICAR Research Complex for NEH Region, Manipur Center, Imphal – 795004, Manipur, India,
E-mail: subhrasaikat@gmail.com

Sumana Sarkhel
Department of Human Physiology, Vidyasagar University, Paschim Midnapore – 721102, West Bengal,
India, E-mail: sumana.sarkhel@yahoo.in

Karuna Shanker
Analytical Chemistry Department, CSIR-Central Institute of Medicinal and Aromatic Plants,
Near Kukrail Picnic Spot, P.O. CIMAP, Lucknow – 226015, Uttar Pradesh, India,
Tel.: +91-522-2718580, Fax: +91-522-2719072, E-mail: kspklko@yahoo.com

A. B. Sharangi
Department of Plantation, Spices, Medicinal, and Aromatic Crops, Faculty of Horticulture,
Bidhan Chandra Krishi Viswavidyalaya (Agricultural University), Mohanpur, Nadia – 741252,
West Bengal, India, E-mail: absharangi@gmail.com

Susheel Kumar Sharma
ICAR Research Complex for NEH Region, Manipur Center, Imphal – 795004, Manipur, India

Jugreet Bibi Sharmeen
Department of Health Sciences, Faculty of Science, University of Mauritius, Réduit – 80837, Mauritius

Kulveer Singh
School of Agriculture, Suresh Gyan Vihar University, Jaipur, Rajasthan – 302017, India

Pratibha Singh
Sophisticated Analytical Instrument Facility, CSIR-Central Drug Research Institute,
Lucknow – 226001, Uttar Pradesh, India

Thangjam Surchandra Singh
ICAR Research Complex for NEH Region, Manipur Center, Imphal – 795004, Manipur, India

Madhumita Srivastava
Analytical Chemistry Department, CSIR-Central Institute of Medicinal and Aromatic Plants,
Near Kukrail Picnic Spot, P.O. CIMAP, Lucknow – 226015, Uttar Pradesh, India

Nupur Srivastava
Analytical Chemistry Department, CSIR-Central Institute of Medicinal and Aromatic Plants,
Near Kukrail Picnic Spot, P.O. CIMAP, Lucknow – 226015, Uttar Pradesh, India

D. V. Swami
Department of Plantation, Spices, Medicinal, and Aromatic Crops, Dr. YSRHU, Venkataramannagudem,
West Godavari, Andhra Pradesh – 534101, India

K. Tamreihao
ICAR Research Complex for NEH Region, Manipur Center, Imphal – 795004, Manipur, India

Tarun Kumar Upadhyay
Parul Institute of Applied Sciences and Animal Cell Culture and Immunobiochemistry Lab,
Parul University, Vadodara, Gujarat – 391760, India, E-mails: tarun_bioinfo@yahoo.co.in;
tarunkumar.upadhyay18551@paruluniversity.ac.in

Akhilesh Kumar Verma
Department of Chemistry, University of Delhi, North Campus, New Delhi – 110007, India,
Phone: 011-27666648, E-mail: akhilesh682000@gmail.com

Leonard L. Williams
Center for Excellence in Post-Harvest Technologies, North Carolina Agricultural and Technical State University, The North Carolina Research Campus, 500 Laureate Way, Kannapolis, NC – 28081, USA, E-mail: llw@ncat.edu

Tiqiao Xiao
Shanghai Synchrotron Radiation Facility (SSRF), Shanghai Advanced Research Institute, Chinese Academy of Sciences, Pudong, Shanghai – 201203, P. R. China

Yanling Xue
Shanghai Synchrotron Radiation Facility (SSRF), Shanghai Advanced Research Institute, Chinese Academy of Sciences, Pudong, Shanghai – 201203, P. R. China

ABBREVIATIONS

2D	two-dimensional
ACE	angiotensin-converting enzyme
AD	Alzheimer's disease
ADA	American Diabetes Association
AEs	adverse events
AFLP	amplified fragment length polymorphism
AFM	atomic force microscopy
AI	alloxan-induced
AIRE	autoimmune regulator
ALT	alanine aminotransferase
AMPK	AMP-activated protein kinase
API	active pharmaceutical ingredient
ASI	acne severity index
AST	aspirate aminotransferase
ATHT	aroma touch hand technique
ATM	African traditional medicine
BCR	benefit: cost ratio
BMI	body mass index
BP	blood pressure
BPSDs	behavioral and psychological symptoms of dementia
BSI	botanical survey of India
CAD	collision-activated dissociation
CAD	computer-aided design
CAGR	compound annual growth rate
CAM	complementary and alternative medicine
CAR	carboxene
CB	cannabinoid
CE	collision energy
CERPA	center for research, planning, and action
CHM	Chinese herbal medicine
CIMAP	center for medicinal and aromatic plants
CINV	chemotherapy-induced nausea and vomiting
CM	critical material attributes
CMAI	Cohen-Mansfield agitation inventory

COC	copper oxychloride
CPP	critical process parameters
CPT-1	carnitine palmitoyl transferase-1
CQA	critical quality attributes
CRP	count and C-reactive protein
CSIR	Council for Scientific and Industrial Research
CST	celastrol
CT	computed tomography
CTM	Chinese traditional medicine
CVD	cardiovascular diseases
CXP	cell exit potential
DBP	diastolic blood pressures
DMAPR	directorate of medicinal and aromatic plants
DMPO	5,5-dimethyl-1-pyrroline-N-oxide
DP	declustering potential
DVB	divinylbenzene
EBP	enhancer-binding protein
EGCG	epigallocatechin-3-gallate
EI	emergence index
EOs	essential oils
EP	entrance potential
EPF	herbaepimedii flavonoids
ESR	electron spin-resonance
ET	*Eucalyptus tereticornis*
EXAFS	extended X-ray absorption fine structure
FBG	fasting blood glucose
FIA	flow injection analysis
FRHLT	foundation for the revitalization of local health tradition
GACP	guidelines on good agricultural and collection practices
GAD	generalized anxiety disorder
GAPs	good agricultural practices
GC	gas chromatography
GC-MS	gas chromatography-mass spectrometry
GDM	gestational diabetes mellitus
GE	germination energy
GK	glucokinase
GMPs	good manufacturing practices
GR	germination recovery
GWAS	genome-wide association studies

HAMA	Hamilton anxiety scale
HBOA	4-hydroxy-2-benzoxazolone
HCA	hydroxy citric acid
HDL	high-density lipoprotein
HePG	hepatocellular carcinoma cell line
HLTE	hind limb tonic extensions
HPLC	high-performance liquid chromatography
HPTLC	high-performance thin-layer chromatography
HPX	hypoxanthine
ICAR	Indian Council of Agricultural Research
ICFRE	Indian Council of Forestry Research and Education
ICMR	Indian Council of Medical Research
IHM	Indian herbal medicine
IMCU	intermediate care unit
iNOS	inducible nitric oxide synthase
ISM&H	Indian System of Medicine and Homeopathy
ISO	International Organization for Standardization
ISSR	inter simple sequence repeats
ITS2	internal transcribed spacer
IUCN	international union for conservation of nature
LC-MS	liquid chromatography-mass spectrometry
LOD	limit of detection
LOQ	limit of quantitation
LOS	lipoprotein oxidation susceptibility
LSAs	lateral surface area
MAC	mono carbonyl analogs of curcumin
MAHD	microwave-assisted hydrodistillation
MAPs	medicinal and aromatic plants
MAS	marker-assisted selection
MES	maximal electroshock
MIDAS	migraine disability assessment scores
MODY	maturity-onset diabetes of the young
MPCA	medicinal plants conservation areas
MPCDA	medicinal plants conservation and development areas
MRI	magnetic resonance imaging
MSI	mass spectrometry imaging
MSP	minimum support price
NaF	sodium fluoride
NCD	noncommunicable disease

NCRAE	natural chicoric acid extract
NDDS	novel drug delivery system
NE	northeast
NEH	north eastern Himalayan
NEHU	North-Eastern Hill University
NIH	National Institutes of Health
NMPB	National Medicinal Plant Board
NO	nitric oxide
NSAIDs	non-steroidal anti-inflammatory drugs
OGTT	oral glucose tolerance test
PCS	photon correlation spectroscopy
PDMS	polydimethylsiloxane
PE	phosphatidylethanolamine
PEPCK	phosphoenolpyruvate carboxykinase
PET	positron emission tomography
PG	prostaglandin
PPAR	peroxisome proliferator-activated receptor
PPAR-g	peroxisomes proliferating activated receptor-g
PTs	pentacyclic triterpenes
PTZ	pentylenetetrazole
PUFA	polyunsaturated fatty acids
QBD	quality by design
R&D	research and development
RAPD	random amplified polymorphic DNA
RBF	round bottom flask
RFLP	restriction fragment length polymorphism
RIs	retention indices
ROS	reactive oxygen species
RRL	regional research laboratories
SAIDs	steroidal anti-inflammatory drugs
SAR	structure-activity relationship
SBP	systolic blood pressures
SEM	scanning electron microscopy
SHRs	spontaneously hypertensive rats
SNP	single nucleotide polymorphism
SOD	superoxide dismutase
SOSA	superoxide scavenging activity
SPC	soy phosphatidylcholine
SPME	solid-phase microextraction

SREBP	sterol regulatory element-binding protein
SR-FTIR	synchrotron radiation-Fourier transform infrared
SSR	simple sequence repeats
SSRF	shanghai synchrotron radiation facility
STZ-I	streptozotocin induced
STZN-I	streptozotocin nicotinamide induced
TCM	traditional Chinese medicine
Td	trichosanthes dioica
TD-GC-MS	thermal desorption-gas chromatography-mass spectrometry
TEM	transmission electron microscope
TERI	The Energy Resources Institute
TG	total glycerides
TKR	total knee replacement
TLC	total acne lesions counting
TM	traditional medicine
TNF-alpha	tumor necrosis factor-alpha
TPC	total phenolic contents
UAE	ultrasound-assisted extraction
UCP-1	uncoupling protein 1
VAS	visual analog scale
VEGF	vascular endothelial growth factor
VMAT	vesicular monoamine transporter
WBC	white blood cell
WHO	World Health Organization
XAS	X-ray absorption spectroscopy
XOD	xanthine oxidase
XRF	X-ray fluorescence
μ-XRF	X-ray micro fluorescence

FOREWORD

Medicinal and aromatic plants (MAPs) and their derivatives are looked upon not only as a source of affordable wellness and health care but also as important commodity items of national and international trade and commerce. As per WHO estimates, traditional indigenous medicines, mostly plant drugs, cater to the health needs of nearly 80% of the world population. The Asian continent has a long tradition of use of herbal medicines and sustains a very rich diversity of medicinal and aromatic plants. About 8,000 flowering plants, 650 lichens, 650 algae, 200 pteridophytes, and 150 bryophytes are attributed to medicinal and healing properties. Among indigenous systems of medicine (Ayurveda, Siddha, Unani, tribal folklore Ayurvedic), the system alone prescribes 1000 single drugs and over 8,000 compound formulations of recognized merit. Many medicinal and aromatic plants are sources of clinically useful prescription drugs used in modern systems of medicine. Incredible knowledge on phytomedicine is acquired in non-coded form by tribals and rural communities practicing folklore medicine. Serious attempts are made to collect, verify, validate, and add value to such knowledge by conferring intellectual property rights to tribals and "vaidhyas." India is one of the mega-biodiversity centers of the world, with a wealth of 15,000–20,000 medicinal plants species. It harbors two of the 25 hotspots of the world—Eastern Himalayas and Western Ghats; around 70% of medicinal plants species in India are in tropical forests across Eastern Himalayas and the Western Ghats, Vindhyas, Chota Nagpur Plateau, and Aravalis.

The significance and importance of medicinal and aromatic plants have risen in recent years due to changes in lifestyles, and nutrition habits, migration to urban areas, and even inter boundaries.

The present book, *Medicinal Plants: Bioprospecting and Pharmacognosy*, with 22 chapters authored by working scientists and professors in the field, assumes academic and scientific importance. Apple Academic Press is doing a great service by publishing and disseminating the information on bioprospecting and pharmacognosy of medicinal and aromatic plants at a time when new lifestyle diseases are taking a toll.

I congratulate Prof. Amit Sharangi, BCKVV, West Bengal, and Prof. K. V. Peter, President Indian Society of Vegetable Science Varanasi, for conceiving the topic, compilation, and editing this important book.

—M. S. Swaminathan
Founder Chairman, M. S. Swaminathan Research Foundation
Ex-Member of Parliament (Rajya Sabha)
3rd Cross Road, Taramani Institutional Area, Chennai (Madras) – 600113,
Tamil Nadu, India
Phone: +91-44-2254 2790, 2254 1698, Fax: +91-44-2254 1319,
E-mail: founder@mssrf.res.in, swami@mssrf.res.in

PREFACE

The first wealth is health.
−Emerson

Nutrition is the only remedy that can bring full recovery and can be used with treatment. Remember, food is our best medicine.
−Bernard Jensen

Let food be thy medicine and medicine be thy food.
−Hippocrates

The above quotes link medicinal plants to health, wellness, and nutrition. The much-read *Hortus Malabaricus*, conceived by Hendrik van Rheede in 1678–1693, comprising 12 volumes, gave a detailed account of flora, 742 plants of health and wellness value. The Food and Agriculture Organization (FAO) reported over 50,000 plants across the world with medicinal values and uses. The FAO defined a medicinal plant as the one used to maintain health, to be administered for a specific condition in modern medicine or in traditional medicine (TM). The Royal Botanical Gardens, Kew, UK, listed 17,810 plant species with medicinal uses.

Medicinal plants and their derivatives are looked upon as sources of affordable health care but also as important commodity items of international trade and commerce. The World Health Organization (WHO) lists about 8000 flowering plants, 650 lichens, 650 algae, 200 pteridophytes, and 150 bryophytes having medicinal properties. WHO estimates that traditional medicines, mostly plant-based drugs, cater to the health needs of nearly 80% of the world population. The oriental systems of natural medicine-folklore, Ayurveda, Siddha, Unani, tribal, Tibetan, Chinese, make use of plant-based drugs for health and wellness. The oriental system focuses on protective and preventive medicines rather than curative, which leaves few side effects and allergens. In addition, they are natural products, non-narcotic, easily accessible at affordable prices, and eco-friendly.

Medicinal plants are increasingly being recognized as a source of significant livelihood opportunities for many rural communities, especially primitive forest-dwellers, landless poor, and marginalized farmers. Medicinal plants and their by-products constitute an important part of the foreign trade in major growing countries, including India. The global medicinal plants' industry is valued at over US$ 60 billion, mainly in the form of pharmaceuticals (US$ 40 billion), spices and herbs (US$ 5.9 billion), natural cosmetics (US$ 7 billion), and essential oils (US$ 4 billion) and growing at 7% per year and expected to reach US$ 5 trillion by 2050.

There are challenges to the maintenance, collection, conservation, value addition, and products development in the regime of climate change, encroachment and destruction of natural forest habitats, new lifestyles, migration, and the emergence of viral diseases like COVID-19. For instance groundwater tables going down and seawater incursion occurs, and the natural habitat of medicinal plants is disturbed.

The present edited book *Medicinal Plants: Bioprospecting and Pharmacognosy* is a compilation of 22 chapters authored by 62 well-known scientists working at reputed research institutes and universities in five countries. Bioprospecting of medicinal plants tries to look forward to the potential uses of the present and future. Pharmacognosy reveals descriptive pharmacology dealing with crude drugs and samples. Medicinal and aromatic plants (MAPs), like fennel, basil, clove, turmeric, Indian ginsing, asparagus, Khejri, and many herbs are narrated for therapeutic uses like antirheumatics, anti-asthmatics, anti-diabetics, carminatives, diuretics, febrifuges, and hypotensive.

We are grateful to all the 62 contributors for their time, patience, and academic acumen. We appreciate the publishers Apple Academic Press and Taylor and Francis for support, guidance, and publication.

—Editors

CHAPTER 1

MEDICINAL PLANTS: PERSPECTIVES AND RETROSPECTIVES

D. V. SWAMI,[1] M. ANITHA,[1] M. CHANDRA SURYA RAO,[2] and A. B. SHARANGI[3]

[1]Department of Plantation, Spices, Medicinal, and Aromatic Crops, Dr. YSRHU, Venkataramannagudem, West Godavari, Andhra Pradesh – 534101, India, E-mail: anithamajji01@gmail.com (M. Anitha)

[2]MS Swaminathan School of Agriculture, Centurion University of Technology and Management, Odisha-761211, India

[3]Department of Plantation, Spices, Medicinal, and Aromatic Crops, Bidhan Chandra Krishi Viswavidyalaya, Mohanpur, Nadia, West Bengal – 741252, India

ABSTRACT

Medicinal plants or medicinal herbs have been used for humankind to cure different ailments since long back. It has a fascinating history intertwined with the culture, tradition, and well-being of human civilizations across the world. Plants synthesizing secondary metabolites known as phytochemicals were identified to use in different therapeutic actions. These phytochemicals are essentially the active constituents present in different parts of the medicinal plants with immense biological properties. With all these attributions over the time and wisdom of human civilization, these special groups of plants and their products have been gradually elevated from their folkloric usage to modern medicinal essentialities. Phyto-chemical contents and pharmacological actions of the plants need to be reassessed thoroughly by means of scientific research keeping their efficacy and safety as the main focus. Both for biodiversity enrichment and increased human empowerment, widespread growing, and processing of medicinal plants is altogether necessary.

Phytochemical and biochemical research with an incessant attempt for the revitalization of natural drugs and its legacy for the well-being of humanity at large is precisely the need of the hour.

1.1 INTRODUCTION

Humans mostly depend on nature for basic needs like cloth, shelter, and food in addition to flavored items, drugs, insecticides, fertilizers, and so on. Especially before the introduction of chemical medicines or synthetic medicines, man relied on the therapeutic and restorative properties of medicinal plants. To the increasing global population, plants having medicinal properties play an important role in providing health care systems to ailing people across the world. Traditional medicine (TM) owes a lot to medicinal plants, which are often regarded as its moral fiber. On average, more than 3.3 billion people in developing countries utilize medicinal plants for regular consumption. In India and China, the usage of herbs as medicine has a continuous and consistent history. Recognition of medicinal plants, their drug identification, and further development through cultivation need financial support. Its role after drug development to aid in the industrialization of developing nations is very much defined (WHO, 1998).

The remarkable contribution of medicinal plants in the preparation of fine chemicals, cosmetics, pharmaceutical drugs, industrial raw materials, etc., to aid in diversified industries as commercially acclaimed. Experimental findings and accumulated wisdom over hundreds to thousands of years explored the beneficial characteristics of such plants. In about 2600 BC, the earliest reports were carved on cuneiform clay tablets in Mesopotamia. Identified materials from these tablets were oils of *Commiphora* species (Guggul), *Cedrus* species (Cedar), *Glycyrrhiza glabra* (Liquorice), *Papaver somniferum* (Poppy capsule), and *Cupressus sempervirens* (Cypress). These medicinal plant species are still being used today for the diverse range of cure of diseases, including cold and cough to inflammation and parasitic infections (Fakim, 2006). Southeast Asian countries like China, India, Japan, Pakistan, Sri Lanka, and Thailand are rich in TM practice. Out of the total medicinal consumption in China, about 40% is attributed to traditional tribal medicines, whereas, in Japan, the demands of herbal medicinal preparations exceed those of mainstream pharmaceutical products.

Production of safe medicine is mostly dependent on medicinal plant species (Hamburger and Hostettmann, 1991). Today we have plenty of contemporary drugs, but still, it is genuinely urgent to discover, rediscover, and develop newer therapeutic drugs to overcome the newly evolved diseases. It is identified that acceptable therapy is available only for about 30% of human ailments. Hence, it is imperative to go for new drug discovery at the utmost. The major advantages of traditional herbal medicines in modern-day drug industries are their minor side effects as well as the synergistic activity of different compounds in combination. Moreover, they are easily accessible, within reach of the common man, are time-tested, and thus considered to be much safer than modern synthetic drugs. For the same reasons, the World Health Organization (WHO) endorses and promotes the use of herbal drugs in different national health care programs. The extensive research works on the pharmacological activity of phytochemicals offer effective solutions to certain diseases on which the synthetic drug industry has failed to afford. Examples for such type of research work are on plant species like *Artimisia annua, Cathranthus roseus, Taxus species, Lantana camara, Bacopa species,* etc. Certain plant species which were earlier considered as poisonous or useless, are now identified to contain compounds of high drug value and are considered as medicinal herbs of great significance is *Lantana camara.*

1.2   HISTORY

The early history of human healthcare is precisely the history of herbal medicine. The first book written about plant species having medicinal value is the texts of the *Ebers Papyrus* (by George Ebers written in 1500 BC), in which the names of many medicinal plant species had appeared (Ackerknecht, 1973). Herbs and spices, used mainly in culinary preparations, and several weed species can be used as herbal medicines, such as clove, cinnamon, pepper, cardamom, turmeric, ginger, many seed spices in one hand, and nettle, dandelion, and chickweed in other (Stepp, 2004). Paleolithic people had knowledge about traditional herbal medicine, as confirmed through the plant samples from prehistoric burial sites are among the lines of evidence that. For instance, the 60,000-year-old Neanderthal burial site, "Shanidar IV" in northern Iraq, had yielded large amounts of pollen from eight plant species, of which seven species are now used as herbal remedies. A mushroom, found in a body of 5,000 years old, was probably used against whipworm (Capasso, 1998).

Herbalism was flourished in the Islamic world, particularly in Baghdad and in Al-Andalus. Among many works on medicinal plants, Abulcasis (936–1013) of Cordoba wrote *The Book of Simples*, and Ibn al-Baitar (1197–1248) recorded hundreds of medicinal herbs such as aconitum, nux vomica, and tamarind in his *Corpus of Simples*. Avicenna, in his written document *The Canon of Medicine*, incorporated many plants in 1025. Further, the authors Abu Rayhan, Biruni, Ibu Zuhur, and Peter of Spain (*https://en.wikipedia.org/wiki/Medicinal_plants*) popularized pharmacopeia. In the Greek civilization, Hippocrates (470–471 BCE) was the first to reject divine causality and developed a new approach to cure diseases based on scientific scrutiny of the human body. Hippocrates is nowadays considered the Father of Medicine. His work was based on religion and, in opposition with the mainstream Aesclepian beliefs, marked the first split between science-based and religion-based medicine. The *Hippocratic Oath* is a moral orientation and dictum in the medical community worldwide. Galen, a Greek physician, afterward contributed to the growth of Greek medical wisdom contained by the Roman Empire, which became the leading mention for more than a millennium (Tipton, 2014).

The Chinese book by Emperor Shen Nung circa 2500 BC, on roots and grasses named *Pen T'Sao*, mentioned about 365 drugs (dried parts of different medicinal plants). Many of them are used nowadays, e.g., *Rhei rhisoma*, camphor, *Thea folium, Podophyllum*, the great yellow gentian, ginseng, jimson weed, cinnamon bark, and ephedra (Wiart, 2006). The Ebers Papyrus from ancient Egypt describes over 800 prescriptions referring to 700 herbal medicines like pomegranate, castor oil, aloe, senna, garlic, onion, fig, willow, coriander, etc. Wormwood (*Artemisia*) and common centaury (*Centaurium umbellatum* Gilib) were used against fever, garlic against intestine parasites, opium, henbane, deadly nightshade, and mandrake were used as narcotics, sea onion, celery, parsley, asparagus, and garlic as diuretics, oak, and pomegranate as astringents (Gorunovic, 2001). Dioscorides (famous Greek physician), who worked in the Roman army, documented more than 1,000 recipes for the preparation of different herbal medicines using 600 medicinal plant species in *De Materia Medica* book (60 AD). This formed the basis for medical pharmacopeias for about 1,500 years. Pharmacologically active substances in nature are searched and identified by drug researchers through the use of ethnobotany, and hundreds of useful compounds have been discovered. These compounds include aspirin, digoxin, quinine, and opium which are essentially plant-based and mostly belong to four major biochemical classes, namely alkaloids, glycosides, polyphenols, and terpenes (*https://en.wikipedia.org/wiki/Medicinal_plants*).

In herbal medicine, different medicinal plant species are used for the study of their medicinal behavior and benefits from various plant parts like fruit, seed, stem, bark, flower, leaf, stigma, root, gums, as well as non-woody portions (The term herb commonly referring to all of these). The specific uses of plant species are manifold like food, medicine, or perfume and also involve diversified activities like spiritual, religious, cultural, and social (https://www.nhp.gov.in/introduction-and-importance-of-medicinal-plants-and-herbs_mtl). The isolation of serpentine during 1953 from *Rauwolfia serpentina* root was remarkable in the history of hypertension treatment and lowering of blood pressure (BP). During 1971–1990 fresh phytochemicals, i.e., artemisinin, zguggulsterone, ginkgolides, lectinam, E-guggulsterone, teniposide, ectoposide, plaunotol, and nabilone came into existence globally. The medicines appeared during 1991–1995 include irinotecan, toptecan, paclitaxel, and gomishin, etc. The Vinblastine was used for the treatment of leukemia in children, Hodgkins choriocarcinoma, non-Hodgkins lymphomas was isolated from the *Catharanthus roseus* (Jones, 1998). Development of morphine on an industrial scale by E. Merck, Germany in 1826 sets the foundation of commercialization of plant-derived drugs (Galbley and Thiericke, 2000).

In Bible and the Talmud (a Jewish book), there are memorandum of aromatic plants like myrtle. Indian holy book, the Vedas, mentioned about handling and curing of illness through medicinal plants. Numerous spices viz, pepper, cardamom, turmeric, etc., popularized over the world were actually originated from India (Tucakov, 1971). "The Rig-Veda, perhaps the oldest repository of human knowledge written in 4500–1600 BC, claims about 99 medicinal plants. The Yajurveda is having description of 82 plants and the Sam Veda too have the description of medicinal plants. Atharva Veda deals with 288 plants having medicinal value and was used for deadly diseases" (Kapoor, 2003). Other early works on the medicinal value of different plant species are: Charaka Samhita, Susruta Samhita, Vagbhata I, Vagbhata II, Vagbhata III, Madhavakara, Cakrapanidatta, Sarangadhara, and Bhava Misra.

1.2.1 MEDICINAL HERBS AND TRADITIONAL MEDICINE (TM)

The WHO defines traditional medicinal plants as natural plant materials mainly used for the treatment of diseases without or minimal processing at a local or regional scale (Tilburt and Kaptchuk, 2008). Traditional herbal medicines have been used by the developing and developed countries for a considerable period only due to their having comparatively less side effects (Czygan, 2004). Various other traditional drugs are now being widely used in Asia, Africa, and Latin America to meet basic health needs and are often referred to as complementary or alternative medicine. In the United States, the National Institutes of Health (NIH) uses the complementary and alternative medicine (CAM) to address the health systems, practices, and products. Traditional Chinese Medicine (TCM), amongst all traditional medical systems, is currently the most admired system followed by Indian medicine across the world. Medicinal plants are an obvious and unique input used among all treatments in TM systems (Liu, 2011).

1.2.2   MEDICINAL PLANTS AND CONVENTIONAL MEDICINE

The significance of medicinal plants and their products is gradually more accredited and the public reliance is persistently gaining ground (Zargari, 1992). The clinical, pharmaceutical, and chemical studies of these plant-derived traditional drugs fine-tuned many accepted drugs of earlier days or olden days viz., Aspirin (from willow bark), Digoxin (from Foxglove), Morphine (from Opium poppy), Quinine (from Cinchona skin) and Pilocarpine (from Maranham Jaborandi). Currently, it is anticipated that over 50% of the available drugs are somehow originated from medicinal plants (Yarnell and Abascal, 2002; Harvey, 2008). Phytotherapy is widely being used across the world with a continuously upward trend. Therefore, the worldwide preference of synthetic compounds has been twisted to herbal drugs, as a revert to the nature to turn away diseases and pains (Fabricant and Farnsworth, 2001).

1.2.3   DRUG DISCOVERY OF NATURAL COMPOUNDS

Plant materials are initially tested to find out their pharmaceutical purposes, if any. The extract is fractioned, the active compound is isolated and identified and may be used for further research when they are found pharmaceutically promising during testing. Bioassay-guided fractionation is followed throughout each step of decomposition and isolation. Every so often, a direct product isolation method is also used despite the consequences of bioactivity.

But this procedure can sometimes be sluggish and fruitless, without securing isolation of lead compounds from screening (Sarker and Nahar, 2013).

1.3   DISTRIBUTION OF MEDICINAL PLANTS

India has a geographic area of about 329 million hectares which is 2.4% of world's total area, but comprising with 8% of global diversity. It is fortunately endowed with such a wide spectrum of biodiversity basically due to three foremost bio-geographic realms, the Indo-Malayan, Eurasian, and Afro tropical. India is acknowledged for one of 12 mega diversity hot spot regions of the world. Other countries included are Brazil, Columbia, China, South Africa, Mexico, Venezuela, Indonesia, Ecuador, Peru, USA, and Bolivia (Scippmann, 2002). Medicinal plants were distributed in diverse habitats, in the Indian subcontinent, nearly 70% of these found in tropical forests of both Eastern and Western Ghats, Chota Nagpur plateau, Aravalis, Vindhyas, and the Himalayas. Among the Himalayas, Kashmir Himalayan region, settled within the Northwestern folds is recently designated as global biodiversity hotspot of the Himalayas (Mittermeier et al., 2005). Indian forests comprise 90% of medicinal plant species diversity, whereas 10% of known medicinal plants are restricted to non-forest habitats.

Some of the most important medicinal plant species present in Kashmir, Himalaya region are *Dioscorea deltoidea, Rheum Emodi, Arnebia benthamii, Inula racemosa, Datura stramonium Aconitum heterophyllum, Artemisia spp., Podophyllum hexandrum, Juniperus macropoda, Hypercum perforatum, Hyoscyamus niger, Saussurea spp., Picrorhiza kurroa,* etc. Important aromatic plant species include in this area are Caraway (*Carum carvi*), Saffron (*Crocus sativus*), Siya zira (*Bunium persicum*), Garlic (*Allium sativa*), Coriander (*Coriandrum sativum*), Mint (*Mentha spp.*), Fennel (*Foeniculum vulgare*), and Hare's foot (*Trigonella foenum-graecum*). Hamilton (2003) reported that 44% of flora present in India is used for medicinal purpose.

1.4   GLOBAL SCENARIO

There is an extensive global trade for traditional herbal medicine. But lack of proper knowledge to identify the medicinal value of individual plants and paucity of reliable statistics make it difficult to turn this trade international in real sense. Products prepared from medicinal plant species often include gums, spices, teas, infusions, cosmetics, and insecticides.

It has been said that as many as 35,000–70,000 of plant species have been used for medicinal purposes (Farnsworth et al., 1992). Tropical and sub-tropical continents, like Africa and South East Asia, majority of people resort to traditional herbal medicine for the majority of their primary healthcare needs. There is also a strong tradition of using herbal medicine in parts of Europe, like Germany, France, and Eastern Europe. The herbal sector is growing day by day, increasing by 12–15% by value per year in countries like the UK, USA, and Italy (Abrahams, 1992). Based on a review of a recent consultancy report by Mc Alpine Thorpe and Warrier (1992) more than, 2000 and 220 herbal medical companies are present in Europe and the USA, respectively; this review states that Germany is having largest market for herbal medicine in global wide, with annual sales of $1.2 billion representing 25% of the national pharmaceutical market. The USA is the next largest market with sales of $480 million. Several studies have reported international trade in medicinal and aromatic plants (MAPs) at a value of 1,224 million US$, with Japan and USA as top consumers and China and India as the largest producers, followed by Hong Kong, USA, Germany, Rep. of Korea, Canada, and Poland. Recent reports suggest five major trade centers of MAPs, worldwide, viz. USA, Hong Kong, Germany, Rep. of Korea, and China. The total trades in MAPs have increased from US$ 2.4 billion in 1996 to US$ 6.2 billion in 2013 with an annual growth rate of 5.4% in the past 18 years. It is reported that a growth rate of 10.7% is registered in this segment in recent years. As per trade value, USA, and Hong Kong are the largest importers accounting 13.5% and 13.3%, respectively, followed by Japan and Germany (9.1% each).

Recently, WHO reported that 80% of people worldwide rely on traditional herbal medicines for their primary health care needs and around 21,000 plant species have the potential as medicinal plants. As per data available, over 75% of the world population relies mainly on plants and plant extracts for their health needs. In the United States, plant drugs were earlier found to constitute lesser percentages of the total drugs, but gradually in an increasing trend. Whereas, in countries like India and China, the contribution of the same is comparatively high. Thus, the medicinal plants species play a major role in the economy of many countries in the world (https://www.nhp.gov.in/introduction-and-importance-of-medicinal-plants-and-herbs_mtl) (Table 1.1).

TABLE 1.1   Status of Useful Medicinal Plant Species Present in the World

Country	Medicinal Plant Species	Percentage Contribution Over Total Number of Plant Species
China	4,941	18.9
India	3,000	20.0
Indonesia	100	4.4
Malaysia	1,200	7.7
Nepal	700	10.0
Pakistan	300	6.1
Philippines	850	9.5
Sri Lanka	550	16.6
Thailand	1,800	15.5
Vietnam	1,800	17.1
USA	2,564	11.8
World	72,000	

Source: Hamilton (2003).

On an average 72,000 plant species are used for medicinal purpose (Tables 1.1 and 1.2) in global scale. According to International Union for Conservation (IUCN), 1,500 species are documented as medicinal plant species, 3,000 medicinal plant species are globally traded and 900 species are cultivated (Scippmann et al., 2006).

TABLE 1.2   Medicinal Plant Species Recorded from Different Countries

Country or Region	Identified Medicinal Plants Species Number
China	11,146
India	7,555
Mexico	2,237
North America	2,572
World wide	52,896

Source: Hamilton (2003).

Around 70–90% of the medicinal plants are collected from the wild. 50–70% of medicinal plant biomass is sourced from wild collections only. By collecting medicinal plant species from wild making, they threatened (Rao and Rajput, 2010).

1.5   INDIAN SCENARIO

India is one of the top mega diversity centers of the world with a distinctive wealth of 15,000–20,000 medicinal plant species. Out of 25 hot spots available in the world, India harbors two, namely, Eastern Himalayas and Western Ghats. Around 70% of medicinal species in India are found in the tropical forests extended across Eastern and Western Ghats, *Vindhyas*, Chota Nagpur Plateau and *Aravalis*. Rest 30%, usually obtained in temperate and alpine areas of higher attitudes, are found more potent in their medicinal activity. Habit analyzes of enlisted medicinal species found in India indicate that about 1/3rd are trees, 1/3rd shrubs, and climbers and the remaining, herbs, and grasses. Fabaceae, Poaceae, Asteraceae, Euphorbiaceae, Rubiaceae, Acanthaceae, Apocynaceae, Convolvulaceae, Malvaceae, Solanaceae, and Cucurbitaceae are the foremost plant families contributing to medicinal plant wealth. India precisely encompass 10 bio-geographical zones, i.e., Trans Himalayan zone, Himalayan zone, Desert zone, Semi-arid zone, Western Ghats, Deccan Peninsula, Gangetic Plains, North East India, Andaman, Nicobar, and Laccadive islands and Coastal zone. A few key medicinal species representing these zones are *Ephedra gerardiana, Aconitum* sp., *Citrullus* sp., *Commiphora wightti, Coscinium fenestratum, Pterocarpus santalinus, Rauvolfia serpentina, Smilax* sp., *Calophyllum inophyllum* and *Rhizophora* sp.

So far as the medicinal and aromatic plant-based commodities are concerned, India is the second-largest exporter after China. India's major export in MAPs include, *Psyllium* (seed+husk), Senna leaves and pods, Galangal rhizomes, Zedoary roots, Sandalwood chips and dust, *Vinca rosea* leaves, tukmaria (*Ocimum basillicum*), etc., whereas, Cubeb, Chirata, and Garcinia are the major ones that are imported (Table 1.3).

TABLE 1.3   Area, Production, and Productivity of Important MAPs Commercially Cultivated in Different States in India

Crops	Area (ha)	Production (tons)	Productivity (kg ha^{-1})
Kerala			
Plumbago (*Plumbago rosea*)	40	400	10,000 (fresh root)
Aromatic ginger (*Kaempferia galangal*)	40	100	2,500 (dry rhizome)
Vetiver (*Vetiveria zizanioides*)	200	1,100	5,500 (root)
Citronella species	80	96	120 (oil)

TABLE 1.3 *(Continued)*

Crops	Area (ha)	Production (tons)	Productivity (kg ha^{-1})
Round-rooted galangal (*Kaempferia rotunda*)	12	120	10,000 (fresh rhizome)
Rajasthan			
Opium poppy (*Papaver somniferum*)	8,461	506.00	59.38 (latex)
Isabgol (*Plantago ovata*)	81,538	41,721.00	512
Henna (*Lawsonia inermis)*	42,339	26,027.00	614
Bishop's Weed (*Trachyspermum ammi*)	10,753	5,784.00	538
Fenugreek (*Trigonella foenum-graecum*)	45,138	54,559.00	1,208
Indian Ginseng (*Withania somnifera*)	2,010	1,620.00	806
Safed musli (*Chlorophytum borivilianum*)	1,012	316.00	312
Rose (*Rosa* spp.)	1,100	13,200.00	12,000
Garden Cress (*Lepidium sativum*)	8,450	2,704.00	320
Chhattisgarh			
Lemongrass (*Cymbopogon flexuosus*)	2,248	–	51,261
Vetiver (*Vetiveria zizanioides*)	1,022	–	11,987
Aloe (*Aloe barbadensis*)	784	–	7,139
Safed musli (*Chlorophytum borivilianum*)	293	–	190
Sweet flag (*Acorus calamus*)	148	–	528
Snakeroot (*Rauvolfia serpentina*)	29	–	531
Citronella (*Cymbopogon* species)	3,289	–	12,140
Indian Ginseng (*Withania somnifera*)	176	–	236
Patchouli (*Pogostemon cablin*)	200	–	76
Senna (*Senna angustifolia*)	24	–	26
Rosha grass (*Cymbopogon martinii* var *motia*)	1,631	–	2,939
Others	2,279	–	4.360

TABLE 1.3   *(Continued)*

Crops	Area (ha)	Production (tons)	Productivity (kg ha⁻¹)
Andhra Pradesh			
Aloe (*Aloe barbadensis*)	60.81	1,064.21	17,500 (leaf)
King of bitters (*Andrographis paniculata*)	120.00	264.00	2,200 (herbage)
Satavary (*Asparagus racemosus*)	20.00	875.00	43,750 (fleshy root)
Senna (*Senna angustifolia*)	17.54	35.09	2,000 (leaf, flower, and pod)
Coleus (*Coleus barbatus*)	752.19	1,034.26	1,375 (Root)
Glory lily (*Gloriosa superba*)	8.22	24.66	3,000 (fleshy root)
Tulsi (*Ocimum sanctum*)	62.00	387.50	6,250 (herbage)
Long pepper (*Piper longum*)	1400.00	2,100.00	1,500 (Fruit and root)
Snake root (*Rouvolfia serpentina*)	12.00	30.00	2,500 (root)
Indian ginseng (*Withania somnifera*)	1,250.73	1,188.19	950 (root)
Sweet flag (*Acorus calamus*)	2.00	17.50	8,750 (root)
Velvet bean (*Mucuna pruriens)*	83.67	177.80	2,125 (seeds)
Indian gooseberry (*Emblica officinalis*)	91.26	182.53	2,000 (fruit)
Neem (*Azadirachta indica*)	16.00	244.80	15,300 (leaf)
Ashoka (*Saraca asoca*)	269.99	–	–(bark)

Source: State Departments/DMAPR, Anand (2011–2012).

1.6   SOCIO-CULTURAL ASPECTS

Almost every group of around 2,000 ethnic groups in the world has its own traditional medical knowledge and experiences (Liu et al., 2005). The technologies for domestication are to be developed and be attuned to the specific social values and livelihood assets of intended groups (Weirsum, 1997). Main scope of cultivating medicinal plants is its contribution towards poverty alleviation. Pioneering the domestication of medicinal plants should not be considered as a mere process of transfer of professionally developed cultivation techniques, but rather as a process of change in institutionally ingrained local resource use and management practices. In Kenya, Maasai tribe heavily depends on indigenous medicine as primary healthcare (Kiringe,

2005). Around 90% of their people rely on herbal medicine only and have immense knowledge on ethnomedicinal practices to treat and handle assorted illness both in humans as well as livestock. The existence and survival of TM depends on the diversity of plant species and associated acquaintance concerning their usage as medicine in local people. So, traditional as well as knowledge regarding plant species are vital to the herbal medicine trade and pharmaceutical industry.

The Ayurvedic system of medicine was accomplished in Indian continent, where three humors-phlegm, bile, and flatulence along with those of hot and cold are believed to be crucial. Chinese system of medicine also works in the same principle, and it is supposed that the balance between hot and cold of the body is the base of health. For example, when a man is fainted with sunstroke, a food item like plant soup is given which are cold to the body. And, for instance, when a mother gives birth to a child, she has to eat heat-treated products like meat. In some cultures, there is a religious belief that supernatural powers and spirits will affect the human body and those *Gods* or *Spirits* were the major cause of illness (Ember et al., 2015). Plants which are medicinally important are included in Indian cultural and religious rituals, e.g., *Ficus religiosa, Azadirachta indica, Cynodon dactylon, Artemesia sp, Calotropis gigantea,* etc. In some festivals associated with Hindu belief, plants which are medicinally valuable symbolize God and sacredness, e.g., *Aegle marmelos* (bael), *Ocimum sanctum* (tulasi) (Prakash, 2013). The particular implication of socio-cultural aspects is that medicinal plants conservation improves rural livelihoods, culture, and economy (Hamilton, 2004).

1.7 FOLKLORE, TRADITIONAL MEDICINE (TM), AND USES

The WHO first officially recognized the importance of TM as a source of one of the primary health care systems in 1978 at its Alma Ata Conference (Dey et al., 2007). TM as an easy way of curing of diseases/healing wounds has long been followed by the tribes or communities using locally accessible medicinal herbs flora coupled with their traditional wisdom and passing the same down to new generations year after year. It is by far the oldest form of health care in the world taking care of prevention and treating of physical as well as mental illness. Different societies are historically developed using various healing methods to combat a variety of life-threatening diseases. TM still plays a pivotal role in many countries and is known as complementary and alternative, or ethnic medicine (WHO, 2000). But appropriate processing and dose regulation through clinical trials is required to acquire drug efficacy to minimize side effects and to increase its precision over particular disease as well.

Usage of TM is mostly prevalent in rural areas in different parts of the world. Rural people have immense knowledge in folklore and ethno-medicine. Individual tribes and ethnic communities in diverse parts of the world conserved different versions of native or customary knowledge (Bruchac, 2014). There is an estimation that on an average 25,000 effective plant-based formulations, is used in folklore and is known by rural communities of India. On an average, 1.5 million people worldwide are practicing the traditional medicinal system using different medicinal plant species for preventive and curative purposes. India is one of the richest sources for TM in the world. It is reporting that an average of 7,800 medicinal drug manufacturing units in India are using around 2,000 tons of herbs as raw material annually and the largest users are India and China (Ramakrishnappa, 2002; Rawat, 2002). Medicinal plant species are mostly used in unprocessed, unrefined, or semi-processed form, often as mixtures in the pharmaceutical industry (Hamilton, 1992).

TCM is also a popular system, followed by Indian medicine across the world. In Western countries, Oriental Medicine refers to Chinese, Japanese, and Korean medicines preferred by immigrants from Korea, while "Asian medicine" often includes TCM, India (Ayurveda) and Tibetan medicine. Among different treatments in traditional systems, medicinal plants are most frequently used (Liu, 2011). In the United States, the NIH uses the CAM to recuperate health systems, practices, and products.

Localized knowledge and experience about TM gained through generations includes distribution, ecology, types, methods of management and methods of extracting the drugs from useful medicinal plant species. The precision of wisdom and are fast disappearing due to lack of written documents, the death of seniors, migration of people due to flood, drought, and social problems, urbanization, and an influx of different cultures (Regassa, 2013). TM is also constantly threatened by changing life style, demography, and exposure to western culture dominating with allopathic system of medicine (using synthetic drugs). However, the practitioners of TM have normally strict traditional values which include taboos, superstitions, norms, and cultural beliefs related to the harvesting of medicinal plants, and, therefore, they contributed much towards the conservation and diversification of medicinal plant species (Kambizi and Afolayan, 2006). All these contribute to the sustainability of this practice at least partially.

Specific uses of TM:

- Plants like tulsi, aloe, turmeric, and ginger are used in our daily life as home remedies and also used to prepare anticancer and anti-obesity drugs. Some of them are acknowledged for their therapeutic values, e.g., green tea, walnuts, pepper, mint, etc. Some plant species and their extracts are considered as vital resources for active ingredients.
- Herbs like basil, fennel, chives, cilantro (coriander), mint, thyme, oregano, fenugreek, dill, rosemary, variegated sage, etc., are medicinally important antipyretic, antifungal, and antibacterial properties along with nutritional value, can be planted in kitchen. These are very easy to grow and smell amazingly having insect repellent properties.
- Some plant species are used as blood purifiers to modify or transform a long-standing disease by eliminating the metabolic toxins and also by removing the free radicals through radical scavenging activity, e.g., turmeric, aloe. These types of plants are also known as 'blood cleansers.' e.g., green tea. Certain herbs improve the immunity, some can alleviate fever due to its antipyretic properties, e.g., kalmegh.
- Wood and bark plants like sandalwood and cinnamon have astringent properties.
- Spices like cardamom, coriander, and ginger possess appetizing qualities and they also remove the gas from the stomach.
- Plants like kalmegh, sarpagandha, and sage act against poisons and snake bites.
- Herbs like rosemary, thyme, coriander, kasuri methi, basil, mint, oregano, etc., give a pleasant aroma to food, rich in nutritive values and possess antioxidant, antibacterial, and also antibiotic properties that inhibiting growth of harmful bacteria.
- Ginger, tulasi, cloves, etc., are used in preparation of cough syrups because they are known for their expectorant property, which means they eject mucus from the bronchial system.
- Opium latex is used in cough syrups as sedative drug (sleep-inducing) and regarded for its narcotic property. But opium seeds, free of narcotic properties, are rich in unsaturated fatty acids like linoleic acid.

- Fenugreek seed mucilage (galactomannan), aloe mucilage (gluco-mannan), are identified for their anti-obesity and diabetic properties. Mostly aloe known as sunburn plant, to treat burns and it is famous for cosmetic preparations, e.g., aloe gel, soaps, moisturizers, etc.
- Aloe juice extract, in combination with other medicinal fruits like amla and jamun, is used as a blood purifier.
- Triphala, a famous herbal Rasayana, made up of equal parts of amla (*Emblica officinalis*), bibhitaki (*Terminalia bellerica*), haritaki (*Terminalia chebula*), and rich in phenolic compounds are believed to be having properties like carminative, anti-diabetic, stimulate immune system, etc.
- Solanaceous plant-like belladonna and datura having narcotic proper-ties are mainly supportive in treating nervous disorders. Especially belladonna, containing 1-hyoscine, acts as a truth confessor to find criminals.
- Aloe gel and senna leaves are having laxative properties and are cathartic in nature. Isabgol husk is rich in mucin and mucopolysac-charides helpful in treating dysentery.
- Plants like pyrethrum (pyrethrins) and *Acorus calamus* (asarones) having insecticidal properties.
- Some crops like saffron (stigma), turmeric (curcumin), marigold (lutein) are useful as natural food colors because they are rich in carotene.
- Certain herbs are stimulants to increase the activity of system or an organ, for example, herbs like chilli (capsaicin and capsanthin), camphor, eucalyptus, and guggul. Especially crops like chilli and guggul having anti-cholesterol properties lower total cholesterol levels for treating against obesity.
- Herbs such as chamomile, calamus, ajowan, basil, cardamom, chry-santhemum, coriander, fennel, peppermint, and spearmint, cinnamon, ginger, and turmeric are helpful in promoting good blood circulation. So, they are used as cardiac stimulants.
- Herbal teas are prepared from herbs like lemongrass, tulasi, green tea and flowers like chrysanthemum, chamomile, rose, rosette, etc., are having carminative, antioxidant, radical scavenging, and astrin-gent properties and also stimulate the nervous system hence used in insomnia treatment (https://www.nhp.gov.in/introduction-and-importance-of-medicinal-plants-and-herbs_mtl) (Table 1.4).

TABLE 1.4 Source of Different Phytochemicals and Their Pharmacological Activity

SL. No.	Drugs from Plants	Source	Family	Medicinal Activity
1.	Atropine	*Atropa belladona*	Solanaceae	Anti-muscarinus
2.	Codeine, Morphine	*Papaver somniferum*	Papaveraceae	Analgesic, sedative
3.	Digoxin	*Digitalis lanata*	Scorphulariaceae (Plantaginaceae)	Cardiovascular
4.	Ephedrin	*Ephedra vulgaris*	Ephedraceae	Anti-asthma
5.	Podophyllotoxin	*Podophyllum pettarum*	Berberidaceae	Anticancer
6.	Quinine	*Cinchona species*	Rubiaceae	Anti-malarial
7.	Reserpine	*Rauwolfia serpentina*	Apocynaceae	Hypotension and anticholinergic
8.	Taxol	*Taxus species*	Taxaceae	Anticancer
9.	Vinblastine Vincristine	*Catharanthus roseus*	Apocynaceae	Anticancer
10.	Andrographolides	*Andrographis paniculata*	Acanthaceae	Antipyretic
11.	Sennosides and anthraquinones	*Cassia species*	Fabaceae (Caesalpinioideae)	Laxative and Cathartic
12.	Abrin (toxalbumin)	*Abrus precatorius*	Fabaceae (Papilionaceae)	Uterine stimulant, abortifacient
13.	Withaferin	*Withania somnifera*	Solanaceae	Anticancer, for Alzheimer and anxiety
14.	Phyllanthin and hypophyllanthin	*Phyllanthus niruri*	Phyllanthaceae	Against Hepatitis B virus
15.	Artemisinin	*Artemisia annua*	Asteraceae	Antimalarial
16.	Vasicine	*Adhatoda vasica*	Acanthaceae	Bronchiodilatory expectorant
17.	Coumarins (xanthotoxol), flavonoids (rutin and marmesin)	*Aegle marmelos*	Rutaceae	Stomachic, anti-diarrheal
18.	Anthraquinone glycosides	*Aloe barbadensis*	Lilliaceae (Agavaceae)	Purgative, anti-inflammatory
19.	Methyl cinnamate, cineole, d-pinene	*Alpinia galanga*	Zingiberaceae	Carminative, circulatory stimulant, anti-inflammatory
20.	Curcumin	*Curcuma longa*	–	Hypolipidemic

Source: Khare (2007).

Based on the region where they are adapted as folklore medicine, herbalism is classified into four types namely, Ayurvedic, Chinese, African, and Western herbalism (Naseem et al., 2014):

1. **Ayurvedic Herbalism:** The word *Ayurveda* is derived from Sanskrit word *Ayu,* meaning 'life' and *veda,* meaning 'science.' Hence, Ayurveda means 'science of life.' This 500 years old system has been originated from Indian medicines and also practiced in adjoining countries like Sri Lanka.
2. **Chinese Herbalism:** This herbalism or herbal medicine is also well-known as TCM. It utilizes the principles of *yin* (cooling) or *yang* (stimulating) and are used frequently in combination to achieve synergy.
3. **African Herbalism:** It is one of the oldest and holistic approaches connecting body and mind together.
4. **Western Herbalism:** It emphasizes the properties of herbs on body systems of individual entity. For example, herbs may be used in individuals for their anticipated anti-inflammatory, expectorant, antispasmodic or immune-stimulatory properties.

1.8   INDIAN SYSTEM OF MEDICINE

India has often been regarded as the *Medicinal Plants Garden of the World* because of having diverse climatic zones containing various numbers of medicinal plants. The Vedas and the other historic treatises like Kama sutra, Charaka Samhita and Sushrutha Samhitha described the therapeutic applications of different plants focusing on their description, protocols for different medicine preparation, application singly or in combination, etc. India has a unique position worldwide with scores of recognized traditional systems of medicines viz., Ayurveda, Siddha, Unani, Homeopathy, Yoga, and Naturopathy were originated (Kumar et al., 2015). AYUSH systems (standing for Ayurveda, Yoga, Unani, Siddha, and Homoeopathy) codified around 8,000 herbal remedies from amongst a diverse group of natural resources. Ayurveda, Unani, Siddha, and Folk (tribal) medicines are actually the four pillars of indigenous medicines. Among these systems, Ayurveda and Unani medicine are most developed and extensively accomplished in India (*https://www.nhp. gov.in/introduction-and-importance-of-medicinal-plants-and-herbs_mtl*).

Ayurveda is mentioned as an ancient health care system and which was evolved in India about 5,000 years ago. As per the ancient literature of India,

Ayurveda was accomplished and reached its peak during the Vedic period. In some countries, it was and is still being used as complementary medicine along with other types of medicine or other TM. This system of medicine having the objectives like to safeguard, support, and uphold good health and prevent diseases through maintaining healthy way of life. Originated from Sanskrit word, AYURVEDA means "science of life." About 7,500 plants are used in local health traditions in most rural and tribal villages of India. Herbal medicine treatment is the most admired form of Traditional Medical System (Sarker and Nahar, 2007).

Great ancient authors namely Charaka, Susruta, and Vahata put on record some of the classical Ayurvedic texts, namely, Charaka Samhita, Susruta Samhita and Astanga-Hridaya-Samhita, respectively. In ancient works, it may come to about 700 plants have medicinal properties on a rough calculation, excluding the unidentified food grains, divine drugs, and poisonous plants. On an average of 1,200 Sanskrit names of plants were mentioned in the above books, approximately around 1,270 names in Sushrutha Samhitha, 1,100 plant names in Charaka Samhita and 1,150 names in Astanga-Hridaya-Samhita, respectively (Moos, 1982) (Figures 1.1 and 1.2).

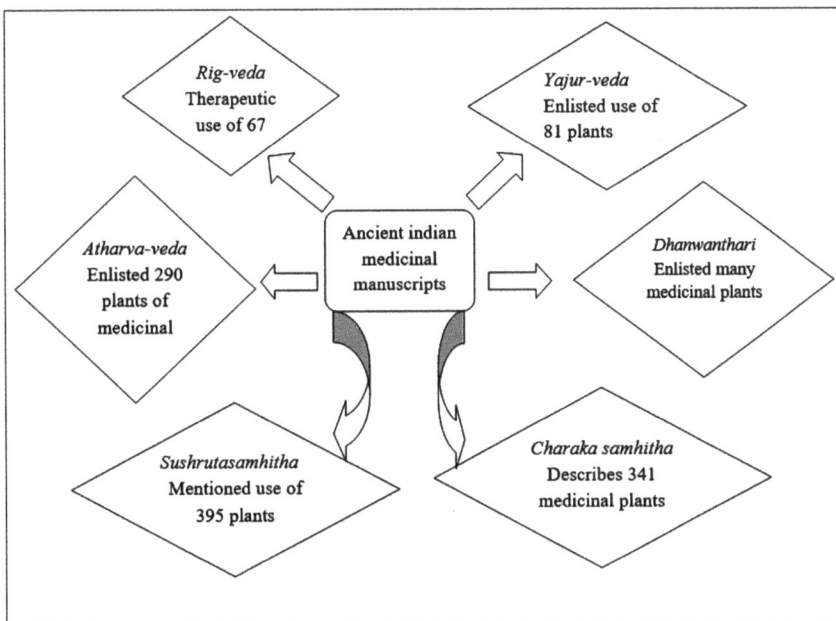

FIGURE 1.1 Different ancient Indian medicinal manuscripts (Adhikari and Paul, 2018).

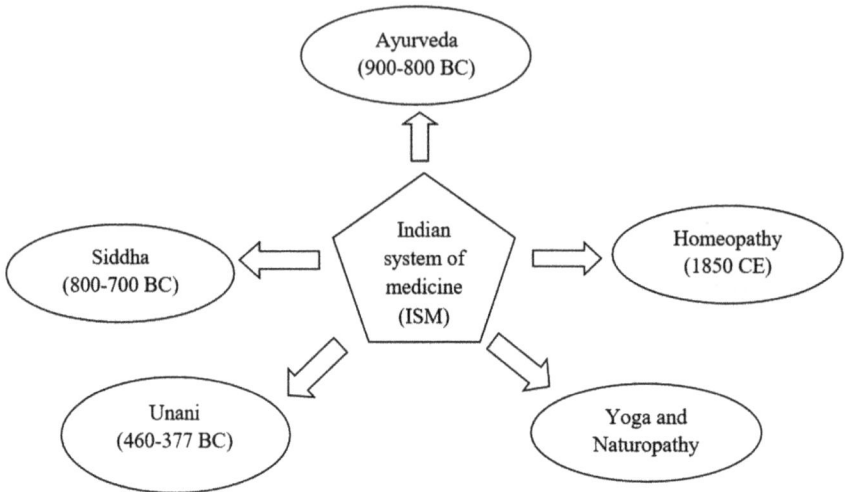

FIGURE 1.2   Different medicinal systems followed in India (Adhikari and Paul, 2018).

Another ancient Greek holistic medical system, Unani, is having a fascinating history traced back to 2,500 years (Lore et al., 2013). Since the mid-1970s, when the WHO began to place a greater spotlight on TM, Unani has engrossed considerable attention all over the world, particularly in the Indian sub-continent, wherein it is slowly integrated into the national health care system (Jabin, 2011).

Unani medicinal system is a comprehensive medication where single, formulation, or crude form is preferred to miraculously deal with diseases. This system acutely addresses gastrointestinal, nervous, and cardiovascular disorders. Siddha medicinal system is developed ever since the earliest human culture in India, around 10,000 BCE-4000 BCE. Like Ayurveda, it is developed through everyday skills of utilizing natural wealth for maintaining superior health having its fundamental confinement in South India only. This practice of medicine is based principally on *Saiva* philosophy wherein the word "Siddha" denotes "holy harmony" or "attaining excellence" or "recognized fact." Accordingly, "Siddhars" were supernatural beings who obtain intellectual powers by constant practice of Siddha. Its truth-seeking design is to sustain human well-being towards succeeding the eternal bliss. It believes "food is medicine, medicine is food" and "sound mind makes a sound body" (Sathasivampillai et al., 2017). Yoga is a Sanskrit word, originated from India. It explores defensive and remedial aptitudes as a training work out for people to develop mindfulness. Dialectical conduct therapy has its fundamental practicalities in cognitive behavior rehabilitation. A different representation of mindfulness happens to be the cognitive therapy practices, identified as care based subjective management (Gordon, 2013).

Naturopathy is an exacting type of system in which vital drugs balance age-old curative ethnicity with reasonable advancement and up to date research. It is guided by an exciting agreement of the regulation that perceives the body's inborn healing competence, emphasizes disease preclusion, and urges outstanding accountability to get perfect well-being. Naturopathic presupposes that the disease is seen as a process of disorder to comfort and subsequent recovery with regard to natural healing systems (Figure 1.3) (Grabia and Ernst, 2003).

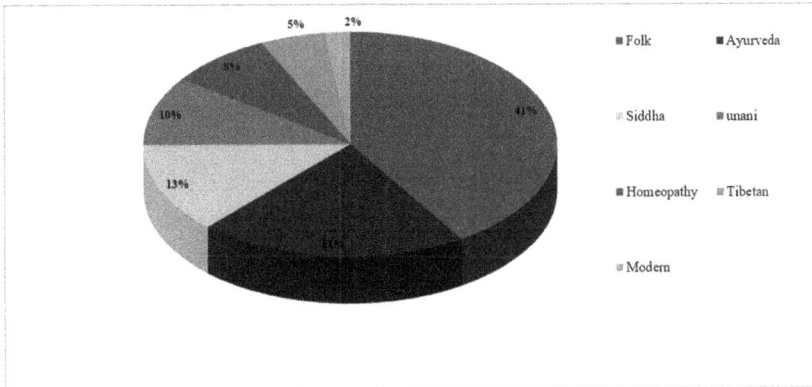

FIGURE 1.3   Percentage of plants used in different medicinal systems (Adhikari and Paul, 2018).

The principle of Homoeopathy stays as one of the most controversial therapeutic practice and familiar from Hippocrates of Greece around 450 BCE. The existing practice of Homoeopathy is better documented by a German doctor, Dr. Samuel Hahnemann (1755CE–1843CE). The word "Homoeopathy" has been originated from Greek words, "Homois" which means similar and "pathos" which means suffering. It is essentially a thera-peutic technique utilizing scheduling of substances whose impact match the appearance of illness of individual patient when regulated to healthy indi-vidual person (Ernst, 1997). Since 1995, a special department called Indian System of Medicine and Homoeopathy (ISM&H) was continued. AYUSH was the new name of ISM&H as it was altered in 2003 standing apart from Department of Ministry of Health and Family Welfare, Government of India.

Sowa-Rigpa is the living, documented medical tradition and one of the oldest systems of medicine derived from Bhoti language which means 'knowledge of healing.' It is more admired in regions like Himalayan societies particularly in states like Jammu and Kashmir (Ladakh region), Himachal Pradesh (Lahoul and Spiti region), West Bengal (Darjeeling region), Sikkim, and Arunachal Pradesh, etc. This system of medicine is having similarity with the Ayurvedic Principles of India since many texts (>75%) are taken from one of the most famous treatises named Ashtanga Hridaya. Plant medicines viz., Triphala, Ashoka, Ashwagandha, Guggul, Haridra are frequently used in this system (*www.ayush.gov.in*).

1.9 TRADITIONAL CHINESE MEDICINE (TCM)

Traditional Chinese medicine (TCM), which is the quintessence of Chinese cultural heritage, had a long history of 5,000 years as China and had made an everlasting contribution to the Chinese Nation survival capacity and producing generations and their prosperity. It was the leading form of medicinal system in China, especially for the most glorious era of the Han dynasty (206 BC–AD 220) (Dong, 2013). TCM was further improved during the Ming dynasty (AD 1368–1644). In China, western medicine was introduced in the 16th century, but it did not endure any further development till 19th century. In 1840, during opium wars, western medicine was gradually developed and also due to political revolution, some revolutionists discarded TCM because it was considered to be a feudal culture. But later in the 20th century, especially during the 1950s Chinese government recognized the importance of TCM and started progression by policies (Mao, 1993). Standard processing protocol (GMP) and dose guidelines are immediately looked-for in TCM to advance drug efficacy and decrease drug side effects or toxicity (Yuan et al., 2016).

Chinese herbal medicine (CHM) is currently used by 1.5 billion people worldwide (Qi et al., 2013). Basically, TCM is based on Yinyang and Wuxing concepts. It should be noted that in TCM, several herbs and ingredients are combined based on strict rules to form prescriptions, which are referred to as formulas (*fang ji* in Chinese). A classic formula is composed using of four elements—the "monarch," "minister," "assistant," and "servant"—according to their different roles, each of which consists of one to several drugs. Ideally, these drugs are composed of at least one organic group to produce the preferred curative outcome and diminish unfavorable reactions (Zhang, 2013).

Initially, medicine was an applied, sensible, and efficient skill, which was based upon observation experience and philosophical speculations. It was thought that health is actually the maintenance of body and mind by a relative balance, not only internally but also with the external environment (Tian, 2000). So, diagnosis is based on methods (like inspection on listening and smelling, inquiring, pulse-taking, and palpitation) and treatment methods (like herbal remedies, acupuncture, cupping, systematic exercise, breathing exercise therapy, massage, hydrotherapy, etc.), aiming at identification of the imbalances present and then restore it to normal.

1.10 POTENTIAL PROSPECTS

MAPs are fast emerging in the Indian agriculture scenario having several direct and indirect implications. Firstly, traditional health system under Ayurveda, Yoga, Unani, Siddha, and Homeopathy has still been admired today due to holistic curing and augmented consciousness for using natural products. It has spurred the demand for medicinal plant species and herbs throughout the globe. Secondly, indiscriminate collection as well as exploitation of medicinal herbs and plants species from the natural habitat under minimal supervised environment leads to declining diversity at a faster rate. This over-exploitation of medicinal plant species, of course, has its own positive dimension leading to the commercial cultivation of those species under field conditions. Lastly, medicinal, and aromatic plant species have better opportunities in trade and industry compared to other horticulture counterparts. Thereby, a further substantial demand from pharmaceutical industries for these unique raw materials ultimately fetches higher remunerative to the cultivators, collectors, and associated stakeholders. All these will lead to the emergence of medicinal and aromatic crops as an alternative to the traditional uneconomic crops (Mohapatra, 2018).

Many medicinal species being pseophytic (shade-loving) climbers, they can easily be accommodated as under-story of different forests. They can also grow in marginal and poor soils with poor soil moisture status. Thereby, they can assist in the replenishment of green cover of the existing degraded forests. Hence, there is a great scope of production and conservation of native MAPs in the understory of degraded forests without reducing area under agriculture production for meeting the food priorities of the escalating global population (Kumar et al., 2017). The use of TM is not restricted to countryside, low-income groups, but also prevails in urban and peri-urban areas. The trade-in TMs forms part of a 'hidden economy' with a turnover to the tune of multimillion-dollar in many developing countries like southern Africa (Cunningham 1989).

It is also important to identify the medicinal plant cultivation as a means for conservation by local people. It leads to biodiversity conservation and poverty alleviation as well. But importance of cultivation and its direct impact on the conservation of threatened species and its scope should be further considered within a more general framework of intensifying cultural values of biodiversity and thus creating an affirmative approach towards biodiversity conservation (Wiersum et al., 2006).

Continuous growing of economic importance of medicinal plants species and plant-based pharmaceuticals in developing countries and mostly are indigenous to these countries. So, they have to identify the importance of medicinal plants and motivate the policymakers to sustain the funding of research on medicinal plants species will boost foreign exchange of developing countries and also increase the national health system by curing of endemic diseases. And further improves the healthcare delivery system by making available essential pharmaceuticals at affordable prices to the majority of the population (Bukar et al., 2016).

Human societies are in close contact with nature since the beginning of human origin and used ingredients obtained from nature to obtain food and medicine (Lorigooini et al., 2018). As human lifestyle is running far away or avoiding from nature and without remembering that we cannot continue to exist without nature. As medicinal plant species are products from nature and eco-friendly and locally available and are giving less side effects than compared to synthetic drugs. Although medicinal plant species and spice crops has been using for their medicine, flavoring, and aromatic qualities for centuries, need a physician help in some cases especially in usages of narcotic crops like opium, datura, and belladonna.

There will be a promising future of cultivating and using medicinal plant species in lucrative ways for the reason that there are about half a million plants around the world, most of them still investigated and unexplored in terms of hidden potential. Further, it can be crucial in the treatment of ill health and studies correlating past, present, and future (Singh, 2015). To enrich biodiversity and to increase human empowerment, widespread growing and processing of medicinal plants are necessary. Phytochemical and biochemical research with an incessant venture for the revival of natural drugs and its legacy for the well-being of the society at large is precisely the need of the hour.

KEYWORDS

- **biodiversity**
- **folklore medicine**
- **medicinal plants**
- **phytochemicals**
- **traditional Chinese medicine**
- **traditional medicine**
- **World Health Organization**

REFERENCES

Abrahams, P., (1992). *Herbal Sales Set to Grow.* Financial Times. London, UK.

Ackerknech, E. H., (1973). *Therapeutics, from the Primitives to the 20th Century.* New York: Hafner Press.

Adhikari, P. P., & Paul, S. B., (2018). History of Indian traditional medicine: A medical inheritance. *Asian Journal of Pharmaceutical and Clinical Research, 11*(1), 421–426.

Anonymous, (2011–12). *Annual Report.* State Department, Directorate of Medicinal and Aromatic Plant Research, Anand.

Bruchac, M., (2014). Indigenous knowledge and traditional knowledge. In: Smith, C., (ed.), *Encyclopedia of Global Archaeology* (pp. 3814–3824). New York: Springer.

Bukar, B. B., Dayom, A. W., & Uguru, M. O., (2016). The growing economic importance of medicinal plants and the need for developing countries to harness from it: A mini-review. *IOSR Journal of Pharmacy, 6*(5), 42–52.

Capasso, L., (1998). 5300 years ago, the Ice Man used natural laxatives and antibiotics. *Lancet, 352*(9143), 1864. http://linkinghub.elsevier.com/retrieve/pii/S0140-6736(05)79939-6 (accessed on 01 November 2021).

Cunningham, A. B., (1989). Herbal medicine trade: A hidden economy. *Indicator South Africa, 6*(3), 51–54.

Dey, A. N., Datta, S., & Maitra, S., (2007). Traditional knowledge on medicinal plants for remedy of common ailments in northern part of West Bengal. *The Indian Forester, 133*(11), 1535–1544.

Dong, J. C., (2013). The relationship between traditional Chinese medicine and modern medicine. *Evid. Based Complement. Altern. Med.*, Article ID: 153148, 1–10, http://dx.doi.org/10.1155/2013/153148.

Ember, C. R., Ember, M., & Peregrine, P. N., (2015). *Anthropology* (14th edn.). Pearson Education Asia, Replica Press India. ISBN: 9780205957187.

Ernst, E., (1997). Homoeopathy: Past, present and future. *Br. J. Clin. Pharmacol, 44*, 435–437.

Fabricant, D. S., & Farnsworth, N. R., (2001). The value of plants used in traditional medicine for drug discovery. *Environ Health Perspect, 109*(1), 69–75.

Fakim, A. G., (2006). Medicinal plants: Traditions of yesterday and drugs of tomorrow. *Molecular Aspects of Medicine, 27*, 1–93.

Farnsworth, N. R., Akerele, O., Heywood, V., & Soejarto, D. D., (1992). Global importance of medicinal plants. In: Akerele, O., Heywood, V., & Synge, H., (eds.). *Conservation of Medicinal Plants* (pp. 25–51). Cambridge Univ. Press, Cambridge, UK.

Franz-Christian, C., (2004). In: Wichtl, M., & Norman, G. B., (eds.), *Herbal Drugs and Phytopharmaceuticals: A Handbook for Practice on a Scientific Basis* (3rd edn., p. 708). Boca Raton, CRC Press. ISBN: 9780849319617.

Galbley, S., & Thiericke, R., (2000). *Drug Discovery from Nature, Series: Springer Desktop Editions in Chemistry* (Vol. XIX, p. 347). Springer, Berlin. ISBN:978-3-540-66947.

Gordon, T., (2013). Theorizing yoga as a mindfulness skill. *Procedia-Soc Behav Sci., 84*, 1224–1227.

Gorunovic, M., & Lukic, P., (2001). *Pharmacognosy* (pp. 1–785). Belgrade University, Faculty of Pharmacy,

Grabia, S., & Ernst, E., (2003). Homeopathic aggravations: A systematic review of randomized, placebo-controlled clinical trials. *Homeopathy, 92*(2), 92–98.

Hamburger, M., & Hostettmann, K., (1991). Bioactivity in plants: The link between phytochemistry and medicine. *Phytochemistry, 30*, 3864–3874.

Hamilton, A. C., (2004). Medicinal plants, conservation and livelihoods. *Biodiversity and Conservation, 13*, 1477–1517. https://en.wikipedia.org/wiki/Medicinal_plants (accessed on 01 November 2021).

Hamilton, A., (1992). International trade in medicinal plants: Conservation issues and potential roles for botanic gardens. *1992 Conference at Botanic Gardens Conservation Congress at Rio de Janeiro, Brazil.*

Hamilton, A., (2003). *Medicinal Plants and Conservation: Issues and Approaches (online).* UK, WWF, Portable Document Format. Available from Internet: http://www.org.uk/filelibrary/pdf/medplantsandcons.pdf (accessed on 01 November 2021).

Harvey, A. L., (2008). Natural products in drug discovery. *Drug Discov. Today, 13*(19, 20), 894–901. doi: 10.1016/j. drudis.2008.07.004.

Jones, W. B., (1998). Alternative medicine-learning from the past examining the present advancing to the future. *J. American Medical Assoc., 280*, 1616–1618.

Kambizi, L., & Afolayan, A. J., (2006). Indigenous knowledge and its impact on medicinal plant conservation in Guruve, Zimbabwe. *Indilinga Afr. J. Ind. Knowl. Syst., 5*(1), 26–31.

Kapoor, S., (2003). *Ancient Indian Sciences: Technical and Scientific Literature and Practices in Ancient India* (Vol. 1). Cosmo Publications, India. ISBN-13: 978-8177552942.

Khare, C. P., (2007). *Indian Medicinal Plants: An Illustrated Dictionary* (1st edn., p. 900). Springer Publication, New York, USA. ISBN: 978-0387706405.

Kiringe, J. W., (2005). Ecological and anthropological threats to ethnomedicinal plant resources and their utilization in Maasai communal ranches in the Amboseli region of Kenya. *Ethnobotany Research and Applications, 3*, 231–241.

Kumar, N., Wani, Z. A., & Dhyani, S., (2015). Ethnobotanical study of the plants used by the local people of Gulmarg and its allied areas, Jammu & Kashmir, India. *International Journal of Current Research in Bioscience and Plant Biology, 2*(9), 16–23.

Kumar, R., Sanwal, C. S., Dobhal, S., Kerkatta, S., & Bhardwaj, S. D., (2017). Production and conservation of medicinal plants in understorey of degraded chir pine forests using sustainable techniques. *Current Sci., 112*(12), 2386–2391.

Liu, W. J. H., (2011). *Traditional Herbal Medicine Research Methods: Identification, Analysis, Bioassay, and Pharmaceutical and Clinical Studies* (p. 477). John Wiley Sons Inc.

Liu, Y., Dao, Z., Liu, Y., & Long, C., (2005). Medicinal plants used by the Tibetan in Shangri-la, Yannan, China. *Ethnobiol. Ethnomed., 5*, 15.

Lorigooini, Z., Jamshidi-Kia, F., & Mini-Khoei, H., (2018). Medicinal plants: Past history and future perspective. *J. Herbmed. Pharmacology, 7*(1), 1–7.

Mao, Z., (1993). *Traditional Chinese Medicine is a Great Treasury* (Vol. VII). Collected Works of Mao Zedong, The Central Documents Research Institute, Beijing.

McAlpine, T., & Warrier, (1992). *Competitive Positioning: Who's Doing What in the Herbal Medical Industry*. Consultancy report. Private publ. UK.

Mittermeier, R. A., Gil, R. P., Hoffman, M., Pilgrim, J., Brooks, T., Mittermeier, C. G., Lamoreux, J., & Fonseca, G. A. B., (2005). *Hotspots revisited: Earth's Biologically Richest and Most Endangered Terrestrial Ecoregions* (p. 392). University of Chicago Press, Boston.

Mohapatra, U., Rudrapur, S., Deepa, B. H., & Mohapatra, S., (2018). Medicinal and aromatic plants sector in Karnataka: An economic perspective and SWOT analysis. *J. Pharmacognosy and Phytochem, 3*, 232–235.

Moos, N. S., (1982). Identification and cultivation of medicinal plants mentioned in ayurvedic classics. *Ancient Science of Life, 1*(4), 224–228.

Naseem, U., Zahoor, M., Khan, F. A., & Khan, S., (2014). A review on general introduction to medicinal plants, its phytochemicals and role of heavy metal and inorganic constituents. *Life Science Journal, 11*(7), 520–527.

Prakash, P. S., (2013). Religious culture and medicinal plants: An anthropological study. *Dhaulagiri Journal of Sociology and Anthropology, 7*, 197–224.

Qi, F. H., Wang, Z. X., Cai, P. P., Zhao, L., Gao, J. J., Kokudo, N., Li, A. Y., Han, J. Q., & Tang, W., (2013). Traditional Chinese medicine and related active compounds: A review of their role on hepatitis B virus infection. *Drug Discov. Ther., 7*, 212–224.

Ramakrishnappa, K., (2002). Impact of cultivation and gathering of medicinal plants on biodiversity: Case studies from India, In: *Biodiversity and the Ecosystem Approach in Agriculture, Forestry and Fisheries*. https://www.fao.org/3/aa021e/aa021e00.htm (accessed on 01 November 2021).

Rao, B. R. R., & Rajput, D. K., (2010). Global scenario of medicinal plants. In: *Proceedings of National Conference on Conservation of Medicinal Plants- Herbal Products and Their Uses* (pp. 17–20). Arts and Science College for Women, Hyderabad, India.

Rawat, R. B. S., (2002). Medicinal plants sector in India with reference to traditional knowledge and IPR issues. *Paper Presented at International Seminar for the Protection of Traditional Knowledge.* New Delhi.

Regassa, R., (2013). Assessment of indigenous knowledge of medicinal plant practice and mode of service delivery in Hawassa City, Southern Ethiopia. *J. Med. Plant. Res., 7*(9), 517–535.

Sarker, S. D., & Nahar, L., (2007). *Chemistry for Pharmacy Students General, Organic and Natural Product Chemistry* (pp. 283–359). John Wiley and Sons, England.

Sarker, S. D., & Nahar, L., (2013). *Chemistry for Pharmacy Students: General, Organic, and Natural Product Chemistry* (pp. 1–383). John Wiley Sons Inc.

Sathasivampillai, S. V., Rajamanoharan, P. R., Munday, M., & Heinrich, M., (2017). Plants used to treat diabetes in Sri Lankan Siddha medicine - an ethnopharmacological review of historical and modern sources. *J. Ethnopharmacol., 198*, 531–599.

Scippmann, U., Leaman, D. J., & Cunningham, A. B., (2002). Impact of cultivation and gathering of medicinal plants on biodiversity: Global trends and issues. In: *Biodiversity and the Ecosystem Approach in Agriculture, Forestry and Fisheries* (pp. 1–21). FAO.

Scippmann, U., Leaman, D., & Cunningham, A. B., (2006). Comparison of cultivation and wild collection of medicinal and aromatic plants under sustainable aspects. In: Ro, R. J., Craker, L. E., & Lange, D., (eds.). *Medicinal and Aromatic Plants* (pp. 75–95). Springer, The Netherlands.

Singh, R., (2015). Medicinal PLANTS: A review. *Journal of Plant Sciences. Special Issue: Medicinal Plants, 3*(1), 50–55.

Stepp, J. R., (2004). The role of weeds as sources of pharmaceuticals. *Journal of Ethnopharmacology, 92*(2, 3), 163–166. doi: 10.1016/j.jep.2004.03.002.

Tian, J., (2000). The developing history and present situation of traditional Chinese medicine. In: *Traditional Chinese Medicine: Past, Present and Future, The Role of Traditional Medicine in Primary Health Care in China* (pp. 1–80).

Tilburt, J. C., & Kaptchuk, T. J., (2008). Herbal medicine research and global health: An ethical analysis. *Bull. World Health Organ., 86*(8), 594–599.

Tipton, C. M., (2014). The history of "Exercise Is Medicine" in ancient civilizations. *Adv. Physiol. Educ., 38*, 109–117.

Tucakov, J., (1971). *Healing with Plants – Phytotherapy* (pp. 180–190). Beograd: Culture.

Wiart, C., (2006). *Ethnopharmacology of Medicinal Plants* (pp. 1–50.). Humana Press, New Jersey.

Wichtl, M., (2004). *Herbal Drugs and Phytopharmaceuticals: A Handbook for Practice on a Scientific Basis.* Boca Raton, CRC Press.

Wiersum, K. F., (1997). From natural forest to tree crops, co-domestication of forests and tree species: An overview. *Netherlands J. Agri. Sci., 45*(4), 425–438.

Wiersum, K. F., Dold, A. P., Husselman, M., & Cocks, M., (2006). Cultivation of medicinal Plants as a tool for biodiversity conservation and poverty alleviation in the Amatola region, South Africa. In: Bogers, R. J., Craker, L. E., & Lange, D., (eds.), *Medicinal and Aromatic Plants* (pp. 43–57). Springer (Netherlands).

World Health Organization (WHO), (1998). *Regulatory Situation of Herbal Medicines: A Worldwide Review* (pp. 1–5). Geneva, Switzerland.

World Health Organization, WHO, (2000). *General Guidelines for Methodologies on Research and Evaluation of Traditional Medicine* (pp. 1–74). World Health Organization: Geneva, Switzerland.

Yarnell, E., & Abascal, K., (2002). Dilemmas of traditional botanical research. *Herbal Gram., 55*, 46–54.

Yuan, H., Ma, Q., & Piao, G., (2016). The traditional medicine and modern medicine from natural products. *Molecules, 21*, 559. doi:10.3390/molecules21050559.

Zargari, A., (1992). *Medicinal Plants* (889). Tehran University Press.

Zhang, A., Sun, H., Qiu, S., & Wang, X., (2013). Advancing drug discovery and development from active constituents of *Yinchenhao tang*, a famous traditional Chinese medicine formula. *Evid. Based Complement. Altern. Med.*, Article ID: 257909. http://dx.doi.org/10.1155/2013/257909.

CHAPTER 2

TRADITIONAL MEDICINE IN HEALTH CARE AND DISEASE MANAGEMENT

SUMANA SARKHEL

Department of Human Physiology, Vidyasagar University, Paschim Midnapore – 721102, West Bengal, India, E-mail: sumana.sarkhel@yahoo.in

ABSTRACT

Since the advent of human civilization, human beings have explored nature for their sustenance and survival. Traditional medicine (TM) is based on the beliefs and experiences of indigenous culture. Chinese, Indian, and African traditional medicine (ATM) are very popular. These medicinal systems are based on a holistic discipline that uses indigenous herbalism with spirituality. The practice of TM is an amalgamation of age-old knowledge, culture, experience, and faith that have percolated from generation to generation. In an era of modern medicine, about 70–80% population worldwide depends on TM. TM, however is an underestimated part of health services. The present chapter is an attempt to investigate the diversity and richness of phytotherapy and how it has influenced medicinal practices worldwide.

2.1 INTRODUCTION

The World Health Organization (WHO) estimates about 4% of the world's population die annually of different forms of diseases regardless of their level of civilization. Unhygienic practices, under-nutrition, poor communication, and lack of basic amenities like portable water, good roads keep communities worldwide in a perpetual state of risk and help to accelerate disease episodes. Traditional medicinal systems are widely accepted worldwide. The WHO has defined ethnomedicine as the indigenous knowledge, skills, and practices in different cultures (WHO, 2008). Among American traditional folk healers, herbal remedies, cupping, and leeching practices are common (Baxandall, Gordon, and Reverb, 1995). Bio-archeological and paleogenetic techniques assuredly became important tools for those who wish to write the history of disease from a global or long-term perspective, and were particularly important where manuscript and other documentary sources are fragmentary or ambiguous.

2.2 TRADITIONAL MEDICINAL SYSTEMS IN DIFFERENT PARTS OF THE WORLD

Traditional medicine (TM) aims to integrate societal and cultural heritage of different communities worldwide. TMs, sometimes known as complementary or alternative medicine, are being used in different parts of the world (Abdullahi, 2011; World Health Organization, 2000). The Chinese traditional medicinal system has been adopted in different cultures. The importance of acupuncture, herbal massage, exercise, needle therapy, rub (*Tui na*) is widely accepted. Several such therapies have alleviated problems like chronic pain, headache, hormonal imbalance and improved liver health and cognitive performance. *Tai chi* is an ancient Chinese practice of slow movements and focuses on breath. Similarly, moxibustion is a therapeutic approach where dried herbs are burned near the skin (Qi et al., 2013; Dobos et al., 2005; Fabricant and Farnsworth, 2001). In Nepal, the government has advocated the importance of TM in Nepalese health care policy in the year 1950s (Cameron, 2008). African traditional healthcare system is a comprehensive, widely acclaimed practice. In countries like Zambia, Ghana children suffering from malaria use traditional remedies for cure.

In India, use of TMs like *Sarpagandha, Haritaki, Kalmegh, Tejpatra* are in practice. In *Ayurveda,* the concept of Pharmacodynamics is based on *Panchamahabhoota* which forms the essence of physiological systems. Kampo medicine of Japan, aroma and steam therapy, Reiki, hydrotherapy, Thai massage, leech therapy, physiotherapy are practiced in different parts of the world. Japanese TM advocated the Chinese practices of needle therapy and moxibustion, although *Kampo* medicinal system is widely used (Goyal, Singh, and Sibinga, 2014; Ito et al., 2017; Prasad, 2002).

2.3   MODES OF TREATMENT IN TRADITIONAL MEDICINE (TM)

Plants, minerals, and animals are the major natural resources used in TMs worldwide. The ancient practices of *Unani, Ayurveda, Siddha* have their deep roots in Indian medicinal system. In African traditional medicine (ATM) the midwives used indigenous plants to aid childbirth. In different parts of South Africa, Zimbabwe, and Mozambique, there are small markets selling herbal medicine. TM is culturally bound and guided by indigenous ancient knowledge of herbs. Human civilization have always faced challenges in health and harnessed different natural resources to overcome it. There is a need to harmonize traditional knowledge with modern medicine globally. There are different modes of traditional treatment like poultice, infusion, acupuncture, moxibustion, bone setting, etc., which have been extensively practiced. In China 100,000 herbal formulations are recommended for clinical use. Several herbal remedies are isolated and identified for biological activity. The concepts of *Rasayana, Panchakarma, Shirodhara, Shirobasti* are prevalent Ayurvedic practices in India (Figure 2.1).

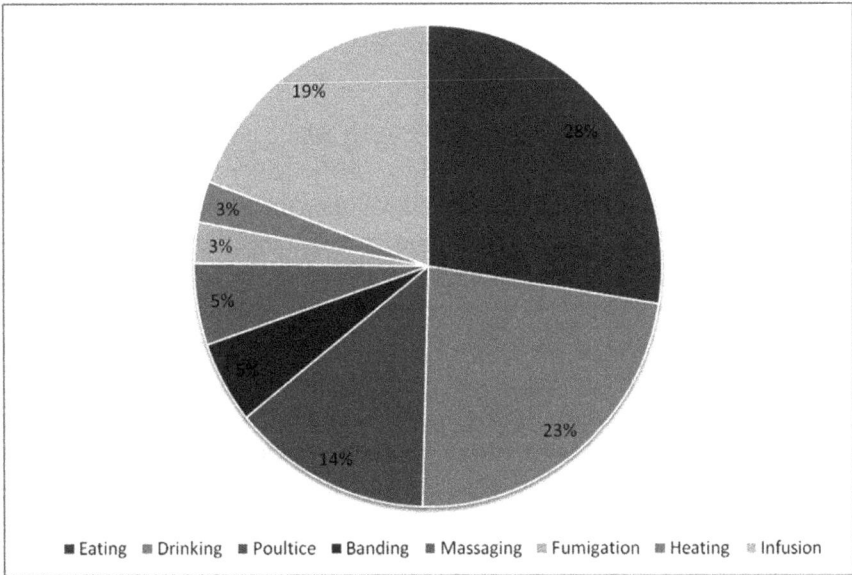

FIGURE 2.1   Types of healing strategies used in traditional medicine.

2.4 TRADITIONAL MEDICINAL SYSTEMS IN INDIA

The Vedic literature is the source of medicinal practice in India. Ayurveda also redefines the science of life and provides the footprint for living a long healthy life. Rural India has adopted TM as their primary health care. The subcontinent harbors nearly 2,500 medicinal plants which have been used by its tribal population in the promotion of health. There are 1,500 herbals that are sold as supplements. In the tribal societies of India, there is a common faith that there is a relation between illness and religion. They adopt various herbal remedies for sustainable living. However, with globalization and potential threats to their survival, this traditional knowledge is been eroded. These nomadic or semi nomadic populations are gradually losing access to their medicinal systems. There is an urgent requirement for the documentation of these traditional resources which have been inculcated in the tribal life of India for generations and has been harnessed from time to time. In Ayurveda, it is believed that a balance of *Vata, Pitta, and Kapha* leads to healthy state and their disturbance leads to diseases. Thus, the scaffolds of modern medicine have been promoted on the theories and beliefs of ancient Indian medicinal practices (Table 2.1).

2.5 CONCLUSION

TM is a time and culture bound knowledge of ethnic populations throughout the world. Every civilization had to face challenges related to health and diseases and every culture imbibed and developed their own and unique practice of medicine. With the advent of modern medicine, there was a competition between the locally available herbal medicines and the modern drugs. Indigenous medicine and TM men thus lost grounds in urban civilizations. But TM still persisted in the face of such global competition. About 80% of the people throughout the world practice traditional medicinal systems in one form or other. Harmonizing traditional and modern medicine is the major requirement of today's world where the potential threats of diseases still persist in the façade of conventional modern drugs. Although the health-related challenges are addressed with modern drugs but the imprints of TMs in prescribed practices of medicine could not be underestimated. Herbs and herbal remedies are staging a comeback and herbal "renaissance" is imminent.

TABLE 2.1 Traditional Uses of Medicinal Plants by Indian Communities

Scientific Name of the Plant	Tribal Name	Common Name	Part Used	Method(s) of Administration
Achyranthes aspera Linn.	*Rechari, Buridatrum,* (Lo.); *Chir-Chir* (Or.); *Sittirkad* (Sa.)	*Prickly chaff flower*	Fruit, Root	*Lodhas* give the paste of 3–5 roots to women thrice a day for stopping bleeding after abortion. Santals use fresh root about 9 cm long stick for causing abortion. They apply macerated roots to get relief of pain from scorpion strings.
Acorus calamus Linn.	*Nai-nag lea, panibach* (Lo).	*Sweet flag*	Root	Lodhas give root paste about 10 gm with that black pepper (*piper longum*) (3:1) in the treatment of chickenpox.
Alstonia scholaria Linn.	*Chatini-daru,* (Lo.); *Kunumung* (Sa.).	*Dita bark*	Root, leaf, bark	Lodha women apply root paste about 7 gm with paste of 7 long pepper for treatment of Thunka (Mastitis). Paste of stem bark and black peppers as cure for rheumatic (joint) swelling.
Andrographis paniculata Brum	*Bhui-nimb* (Lo.).	*Creat*	Root, leaf	Lodhas prescribe root paste about 10 gm against general debility of children and give plant decoction 15 ml in treatment of fever. Santals take juice about 5 ml, for 2–3 days, after meals, in colic pain.

TABLE 2.1   *(Continued)*

Scientific Name of the Plant	Tribal Name	Common Name	Part Used	Method(s) of Administration
Aristolochia indica Linn	*Isher-mul* (Lo.); *Bhedi-janet* (Mu.).	*The Indian birthwort*	Bark, root	Lodhas prescribe root paste (3–5 roots) with paste of 7 long peppers as antidote to snake venom.
				Stem bark paste with extract of Haluhulu (*Curcuma longa*) (3:1) in the treatment of allergic eruption. Women use a piece of root for causing abortion up to 3–4 months of pregnancy.
Azadirachta indica A. juss	*Nim-daru* (Lo); *Bokom-dare*(sa.).	*Nemm tree, Margosa tree*	Root bark, stem bark, flower, leaf	Santals prescribe dry flower powder as anthelmintic. They use leaf decoction for washing septic wounds.
Bombax ceiba Linn.	*Edel-daru* (Lo.); *simul-dare*(sa.).	*Silk cotton tree*	Root, flower	Lodhas women take paste of fresh roots of young plant with unbioled cow milk (1:2) to regulate irregular menstruation.
				Santal apply flower paste on smallpox wounds.
Bridela tomenta Blume	*Kaj* (Lo.)	*Pikpoktsai bridelia*	Stem bark	Lodhas take ash (prepared by burning stem bark) as antacid and they give stem bark decoction with country liquor (1:1) as antidote to snake venom.
Calotropis gigantea Linn.	Orakka kulatos, Swet-akand (Lo) *patla dudha* (Mu); *Ark* (Or.): *parkasa* (Sa.)	*Tembega*	Root, leaf	Lodhas prescribe root decoction with paste of long peppers (3:1) to women in the treatment of leucorrhea. They apply dried root powder with country liquor (5:2) leprotic wounds.
				They apply fomented leaves against enlargement of livers.

TABLE 2.1 (Continued)

Scientific Name of the Plant	Tribal Name	Common Name	Part Used	Method(s) of Administration
Curcuma amada Roxb	Ke-a-sanga (Lo.); Ban-haldi (Sa.).	Mango ginger	Whole plant	Lodhas prescribe rhizome decoction 20 ml twice in a day against cold and cough. They apply rhizome infusion as liniment in pain.
Emblica officinalis Gaertn.f.	Miral-daru (Lo.); Amla (Or.); Aouhal (Sa.).	Emblic myrobalan; Indian gooseberry.	Leaf, fruit, root	Lodhas put fresh leaf juice with diluted solution of common salt (2:1) as drop-in eyes for improving weak eyesight. Santal use powder of the male flowers as snuff in Nasa (nasal hemorrhage). They give ripe fruits about 12 gm to with common salt (3:1) against gripe. Other ethnic communities use fresh fruit and root paste 15 gm as a cure for jaundice.
Ficus benghalensis Linn	Baridaru (Lo.); Bara (Or.); Bargch (Sa.);	Banyan tree	Stem bark, leaf	Stem bark decoction about 10 ml to women prescribed the decoction with paste of ginger (3:1) for the treatment of diabetes. Santals apply leaf juice with Kusum seed oil (3:1) as a cure for burn wounds.
Hemidesmus indica Linn	Atkir, Anantamul, palumala (Lo.); Trajamala (Mu.); Ladugara (Or.); Gargeri, Anal sing (Sa.).	Indian Sarsaparilla	Root, seed	Lodhas prescribe root paste about 10 gm for treatment of leukoderma and apply that paste with common salt (3:2) as cure for eruptions of tongue of children. They prescribe root decoction with paste of Huring atkir (asparagus racemosus) and paste of long peppers (3:2:1) in treatment of gonorrhea and give the decoction with paste of kangi (Eleusine coracana) seed paste and milk (3:2:1) to children as a cure for diarrhea.

TABLE 2.1 *(Continued)*

Scientific Name of the Plant	Tribal Name	Common Name	Part Used	Method(s) of Administration
Jatropha curcas Linn	*Bir-jara; gab-jara* (Lo); *kula-jara* (Mu.): *bag-rendi* (Sa.)	*Physic nut, Purging nut*	Latex	Lodhas used in the treatment of leucorrhea. They apply latex as a cure for eczema. Oranos use fresh latex with common salt (1:1) for mixing loose teeth.
Mikania micrantha H.B.K	*German-lor* (Lo).	*Climbing hemp weed.*	Leaf	Lodhas and Oranos apply crushed fresh leaves on fresh cuts for stopping bleeding. Other ethnic communities put fresh leaf juice as drop-in nostril as a cure for epilepsy.
Moringa oleifera Linn	*Doro, Mung-ara* (Lo.); *Munga-sag*(Sa.)	*Drum stick tree; Horseradish tree.*	Root; Stem bark; Leaf	Lodhas gives dried root powder with cow milk (3:2) treatment of hysteria. They apply stem bark as a cure for Rangbad (a kind of skin disease of children) and put leaf paste as poultice on swelling legs.
Mucuna pruriens Linn.	*Alkusi* (Lo.); *Itika* (Sa.)	*Common Cowitch; Cowhage*	Root	Lodhas prescribe root decoction with paste of long peppers (2:1) for treatment of delirium. They give seed decoction with common salt (2:1) for the treatment of coma.
Oryza sativa Linn	*Dhan* (Lo. and Sa.)	*Rice, Paddy*	Root	Lodhas prescribe fresh root paste with paste of long peppers (3:2) for treatment of measles. They give gain powder with palm sugar (3:2) antidote to Kuchilia (Strychnos nux-vomica) seed poison.
Ricinus communes Linn	*Digherandi* (Or.).	*Castor, Castor seed*	Leaf, seed	Lodhas give leaf decoction and unbioled eggs (3:2) to children for treatment of night blindness and apply leaf paste on forehead as cure for headache. Santals apply fresh Youngs leaf as poultice on boils.

TABLE 2.1 *(Continued)*

Scientific Name of the Plant	Tribal Name	Common Name	Part Used	Method(s) of Administration
Terminalia arjuna Roxb.	*Gara-hatna; Kahua* (Lo.); *Behera* (Sa.)	*Arjun tree; white murdah; White-wingedmyrobalan.*	Stem bark	Lodhas prescribe stem decoction with goat milk to women (3:2) as a cure for debility. Oraons give stem decoction about 15 ml for treatment of heart diseases. Santals use ash (prepare by burning stem bark) as tooth powder for caries in teeth. They give decoction of stem bark about 20 ml for treatment of malarial fever.
Tinospora cordifolia Thoms	*Titmaal; Nim-gulancha* (Lo.); *Srasati loar* (Or.); *Cunchi* (Sa.)	*Gulancha tinospora; Cow protector; Moon creeper; Bile killer*	Stem	Lodhas prescribe stem decoction with paste of long peppers (3:1) for healing bone fracture. Santals prescribe paste of aerial root tips decoction of long pepper (5:3) against gastralgia (Stomachache) and give decoction of root tips with common salt (3:1) to women against irregular menstruation flow.

KEYWORDS

- hydrotherapy
- indigenous cultures
- pharmacodynamics
- phytotherapy
- traditional medicine
- Sarpagandha

REFERENCES

Abdullahi, A. A., (2011). Trends and challenges of traditional medicine in Africa. *Afr. J. Tradit. Complement. Altern. Med., 8*, 115–123.

Baxandall, R. F., Gordon, L., & Reverb, S., (1995). *America's Working Women: A Documentary History, 1600 to the Present* (p. 50). W. W. Norton and Company.

Cameron, M., (2008). Modern desires, knowledge control, and physician resistance: Regulating Ayurvedic medicine in Nepal. *Asian Medicine., 4*, 86–112.

Dobos, G. J., Tan, L., Cohen, M. H., McIntyre, M., Bauer, R., Li, X., & Bensoussan, A., (2005). Are national quality standards for traditional Chinese herbal medicine sufficient? Current governmental regulations for traditional Chinese herbal medicine in certain Western countries and China as the eastern origin country. *Complement. Ther. Med., 13*, 183–190.

Fabricant, D. S., & Farnsworth, N. R., (2001). The Value of Plants Used in Traditional Medicine for Drug Discovery. *Environ. Health Perspect., 109*, 69–75.

Goyal, M., Singh, S., & Sibinga, E. M., (2014). Meditation programs for psychological stress and well-being: A systematic review and meta-analysis. *JAMA Internal Medicine, 174*(3), 357–368.

Ito, M., Maruyama, Y., Kitamura, K., et al., (2017). Randomized controlled trial of juzen-taiho-to in children with recurrent acute otitis media. *Auris Nasus Larynx, 44*(4), 390–397.

Prasad, L. V., (2002). In: *Indian System of Medicine and Homoeopathy Traditional Medicine in Asia* (pp. 283–286). New Delhi: WHO- Regional Office for southeast Asia.

Qi, F. H., Wang, Z. X., Cai, P. P., Zhao, L., Gao, J. J., Kokudo, N., Li, A. Y., et al., (2013). Traditional Chinese medicine and related active compounds: A review of their role on hepatitis B virus infection. *Drug Discov. Ther., 7*, 212–224.

World Health Organization, (2000). *General Guidelines for Methodologies on Research and Evaluation of Traditional Medicine*. World Health Organization; Geneva, Switzerland.

World Health Organization (WHO). (2008). World Health Organization. Definitions. In: *Traditional Medicine Strategy: 2014-2023*. WHO Library Cataloguing-in-Publication Data. p.15. Printed in Hong Kong SAR, China. http://www.who.int/medicines/areas/traditional/definitions/en/ (accessed 23 November 2021).

CHAPTER 3

HERBAL DRUG DISCOVERY AGAINST INFLAMMATION: FROM TRADITIONAL WISDOM TO MODERN THERAPEUTICS

SHALINI DIXIT,[1] KARUNA SHANKER,[1] MADHUMITA SRIVASTAVA,[1] PRIYANKA MAURYA,[1] NUPUR SRIVASTAVA,[1] JYOTSHNA,[1] and DNYANESHWAR U. BAWANKULE[2]

[1]*Analytical Chemistry Department, CSIR-Central Institute of Medicinal and Aromatic Plants, Near Kukrail Picnic Spot, P.O. CIMAP, Lucknow – 226015, Uttar Pradesh, India, Tel.: +91-522-2718580, Fax: +91-522-2719072, E-mail: kspklko@yahoo.com (K. Shanker)*

[2]*Molecular Bioprospection Department, Central Institute of Medicinal and Aromatic Plants, Near Kukrail Picnic Spot, P.O. CIMAP, Lucknow – 226015, Uttar Pradesh, India*

ABSTRACT

Inflammation is the primary response of the body to deal with the hallmarks such as pain, redness, swelling, fever, and injuries. Though it is a short-term adaptive response but crucial part of tissue restoring process and it includes integration of many complex signals in different cells and that too in the organ. Prolonged symptoms of inflammation lead to chronic pathological conditions which can be managed by specific therapeutics. Inflammation is a key feature of many diseases such as obesity and type 2 diabetes atherosclerosis, malaria, rheumatoid arthritis, and infections. Beyond doubt, natural products play an imperative role in the management and treatment of some diseases and symptoms and complications in chronic disease, particularly autoimmune. Extensive pre-clinical and clinical research on phytomolecules viz. curcumenoides, parthenolide, cucurbitaceous, 1, 8-cineole, etc., is well documented for their anti-inflammatory effect. Additionally, some pre-clin-ical and clinical studies on the standardized plant extract, e.g., *T. wilfordii* extract for rheumatoid arthritis; *Cannabis sativa* for anti-nociceptive actions; baccosides enriched for diabetes and phytosomes viz., silybin, lyprinoland bromelain. Further, in the same progression, there is still a requirement to find some more new lead from the natural sources. This review article updated the latest research progresses of most promising anti-inflammatory drugs from plant origin. Traditional and modern usage plant drugs intended for anti-inflammatory actions will also be discussed in order to drug development prospects. In this review article, we have summarized traditional folk medic-inal plants used as anti-inflammatory agents, synthetically derived natural products, and the bioactive agents isolated from plants going through clinical trials have also been discussed. The essential pharmacophoric characteristics of selected lead compounds will also be discussed for their qualification as an investigational new drug for the management of inflammation caused by the specific disease. Anti-inflammatory activities were found in some papers and basic research was described alongside both experimental and clinical findings. A brief account of plants derived from *Ayurveda* and compounds isolated with their derivatives are discussed in this review. Structure-activity relationship (SAR) is also discussed to find a basic idea about what kind of structures responsible for the anti-inflammatory activity.

3.1 INTRODUCTION

Inflammation is the immediate response of the immune system to any infec-tion and injury. Inflammation is the initial stage is a beneficial event to host that leads to removal of offending factors, restoration of tissue repair, and normal physiological function, however latter if prolonged due to persistent stimuli, it may result in unfavorable response causing derangement of normal physiological and restoration process. In general, normal inflammation is rapid and self-limiting, but prolonged inflammation causes various chronic disorders (Sarkar et al., 2016). The inflammatory response may be acute or chronic. Acute inflammation is rapid and self-limiting and it is easy for host defenses to return the body to homeostasis but under specific conditions. This could lead into a chronic state that is prolonged inflammation which is characterized by the excessive release of inflammatory cells and cytokines, a malfunction in cellular signaling and loss of barrier function, thereby becoming a causative factor in the pathogenesis (Pan, Lai, and Ho, 2010).

Such persistent inflammation is associated with a wide range of chronic human conditions and diseases including sepsis, allergy, atherosclerosis, cancer, arthritis, metabolic disorders, and autoimmune diseases (Calder et al., 2009; Libby, 2007).

Plants are progressively used in the treatment of diseases as complementary medicine. Natural products or natural product derivatives represent a great molecular and structural diversity over synthetic compounds. About 60% of new chemical entities are derived from or based on natural products reported from 1981 to 2006 (Newman and Cragg, 2016). Therefore, natural products play a leading role in the discovery and development of leads for treating human diseases. Wide literature is available discussing the treatment of inflammation remission, including the role of several pharmacophores which belongs to natural and of their synthetic counterpart or completely of synthetic origin.

There are ample class of compounds reported from natural products for suppressing inflammation including steroids, non-steroidal anti-inflammatory drugs (NSAIDs) and immune-suppressants. These diverse chemical compounds are reported to possess adverse effects. Steroidal anti-inflammatory drugs (SAIDs) are used for the management of rheumatoid arthritis, adverse effects which lead some serious physiological disorders viz. Cushing habit (appearance with a rounded face, supraclavicular hump, obesity, thin limbs), hyperglycemia, hypertension, muscular weakness, increased susceptibility to infection, osteoporosis, glaucoma, and psychiatric disturbances, etc. Similarly, the side effects associated with the use of NSAIDs are gastrointestinal ulceration and bleeding, platelet dysfunction due to the inhibition of COX-1-derived prostanoids, whereas inhibition of COX-2-dependent prostaglandin (PG) biosynthesis accounts for the anti-inflammatory, analgesic, and antipyretic effects. The COX-2 inhibitors also exhibit cardiovascular side effects due to inhibition of prostacyclin formation in the infarcted heart, tipping the balance of prostacyclin/thromboxane, coupled with a diminution in prostacyclin in heart muscle (Jachak, 2006; Gautam and Jachak, 2009). While in dealing with natural products, our aim is to apply minimum effective dose by the highest efficacy with the least adverse effects.

Prolonged uses of synthetic drugs may lead to a difficult situation, and also drug resistance against microbes and parasites can be developed — natural products provided with this benefit of having fewer side effects. Researchers are made to tend towards this side of natural product drug discoveries. There are certain compounds from plant source made to come in the human trails such as curcumin, parthenolide, resveratrol, boswellic acid, betulinic acid, ursolic acid, and oleanolic acid are now studied as possible drugs for the future against inflammatory (Gautam and Jachak, 2009; Kashyap et al., 2016; Sur et al., 2009; Adedapo, Adewuyi, and Sofidiya, 2013). In this review, we will give a brief description related to the plants reported from the traditional system of medicine, the plants extract newly described to have anti-inflammatory activity and pharmaco-logical aspects with the structure of pharmacophores qualified to reach to the clinical trials.

3.2   TRADITIONAL WISDOM

Ayurveda is an ancient Indian system (before 2500 B.C.) known for its preventative actions and holistic approaches to treating diseases. It is a lifestyle practice to go with *Ayurveda* which is a little difficult to maintain for a long time. Thus, to make it in the system, scientists started the reverse pharmacology and tried to find the active ingredients from the sources such as plants, minerals, and the formulations. In *Ayurveda* pharmacological view is comprised of *Vata, Pitta,* and *Kapha,* collectively known as '*Tridoshas.*' These *doshas* are considered as the basic elements of the human body. The basic psycho-biological functions in the body are governed and controlled by these *doshas*. Optimal equilibrium among these three *doshas* represents a healthy body whereas the disturbance in three *doshas* culminates into disease conditions. These *doshas* also explain about human physiology and vary person to person. The disturbance in *vata* leads to receding gums, blood clotting, insomnia, dry skin, paralysis. The *Kapha dosha* imbalances lead to goiter, breast cancer, lung cancer, and obesity, etc. The imbalances in *pitta* lead to hepatitis, urinary tract infections, stress-related diseases, and hypertension (Bhagwandash, 1978).

Approximately, 1250 medicinal plants are reported in *Ayurveda*. *Ayurvedic* formulations are complex mixtures of a number of plants, minerals, and metals. Sarpagandha plant (*Rauwolfia serpentina*) was the first significant contribution in *Ayurveda* with the isolation of alkaloids for the treatment of hypertension, insomnia, and insanity (Ravishankar and Shukla, 2007). It provided a base for the development of anti-hypertensive drug and the first important link between ancient *Ayurvedic* knowledge and modern therapeutic action.

The evidence to support the use of the natural product in medication came into existence in 1805 with the discovery of morphine. There are some plants described in *Ayurveda* as well as in *Ayurvedic Pharmacopeia of India* having inflammatory properties such as *Curcuma officinalis* (Family: Zingibera-ceae), *Aralia nudicaulis* (Family: Araliaceae) (Lee et al., 2011; Oh et al., 2009; Seo et al., 2007; Wang, Li, Ivanochko, and Huang, 2006; Chung et al., 2005; Park et al., 2005; Ryu et al., 1996). These are the plants extensively studied and addressed for their profound pharmacological activities and also been used as traditional medicine (TM) for the treatment of rheumatoid arthritis, ulcerative colitis, pancreatitis, cancer, and osteoarthritis, etc. Plants such as *Bauhinia variegate* (aerial part) found to have promising anti-inflam-matory activity against the lipopolysaccharides, interferon λ induce nitric oxide (NO) and cytokines (Singh, Singh, and Singh, 2016). *Glycyrrhiza glabra* and *Acacia arabica* (Babul) used for respiratory tract infections are mentioned in *Ayurveda* (Aggarwal et al., 2011). The glycosidal fraction of ethanolic extract of unripe pods of *Acacia farnesiana*, *Aegle marmelos* (L.), Correa ex Roxb. (Bael) yields coumarin and marmin from the roots, The plant extract of *Ageratum conyzoides* of family *Asteraceae*, mentioned as Dochunty, *Berberis aristata* of family *Berberidaceae* commonly known as '*Daruharidra*' is an evergreen shrub (Khare, 2008). The mucosal inflamma-tion in the oral tract can be treated with *Agrimonia eupatoria*. The salicylate components of *Aloe barbadensis* Ghritkumaarika (Mill) or Aloe gel reported to inhibit bradykinin, a pain-producing agent. *Blumea lacera* called as Kukundara showed marked anti-inflammatory activity in bradykinin and carrageenin-induced inflammation in rats. *Boerhavia diffusa* Linn, a weed *Rakta-punarnavaa* found throughout India possess anti-inflammatory prop-erty for renal diseases and also possess antiarthritic activity. Ethanolic extract of *M. flagellipes* decreased the edema at the rate of 11.7% and 54.2% in acute inflammation and 7.00% and 42.40% for chronic inflammation at the dose of 10 and 50 mg/kg induced by carrageenan and formalin (Uchegbu et al., 2015). *Magnolia kobas* stem bark inhibits the pro-inflammatory mediators (IL-β, TNFα). The *M. kobas* treatment suppresses TPA induced ear swelling (*in-vitro/in-vivo*) (Kang et al., 2008). 4-O-methylhonokiol novel compound isolated from *Magnolia officinalis* shows anti-inflammatory properties by inhibiting the NF-κB (Oh et al., 2009). The chloroform extract of dried fruits of *Babassu mesocarp* showed significant anti-inflammatory and analgesic properties (Azevedo et al., 2007). Some other plants have also been reported for having anti-inflammatory activities are given in Table 3.1.

TABLE 3.1 Medicinal Plants Having Anti-Inflammatory Activities

SL. No.	Plant Name	Plant Part	Target	Inhibition (%)	References
1.	*Ajuga remota*	Aerial parts	COX-1	90.3 ± 0.8 (Hexane)	
				74.0 ± 0.1 (Methanol)	Matu and Van (2003)
				47.0 ± 2.0 (Water)	
2.	*Conyza schimperiana*	Roots	COX-1	47.0 ± 2.5 (Hexane)	
				65.0 ± 4.5 (MeOH)	
				16.0 ± 2.0 (Water)	Matu and Van
		Aerial parts	COX-1	69.0 ± 5.5 (Hexane)	(2003)
				87.0 ± 3.5 (MeOH)	
				27.0 ± 4.0 (Water)	
3.	*Croton macrostachyus*	Roots	COX-1	37.0 ± 0.5 (Hexane)	
				65.0 ± 3.0 (MeOH)	
				40.0 ± 1.5 (Water)	Matu and Van
		Leaves	COX-1	90.6 ± 1.8 (Hexane)	(2003)
				85.0 ± 3.5 (MeOH)	
				74.0 ± 2.5 (Water)	
4.	*Zanthoxylum sambarense*	Roots	–	86.0 ± 2.0 (Hexane)	
				99.0 ± 1.5 (MeOH)	
				78.0 ± 1.4 (Water)	
		Bark	–	97.5 ± 2.8 (Hexane)	
				87.5 ± 3.8 (MeOH)	Matu and Van (2003)
				64.5 ± 2.9 (Water)	
		Leaves	–	84.6 ± 1.4 (Hexane)	
				92.8 ± 2.6 (MeOH)	
				46.0 ± 2.5 (Water)	
5.	*Maytenus senegalensis*	Roots	–	49.0 ± 2.0 (Hexane)	
				93.0 ± 1.0 (MeOH)	
				84.0 ± 2.5 (Water)	
		Bark	–	40.0 ± 0.8 (Hexane)	
				81.0 ± 1.0 (MeOH)	Matu and Van (2003)
				53.0 ± 2.0 (Water)	
		Leaves	–	32.0 ± 1.9 (Hexane)	
				67.0 ± 0.7 (MeOH)	
				21.0 ± 0.6 (Water)	

TABLE 3.1 *(Continued)*

SL. No.	Plant Name	Plant Part	Target	Inhibition (%)	References
6.	*Plectranthus barbatus*	Roots	–	93.8 ± 0.1 (Hexane)	
				95.6 ± 0.6 (MeOH)	
				34.0 ± 2.5 (Water)	
		Bark	–	70.0 ± 1.4 (Hexane)	Matu and Van (2003)
				87.0 ± 4.5 (MeOH)	
				10.0 ± 1.0 (Water)	
		Leaves	–	88.0 ± 3.5 (MeOH)	
				7.0 ± 1.5 (Water)	
7.	*Galinsoga parviflora*	Aerial parts	–	68.0 ± 4.5 (Hexane)	Matu and Van (2003)
				90.0 ± 1.5 (MeOH)	
				54.0 ± 2.5 (Water)	
8.	*Mondia whitei*	Roots	–	85.0 ± 1.3 (Hexane)	
				93.0 ± 2.0 (MeOH)	
				48.0 ± 5.5 (Water)	Matu and Van (2003)
		Leaves	–	51.0 ± 2.5 (Hexane)	
				93.0 ± 4.0 (MeOH)	
				67.0 ± 2.0 (Water)	
9.	*Oxygonum sinuatum*	Aerial parts	–	91.0 ± 0.1 (Hexane)	Matu and Van (2003)
				91.0 ± 1.9 (MeOH)	
				42.0 ± 1.8 (Water)	
10.	*Spiranthes mauritianum*	Whole plant	–	76.0 ± 2.0 (Hexane)	Matu and Van (2003)
				84 ± 2.0 (MeOH)	
				32.0 ± 3.0 (Water)	
11.	*Zanthoxylum chalybeum*	Roots	–	67.0 ± 1.5 (Hexane)	
				94.8 ± 2.4 (MeOH)	
				73.7 ± 1.4 (Water)	
		Bark	–	57.0 ± 1.0 (Hexane)	Matu and Van (2003)
				89.0 ± 2.3 (MeOH)	
				56.0 ± 1.5 (Water)	
		Leaves	–	58.0 ± 3.0 (Hexane)	
				87.0 ± 3.0 (MeOH)	
				30.0 ± 0.5 (Water)	
12.	*Desmodium gangeticum*	Aerial parts	COX-2	39.5 (Water)	Bisht, Bhattacharya, and Jaliwala (2014)
			COX-1	49.5 (Water)	

TABLE 3.1   *(Continued)*

SL. No.	Plant Name	Plant Part	Target	Inhibition (%)	References
13.	*Abroma augusta*	Roots	COX-1	36.5 (Hexane)	Bisht, Bhattacharya, and Jaliwala (2014)
			COX-2	59 (Hexane)	
14.	*Peltophorum africanum*	Leaves	15 LOX	12.42 (Crude)	Adebayo et al. (2015)
15.	*Zanthoxylum capense*	–	15-LO	14.92 (Acetone)	Adebayo et al. (2015)
16.	*Spatholobus suberectu*	Stem	COX-1	158 (EtOAc)	
			COX-2	–	
			PLA2	54 (EtOAc)	Li et al. (2003)
			5-LO	31 (EtOAc)	
			12-LO	35 (EtOAc)	
17.	*Trachelospermum jasminoides*	Stem	COX-1	35 (EtOAc)	Li et al. (2003)
			PLA2	33 (EtOAc)	
18.	*Tripterygium wilfordi*	Root	COX-1	27 (EtOAc)	
			COX-2	125 (EtOAc)	Li et al. (2003)
			5-LO	22 (EtOAc)	
19.	*Piper kadsura*	Stem	COX-1	251±14 (EtOAc)	
			COX-2	631±44 (EtOAc)	
			PLA2	147±9 (EtOAc)	Li et al. (2003)
			5-LO	85±4 (EtOAc)	
			12-LO	ND(EtOAc)	
20.	*Polygonum multiflorum*	Stem	COX-1	398±10 (EtOAc)	
			COX-2	>1000 (EtOAc)	
			PLA2	691±27 (EtOAc)	Li et al. (2003)
			5-LO	>1000 (EtOAc)	
			12-LO	309±25 (EtOAc)	
21.	*Tinospora sagittata*	Stem	COX-1	19.8±2.7 (EtOAc)	Li et al. (2003)
22.	*Tinospora sinensis*	Root	COX-1	10.0±2.0 (EtOAc)	Li et al. (2003)
23.	*Memecylon talbotianum*	Leaves	LOX	1 (MeoH)	
				1.36 (Crude)	Bharathi, Nadafi, and Prakash (2014)
			XO	12.65 (MeOH)	
				24.19 (Crude)	
24.	*Zingiber officinale*	Rhizome	COX	145.04 (EtOAc)	Siriwatanametanon et al. (2010)

TABLE 3.1 *(Continued)*

SL. No.	Plant Name	Plant Part	Target	Inhibition (%)	References
25.	*Muehlenbeckia latyclada*	–	NF-κB	>200.00 (Hexane)	
				>200.00 (MeOH)	
				83.28 (EtOAc)	
			IL-6	24.95 (Hexane)	
				3.38 (MeOH)	
				36.40 (EtOAc)	Siriwatanametanon et al. (2010)
			IL-1	0.73 (MeOH)	
				3.27 (EtOAc)	
			TNFα	22.59 (Hexane)	
				8.67 (MeOH)	
				0.86 (EtOAc)	
26.	*Gynura pseudochina*	–	NF-κB	159.76 (MeOH)	
				83.20 (EtOAc)	
			IL-6	22.23 (Hexane)	
				28.62 (MeOH)	
				11.63 (EtOAc)	
			IL-1	>50.00 (Hexane)	Siriwatanametanon et al. (2010)
				15.44 (MeOH)	
				15.44 (EtOAc)	
			TNFα	>50.00 (Hexane)	
				1.04 (MeOH)	
				33.28 (EtOAc)	
27.	*Cayratia trifolia*	–	NF-κB	200.00 (Hexane)	
				83.16 (MeOH)	
				200.00 (EtOAc)	
			IL-6	>50.00 (Hexane)	
				19.53 (MeOH)	
				25.47 (EtOAc)	Siriwatanametanon et al. (2010)
			IL-1	>50.00 (Hexane)	
				>50.00 (MeOH)	
				42.04 (EtOAc)	
			TNFα	>50.00 (Hexane)	
				28.45 (MeOH)	
				20.83 (EtOAc)	

TABLE 3.1   *(Continued)*

SL. No.	Plant Name	Plant Part	Target	Inhibition (%)	References
28.	*Basella alba*	–	NF-κB	>200.00 (Hexane)	
				>200.00 (MeOH)	
				83.28 (EtOAc)	
			IL-6	46.74 (Hexane)	
				32.38 (MeOH)	Siriwatanametanon
				36.40 (EtOAc)	et al. (2010)
			IL-1	36.73 (MeOH)	
			TNFα	>50.00 (Hexane)	
				37.68 (MeOH)	
				30.42 (EtOAc)	
29.	*Basella rubra*	–	NF-κB	157.31 (Hexane)	
				139.21 (MeOH	
				162.83 EtOAc)	
			IL-6	44.49 (Hexane)	
				>50.00 (MeOH)	
				38.87 (EtOAc)	Siriwatanametanon
			IL-1	>50.0 (Hexane)	et al. (2010)
				36.49 (MeOH)	
				36.76 (EtOAc)	
			TNFα	>50.0 (Hexane)	
				>50.0 (MeOH)	
				31.72 (EtOAc)	
30.	*Oroxylum indicum*	–	NF-κB	47.45 (EtOAc)	
			IL-6	37.13 (Hexane)	
				>50.0 (MeOH)	
				27.98 (EtOAc)	
			IL-1	>50.0 (MeOH)	Siriwatanametanon
				44.12 (EtOAc)	et al. (2010)
			TNF-α	>50.0 (Hexane)	
				>50.0 (MeOH)	
				20.33 (EtOAc)	

TABLE 3.1 *(Continued)*

SL. No.	Plant Name	Plant Part	Target	Inhibition (%)	References
31.	*Rhina canthusnasutus*	–	NF-κB	138.16 (Hexane)	
				118.03 (MeOH)	
				104.04 (EtOAc)	
			IL-6	>50.0 (Hexane)	
				>50.0 (MeOH)	
				>50.0 (EtOAc)	Siriwatanametanon et al. (2010)
			IL-1	>50.0 (Hexane)	
				>50.0 (MeOH)	
				>50.0 (EtOAc)	
			TNFα	>50.0 (Hexane)	
				>50.0 (MeOH)	
				43.83 (EtOAc)	
32.	*Pouzolzia indica*	–	NF-κB	134.69 (MeOH)	
			IL-6	46.51 (Hexane)	
				>50.0 (MeOH)	Siriwatanametanon et al. (2010)
			TNFα	42.52 (Hexane)	
				>50.0 (MeOH)	
				15.68 (EtOAc)	
33.	*Cissus quadrangularis*	–	COX-1	46.64 ± 0.69 (Hexane)	
				28.18 ± 0.70 (Water)	
				84.94 ± 0.99 (Ethanol)	Shaikh, Pund, and Gacche (2016)
			COX-2	47.92 ± 0.44 (Hexane)	
				24.05 ± 0.64 (Water)	
				81.01 ± 0.62 (Ethanol)	
34.	*Plumbago zeylanica*	–	COX-1	36.25 ± 0.54 (Hexane)	
				41.48 ± 0.62 (Ethanol)	
			COX-2	31.35 ± 0.71 (Hexane)	Shaikh, Pund, and Gacche (2016)
				33.27 ± 0.74 (Water)	
				63.98 ± 0.51 (Ethanol)	

TABLE 3.1   *(Continued)*

SL. No.	Plant Name	Plant Part	Target	Inhibition (%)	References
35.	*Terminalia bellarica*	–	COX-1	48.09 ± 0.56 (Hexane)	
				75.16 ± 0.41 (Water)	
				62.24 ± 0.79 (Ethanol)	Shaikh, Pund, and Gacche (2016)
			COX-2	60.09 ± 0.45 (Hexane)	
				88.79 ± 0.71 (Water)	
				71.14 ± 0.90 (Ethanol)	
36.	*Terminalia chebulla*	–	COX-1	86.32 ± 1.18 (Hexane)	
				72.16 ± 0.93 (Water)	
			COX-2	50.88 ± 0.34 (Hexane)	Shaikh, Pund, and Gacche (2016)
				88.16 ± 0.73 (Water)	
				85.40 ±.97 (Ethanol)	

3.3   SECONDARY METABOLITES: AN ANTI-INFLAMMATORY AGENT

Secondary metabolites are low molecular weight organic compounds produced in plants. The biosynthesis of secondary metabolites is restricted to the selected plant groups and is exhibiting a huge structural diversity. These secondary metabolites which are generally used for the self-defense of plants attracted natural products researchers around the globe. The structures provided a number of pharmacophores compatible with the receptor molecules in the body. A large number of secondary metabolites also qualify the criterion of Lipinski rule to be considered as a drug. As a result, a number of blockbuster molecules provided by the plants as well as the marine source in the area of drug discovery. These compounds are mainly classified as flavonoids, terpenes, glycosides, steroids, and alkaloids. In recent trends, these molecules correspond to valuable contribution in pharmaceutics, cosmetics, and fine chemicals and more recently in nutraceuticals as well (Pichersky and Gang, 2000). We summarized a small understanding of these beautiful defensive compounds in the plant kingdom. Natural products obtained from the plants are summarized in Table 3.2.

TABLE 3.2 Active Anti-Inflammatory Compounds Reported from Plants

SL. No.	Plant	Plant Part	Active Constituents	References
1.	*Luffa cylindrica*	Seed	Cu-1, Cu-3	Muthumani et al. (2010)
2.	*Curcuma domestica*	Rhizome	Curcuminoids, Curcumin	Kuptniratsaikul et al. (2014)
		Aerial Parts	Quercetin 3-rutinoside, Quercetin 3-rhamnosyl-(1→2)-rhamnoside, Quercetin-3-*O*-rhamnoside	Adebayo et al. (2015)
3.	*Allium sativum*	Bulb	*Z*- and *E*-ajoene	Lee et al. (2012)
4.	*Allium cepa*	Bulb	Allicin, α-Amyrin, Ascorbic acid, β-sitosterol, Cycloartenol, Quercetin, Quercetin 3-O-β-D-Glucoside, Essential oils	Upadhyay (2016); Foe et al. (2016)
5.	*Prunus persica*	Stem bark	Acetophenone 6-hydroxy 4-methoxy 2-O-β-Dglucopyranoside (1), Crysophenol 8-O-β-D-glactopyranoside (2), β-Sitosterol, Querceitin.	Raturi et al. (2011)
		Leaves	Saponins	Edrah, Alafid, and Kumar (2013)
6.	*Commiphora mukul*	Gum resin	Cembrenoids, Guggulusterone, Myrrhanone, Myrrhanol	Francis, Raja, and Nair (2004)
7.	*Zingiber officinale*	Rhizome	10-Gingerols, 10-Shojail, Diarylheptanoid, Yakuchinone A, Proanthocyanidin,	Mashhadi et al. 2013; Al-Nahain, Jahan, and Rahmatullah (2014)
8.	*Vitis vinifera*	Leaf	Resveratrol, Quercetin, Catechin, Flavone, Flavonols, Anthocyanin, Gallic acid, Epicatechin	Aoueya et al. (2016)
		Fruit	Anthocyanins, Flavonoids, Resveratrol	Yadav et al. (2009); Xia et al. (2010)

TABLE 3.2   *(Continued)*

SL. No.	Plant	Plant Part	Active Constituents	References
9.	*Ferula assa-faetida*	Oleo-gum-resin	Umbelliprenin (Principle)	Iranshahi et al. (2009)
10.	*Ocimum sanctum*	Leaves	Cirsilineol, Cirsimaritin, Isothymusin, Isothymonin, Apigenin, Rosmarinic acid, Eugenol	Kelm et al. (2000); Prakash and Gupta (2005)
11.	*Rosmarinus officinalis*	Leaves	Triterpenes, Ursolic acid, Oleanolic acid	Altinier et al. (2007); Rahbardar et al. (2017)
12.	*Perilla frutescens*	Leaves	Ursolic acid, Corosolic acid, 3-epicorosolic acid, Pomolic acid, Tormentic acid, Hyptadienic acid, Oleanolic acid, Augustic acid, 3-epimaslinic acid	Banno et al. (2004)
13.	*Eucalyptus globulus*	Whole plant	1,8-cineole	Vecchio, Loganes, and Minto (2016)
14.	*Gentiana dahurica*	–	Roburic acid (principle),10 Iridoid glycosides, Scarban G3, Olivieroside C, Loganic acid, Loganin, Coniferin, Ecdysteroid,	Wang et al. (2013)
15.	Glycyrrhiza glabra	Roots and Rhizome	β-glycyhrritinic acid, Glyderinine	Capasso et al. (1983)
16.	*Achillea fragrantissima*	Whole plant	Cirsiliol	Yoshimoto et al. (1983)
17.	*Silybum marianum* L	Leaves	Silybin, Silydian, and Silychristin,	Gupta et al. (2000)
18.	*Apium graveolens*	Leaves	Apiin (principle)	Mencherini et al. (2007)
19.	*Carica papaya*	Leaves Fruit	Carpain, Pseudocarpain, Dehydrocarpaine I and II, Choline, Papain, Chymopapain, Vitamin C, Vitamins E, β-carotene	Yogiraj et al. (2014)

TABLE 3.2 *(Continued)*

SL. No.	Plant	Plant Part	Active Constituents	References
20.	*Syzygium aromaticum*	Flower bud	Eugenol (principle) Beta-caryophyllene, Crategolic acid, tannins, gallotannic acid, methyl salicylate (painkiller), eugenin, kaempferol, rhamnetin, and eugenitin, oleanolic acid.	Bhowmik et al. (2012)

3.3.1 FLAVONOIDS AND ISOFLAVONOIDS

Flavonoids are known for its valuable contribution against inflammation. Quercetin inhibited COX and LOX pathways at the high concentrations primary target to show anti-inflammatory activity (Mohammed et al., 2014). Luteolin, luteolin 7-glucoside, and genistein inhibit LPS stimulated TNF-α and IL-6 release leading to promising anti-inflammatory activity (Calixto et al., 2004). Apigenin found in *Achillea millefolium* is reported to have anti-inflammatory, antiplatelet properties. It is reported that silymarine (a mixture of flavonoids) isolated from *Silybum marianum* L. exhibits anti-inflammatory activity with inhibition of IL-2 and 4 (Manna et al., 1999). Nepetin, jaceosidin, and hispidulin three flavonoids isolated from dichloromethane extract of *Eupatorium arnottianum* Griseb. were found as active anti-inflammatory agents (Calixto et al., 2004). A flavonoid isolated from *Celosia argentea* L. showed anti-inflammatory activity (Shelar et al., 2010). Acacetin found in *Robinia pseudocacia* have been shown to possess significant anti-inflammatory activity (Djerassi, Connolly, and Faulkner, 1997; Sun et al., 2017). 5-hydroxy-3, 6, 7, 3′, 4′-pentamethoxyflavone isolated from the leaves of *Cordia verbenacea* (Boraginaceae) showed marked anti-inflammatory activity using various experimental models in rats. Aqueous methanolic extract of the bark of *Cinnamomum sieboldii* Meissn. (Lauraceae) yields epicatechin, catechin, procyanidin B2/B4, cinnamonol D1 and D4 possess potent inhibitory activity on the formation of granulation tissue through screening by the fertile egg methods (Otsuka et al., 1982). Zingiberaceae also reported to have anti-inflammatory activity (Harborne, (1989). Hesperidin, an active constituent isolated from *Citrus* plants have significant anti-inflammatory activity on rat paw edema induced by both carrageenan and dextran on carrageenan pleurisy, without producing the side effects that are caused by other classes of anti-inflammatory drugs (Mohammed et al., 2014). About 30 flavonoids isolated from several plants of the composite family were already investigated for anti-inflammatory activities (Jin et al., 2010).

3.3.2 POLY-PHENOLS

Polyphenols represent an important class of natural compounds with unique biological properties. These are mainly present as a dietary supplement in fruits, vegetables, green tea, and white wine, etc. By experimental data on animals and human cell lines, it has been proven that polyphenols help as potent anti-inflammatory agents since they possess scavenging properties towards radical oxygen species and complex forming ability towards proteins. Thus, polyphenols prove very interesting naturally occurring compounds for the treatment and prevention of various diseases like cancer and inflammation. Pro-anthocyanidins present in grape seeds reduce the expression of TNF-α and IKKα/β, shows strong anti-inflammatory activity. Catechins contain a polyphenolic ring mainly present as important biologically active constituents in green tea and are considered as one of the most powerful antioxidants (Somani et al., 2015). Epigallocatechin-3-gallate (EGCG), catechin isolated from green tea plant *Camellia sinensis*, shows therapeutic potential in the treatment of arthritis. Further, it acts as a strong modulator for inflammation by inhibiting the activation of NF-κB and several well established proinflammatory cytokines such as IL-1 and TNFα (Lin et al., 2008).

A polyphenolic compound hydroxytyrosol, from extra virgin olive oil, exhibits strong anti-inflammatory activity by improvement in a model of DSS-induced colitis (Sánchez et al., 2015). Resveratrol mainly present in grapes, wine, and peanut products, etc., is a polyphenolic stilbene which occurs in *cis* or *trans* configuration. Laboratory studies on animals, human cultured cells suggest that it possess therapeutic potential as anti-inflammatory, anti-carcinogenic, anti-oxidants which may further prove relevant for the treatment of chronic diseases (Smoliga, Baur, and Hausenblas, 2011). Another important flavonol, kaempferol [3,5,7-trihydroxy-2-(4-hydroxyphenyl)-4H-1-benzopyran-4-one] has a wide range of pharmacological activities, including antioxidant, anti-inflammatory, anticancer, cardioprotective, neuroprotective, antiallergic, and antidiabetic (Somani et al., 2015).

3.3.3 ALKALOID

Isoquinolines protoberberine (berberine, palmatine, jatrorrhizine, columbamine), bisbenzylisoquinoline (berbamine, oxyacanthine, aromoline) and aporphine (magnoflorine) isolated from the roots, barks, and branches of *Turkish berberis* species have shown good anti-inflammatory activity (Hristova and Istatkova, 1999). Since ancient times bisbenzylisoquinoline alkaloids have been used as major components of some anti-rheumatic remedies. Recently, bisbenzylisoquinoline alkaloids are also reported to possess anti-inflammatory properties by inhibiting synthesis or the action of some pro-inflammatory cytokines. One of the well-known bisbenzylisoquinoline alkaloids is tetrandrine and its analogsberbamine, fangchinoline. Cepharanthine, cycleanine, isotetrandrine isolated from *Stephania cephararantha* exhibited suppressive effects on histamine release (Satoh, Nagai, Ono, and Aoki, 2003). *Aconitum flavum* Hand-Mazz and *A. pendulum* Busch from family Ranunculaceae were found to inhibit the increased vascular permeability induced by acetic acid or histamine and also inhibited carrageenan-induced edema (Tang et al., 1984). O-acetylethanolamine an active constituent isolated from the seeds of *Adenanthera pavonina* Linn. contains an anti-inflammatory activity. A piperidine alkaloid betonicine distributed among various plants viz. *Betonica officinalis*, *Marrubium vulgare*, *Stachys sylvatica* (Labiatae), *Achillea moschata*, and *A. millefolium* (Compositae) is found to significantly inhibit carrageenan-induced hind paw edema (MacLean, 1985).

3.3.4 TERPENES

A number of triterpenes of oleanane, ursane, and euphane series have been isolated from the gum-resin of *Boswellia serrata* is used in *Ayurveda* for the treatment of osteoarthritis, juvenile rheumatoid arthritis. The four major pentacyclic triterpenic acids, i.e., β-boswellic acid, acetyl-β-boswellic acid, 11-keto-β-boswellic acid (most potent) and acetyl-11-keto-β-boswellic acid are mainly responsible for the inhibition of pro-inflammatory enzymes (Siddiqui, 2011). Andrographolide, and neoandrographolide isolated from the methanolic extract of *Andrographis paniculata*, inhibit LPS-stimulated NO production in a concentration-dependent manner (Batkhuu et al., 2002). The chloroform extract of the stem has also shown statistically significant anti-inflammatory activity against carrageenan-induced edema (Radhika et al., 2009). The seeds of *Aesculus indica* possess anti-inflammatory activity due to the presence of aescin, aesculuside A and B (triterpene glycoside) (Singh, Agrawal, and Thakur, 1987). The essential oils (EOs) of many species of the genus Eucalyptus (Myrtaceae), *Cordia verbenacea* (Boraginaceae), *Lippia sidoides* leaves (Verbenaceae), *Lippia gracilis* Schauer leaves (Verbenaceae), and *Zizyphus jujube* seeds are well established for their analgesic and anti-inflammatory effects. Camphor an active constituent isolated from *Matricaria parthenium* (Compuestas) has pronounced anti-inflammatory activity in rat paw edema studies (Saxena et al., 1982; Chaturvedi et al., 1974; Pitre and Srivastava, 1987; Rudakov, 1976).

Chrysanthemum indicum is widely used to treat immune-related and infectious disorders in East Asia for a long time. Flower oil contains 1,8-cineole, germacrene D, camphor, α-cardinal, camphene, pinocarvone, β-caryophyllene, 3-cyclohexane-1-on, and γ-curcumene. Octulosonic acid derivative, chrysannol A, isolated from *Chrysanthemum indicum* flowers has also shown *in-vitro* anti-inflammatory effects. Results are important in terms of the development of *C. indicum* as an anti-inflammatory functional food (Hwang and Kim, 2013; Luyen et al., 2015). The most valued and ancient among medicinal plants *G. biloba* of family Ginkgoaceae rediscover its existence as important pharmacological compounds and their therapeutic effects. The worldwide sales of ginkgo leaf products are difficult to estimate but believed to be worth around half a billion USD or more (Isah, 2015). The main constituent of oil coriander linalool from *Coriandrum sativum* (Umbelliferae) exhibits anti-inflammatory action. The bioactive constituent α and β pinene of *Bupleurum fructicosum* L. (Umbelliferae) essential oil have shown significant anti-inflammatory activity in carrageenan-induced rat paw edema model (Perez, 2001). Lupeol, a novel dietary triterpene (also known as Fagarsterol) present in white cabbage, green pepper, strawberry, olive, mangoes, and grapes is reported to possess beneficial effects as anti-inflammatory and anti-cancer (Mohammad, 2009).

3.3.5 STEROLS

Pentacyclic triterpenes (PTs) as aglycones of saponins have been used as anti-inflammatory remedies in folk medicine (Safayhi and Sailer, 1997). *Betula alba*, *B. pendula*, *B. pubescent,* and *B. platyphylla* containing betulin as an active biological constituent. Studies reported on the activity of methanolic extract from the rhizomes of *N. nucifera*, as well as betulin and betulinic acid, revealed a marked inhibition of the carrageenan and serotonin-induced rat paw edema. The fruit juice of *Ecballium elaterium* L.A Cucurbitacin. (Family-Cucurbitaceae) used as Turkish folk medicine for the treatment of sinusitis has been investigated for its anti-inflammatory activity (Perez, 2001). Plant sterols and n-3 polyunsaturated fatty acids (PUFA) reduces systemic inflammation as well as are cardioprotective in hyperlipidemic individuals (Micallef and Garga, 2009). Oleanolic acid 3-glucoside Isolated from *Randia dumetorum* Lam. (Rubiaceae) seeds showed significant anti-arthritic activity in the exudative and proliferative phases of inflammation in rats (Perez, 2001). *Cyperus rotundus* (Cyperaceae) and *Bryophyllum pinnatum* (Crassulaceae) contain β-sitosterol which shows anti-inflammatory and antipyretic activities which have been studied on carrageenan-induced edema, cotton pellet implantation, and Brewer's yeast-induced pyrexia in rats. β-Sitosterol was found to possess potent anti-inflammatory activity against both tests, similar to hydrocortisone and oxyphenbutazone (Perez, 2001).

3.3.6 SAPONINS

Saponins are steroids or triterpenoid glycosides which are commonly present in plants or plant products having diverse biological action. Various saponins have been isolated from plants with well addressed anti-inflammatory activity. A triterpene saponin from *Bupleurum rotundifolium* proved to be effective against TPA (12-O-tetradecanoylphorbol-13-acetate)-induced ear edema in mice (Navarro et al., 2001). According to folk medicine extract of *Yucca schidigera* have anti-arthritic and anti-inflammatory effects. Presence of 10% of steroidal saponins in its stem dry mater makes the plant one of the richest commercial sources of saponins (Cheeke, Piacente, and Oleszek, 2006).

Buddleja saponin IV, an anti-inflammatory compound isolated from *Pleurospermum kamtschatidum* inhibits the expressions of iNOS, COX-2, TNF-α, IL-1β, and IL-6 by blocking NF-κB activation (Won et al., 2006). α-hederin and hederasaponin-C of *Hedera helix*, and hederacolchisides-E/F of *H. colchica* origin have inhibited carrageenan-induced acute paw edema in rats. The anti-inflammatory effects of the compounds are reported due to blocking of bradykinin or other inflammation mediators. The structure-activity relationship of saponins suggests that sugars at C_3 position and Rha7-Glc1-6Glc moiety at C_{28} position are essential for the acute anti-inflammatory effect (Gepdiremena et al., 2005).

3.4 NATURAL PRODUCT INSPIRED SCAFFOLD DESIGNING

Nature provides an inexhaustible array of compounds for medicinal, nutra-ceutical, and pharmaceutical purposes in the form of naturally occurring bioactive constituents or by providing leads for semi-synthetic targets. The screening of the potential leads for further drug designing by semi-synthesis or total synthesis approaches has derived as a new tool for the discovery of novel active leads for anti-inflammatory compounds. Curcumin, a well-known biologically active compound possesses a wide range of pharmacological activities including anti-inflammatory. Studies revealed the pharmacological potential of curcumin analogs. Based on the remarkable anti-inflammatory activity biologically active leads could be generated (Figure 3.1) (Bukhari et al., 2013). The potential anti-inflammatory activity of overall 33 alkylated and prenylated mono carbonyl analogs of curcumin (MACs) have shown the inhibition of expression of TNF-α and in LPS-induced RAW 264.7 macro-phages (Figure 3.2) (Liu et al., 2014). A curcumin derivative namely (2E,5E)-2,5-bis(4-(3-(dimethylamino)-propoxy)benzylidene)cyclopentanone   has shown significant inhibition in plasma concentration NO, TNF-α, and IL-6 in lipopolysaccharide-challenged mice, and also inhibited the increase of hepatic inflammatory gene transcription, thus improved pulmonary damages (Figure 3.3) (Wang et al., 2012).

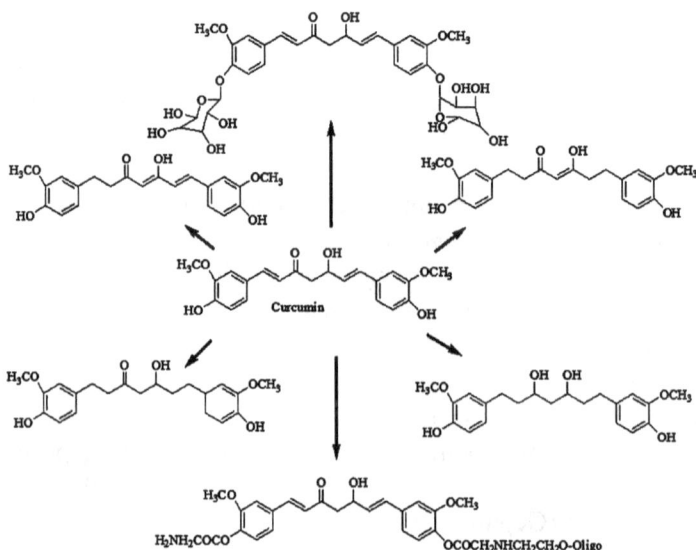

FIGURE 3.1   Curcumin derivates and their analogs.

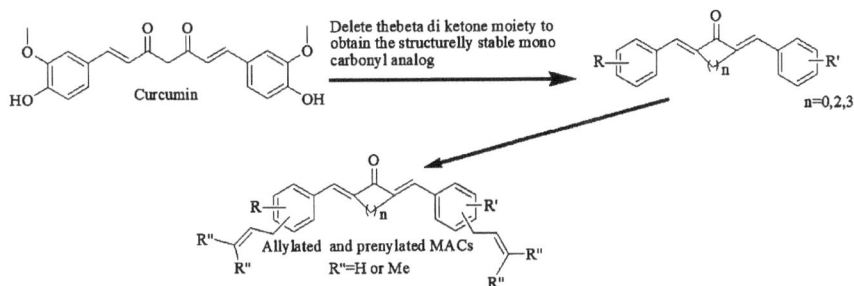

FIGURE 3.2 Alkylated and prenylated mono-carbonyl analogs of curcumin.

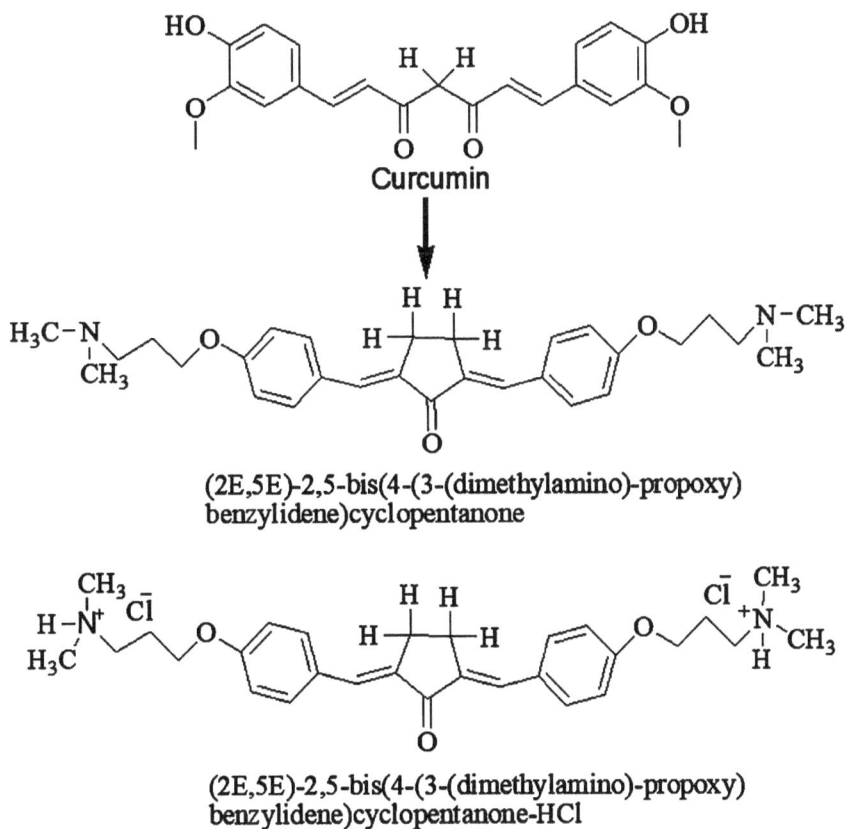

(2E,5E)-2,5-bis(4-(3-(dimethylamino)-propoxy)
benzylidene)cyclopentanone

(2E,5E)-2,5-bis(4-(3-(dimethylamino)-propoxy)
benzylidene)cyclopentanone-HCl

FIGURE 3.3 Mono-carbonyl analog of curcumin.

In *Ayurvedic* system of medicine, *Cleome viscosa* (Family: Capparida-ceae) commonly called as Wild mustard is known to be effective in inflam-mations. Polyhalogenated derivatives of cleomiscosin, methyl ether found to exhibit anti-inflammatory potential *in vitro* primary macrophages cell culture system (Figure 3.4) (Mali, 2010; Sharma et al., 2012).

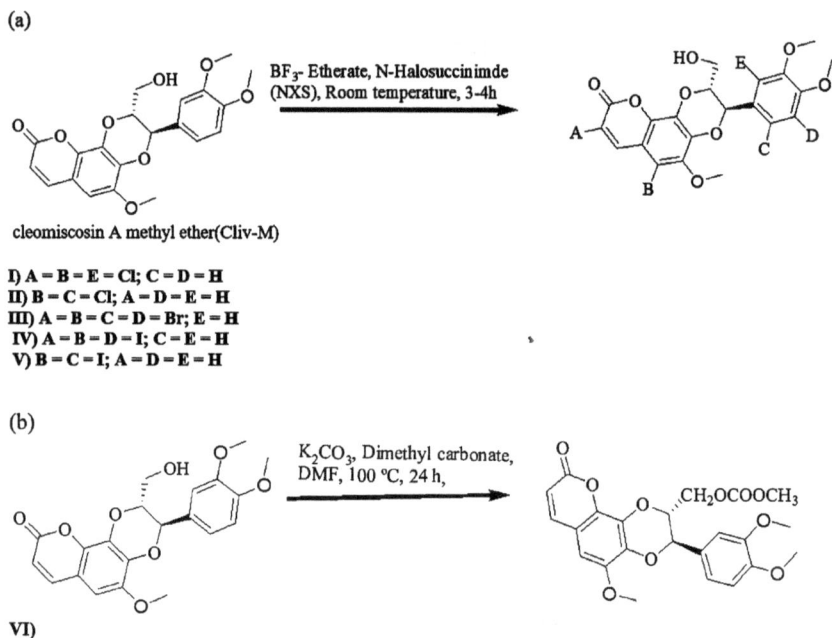

(a)

cleomiscosin A methyl ether(Cliv-M)

I) A = B = E = Cl; C = D = H
II) B = C = Cl; A = D = E = H
III) A = B = C = D = Br; E = H
IV) A = B = D = I; C = E = H
V) B = C = I; A = D = E = H

(b)

VI)

FIGURE 3.4   (a) Synthesis of five new cleomiscosin A methyl ether derivatives; (b) synthesis of cleomiscosin A methyl ether.

Acanthus ilicifolius is a traditional Chinese herb-drug having 4-hydroxy-2-benzoxazolone (HBOA) as the major bioactive benzoxazolones compounds. Total nine derivates of HBOA have been synthesized and examined for their anti-inflammatory activity by using carrageenan-induced rat paw edema test (Figure 3.5) (Zheng et al., 2015). (+)-Balasubramide is an eight-membered lactam compound obtained from the leaves of the Sri Lankan plant *Clausena India*. Li et al. prepared (+)–Balasubramide and its derivatives. All compounds were undertaken to test their *in vitro* antineuro-inflammatory effects against LPS-induced pro-inflammatory cytokine TNFα expression in microglial cells (Figure 3.6) (Li et al., 2016).

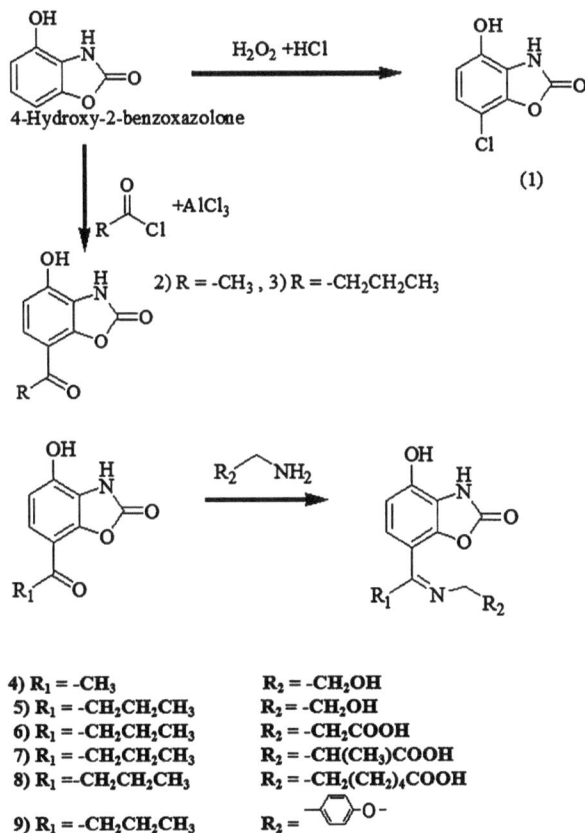

4-Hydroxy-2-benzoxazolone

H_2O_2 +HCl

(1)

+AlCl$_3$

2) R = -CH$_3$, 3) R = -CH$_2$CH$_2$CH$_3$

R_2 NH$_2$

4) R$_1$ = -CH$_3$ **R$_2$ = -CH$_2$OH**
5) R$_1$ = -CH$_2$CH$_2$CH$_3$ **R$_2$ = -CH$_2$OH**
6) R$_1$ = -CH$_2$CH$_2$CH$_3$ **R$_2$ = -CH$_2$COOH**
7) R$_1$ = -CH$_2$CH$_2$CH$_3$ **R$_2$ = -CH(CH$_3$)COOH**
8) R$_1$ =-CH$_2$CH$_2$CH$_3$ **R$_2$ = -CH$_2$(CH$_2$)$_4$COOH**

9) R$_1$ = -CH$_2$CH$_2$CH$_3$ **R$_2$ =**

FIGURE 3.5   Syntheses of 4-hydroxy-2-benzoxazolone derivates.

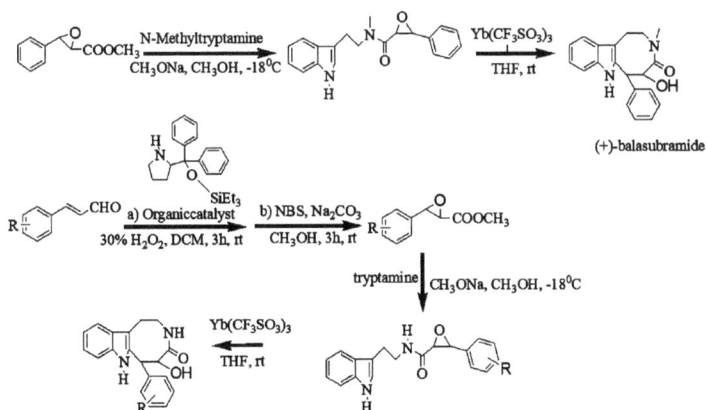

FIGURE 3.6   Syntheses of (+)-Balasubramide and their derivatives.

Wide literature available throughout the world has now proven the uses of cloves in a toothache, headache, and respiratory disorders and in many more ailments. Oleanolic acid, one of the constituents of the cloves of *Syzygium aromaticum* is a triterpenoid known for its anti-inflammatory and anti-cancer properties (Lee et al., 2013).3-acetoxyoleanolic acid 3-acetoxy-28-methylester oleanolic acid was synthesized by oleanolic acid isolated from *S. aromaticum* was evaluated for their anti-inflammatory properties using the serotonin and fresh egg albumin-induced inflammatory test models in male Wistar rats weighing from 250 to 300 g (Figure 3.7). Significant results were obtained for semisynthetic analogs 3-acetoxyolea-nolic acid and 3-acetoxy, 28-methylester. Oleanolic acid was found to exhibit anti-inflammatory properties in the albumin and serotonin-induced inflammatory test (Nkeh et al., 2015). In traditional Mexican medicine, *Verbesina persicifolia*, a medicinal plant commonly known as 'huichin,' has been used to treat a variety of diseases. One more compound, i.e., 4β-cinnamoyloxy, 1β, 3α-dihydroxyeudesm-7, 8-ene (1) and its derivates namely diacetate (2), hydrogenate (3) and diacetate hydrogenate (4) were synthesized in lab (Figure 3.8). Further, the anti-inflammatory effect was assayed by TPA-induced ear edema test. All derivatives exerts an anti-inflammatory effect significantly lower than that exerted by (1) (Via et al., 2015).

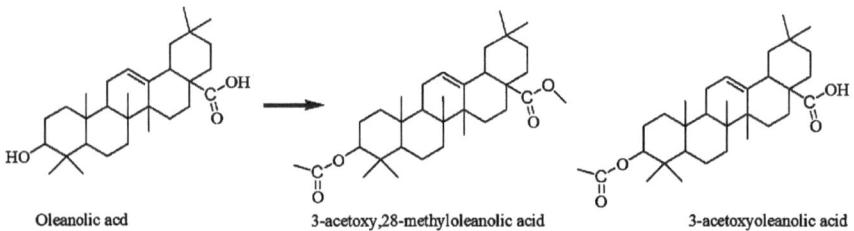

Oleanolic acd   3-acetoxy,28-methyloleanolic acid   3-acetoxyoleanolic acid

FIGURE 3.7   Oleanolic acid and their derivates (3-acetoxyoleanolic acid and 3-acetoxy, 28-methylester oleanolic acid).

The isolation of salicin derivatives from the twigs of *Salix glandulosa* Seemen (Figure 3.9) is reported for their NO inhibitory efficacy in lipo-polysaccharide (LPS)-activated microglial cell (BV-2). The results show that salicin derivatives from *Salix glandulosa* might have potent effect as anti-neuroinflammatory agents (Kim et al., 2015).

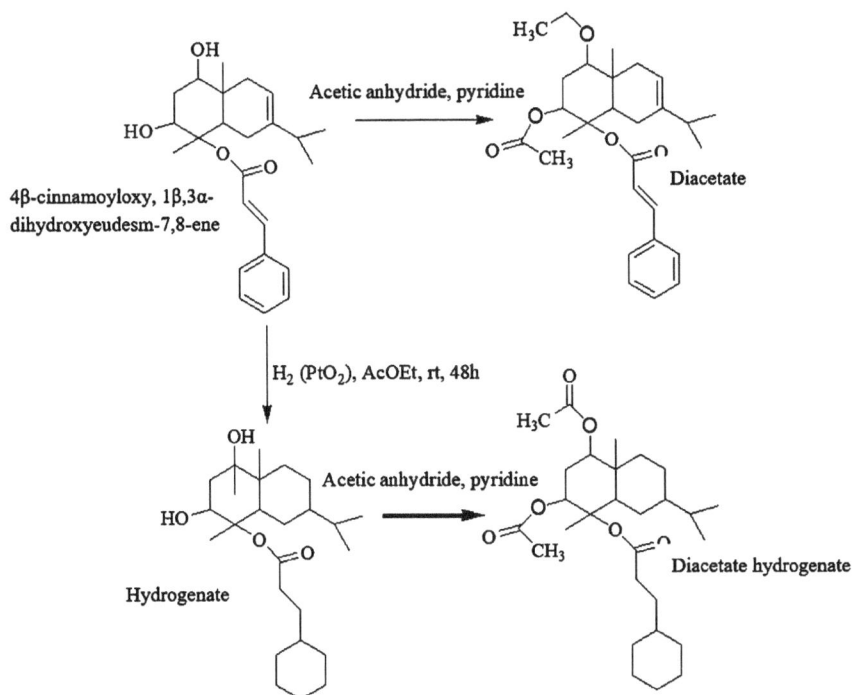

FIGURE 3.8 Synthesis of 4β-cinnamoyloxy, 1β,3α-dihydroxyeudesm-7,8-ene derivatives (diacetate, hydrogenate, and diacetate hydrogenate.

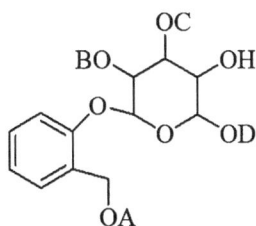

FIGURE 3.9 Salicin derivatives (1–14) where A, B, C, D are H, Ac, benzoyl, etc., groups.

3.5 ANTI-INFLAMMATORY NATURAL PRODUCTS IN CLINICAL TRIALS

Natural products are obtained from a different class of compounds such as alkaloids, flavonoids, terpenoids, saponins, and fatty acids, etc., and are widely distributed in the Plant Kingdom. These secondary metabolites represent a great structural diversity in their basic moiety. Leads obtained from the natural products are counterintuitive as their sources, which is already being used traditionally. Natural products derived leads can be an excellent API (active pharmaceutical ingredient) except for sometimes when its complex structure and bioavailability is a major task. In order to get a detailed understanding of the anti-inflammatory drug development process, the related structure-activity relationship (SAR) and mechanism of action need to understand (Butler et al., 2014).

Since ancient times, natural products have served to treat human diseases. During the '70s and 80's the investigation of natural products reached its height as a source of novel human therapeutics in pharmaceutical industries, which also grabbed the attention of the pharmaceutical landscape to non-synthetic molecules. After that, the number of new chemical entities were introduced in the system in which approximately 49% were natural products, analogs of natural products or natural pharmacophore-based derived mole-cules (Koehn and Carter, 2005). After a tremendous achievement natural products faced a sluggish decline in the last two decades because of the long product development period.

There is a number of plant-derived drugs are in the market, and some are in clinical trial phases such as Flavocoxid extract derived from *Scutellaria baicalensis* (Lamiaceae) and *Acacia catechu* (Mimosaceae) is in Phase I. This is developed by National Institute of Arthritis and Musculoskeletal and Skin Diseases, U.S.A. and Primus Pharmaceuticals. It is found to inhibit COX-1, COX-2, and 5-lipoxygenase. An intravenous chemotherapy agent Paxceed (*micella Paclitaxel*), developed by Agiotech pharmaceuticals is in Phase II. PMI-001 a botanical drug with multiple modes of mechanism and synergistic inhibition of IL-2, α-TNF, COX-2, and iNOS is in III phase of clinical. PMI-005 developed by phytomedicines for rheumatoid arthritis has completed Phase II in clinical trials. PMI-005 orally bioavailable and found to be active against pro-inflammatory cytokines including IL-2, α-TNF (Li and Li, 2011), COX-2 and iNOS. PMI-005 Phase II completed. It is an anti-inflammatory just finished with the II phase of clinical trials. A formula-tion PYN17 from European Chinese plants developed by Phynova to treat chronic hepatitis is in Phase IIa. IP-751 (Ajulemic acid, CT-3) appears to inhibit COX-2, and other inflammatory cytokines, particularly interleukin-1b, TNF-a, and also the peroxisomes proliferating activated receptor-g (PPAR-g) and is partial cannabinoid (CB) receptor agonist (Saklani and Kutty, 2008).

3.5.1 CURCUMINOIDS

Curcumin, bisdemethoxycurcumin and demethoxycurcumin come under curcuminoids in which curcumin is the major component and two other molecules are in less quantity and presence of all three components is the hallmark of the yellow color of *Curcuma longa*. Curcumin, a polyphenolic molecule abundant in India obtained from turmeric (*Curcuma longa*) turmeric has been used traditionally for pain-relieving and inflammation. Curcumin is diferuloylmethane was confirmed during 1970–1980. Structure of curcumin was confirmed by degradative work, boiling with alkali curcumin gives vanillic acid and ferulic acid, fusion with alkali yields protocatechuic acid and oxidation with potassium permanganate yielded vanillin. The presence of olefinic double bond at C3, C4, C3' and C4' as well as the presence of hydroxyl group at C8 and C8' positions is responsible for its anti-inflammatory activity (Mukhopadhyay et al., 1982). Phenolic group of curcumin is the active site when compared with the non-phenolic analogs of curcumin (Venkatesan and Rao, 2000). Most of the curcumin derivatives were designed in place of the hydroxyl group to a methyl group. Studies on the antioxidant properties of ring-substituted analogs of curcumin concluded that phenolic analogs were more active than the non-phenolic analogs. Sterical hindrance by the introduction of two methyl group sat the orthoposition lead the molecule to possess highest antioxidant activity (Selvam et al., 2005).

Pyrazole and isoxazole analogs were synthesized and studied for its antioxidant, COX-1/COX-2 inhibitory and anti-inflammatory activities. Significance enhances of COX-2/COX-1 selectivity and remarkable anti-inflammatory activity in carrageenan-induced rat paw edema assay was found. Pyrazole, isoxazole analogs of curcumin (4 and 7) exhibited higher antioxidant activity than trolox. Molecular docking study revealed the binding orientations of curcumin analogs in the active sites of COX and thereby helps to design novel potent inhibitors.

The SAR studies revealed that curcumin derivative increased the COX-1 activity slightly (80.5–87.0% inhibition), whereas the COX-2 inhibitory activity increased twofold (35–61.0% inhibition). COX-1/COX-2 inhibitory activity of three pyrazole analogs was analyzed by in vitro COX catalyzed PG biosynthesis assay and it was slightly enhanced.

Curcumin was found to have IC_{50} value of 2 lM,10 52 lM11 and 5–10 Lm From the literature it was found that curcumin was investigated for COX inhibitory activity using bovine seminal vesicles, microsomes, and cytosol from homogenates of mouse epidermis showed IC_{50} value of 2 lM,10 52 lM11 and 5–10 Lm. Extensive studies have been reported for curcumin in human volunteers; its anti-inflammatory activity is basically due to inhibition of COX, LOX, iIL, TNFα and NFκB (Yuan et al., 2006).

3.5.2   PARTHENOLIDS

Parthenolide are isolated from *Tanacetum parthenium* L and are major sesquiterpenes lactones. Commonly occurs in leaves and flower heads of feverfew. *Tanacetum parthenium* is locally used by Mexican Indians for infectious diseases for a long time. Its methylene γ-lactone ring epoxide group has neuclophillic nature which enables its fast interaction with the receptor. The interaction between these sites and the receptors can induce oxidative stress and also shows anticancer properties (Mathema et al., 2012; Jain and Kulkarni, 1999; Li et al., 2002).

3.5.3   1-8-CINOLE

Cinole is one of the major constituents of many aromatic plants, also known as eucalyptol/cajeputol. Cineole is a terpene oxide is present in many aromatic plants such as *Lavandula angustifolia*, Eucalyptus oils of *Eucalyptus citriodora*, *Eucalyptus tereticornis* (ET) and *Eucalyptus globulus* (75%), Rosemary (40%), Psidium (40–60%), etc. (Silva et al., 2003). Cineole is reported to have anti-microbial, anti-oxidant, and anti-inflammatory. This major monoterpene of eucalyptus oil inhibits arachidonic acid metabolism and cytokine production in human monocytes. Substitution with the hydrophobic groups or electron-donating groups increase the inhibition. The location of the phenolic ring also plays a major role such as methyl substitution at ortho/para with meta-position in the ring (Dewhirst, 1980).

3.5.4   CUCURBETACIANS

Cucurbitacins are extremely oxygenated, tetracyclic triterpenes containing a cucurbitane skeleton characterized by a 19-(10→9β)-abeo-10α-lanost-5-ene. These are abundant in the Cucurbitaceae family and are also known as the bitter principles, but later they can be seen in other genera also. Cucurbitanes are divided into 12 categories (Yuan et al., 2006; Jayaprakasam, Seeram, and Nair, 2003). Acetyl group position 28(C) is responsible for inhibiting COX-2 and used for inflammation. Dihydrocucurbitacin B, cucurbitacin R, cucurbitacins isolated from the roots of *Cayaponia tayuya*, are found to have decent anti-inflammatory activity (Recio et al., 2004). Cucurbitacins such as cucurbitacin B, D, E, and I were already reported to have significant anti-inflammatory activity.

3.6   CONCLUSION

Over modern drugs, researchers are now focusing on the resurgence of plant-based drugs; in that respect, this review summarized the number of plants from *Ayurveda* which possess anti-inflammatory application either from the formulation or crude drug. Some discoveries also including compounds isolated from *Ayurvedic* plants and pharmacological way of the mechanism are listed. We also have discussed a number of plants used worldwide in their crude form (Extract), to get a basic idea of what are the plants which can be explored extensively for their target molecules responsible for the anti-inflammatory activity. Various studies can be done for hit and trial with the use of modern analytical techniques such as HPLC, NMR, HPTLC, flash chromatography, and UPLC, etc., to identify the lead and study the metabolomics of a compound from the active extract. In this review a brief number of molecules and their derivatives are summarized for a basic understanding of anti-inflammatory compounds, also tried to study the SAR of compounds also illustrated.

KEYWORDS

- **anti-inflammatory**
- **derivatives**
- **medicinal plants**
- **natural products**
- **pharmacophore**
- **structure-activity relationship**

REFERENCES

Adebayo, S. A., Dzoyem, J. P., Shai, L. J., & Eloff, J. N., (2015). The anti-inflammatory and antioxidant activity of 25 plant species used traditionally to treat pain in Southern African. *BMC Complementary and Alternative Medicine, 15,* 159.

Adedapo, A., Adewuyi, T., & Sofidiya, M., (2013). Phytochemistry, anti-inflammatory and analgesic activities of the aqueous leaf extract of *Lagenaria breviflora* (Cucurbitaceae) in laboratory animals. *Revista de Biología Tropical, 61,* 281–290.

Aggarwal, B. B., Prasad, S., Reuter, S., Kannappan, R., Yadev, V. R., Park, B., Kim, J. H., et al., (2011). Identification of novel anti-inflammatory agents from *Ayurvedic* medicine for prevention of chronic diseases: "reverse pharmacology" and "bedside to bench" approach. *Current Drug Targets, 12,* 1595–1653.

Al-Nahain, A., Jahan, R., & Rahmatullah, M., (2014). *Zingiber officinale*: A potential plant against rheumatoid arthritis. *Arthritis,* 1–8.

Altinier, G., Sosa, S., Aquino, R. P., Mencherini, T., Loggia, R. D., & Tubaro, A., (2007). Characterization of topical anti-inflammatory compounds in *Rosmarinus officinalis* L. *Journal of Agriculture and Food Chemistry, 55,* 1718–1723.

Aoueya, B., Sameta, A. M., Fetouia, H., Simmonds, M. S. J., & Bouazizb, M., (2016). Anti-oxidant, anti-inflammatory, analgesic and antipyretic activities of grapevine leaf extract (*Vitis vinifera* in mice and identification of its active constituents by LC–MS/MS analyses. *Biomedicine & Pharmacotherapy, 84,* 1088–1098.

Azevedo, A. P. S., Farias, J. C., Costa, G. C., Ferreira, S. C. P., Aragao, F. W. C., Sousa, P. R. A., Pinheiro, M. T., et al., (2007). Anti-thrombotic effect of chronic oral treatment with *Orbignya phalerata* mart. *Journal of Ethnopharmacology, 111,* 155–159.

Banno, N., Akihisa, T., Tokuda, H., Yasukawa, K., Higashihara, H., Ukiya, M., Watanabe, K., et al., (2004). Triterpene acids from the leaves of *Perilla frutescens* and their anti-inflammatory and antitumor-promoting effects. *Bioscience, Biotechnology, and Biochemistry, 68,* 85–90.

Batkhuu, J., Hattori, K., Takano, F., Fushiya, S., Oshiman, K., & Fujimiya, Y., (2002). Suppression of NO production in activated macrophages *in vitro* and *ex-vivo* by neoandrographolide isolated from *Andrographis paniculata*. *Biological and Pharmaceutical Bulletin, 25,* 1169–1174.

Bhagwandash, V., (1978). *Fundamentals of Ayurvedic Medicine* (p. 228). Konark Publishers, Delhi, India. ISBN: 8122001173.

Bharathi, T. R., Nadafi, R., & Prakash, H. S., (2014). *In vitro* antioxidant and anti-inflammatory properties of different solvent extracts of *Memecylon talbotianum* brandis. *International Journal of Phytopharmacy, 4,* 148–152.

Bhowmik, D., Kumar, K. S., Yadav, A., Srivastava, S., Paswan, S., & Dutta, A. S., (2012). Recent trends in Indian traditional herbs *Syzygium aromaticum* and its health benefits. *Journal of Pharmacognosy and Phytochemistry, 1,* 13–23.

Bisht, R., Bhattacharya, S., & Jaliwala, Y. A., (2014). COX and LOX inhibitory potential of *Abroma augusta* and *Desmodium gangeticum*. *The Journal of Phytopharmacology, 3,* 168–175.

Bukhari, S. N. A., Jantan, I. B., Jasamai, M., Ahmad, W., & Amjad, M. W. B., (2013). Synthesis and biological evaluation of curcumin analogues. *Journal of Medical Sciences, 13,* 501–513.

Butler, M. S., Robertson, A. A. B., & Cooper, M. A., (2014). Natural product and natural product derived drugs in clinical trials. *Natural Product Reports, 31,* 1612–1661.

Calder, P. C., Albers, R., Antoine, J. M., Blum, S., Sicard, B. R., Ferns, G. A., Folkerts, G., et al., (2009). Inflammatory disease processes and interactions with nutrition. *British Journal of Nutrition, 101*, 1–45.

Calixto, J. B., Campos, M. M., Otuki, M. F., & Santos, A. R. S., (2004). Anti-inflammatory compounds of plant origin. Part II. Modulation of pro-inflammatory cytokines, chemokines and adhesion molecules. *Planta Medica, 70*, 93–103.

Capasso, F., Mascolo, N., Autore, G., & Duraccio, M. R., (1983). Glycyrrhetinic acid, leucocytes and prostaglandins. *Journal of Pharmacy and Pharmacology, 35*, 332–335.

Chaturvedi, A. K., Parmar, S. S., Bhatnagar, S. C., Misra, G., & Nigam, S. K., (1974). Anticonvulsant and anti-inflammatory activity of natural plant coumarins and triterpenoids. *Research Communications in Chemical Pathology and Pharmacology, 9*, 11–22.

Cheeke, P., R, Piacente, S., & Oleszek, W., (2006). Anti-inflammatory and anti-arthritic effects of *yucca schidigera*: A review. *Journal of Inflammation, 3*, 1–7.

Chung, Y. S., Choi, Y. H., Lee, S. J., Choi, S. A., Lee, J. H., Kim, H., & Hong, E. K., (2005). Water extract of *Aralia elata* prevents cataractogenesis *in vitro* and *in vivo*. *Journal of Ethnopharmacology, 101*, 49–54.

Dewhirst, F. E., (1980). Structure-activity relationships for inhibition of prostaglandin cyclooxygenase by phenolic compounds. *Prostaglandins, 20*, 209–222.

Djerassi, C., Connolly, J. D., & Faulkner, D. J., (1997). *Dictionary of Natural Products Supplement 4* (Vol. 11, pp. 256–257). Chapman and Hall: Buckingham J. ed. London: CRC Press.

Edrah, S., Alafid, F., & Kumar, A., (2013). Preliminary phytochemical screening and antibacterial activity of *Pistacia atlantica* and *Prunus persica* plants of Libyan origin. *International Journal of Science and Research, 6*, 4–438.

Foe, F. M. C. N., Tchinang, T. F. K., Nyegue, A. M., Abdou, J. P., Yaya, A. J. G., Tchinda, A. T., Essame, J. L. O., & Etoa, F. X., (2016). Chemical composition, *in-vitro* antioxidant and anti-inflammatory properties of essential oils of four dietary and medicinal plants from Cameroon. *BMC Complementary and Alternative Medicine, 16*, 1–12.

Francis, J. A., Raja, S. N., & Nair, M. G., (2004). Bioactive terpenoids and guggulusteroids from *Commiphora mukul* gum resin of potential anti-inflammatory interest. *Chemistry and Biodiversity, 1*, 1842–1853.

Gautam, R., & Jachak, S. M., (2009). Recent developments in anti-inflammatory natural products. *Medicinal Research Reviews, 29*, 767–820.

Gepdiremena, A., Mshvildadzeb, V., Suleymana, H., & Eliasc, R., (2005). Acute anti-inflammatory activity of four saponins isolated from ivy: Alpha-hederin, hederasaponin-C, hederacolchiside-E and hederacolchiside-F in carrageenan-induced rat paw edema. *Phytomedicine, 12*, 440–444.

Gupta, O. P., Singh, S., Bani, S., Sharma, N., Malhotra, S., Gupta, B. D., Banerjee, S. K., & Handa, S. S., (2000). Anti-inflammatory and anti-arthritic activities of silymarin acting through inhibition of 5-lipoxygenase. *Phytomedicine, 7*, 21–24.

Harborne, J. B., (1989). General procedures and measurement of total phenolics. *Methods in Plant Biochemistry, 1*, 1–28.

Hristova, M., & Istatkova, R., (1999). Complement-mediated anti-inflammatory effect of bisbenzylisoquinoline alkaloid fangchinoline. *Phytomedicine, 6*, 357–362.

Hwang, E. S., & Kim, G. H., (2013). Safety evaluation of *Chrysanthemum indicum* L. flower oil by assessing acute oral toxicity, micronucleus abnormalities, and mutagenicity. *Preventive Nutrition and Food Science, 18*, 111–116.

Iranshahi, M., Askari, M., Sahebkar, A., & Adjipavlou, L. D., (2009). Evaluation of antioxidant, anti-inflammatory and lipoxygenase inhibitory activities of the prenylated coumarin umbelliprenin. *Journal of Pharmaceutical Sciences, 17*, 99–103.

Isah, T., (2015). Rethinking *Ginkgo biloba* L.: Medicinal uses and conservation. *Pharmacognosy Review, 9*, 140–148.

Jachak, S. M., (2006). Cyclooxygenase inhibitory natural products: Current status. *Current Medicinal Chemistry, 13*, 659–678.

Jain, N. K., & Kulkarni, S. K., (1999). Antinociceptive and anti-inflammatory effects of *Tanacetum parthenium* L. extract in mice and rats. *Journal of Ethnopharmacology, 68*, 251–259.

Jayaprakasam, B., Seeram, N. P., & Nair, M. G., (2003). Anticancer and anti-inflammatory activities of cucurbitacins from *Cucurbitaandreana. Cancer Letters, 189*, 11–16.

Jin, J. H., Kim, J. S., Kang, S. S., Son, K. H., Chang, H. W., & Kim, H. P., (2010). Anti-inflammatory and anti-arthritic activity of total flavonoids of the roots of *Sophora flavescens. Journal of Ethnopharmacology, 127*, 589–595.

Kang, J. S., Lee, K. H., Han, M. H., Lee, H., Ahn, J. M., Han, S. B., Han, G., et al., (2008). Anti-inflammatory activity of methanol extract isolated from stem bark of *Magnolia kobus. Phytotherapy Research, 22*, 883–888.

Kashyap, D., Sharma, A. S., Tuli, H., Punia, S. K., & Sharma, A., (2016). Ursolic acid and oleanolic acid: Pentacyclic terpenoids with promising anti-inflammatory activities. *Recent Patents on Inflammation & Allergy Drug Discovery, 10*(1), 21–33.

Kelm, M. A., Nair, M. G., Strasburg, G. M., & DeWitt, D. L., (2000). Antioxidant and cyclooxygenase inhibitory phenolic compounds from *Ocimum sanctum* Linn. *Phytomedicine, 7*, 7–13.

Khare, C. P., (2008). *Indian Medicinal Plants: An Illustrated Dictionary.* Springer Science & Business Media, Berlin, Germany.

Kim, C. S., Subedi, L., Park, K. J., Kim, S. Y., Choi, S. U., Kim, K. H., & Lee, K. R., (2015). Salicin derivatives from *Salix glandulosa* and their biological activities. *Fitoterapia, 106*, 147–152.

Koehn, F. E., & Carter, G. T., (2005). The evolving role of natural products in drug discovery: Nature reviews. *Drug Discovery, 4*, 206–220.

Kuptniratsaikul, V., Dajpratham, P., Taechaarpornkul, W., Buntragulpoontawee, M., Lukkanapichonchut, P., Chootip, C., Saengsuwan, J., et al., (2014). Efficacy and safety of *Curcuma domestica* extracts compared with ibuprofen in patients with knee osteoarthritis: A multicenter study. *Clinical Interventions in Aging, 9*, 451–458.

Lee, D. H., Seo, B. R., Kim, H. Y., Gum, G. C., Yu, H. H., You, H. K., Kang, T. H., & You, Y. O., (2011). Inhibitory effect of *Aralia continentalis* on the cariogenic properties of *Streptococcus mutans. Journal of Ethnopharmacology, 137*, 979–984.

Lee, D. Y., Li, H., Lim, H. J., Lee, H. J., Jeon, R., & Ryu, J. H., (2012). Anti-inflammatory activity of sulfur-containing compounds from garlic. *Journal of Medicinal Food, 15*, 992–999.

Lee, W., Yang, E. J., Ku, S. K., Song, K. S., & Bae, J. S., (2013). Anti-inflammatory effects of oleanolic acid on LPS-induced inflammation *in vitro* and *in vivo. Inflammation, 36*, 94–10.

Li, J., Li, J., Xu, Y., Wang, Y., Zhang, L., Ding, L., Xuan, Y., et al., (2016). Asymmetric synthesis and biological activities of natural product (+)-balasubramide and its derivatives. *Natural Product Research, 30*, 800–805.

Li, R. W., Lin, G. D., Myers, S. P., & Leach, D. N., (2003). Anti-inflammatory activity of Chinese medicinal vine plants. *Journal of Ethnopharmacology, 85*, 61–67.

Li, R., & Li, X., (2011). *Methods for Treating Polycystic Kidney Disease (PKD) or Other Cyst Forming Diseases.* Patent U.S, WO211006040A2.

Li, W. M., Giaisi, M., Treiber, M. K., & Krammer, P. H., (2002). The anti-inflammatory sesquiterpene lactone parthenolide suppresses IL-4 gene expression in peripheral blood T cells. *European Journal of Immunology, 32*, 3587–3597.

Libby, P., (2007). Inflammatory mechanisms: The molecular basis of inflammation and disease. *Nutrition Reviews, 65*, S140–S146.

Lin, S. K., Chang, H. H., Chen, Y. J., Wang, C. C., Galson, D. L., Hong, C. Y., & Kok, S. H., (2008). Epigallocatechin-3-gallate diminishes CCL2 expression in human osteoblastic cells via up-regulation of phosphatidylinositol 3-Kinase/Akt/Raf-1 interaction: A potential therapeutic benefit for arthritis. *Arthritis & Rheumatism, 58*, 3145–3156.

Liu, Z., Tang, L., Zou, P., Zhang, Y., Wang, Z., Fang, Q., Jiang, L., et al., (2014). Synthesis and biological evaluation of alkylated and prenylated mono-carbonyl analogs of curcumin as anti-inflammatory agents. *European Journal of Medicinal Chemistry, 74*, 671–682.

Luyen, B. T. T., Tai, B. H., Thao, N. P., Cha, J. Y., Lee, H. Y., Lee, Y. M., & Kim, Y. H., (2015). Anti-inflammatory components of *Chrysanthemum indicum* flowers. *Bioorganic & Medicinal Chemistry Letters, 25*, 266–269.

MacLean, D. B., (1985). Phthalideisoquinoline alkaloids and related compounds. In: *The Alkaloids: Chemistry and Pharmacology* (pp. 253–286). Academic Press. London.

Mali, R. G., (2010). *Cleome viscosa* wild mustard: A review on ethnobotany, phytochemistry, and pharmacology. *Pharmaceutical Biology, 48*, 105–112.

Manna, S. K., Mukhopadhyay, A., Nguyen, T. V., & Aggarwal, B. B., (1999). Silymarin suppresses TNF-induced activation of NF-kappa B, C-Jun N-terminal kinase, and apoptosis. *Journal of Immunology, 163*, 6800–6809.

Mashhadi, N. S., Ghiasvand, R., Askari, G., Hariri, M., Darvishi, L., & Mofid, M. R., (2013). Anti-oxidative and anti-inflammatory effects of ginger in health and physical activity: Review of current evidence. *International Journal of Preventive Medicine, 4*, S36–S42.

Mathema, V. B., Koh, Y. S., Thakuri, B. C., & Sillanpaa, M., (2012). Parthenolide, a sesquiterpene lactone, expresses multiple anti-cancer and anti-inflammatory activities. *Inflammation, 35*, 560–565.

Matu, E. N., & Van, S. J., (2003). Antibacterial and anti-inflammatory activities of some plants used for medicinal purposes in Kenya. *Journal of Ethnopharmacology, 87*, 35–41.

Mencherini, T., Cau, A., Bianco, G., Loggia, R. D., Aquino, R. P., & Autore, G., (2007). An extract of *Apium graveolens* var. dulce leaves: Structure of the major constituent, Apiin, and its anti-inflammatory properties. *Journal of Pharmacy and Pharmacology, 59*, 891–897.

Micallef, M. A., & Garga, M. L., (2009). Anti-inflammatory and cardioprotective effects of n-3 polyunsaturated fatty acids and plant sterols in hyperlipidemic individuals. *Atherosclerosis, 204*, 476–482.

Mohammad, S., (2009). Lupeol. A novel anti-inflammatory and anti-cancer dietary triterpene. *Cancer Letters, 285*, 109–115.

Mohammed, M. S., Osman, W. J., Garelnabi, E. A., Osman, Z., Osman, B., Khalid, H. S., & Mohamed, M. A., (2014). Secondary metabolites as anti-inflammatory agents. *The Journal of Phytopharmacology, 3*, 275–285.

Mukhopadhyay, A., Basu, N., Ghatak, N., & Gujral, P. K., (1982). Anti-inflammatory and irritant activities of curcumin analogues in rats. *Agents and Actions, 12*, 508–515.

Muthumani, P., Meera, R., Mary, S., Devi, P., Kameswari, B., & Priya, B. E., (2010). Phytochemical screening and anti-inflammatory, bronchodilator and antimicrobial activities of the seeds of *Luffa cylindrica. Research Journal of Pharmaceutical, Biological and Chemical Sciences, 1*, 11–22.

Navarro, P., Giner, R. M., Recio, M. C., Manez, S., Cerda-Nicolas, M., & Ríos, J. L., (2001). In vivo anti-inflammatory activity of saponins from *Bupleurum rotundifolium. Life Science, 68*, 1199–1206.

Newman, D. J., & Cragg, G. M., (2016). Natural products as sources of new drugs from 1981 to 2014. *Journal of Natural Products, 79*, 629–661.

Nkeh, C. B. N., Oyedeji, O. O., Oyedeji, A. O., & Ndebia, E. J., (2015). Anti-inflammatory and membrane-stabilizing properties of two semisynthetic derivatives of oleanolic acid. *Inflammation, 38*, 61–69.

Oh, H. L., Lim, H., Cho, Y. H., Koh, H. C., Kim, H., Lim, Y., & Lee, C. H., (2009). HY251, a novel cell cycle inhibitor isolated from *Aralia continentalis*, induces G 1 phase arrest via p53-dependent pathway in HeLa cells. *Bioorganic and Medicinal Chemistry Letters, 19*, 959–961.

Oh, J. H., Kang, L. L., Ban, J. O., Kim, Y. H., Kim, K. H., Han, S. B., & Hong, J. T., (2009). Anti-inflammatory effect of 4-O-methylhonokiol, a novel compound isolated from *Magnolia officinalis* through inhibition of NF-κB. *Chemico-Biological Interactions, 180*, 506–514.

Otsuka, H., Fujioka, S., Komiya, T., Mizuta, E., & Takamoto, M., (1982). Studies on anti-inflammatory agents. VI. Anti-inflammatory constituents of *Cinnamomum sieboldii* Meissn. Yakugaku Zasshi. *Journal of the Pharmaceutical Society of Japan, 102*, 162–172.

Pan, M. H., Lai, C. S., & Ho, C. T., (2010). Anti-inflammatory activity of natural dietary flavonoids. *Food & Function, 1*, 15–31.

Park, H. J., Hong, M. S., Lee, J. S., Leem, K. H., Kim, C. J., Kim, J. W., & Lim, S., (2005). Effects of *Aralia continentalis* on hyperalgesia with peripheral inflammation. *Phytotherapy Research, 19*, 511–513.

Perez, G., (2001). Anti-inflammatory activity of compounds isolated from plants. *The Scientific World Journal, 1*, 713–784.

Pichersky, E., & Gang, D. R., (2000). Genetics and biochemistry of secondary metabolites in plants: An evolutionary perspective. *Trends in Plant Science, 5*, 439–445.

Pitre, S., & Srivastava, S. R., (1987). Pharmacological, microbiological and phytochemical studies on roots of *Aegle marmelos. Fitoterapia, 58*, 194–197.

Prakash, P., & Gupta, N., (2005). Therapeutic uses of *Ocimum sanctum* Linn (Tulsi with a note on eugenol and its pharmacological actions: A short review. *Indian Journal of Physiology and Pharmacology, 49*, 125–131.

Radhika, P., Prasad, R. Y., Sastry, B. S., & Rajya, L. K., (2009). Anti-inflammatory activity of chloroform extract of *Andrographis paniculate nees* stem. *Research Journal of Biotechnology, 4*, 35–38.

Rahbardar, M. G., Amin, B., Mehri, S., Mirnajafi, Z. S. J., & Hosseinzadeh, H., (2017). Anti-inflammatory effects of ethanolic extract of *Rosmarinus officinalis* L. and rosmarinic acid in a rat model of neuropathic pain. *Biomedicine and Pharmacotherapy, 86*, 441–449.

Rani, P. M., Padmakumari, K. P., Sankarikutty, B., Lijo, C. O., Nisha, V. M., & Raghu, K. G., (2011). Inhibitory potential of ginger extracts against enzymes linked to type 2 diabetes, inflammation and induced oxidative stress. *International Journal of Food Sciences and Nutrition, 62*, 106–110.

Raturi, R., Sati, S. C., Sati, H. S., Bahuguna, P., & Badoni, P. P., (2011). Chemical examination and anti-inflammatory activity of *Prunus Persica* Steam Bark. International *Journal of Pharmacy and Pharmaceutical Sciences, 3*, 315–317.

Ravishankar, B., & Shukla, V. J., (2007). Indian systems of medicine: A brief profile. *African Journal of Traditional, Complementary and Alternative Medicines, 4*, 319–337.

Recio, M. C., Prieto, M., Bonucelli, M., Orsi, C., Máñez, S., Giner, R. M., Cerda, N. M., & Ríos, J. L., (2004). Anti-inflammatory activity of two cucurbitacins isolated from *Cayaponia tayuya* roots. *Planta Medica, 70*, 414–420.

Rudakov, G. A., (1976). *Chemistry and Technology of Camphor* (2nd edn., p. 254). Academic Press: London.

Ryu, S. Y., Ahn, J. W., Han, Y. N., Han, B. H., & Kim, S. H., (1996). *In vitro* antitumor activity of diterpenes from *Aralia cordata. Archives of Pharmacal Research, 19*, 77–78.

Safayhi, H., & Sailer, E. R., (1997). Anti-inflammatory actions of pentacyclic triterpenes. *Planta Medica, 63*, 487–493.

Saklani, A., & Kutty, S. K., (2008). Plant-derived compounds in clinical trials. *Drug Discovery Today, 13*, 161–171.

Sánchez, F. S., Villegas, I., Aparicio, S. M., Cárdeno, A., Ángeles, R. M., González, B. A., Marset, A., et al. (2015). Effects of dietary virgin olive oil polyphenols: Hydroxy tyrosyl acetate and 3, 4-dihydroxyphenylglycol on DSS-induced acute colitis in mice. *The Journal of Nutritional Biochemistry, 26*, 513–520.

Sarkar, S., Mazumder, S. J., Saha, S., & Bandyopadhyay, U., (2016). Management of inflammation by natural polyphenols: A comprehensive mechanistic update. *Current Medicinal Chemistry, 23*, 1657–1695.

Satoh, K., Nagai, F., Ono, M., & Aoki, N., (2003). Inhibition of Na+, K+-ATPase by the extract of *Stephania cephararantha* HAYATA and bisbenzylisoquinoline alkaloid cycleanine, a major constituent. *Biochemical Pharmacology, 66*, 379–385.

Saxena, R. C., Nath, R., Palit, G., Nigam, S. K., & Bhargava, K. P., (1982). Effect of calophyllolide, a nonsteroidal anti-inflammatory agent, on capillary permeability. *Planta Medica, 44*, 246–248.

Selvam, C., Jachak, S. M., Thilagavathi, R., & Chakraborti, A. K., (2005). Design synthesis, biological evaluation and molecular docking of curcumin analogues as antioxidant, cyclooxygenase inhibitory and anti-inflammatory agents. *Bioorganic & Medicinal Chemistry Letters, 15*,1793–1797.

Seo, C. S., Li, G., Kim, C. H., Lee, C. S., Jahng, Y., Chang, H. W., & Son, J. K., (2007). Cytotoxic and DNA topoisomerases I and II inhibitory constituents from the roots of *Aralia cordata. Archives of Pharmacal Research, 30*, 1404–1411.

Shaikh, R. U., Pund, M. M., & Gacche, R. N., (2016). Evaluation of anti-inflammatory activity of selected medicinal plants used in Indian traditional medication system *in vitro* as well as *in vivo. Journal of Traditional and Complementary Medicine, 6*, 355–361.

Sharma, S., Chattopadhyay, S. K., Yadav, D. K., Khan, F., Mohanty, S., Maurya, A., & Bawankule, D. U., (2012). QSAR, docking and *in vitro* studies for anti-inflammatory activity of cleomiscosin: A methyl ether derivatives. *European Journal of Pharmaceutical Sciences, 47*, 952–964.

Shelar, D. B., Shirote, P. J., & Naikwade, N. S., (2010). Anti-inflammatory activity and brine shrimps lethality test of *Saraca Indica* Linn leaves extract. *Journal of Pharmacy Research, 3*, 2004–2006.

Siddiqui, M. Z., (2011). *Boswellia serrata*, a potential anti-inflammatory agent: An overview. *Indian Journal of Pharmaceutical Sciences, 73*, 255–261.

Silva, J., Abebe, W., Sousa, S. M., Duarte, V. G., Machado, M. I. L., & Matos, F. J. A., (2003). Analgesic and anti-inflammatory effects of essential oils of *Eucalyptus*. *Journal of Ethnopharmacology, 89, 277–283.*

Singh, B., Agrawal, P. K., & Thakur, R. S., (1987). Aesculuside-B, a new triterpene glycoside from *Aesculus indica*. *Journal of Natural Products, 50*, 781–783.

Singh, V. K., Singh, K. L., & Singh, D. K., (2016). Multidimensional uses of medicinal plant kachnar (*Bauhinia variegata* Linn.). *American Journal of Phytomedicine and Clinical Therapeutics, 4*, 58–72.

Siriwatanametanon, N., Fiebich, B. L., Efferth, T., Prieto, J. M., & Heinrich, M., (2010). Traditionally used Thai medicinal plants: *In vitro* anti-inflammatory, anticancer and antioxidant activities. *Journal of Ethnopharmacology, 130*, 196–207.

Smoliga, J. M., Baur, J. A., & Hausenblas, H. A., (2011). Resveratrol and health - a comprehensive review of human clinical trials. *Molecular Nutrition & Food Research, 55*, 1129–1141.

Somani, S. J., Modi, K. P., Majumdar, A. S., & Sadarani, B. N., (2015). Phytochemicals and their potential usefulness in inflammatory bowel disease. *Phytotherapy Research, 29*, 339–350.

Sun, L. C., Zhang, H. B., Gu, C. D., Guo, S. D., Li, G., Lian, R., Yao, Y., & Zhang, G. Q., (2017). Protective effect of acacetin on sepsis-induced acute lung injury via its anti-inflammatory and antioxidative activity. *Archives of Pharmacal Research, 41*, 1–12.

Sur, R., Martin, K., Liebel, F., Lyte, P., Shapiro, S., & Southall, M., (2009). Anti-inflammatory activity of parthenolide-depleted feverfew (*Tanacetum parthenium*). *Inflammopharmacology, 17*, 42–49.

Tang, X., Lin, Z., Cai, W., Chen, N., & Shen, L., (1984). Anti-inflammatory effect of 3-acetylaconitine. *Acta Pharmacologica Sinica, 5*, 85.

Uchegbu, R. I., Mbadiugha, C. N., Ibe, C. O., Achinihu, I. O., & Sokwaibe, C. E., (2015). Antioxidant, anti-inflammatory and antibacterial activities of the seeds of *Mucuna flagellipes*. *American Journal of Chemistry and Applications, 2*, 114–117.

Upadhyay, R. K., (2016). Nutraceutical, pharmaceutical and therapeutic uses of *Allium cepa*: A review. *International Journal of Green Pharmacy, 10*, S46–S63.

Vecchio, M. G., Loganes, C., & Minto, C., (2016). Beneficial and healthy properties of *Eucalyptus* plants: A great potential use. *The Open Agriculture Journal, 10*, .52–57.

Venkatesan, P., & Rao, M. N. A., (2000). Structure-activity relationships for the inhibition of lipid peroxidation and the scavenging of free radicals by synthetic symmetrical curcumin analogues. *Journal of Pharmacy and Pharmacology, 52*,1123–1128.

Via, L. D., Mejia, M., García-Argáez, A. N., Braga, A., Toninello, A., & Martínez-Vázquez, M., (2015). Anti-inflammatory and antiproliferative evaluation of 4β-cinnamoyloxy, 1β, 3α-dihydroxyeudesm-7, 8-ene from *Verbesina persicifolia* and derivatives. *Bioorganic and Medicinal Chemistry, 23*, 5816–5828.

Wang, J., Li, Q., Ivanochko, G., & Huang, Y., (2006). Anticancer effect of extracts from a North American medicinal plant-wild *sarsaparilla*. *Anticancer Research, 26*, 2157–2164.

Wang, Y. M., Xu, M., Wang, D., Yang, C. R., Zeng, Y., & Zhang, Y. J., (2013). Anti-inflammatory compounds of "Qin-Jiao" the roots of *Gentiana dahurica*. *Journal of Ethnopharmacology, 147*, 341–348.

Wang, Y., Yu, C., Pan, Y., Yang, X., Huang, Y., Feng, Z., Li, X., et al., (2012). A novel synthetic mono-carbonyl analogue of curcumin, a13, exhibits anti-inflammatory effects in vivo by inhibition of inflammatory mediators. *Inflammation, 35,* 594–604.

Won, J. H., Im, H. T., Kim, Y. H., Yun, K. J., Park, H. J., Choi, J. W., & Lee, K. T., (2006). Anti-inflammatory effect of buddlejasaponin IV through the inhibition of iNOS and COX-2 expression in RAW 264.7 macrophages via the NF-kB inactivation. *British Journal of Pharmacology, 148,* 216–225.

Xia, E. Q., Deng, G. F., Guo, Y. J., & Li, H. B., (2010). Biological activities of polyphenols from grapes. Indi*an Journal of Molecular Sciences, 11,* 622–646.

Yadav, M., Jain, S., Bhardwaj, A., Nagpal, R., Puniya, M., Tomar, R., Singh, V., et al., (2009). Biological and medicinal properties of grapes and their bioactive constituents: An update. *Journal of Medicinal Food, 12,* 473–484.

Yogiraj, V., Goyal, P. K., Chauhan, C. S., Goyal, A., & Vyas, B., (2014). *Carica papaya* Linn: An overview. *International Journal of Herbal Medicine, 2,* 1–8.

Yoshimoto, T., Furukawa, M., Yamamoto, S., Horie, T., & Watanabe, K. S., (1983). Flavonoids: Potent inhibitors of arachidonate 5-lipoxygenase. *Biochemical and Biophysical Research Communications, 116,* 612–618.

Yuan, G., Wahlqvist, M. L., He, G., Yang, M., & Li, D., (2006). Natural products and anti-inflammatory activity. *Asia Pacific Journal of Clinical Nutrition, 15,* 143–152.

Zheng, G., Chen, T., Peng, X., & Long, S., (2015). Synthesis, Anti-Inflammatory, and Analgesic Activities of Derivatives of 4-Hydroxy-2 benzoxazolone. *Journal of Chemistry,* 1–5.

CHAPTER 4

FOENICULUM VULGARE MILL: FLAVORING, PHARMACOLOGICAL, PHYTOCHEMICAL, AND FOLKLORE ASPECTS

NAVNEET KISHORE and AKHILESH KUMAR VERMA

Department of Chemistry, University of Delhi, North Campus, New Delhi – 110007, India, Phone: 011-27666648, E-mail: akhilesh682000@gmail.com (A. K. Verma)

ABSTRACT

Foeniculum vulgare Mill is generally known as fennel and considered under the family Apiaceae. Fennel is a flowering biennial herb with its characteristics medicinal and aromatic value. It is extensively spread throughout the world, including India, for its medicinal and economic importance in the traditional system of various localities. This herb has been used in Ayurveda since extensive period in the treatment of various assortments of human ailments. The aerial parts of this plant have significant medicinal value and as an imperative kitchen spice. A fennel seed owns a characteristic aroma flavor which makes it a chief ingredient for the cooking of several dishes. It has also been used in bakery, alcohol industries to make different beverages. Green seeds and bulbs of fennel are eaten cooked or as salads in different parts of Indian states. However, it is a central ingredient of Kashmiri and Guajarati dishes. Apart from the spicy component, fennel is also used to treat several human ailments in traditional medicine (TM) and modern pharmacological aspects due to the presence of countless active secondary metabolites. Literature reports reveals that it has anti-cancer, anti-diabetic, anti-mutagenic, diuretic, anti-bacterial, memory enhancing, anti-inflammatory, hypotensive, antioxidant, anti-thrombotic gastroprotective, and hepatoprotective actions. Phytochemical analysis of fennel seeds discloses that it contains proteins, vitamins, minerals, phenols, phenolic glycosides, and various volatile components. The present chapter summarized the updates on *F. vulgare* including its ethnopharmacological relevance, usage in traditional system, pharmacological aspects, active secondary metabolites, and significant potential as tedious kitchen constituents.

4.1   INTRODUCTION

Medicinal plants are the key source of therapeutic agents for mankind to sustain the smooth and uninfected life from several surrounding factors. It is a universal fact that the ancient populaces were absolutely reliant on plants for their daily needs, including treatment of several disorders. Hence, the discovery of drugs remains rooted in the ancient traditional system of usage of plants in a variety of customs. Although the current research conducted on herbal products/herbal formulations have greatly contributed in the development of pharmacological assessment of plant-based medicine. Mostly the herbal medicines are the parts of the Indian traditional system of medicine as well as other civilizations since ancient periods. The linkage between human and nature have been established from the origin of menfolk itself. The perception regarding the routine usage of plants by human beings rises to heal the countless necessities have also been proved in ongoing research. The reputation of medicinal plants in drug discovery and crude substantial in pharmaceutical sector is on the top rank. So, the medicinal plants could be considered as the plants which provide the defensive action against several diseases that are injurious to human survival. The increasing use of herbal remedies in daily survives have also made a specific attention for the elevated utilization of medicinal plants. The different civilizations have their concise catalog of medicinal plants that are significantly prevents from the countless ailments. The well defined and established folklore system running around the world, which includes the Indian system of medicine (Ayurveda), Chinese traditional medicine (CTM) and African traditional medicine (ATM). A global aspect on plants estimated that two-thirds of all plants grown worldwide have medicinal importance.

Foeniculum vulgare Mill. is commonly known as fennel under the family of flowering plant Apiaceae. It is categorized as a highly aromatic and medicinal plant underneath biennial herb with fluffy foliage like leaves. *F. vulgare* grows up to a height of approximate 2.0 m and having the 10 mm length of its seeds. Currently, it has been tamed widely in various parts of the world nearby the river banks and cultivated for its astonishing flavor (Rani and Das, 2016; Al-Snafi, 2018). According to some botanists, there are two types of fennels, *F. vulgare* var. *dulce* is considered as sweet fennel (Annual or Biennial) *F. vulgare* var. vulgare is categorized as bitter fennel which is perennial. Fennel is used in the treatment of several human ailments since long time and has been used in the formulation of ayurvedic products for various diseases. This herb has been considered as a delighted remedy for the digestive, endocrine, reproduction, and respiration related ailments. Since long time it has been used for curing constipation, cough, diarrhea, and flatulence (Arzoo and Parle, 2017). The fennel has efficient spice value which is attributed due to its penetrating precise odor made fennel as substantial spice. The seeds of fennel have also been used in food industries, bakeries, and production of herbal-based spirits and liqueurs (Timasheva and Gorbunova, 2014). Hence, fennel is well known spice as well as it has admirable medicinal values in the Indian traditional system. In this chapter, we have effort to compile the health benefits, medicinal assets, nutritional value, pharmacological properties and phytochemical profile of fennel. Fennel is keen spice for kitchen and a magical weapon for human health through the protection from several diseases. Fennel seeds are chewed by people in daily life after taking food acts as mouth refresher and also prevented from immoral smell.

4.2 TRADITIONAL USAGE AND ETHNOPHARMACOLOGICAL RELEVANCE

Fennel is also known as "Saunf" in Hindi and used traditionally for the treatment of several human ailments, for cooking, spice for various dishes including other folklore usage from the earliest period. Saunf seeds are chewed for the cure of mouth cancer, bloody gums, to remove bad smell from the mouth and as a mouth freshener. Saunf seeds are considered as the best remedy for constipation by the stimulation of intestinal clearness and to discharge gas unruly. Saunf is a very good remedy for diarrhea, gastralgia, stomach pain and stomach swelling in folklore therapies. It has been considered as the natural antiemetic appetite suppressant and metabolic booster. The regular use of fennel also avoids the obesity. The regular use of fennel tea is supportive in weight loss. It causes the frequent urination via the enhancement working of kidney and regulates the blood pressure (BP). It is also useful in the detoxification and purification of blood. Fennel is good for colon, eye, hair, liver, and skin. Decoction of fennel is used to wash eye ailments including itching and conjunctivitis. The amazing aroma properties of fennel used to mind relaxation and eradicate stress. It has an imperative medicine to women in the medication for leucorrhea, stimulation of milk and repetitive abortion. Fennel is very cheap, easily available and significantly condenses the cold, cough, and fever. It is applied externally on paining joint to help in arthritis due to its anti-inflammatory action. A poultice made from roots of fennel traditionally applied on the bites of mad dogs and mosquito's bites. Decoction from the leaves is very significant for the snake bite to remove the venom as well as counterbalance the poison of vegetables.

4.3   NUTRITIVE CHEMICAL COMPOSITION OF FENNEL

Fennel has very good nutritional value due to the presence of essential minerals, different amino acids required for human body, vitamins, and complex constitution of essential oils (EOs). The minerals, vitamins, amino acid and EOs present in fennel which provides the higher nutritional value have been mentioned in Table 4.1. The percentage-wise composition recorded in fennel is carbohydrates (42.3%), fat (10%), fiber (18.5%), minerals (13.4%) and protein (9.5%). All the parts of this herb are widely used in various traditions in cookery throughout the world. Cooked green seeds are a very good and bulbs, roots, young stems, and green seeds are eaten raw as salad, in side dishes, pastas, and other vegetable dishes.

TABLE 4.1   Significant Nutritional and Chemical Composition of Fennel

Minerals	Vitamins	Amino Acids	Volatile Oils	Terpenoids
Aluminum (Al)	Choline	Alanine	Anisic acid	Carotene
Boron (B)	Folate	Arginine	Anisic aldehyde	β-amyrcene
Calcium (Ca)	Niacin	Aspartic acid	Anisic-ketone	α-phellandrene
Chromium (Cr)	Vitamin A	Cystine	Camphene	Camphor
Cobalt (Co)	Vitamin B_1	Glutamic acid	Cis-anethole	1-8-cineole
Copper (Cu)	Vitamin B_6	Glycine	Diterpene	α-terpineol
Iodine (I)	Vitamin B_2	Histidine	Estragole	D-limonene
Iron (Fe)	Vitamin B_3	Leucine	Fenchone	Dipentene
Magnesium (Mg)	Vitamin B_5	Lysine	Limonene	γ-terpinene
Manganese (Mn)	Vitamin B_9	Isoleucine	Methyl chavicol	Linalool

TABLE 4.1   *(Continued)*

Minerals	Vitamins	Amino Acids	Volatile Oils	Terpenoids
Nickel (Ni)	Vitamin C	Methionine	α-pinene	Terpinen-4-ol
Phosphorous (P)	Vitamin E	Phenylalanine	β-pinene	α-thujene
Potassium (K)	Vitamin K	Proline	Trans-anethole	3-carene
Silicon (Si)	–	Serine	–	Sabinene
Selenium (Se)	–	Threonine	–	Myrcene
Sodium (Na)	–	Tryptophan	–	α/β-terpinene
Tin (Sn)	–	Tyrosine	–	p-cymene
Zinc (Zn)	–	Valine	–	Terpinolene

4.4   PHARMACOLOGICAL PROPERTIES OF FENNEL

The pharmacological properties of fennel have been disclosing in several previous in vitro and in vivo studies which include cytotoxicity, antiviral, antipyretic, analgesic, apoptotic, antinociceptive, antiallergic, antithrombotic, antibacterial, cytoprotective, antimutagenic, anticancer, antitumor, anti-inflammatory, cardiovascular, hepatoprotective, antioxidant, anti-spasmodic, antistress hypoglycemic, (Kooti et al., 2015) hypolipidemic, chemo-modulatory, and has memory enhancement potential by reduction in stress (Badgujar et al., 2014). *F. vulgare* is acts as a natural galactagogue and inspire the production of milk in the mothers during lactation (Anubhuti et al., 2017). A water decoction made from the leaves and roots from the fennel herb help in snake bites. It is also useful in the neutralization of vegetables poisons including mushrooms toxins (Shahat et al., 2011). The infusion of fruits is very significant for the whole alimentary canal to devoid from gaseous problems. Young shoots are helpful in respiratory diseases. Fruit juice is substantial stimulant for the improvement in eyesight. A poultice is applied on the breast to release swelling in nursing mothers at through feeds to babies. Roots infusion is used for the treatment of toothaches and urinary disorders. A hot infusion of fruits and roots is significant herbal drink for amenorrhea (Timasheva et al., 2014).

However, the fennel is used for sustaining human's physical and psychological wellness. *F. vulgare* has sweet seeds with distinctive aroma flavor and make its significant presence in several food products like fish dishes, meat, bakery products, ice creams, herb mixtures, and alcoholic beverage products (Rather et al., 2016). Herbal tea made from fennel or direct infusion of fennel seeds is a famous traditional remedy to treat several gastric ailments as well as respiratory tract problems in Asia and Europe. Fennel is an economically important crop and traded worldwide for its valuable medicinal and spicy magnificence (He and Huang, 2011). In traditional Chinese medicine (TCM), fennel is used for the ancient time for the treatment of dyspeptic disorders as well as in daily food named as Xiaohuixiang in China. On the basis of efficient phytochemical profile and nutritional value of fennel herb provides significant decent properties on human body as well as reduction of the risk of various diseases, it has been considered as functional food (Table 4.2) (Rajic et al., 2018).

TABLE 4.2   Anti-Microbial Activity Against Various Microbial Species

SL. No.	Microbial Species	Type	References
1.	*Agrobacterium tumefaciens*	Bacterial	Khan (2017)
2.	*Alternaria alternate*	Fungal	Kushwah et al. (2016)
3.	*Aspergillus flavus*	Fungal	Kushwah et al. (2016)
4.	*Aspergillus niger*	Fungal	Kushwah et al. (2016)
5.	*Aspergillus ochraceus*	Fungal	Singh et al. (2006)
6.	*Aspergillus oryzae*	Fungal	Singh et al. (2006)
7.	*Bacillus cereus*	Bacterial	Khan (2017)
8.	*Bacillus megaterium*	Bacterial	Khan (2017)
9.	*Bacillus pumilus*	Bacterial	Bano et al. (2016)
10.	*Bacillus subtilis*	Bacterial	Al-Snafi (2018)
11.	*Candida albicans*	Fungal	Skrobonj et al. (2013)
12.	*Curvularia lunata*	Fungal	Al-Snafi (2018)
13.	*Enterococcus faecalis*	Bacterial	Al-Snafi (2018)
14.	*Enterococcus hirea*	Bacterial	Dahak and Taourirte (2013)
15.	*Escherichia coli*	Bacterial	Dahak and Taourirte (2013)
16.	*Fusarium graminearum*	Fungal	Kushwah et al. (2016)
17.	*Fusarium moniliforme*	Fungal	Kushwah et al. (2016)
18.	*Fusarium oxysporum*	Fungal	Al-Snafi (2018)
19.	*Klebsiella pneumoniae*	Bacterial	(Abbas (2016)
20.	*Lactobacillus acidophilus*	Bacterial	Kushwah et al. (2016)
21.	*Listeria monocytogenes*	Bacterial	Bano et al. (2016)
22.	*Micrococcus luteus*	Bacterial	Kushwah et al. (2016)
23.	*Penicillium citrium*	Fungal	Singh et al. (2006)

TABLE 4.2 *(Continued)*

SL. No.	Microbial Species	Type	References
24.	*Penicillium madriti*	Fungal	Singh et al. (2006)
25.	*Penicillium viridicatum*	Fungal	Singh et al. (2006)
26.	*Proteus mirabilis*	Bacterial	Zellagui et al. (2011)
27.	*Proteus vulgaris*	Bacterial	Roby et al. (2013)
28.	*Pseudomonas aeruginosa*	Bacterial	Dahak and Taourirte (2013)
29.	*Pseudomonas pupida*	Bacterial	Khan (2017)
30.	*Pseudomonas syringae*	Bacterial	Khan (2017)
31.	*Rhizoctonia solani*	Fungal	Kushwah et al. (2016)
32.	*Rhizopus stolonifera*	Fungal	Skrobonj et al. (2013)
33.	*Salmonella typhi*	Bacterial	Khan (2017)
34.	*Salmonella typhimurium*	Bacterial	Khan (2017)
35.	*Shigella boydii*	Bacterial	Khan (2017)
36.	*Shigella flexneri*	Bacterial	Skrobonj et al. (2013)
37.	*Shigella dysenteriae*	Bacterial	Khan (2017)
38.	*Shigella shiga*	Bacterial	Khan (2017)
39.	*Staphylococcus albus*	Bacterial	Khan (2017)
40.	*Staphylococcus aureus*	Bacterial	Khan (2017)
41.	*Staphylococcus epidemidis*	Bacterial	Zellagui et al. (2011)
42.	*Streptococcus hemolyticus*	Bacterial	Khan (2017)
43.	*Streptococcus pneumoniae*	Bacterial	Roby et al. (2013)
44.	*Staphylococcus saprophyticus*	Bacterial	Zellagui et al. (2011)

A hydroalcoholic abstract from the fruits of fennel can be consumed by food industries without elimination of solvent. However, the hydroethanolic extraction of fruits of fennel contains a higher degree of flavonoid and phenols metabolites which is responsible for the excellent anti-oxidant potential. Despite the amazing culinary and significant nutritional power, fennel has also several pharmacological properties. A study about the anti-bacterial action of fennel has been evaluated from the different extract in water and in organic solvents. The results displayed the good zone of inhibition (11–25 mm) against the bacterial species *Enterococcus faecalis*, *Staphylococcus aureus* and *Escherichia coli* (Kaur and Arora, 2009). The highest total phenolic contents (TPC) were observed from the methanol extract of fennel seeds (22.93 mg GAE/g) which showed significant total antioxidant potential with the value of 1.63 ± 0.19 µg/mL in the evaluation of phosphor-molybdenium method. The water extract also displayed excellent radical scavenging potential with an IC_{50} value of 207.94 ± 83.38 µg/mL in DPPH assay. The antimicrobial potential of aqueous methanol extract against *Bacillus megaterium* showed the zone of inhibition at a range of 12.29 ± 1.34 mm (Beyazen et al., 2017). The anti-microbial potential of chloroform-methanol (1:1) extract from the aerial parts of fennel was evaluated against six bacterial strains namely *Escherichia coli* (ATCC 25922), *Proteus mirabilis, Proteus vulgaris, Staphylococcus blanc* (ATCC 27853), *Staphylococcus epidemidis* and *Staphylococcus saprophyticus*) and three fungal strains namely *Aspergillus versicolor, Aspergillus fumigatus* and *Penicillium camemberti*). The results showed the significant zone of inhibition with a range of 6.0 to 11.66 mm for all the microbial strains at a concentration of 0.25 mg/mL (Zellagui et al., 2011).

A study conducted by Zaahkouk et al. on anticancer potential of fennel extract against three types of cancer cells, namely human breast cancer cell line (MCF-7), human hepatocellular carcinoma cell line (HePG-2), and colon carcinoma cell line (HCT-116). The results showed that all the extracts were significant anticancer properties with the IC_{50} values were observed 24.5±.08, 28.7±.04 and 59.8±.09 µg/ml for MCF-7, HEPG-2 and HCT-116, respectively (Zaahkouk et al., 2015). Another study carried out on anticancer potential of EOs of fennel against different five types namely, cervical cancer (HeLa), human epithelial colorectal adenocarcinoma cells (Caco-2), human breast cancer cell line (MCF-7), human acute lymphocytic leukemia (CCRF-CEM) and human acute lymphocytic leukemia resistant to doxorubicin (CEM/ADR5000) cancer cell lines. The result showed the IC_{50} values 207, 75, 59, 32 and 165 mg/L for HeLa, Caco-2, MCF-7, CCRF-CEM, and CEM/ADR5000 cell lines, respectively (Sharopov et al., 2017). The EOs from fennel are also used as the insect repellent due to the presence of (+)-fenchone and E-9-octadecenoic acid in fruits oil. These components are very toxic for insects and non-toxic to the human beings (Ahn et al., 2007).

4.5 COMPOSITION OF ESSENTIAL OILS (EOS)

The essential oil obtained from the fennel have a significant role in the preparation of perfumes, liqueurs, breads, cakes, and cookies as a flavoring negotiator (Gorni et al., 2017). Phytochemical composition of fennel led to the presence of several volatile compounds, phenolics, flavonoids, and fatty acids. Various bioactive secondary metabolites have been isolated and iden-tified from the fennel plant. Many promising constituents have been found to display different biological potential. The fennel herb contains phyto-constituents belonging to the class of coumarin, furocoumarins, terpenes, terpenoids, phenolic acids, flavonoids, and flavonoid glucosides which are responsible for the diverse range of pharmacological properties (Badgujar et al., 2014). The GC-MS analysis from the EOs from fennel contains rich composition of estragole, fenchone, limonene, and several monoterpenes' constituents (Telci et al., 2009). Herbal products and EOs made from the fennel fruits displayed significant analgesic, antispasmodic action, anti-oxidant, and diuretic properties. The EOs obtained from the mature fruits of fennel used in the formulation of pharmaceutical products and cosmetic products due to its complex chemical composition. However, the varia-tion in the composition of EOs of fennel has been encountered in different research analysis. It can be described due to the different environmental and climatic conditions, collection time, lifespan of plants and most prominently cultivation type either they grown naturally or planted under the controlled behaviors (Aprotosoaie et al., 2010).

4.6   PHYTOCHEMICAL PROFILE OF FENNEL

These pharmacological potentials are accredited to the presence of diverse class of active metabolites. The bioactive compounds belong to a class of coumarins, fatty acids, flavonoids, flavonoids glycosides, phenolic acids, sterols, saponins, cinnamic acid derivatives, monoterpenoids, sesquiter-penes, triterpenoids, cardiac glycosides, tannins, and some other phenylpro-panoids are residing in fennel herb. There are some bioactive metabolites are mentioned in figure. The chemical composition of fennel revealed that it contains approximately 20% of fatty acid and petroselinic acid is consid-ered as representative of fennel oil fatty acid. The fatty acid composition of acetone extract from fennel displayed that it contains linoleic acid (54.9%), oleic acid (5.4%) and palmitic acid (5.4%) as major components (Figure 4.1) (Cosge et al., 2008).

An aliphatic ketone, 10-nonacosanone has been identified as the precise biomarker in fennel seeds whereas trans-anethole is considered as major constituent in volatile oil obtained from fennel. The composition of EOs from fennel is varied from place to place as well as species to species from all over the world (Bahmani et al., 2016). In a recent study on estragole isolated from the essential oil of fennel was tested on human hepatoma cell line (HepG2) by MTT cytotoxicity assay. Result showed that the metabolite estragole under investigational conditions was unable to induce DNA damage and apoptosis (Villarini et al., 2014). For the search of anticancer bioactive metabolites from medicinal plants, in our research group, the ethanol extract of fennel was found to display the significant anticancer potential against HeLa cells with an IC_{50} value of 19.97 µg/mL (Figure 4.2).

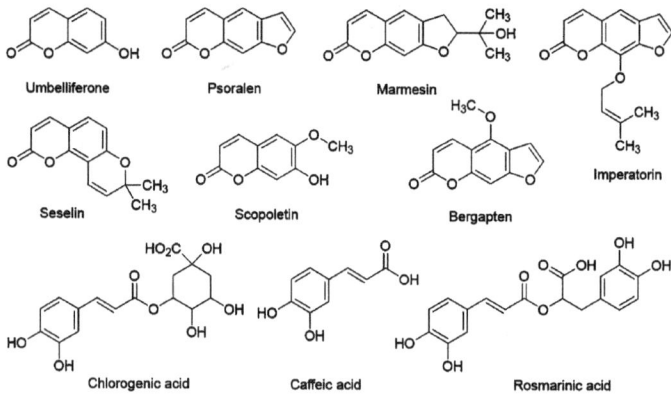

FIGURE 4.1 Bioactive metabolites identified from fennel plant.

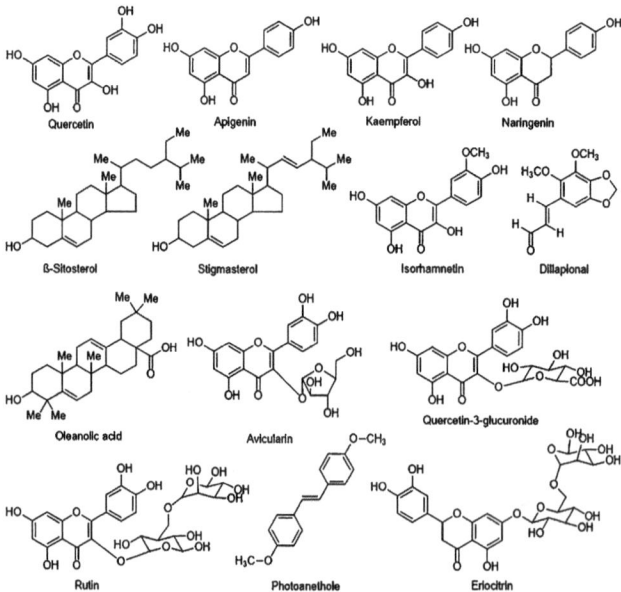

FIGURE 4.2 Bioactive metabolites identified from fennel plant.

The further investigation led to the isolation of two active metabolites, namely syringin and 4-methoxycinnamyl. These both compounds exhibited anticancer activity against DU145, HeLa, and MCF-7 cell lines. 4-methoxycinnamyl displayed significant action with the IC_{50} values of 22.10, 7.82 and 14.24 µg/mL against DU145, HeLa, and MCF-7 cell lines, respectively. The mechanistic studies also showed there was no apoptotic effect at a concentration of 10 µg/mL after 48 h in cell cycle analysis (Lall et al., 2015).

4.7   SOME MISCELLANEOUS USAGE OF FENNEL HERB

Fennel is one of the most important constituents as mouth freshener in the manufacturing of various natural toothpastes. Fennel powder effectively avoids the fleas from houses and food stalls. The flowers and leaves afforded the yellow and brown dyes, respectively. The oil obtained from fennel is used in the formulation of condiments, creams, liquors, fragrances, and soaps to enhance aroma. A juice obtained from the fennel is used to make cough syrups. A composition of anise, fennel, and wormwood afforded an eminent drink initially for its medicinal values, but later it converts in to a famous alcoholic drink named as Absinthe. The preparation of bread, cakes, cookies, and pastries includes the fennel aroma. Leaves are taken as salad as well as in various dishes of fish, meat, and vegetables. Seeds are significantly used in the cooking of several fish, meat, and pork recipes. Fennel is also used in several classical Italian recipes. Seeds are also used in desserts and drinks. It is also used to make health beneficial tea.

4.8   SOME MAGICAL FACTS CONCERNING FENNEL HERB

Apart from the traditional and medicinal usage of the fennel plant, there are some exciting facts about the fennel should be considered here. The production of fennel in India is the highest through all over the world. Male and female fennel can only be identified from the seeds. Fennel has allergic properties to insects, and it is used to keep away flies from horses. Fennel played a very significant role in the enhancement of eye-sight. In traditional culture, it is supposed that the specific aroma of fennel retains the effect of devil and witchcraft away.

4.9   FUTURE PROSPECTIVE

Fennel is one of the highly aromatic medicinal herbs with its astonishing flavor. The home-made recipes and traditional formulations from fennel have extra plenteous devotion in food industry which is continued since ancient times. There are several bioactive metabolites have been identified which displayed significant pharmacological potentials. Oil obtained from fennel has excellent antimicrobial potential. It is a clear liquid contains several primary and secondary metabolites. Various extracts in different solvents showed good pharmacological potentials. The mentioned reports on traditional, pharmacological, ethnopharmacological, and phytochemical profile, it is clear that there is hitherto scantiness of scientific investigation in respect to mode of action inside the human body. However, many more unidentified metabolites accountable for the biological properties should be further explored. Hereafter, the more exploration needed for the credentials of mysterious metabolites and their respective bioactivity. Hence, further exploration may lead to the interest of many researchers/readers to achieve this herb to know about the unseen facets of the fennel plant.

4.10   CONCLUSION

Fennel is well known spice as well as it has admirable medicinal values in the Indian traditional system. It is used in the treatment of several human ailments. It has also been used in the formulation of ayurvedic products. Apart from its medicinal value, it has efficient spice value which is attributed due to its penetrating precise odor made fennel as substantial spice. The seeds of fennel have also been used in food industries, bakeries, and production of herbal-based spirits and liqueurs. However, this herb is distinguished for its therapeutic values and data from nutritional value has been considered as resourceful nourishments. The fennel seeds have unique oil composition which is used in the formulation of several routine products for human life. This oil also enhances the aroma of these daily consumable house hold products. The juice attained from the aerial parts of fennel is efficiently used to treat cough. In this chapter we have effort to compile the health benefits, medicinal assets, nutritional value, biological properties and phytochemical profile of fennel. Fennel is the main ingredient of spices in Indian kitchen which imparts the wonderful aroma in foods. The three main ingredients present in fennel oil, namely, estragole, fenchone, and limonene responsible for strong antifungal potential. Hence, apart from the several pharmacological properties, it is also very effective in skin improvement. The seeds of fennel are chewed after meal for good digestion.

KEYWORDS

- cuisine
- fennel
- *Foeniculum vulgare*
- medicinal properties
- phytochemicals
- prostaglandin

REFERENCES

Abbas, T. F., (2016). Detection the biological activity of aqueous extract of Shamar plant seeds *Foeniculum vulgare* mill. *Muthanna Med. J., 3*, 49–55.

Ahn, Y. J., Kim, D. H., & Kim, S. I., (2007). *Mosquito Repellent Isolated from Foeniculum vulgare Fruit.* United States Patent. Patent No.: US 7,179,479 B1.

Al-Snafi, A. E., (2018). The chemical constituents and pharmacological effects of *Foeniculum vulgare*: A review. *IOSR Journal of Pharmacy, 8*, 81–96.

Anubhuti, P., Rahul, S., & Kant, C. K., (2011). Standardization of fennel (*Foeniculum vulgare*), Its oleoresin and marketed ayurvedic dosage forms. *Int. J. Pharma. Sci Drug Res., 3*, 265–269.

Aprotosoaie, A. C., Spac, A., Hancianu, M., Miron, A., Tanasescu, V. F., Dorneanu, V., & Stsnescu, U., (2010). The chemical profile of essential oils obtained from fennel fruits (*Foeniculum vulgare* mill.). *Farmacia, 58*, 46–53.

Arzoo, & Parle, M., (2017). Fennel: A brief review. *European Journal of Pharmaceutical and Medical Research, 4*, 668–675.

Badgujar, S. B., Patel, V. V., & Bandivdekar, A. H. (2014). *Foeniculum vulgare* mill: A review of its botany, phytochemistry, pharmacology, contemporary application, and toxicology. *BioMed. Research International, 2014*, 1–32. Article ID 842674.

Bahmani, K., Darbandi, A. I., Alfekaiki, D. F., & Sticklen, M., (2016). Phytochemical diversity of fennel landraces from various growth types and origins. *Agronomy Research, 14*, 1530–1547.

Bano, S., Ahmad, N., & Sharma, A. K., (2016). Phytochemical investigation and evaluation of anti-microbial and anti-oxidant activity of *Foeniculum vulgare* (fennel). *Int. J. Pharma Sci. Res., 7*, 310–314.

Beyazen, A., Dessalegn, E., & Mamo, W., (2017). Phytochemical screening, antioxidant and antimicrobial activities of seeds of *Foeniculum vulgare* (ensilal). *World J. Pharm. Sci., 5*, 198–208.

Cosge, B., Kiralan, B., & Gurbuz, B., (2008). Characteristics of fatty acids and essential oil from sweet fennel (*F. vulgare* Mill. var. dulce) and bitter fennel fruits (*F. vulgare* Mill. var. vulgare) growing in Turkey. *Nat. Prod. Res., 22*, 1011–1016.

Dahak, K., & Taourirte, M., (2013). Comparative study of in vitro antimicrobial activities of *Foeniculum vulgare* mill. (Umbelliferae) extract. *Online J. Biological. Sci., 13*, 115–120.

Gorni, P. H., Brozulato, M. O., Lourencao, R. S., & Konrad, E. C. G., (2017). Increased biomass and salicylic acid elicitor activity in fennel (*Foeniculum vulgare* miller). *Braz. J. Food Technol., 20*, e2016172.

He, W., & Huang, B., (2011). A review of chemistry and bioactivities of a medicinal spice: *Foeniculum vulgare. J. Med. Plants Res., 5*, 3595–3600.

Kaur, G. J., & Arora, D. S., (2009). Antibacterial and phytochemical screening of *Anethum graveolens*, *Foeniculum vulgare* and *Trachyspermum ammi. BMC Complementary and Alternative Medicine, 9*, 30.

Khan, N. T., (2017). In vitro antibacterial activity of *Foeniculum vulgare* seed extract. *Agrotechnology, 6*, 162.

Kim, Y. J., Kim, B. H., Lee, S. Y., Kim, M. S., Park, C. S., Rhee, M. S., Lee, K. H., & Kim, D. S., (2006). Screening of medicinal plants for development of functional food ingredients with antiobesity. *Applied Biological Chemistry, 49*, 221–226.

Kooti, W., Moradi, M., Ali, A. S., Sharafi-Ahvazi, N., Asadi-Samani, M., & Ashtary-Larky, D., (2015). Therapeutic and pharmacological potential of *Foeniculum vulgare* mill: A review. *Journal of Herbmed Pharmacology, 4*, 1–9.

Kushwah, P., Patel, R., Midda, A., & Kayande, N., (2016). Pharmacological review on *Foeniculum vulgare. Int. J. Advanced Sci. Res., 1*, 40–42.

Lall, N., Kishore, N., Binneman, B., Twilley, D., Venter, M., Plessis-Stoman, D., Boukes, G., & Hussein, A., (2015). Cytotoxicity of syringin and 4-methoxycinnamyl alcohol isolated from *Foeniculum vulgare* on selected human cell lines. *Nat. Prod. Re.s, 29*, 1752–1756.

Rajic, J. R., Dordevic, S. M., Tesevic, V. V., Zivkovic, M. B., Dordevic, N. O., Paunovic, D. M., Nedovic, V. A., & Petrovic, T. S., (2018). The extract of fennel fruit as a potential natural additive in the food industry. *J. Agricultural Sci., 63*, 205–215.

Rani, S., & Das, S., (2016). *Foeniculum vulgare*: Phytochemical and pharmacological review. *Int. J. Advanced Res., 4*, 477–486.

Rather, M. A., Dar, B. A., Sofi, S. N., Bhat, B. A., & Qurishi, M. A., (2016). *Foeniculum vulgare*: A comprehensive review of its traditional use, phytochemistry, pharmacology, and safety. *Arabian J. Chem., 9*, S1574–S1583.

Roby, M. H. H., Sarhan, M. A., Selim, K. A., & Khalel, K. I., (2013). Antioxidant and antimicrobial activities of essential oil and extracts of fennel (*Foeniculum vulgare* L.) and chamomile (*Matricaria chamomilla* L.). *Ind. Crops Prod., 44*, 437–445.

Shahat, A. A., Ibrahim, A. Y., Hendawy, S. F., Omer, E. A., Hammouda, F. M., Abdel-Rahman, F. H., & Saleh, M. A., (2011). Chemical composition, antimicrobial and antioxidant activities of essential oils from organically cultivated fennel cultivars. *Molecules, 16*, 1366–1377.

Sharopov, F., Valiev, A., Satyal, P., Gulmurodov, I., Yusufi, S., Setzer, W. N., & Wink, M., (2017). Cytotoxicity of the essential oil of fennel (*Foeniculum vulgare*) from Tajikistan. *Foods, 6*, 73–83.

Singh, G., Maurya, S., & Lampasona, M. N., (2006). Chemical constituents, antifungal and antioxidative potential of F. vulgare volatile oil and its acetone extract. *Food Control*, 745–752.

Skrobonj, J. R., Delic, D. N., Karaman, M. A., Matavulj, M. N., & Bogavac, M. A., (2013). Antifungal properties of *Foeniculum vulgare*, *Carum carvi* and *Eucalyptus* sp. essential oils against *Candida albicans* strains. *Jour. Nat. Sci. Matica. Srpska. Novi. Sad., 124*, 195–202.

Telci, I., Demirtas, I., & Sahin, A., (2009). Variation in plant properties and essential oil composition of sweet fennel (*Foeniculum vulgare* mill.) fruits during stages of maturity. *Ind. Crops Prod., 30*, 126–130.

Timasheva, L. A., & Gorbunova, E. V., (2014). A promising trend in the processing of fennel (*Foeniculum vulgare* Mill.) whole plants. *Foods and Raw Materials, 2*, 51–57.

Villarini, M., Pagiotti, R., Dominici, L., Fatigoni, C., Vannini, S., Levorato, S., & Moretti, M., (2014). Investigation of the cytotoxic, genotoxic, and apoptosis-inducing effects of estragole isolated from fennel (*Foeniculum vulgare*). *J. Nat. Prod, 77*, 773–778.

Zaahkouk, S. A. M., Aboul-Ela, E. I., Ramadan, M. A., Bakry, S., & Mhany, A. B. M., (2015). Anti-carcinogenic activity of methanolic extract of fennel seeds (*Foeniculum vulgare*) against breast, colon, and liver cancer cells. *Int. J. Advanced Res., 3*, 1525–1537.

Zellagui, A., Gherraf, N., Elkhateeb, A., Hegazy, M. E. F., Mohamed, T. A., Touil, A., Shahat, A. A., & Rhouati, S., (2011). Chemical constituents from Algerian *Foeniculum vulgare* aerial parts and evaluation of antimicrobial activity. *J. Chil. Chem. Soc, 56*, 759–763.

CHAPTER 5

OCIMUM BASILICUM: A MODEL MEDICINAL INDUSTRIAL CROP ENRICHED WITH AN ARRAY OF BIOACTIVE CHEMICALS

SUNITA SINGH DHAWAN,[1] PANKHURI GUPTA,[1] and RAJ KISHORI LAL[2]

[1]Biotechnology Division, CSIR-Central Institute of Medicinal and Aromatic, Lucknow, Uttar Pradesh, India, E-mails: sunsdhawan@gmail.com; sunita.dhawan@cimap.res.in (S. S. Dhawan)

[2]Division of Genetics and Plant Breeding, CSIR-Central Institute of Medicinal and Aromatic, Lucknow, Uttar Pradesh – 226015, India

ABSTRACT

Tulsi is an annual and perennial aromatic and medicinal herb from the Lamiaceae family. It is traditionally used for the preparation of various Ayurvedic formulations, culinary, and medicinal herbs. It relieves from stress, restore, and improve body immunity and digestion. It is good for digestive and nervous systems, stomach pain, cramp, and digestive disorders. The leaves are carminative, aromatic, galactogog, tonic, and stomachic antispasmodic. They are also used for the treatment during migraine, influenza, nausea, abdominal cramps, poor digestive system, diarrhea, insomnia, and stress. The essential oil of sweet basil is used in aromatherapy that contains linalool methyl chavicol, methyl cinnamate, eugenol, etc. It is also used for acne, insect, and snake bites and also in skin fungal diseases. Leaves can be harvested during the whole year and used as fresh or dried powdered. The mucilaginous seed is used for the treatment of dysentery, chronic diarrhea and gonorrhea. It is rich in Vitamin A and roots are very useful for the treatment of abdominal pain, cramps, and bloating in children.

Ocimum are having phenylpropenes and terpene that accumulates and synthesized in peltate glandular trichomes and their composition and content depend upon different plant developmental stages. *Ocimum* has ovate leaves and pubescent quadrangular branches in structure, which are compactly enclosed with non-glandular and glandular trichomes. The non-glandular trichomes and the glandular trichomes secret lipophilic substances like flavonoids, waxes, lipids, and terpenes protect against many factors like extreme temperatures, excessive water loss, pathogens, herbivores, ultraviolet-B radiation. It has a protective function against many abiotic and biotic factors such as cold. Plant extracts are very effective against internal parasites and are bactericidal. All the Ocimum varieties/genotypes have different chemical composition. In this chapter, a brief account of sweet basil has been discussed and compiles all available commercial genotypes and varieties of *Ocimum* species available for commercial cultivation in India and to explain the medicinal properties, uses, essential oil components and their importance in the world of herbal medicine and trade.

Genome sequencing done by Next-generation sequencing (NGS) platforms of sweet basil has changed the impact of sequencing of plant genes, genomes, and their regulation. It will also help in identifying the target for development of trichomes and also establish novel tools for molecular breeding for generation of new and improved genotypes or varieties of *Ocimum* plant.

5.1   INTRODUCTION

Ocimum (Lamiaceae family) is also known as basil or tulsi. It has many medicinal properties and pharmaceutical applications. There are several types of *Ocimum* available in India, including more than 100 species. It is widely found throughout temperate regions in the world with the most number of species (Dzoyem et al., 2017; Shah et al., 2018). Modern scientific research in *Ocimum* today demonstrates the many psychological and physiological benefits of tulsi consumption and demonstrates the wisdom of Ayurveda, which celebrates tulsi as a plant that can be worshipped, ingested, made into tea and used in daily life for medicinal and spiritual purposes (Cohen, 2014; Jamshidi and Cohen, 2017). It is highly useful for the treatment of heart disease, stomach disorders, headaches, hepatitis, malaria, tuberculosis, swine flu and dengue. For dental health treatment and for healthy gums leaf powder and essential oil of Ocimum are highly beneficial. Ocimum plants are also used as flies, mosquitoes, and insect repellant. Its essential oil can be used to control malaria by decreasing the growth of mosquitoes (Upadhyay, 2017). The genetic germplasm available in CSIR-CIMAP is comprised of many species of Ocimum (Lal et al., 2018).

5.2 IMPORTANT VARIETIES/CULTIVARS DEVELOPED BY CSIR CIMAP AND AVAILABLE GERMPLASM COLLECTION

Varieties/cultivars developed for various industries as well as with specific chemotypic characteristics for higher yields of essential oil, major industrial metabolites and improved tolerance towards abiotic and biotic stresses by CSIR-CIMAP are discussed in subsections.

5.2.1   RAMA TULSI

➤   Common name: Light holy basil
➤   Scientific name: *Ocimum sanctum.*
   Rama tulsi has many important properties like antioxidant and anti-aging. It is mostly recognized for its ayurvedic importance and traditional medicinal values. Its leaves are used to cure stomach infection, seasonal flu, cold, and cough. This crop culti-vation gives a gross profit of about Rs. 65,000–85,000/hectare to farmers and also used by many pharma industries (available: https://www.lawnkart.com/blogs/top-plants/did-you-know-we-have-4-types-of-tulsi-growing-in-india).

Varieties of *Ocimum sanctum* developed by CSIR-CIMAP, Lucknow (Table 5.1):

1.   **CIM-Ayu:** Even during the rainy season, the CIM-Ayu variety developed by CSIR-CIMAP (Figure 5.1) produce 16 quintals of dry leaves or 110 kg per ha of eugenol rich oil (83%). The variety is grown annually in the Indian states of Uttar Pradesh, Gujarat, Karnataka, etc., for essential oil and dry leaf used in herbal tea in about 4,000 ha (Bahl et al., 2018). Even during the rainy season, it also produces eugenol (at least 47%) compared to 5.0% in other strains in the essential oil (Lal et al., 2003). In *O. sanctum* (CIM Ayu-eugenol rich variety) leaf transcriptomics data were reported, and

identification of transcription factors and pathway genes involved in the biosynthesis pathway of phenylpropanoid/ terpenoids were done (Table 5.2). Molecular markers of EST-SSRs were also analyzed to facilitate the marker-assisted breeding of this variety CIM-Ayu (Rastogi et al., 2014).

2. **CIM-Angana:** Developed by selecting the half-sib progeny. The plant is different by its purple stem with green leaves (Figure 5.2), which become purplish during cold. CIM-Angana produces a dry herb yield of leaf (14 q/ha) or an essential oil yield of 90 kg/ha, which contains eugenol 40% and germacrene-D with 16% (Lal et al., 2008).

TABLE 5.1   Chemical Diversity Among Different Varieties of *Ocimum* Species

SL. No.	Variety	Ocimum Species	Major Constituents
1.	CIM-Ayu	*Ocimum sanctum*	Eugenol (~83%) and β-elemene (~7%)
2.	CIM-Angana	*Ocimum sanctum*	Eugenol (~40%) and germacrene-D (~16%)
3.	CIM Kanchan	*Ocimum tenuiflorum*	Methyl eugenol (~70%) and β-caryophyllene (~15%)
4.	CIM-Saumya	*Ocimum basilicum*	Methyl chavicol (~60%) and (-) linalool (~24%)
5.	CIM-Surabhi	*Ocimum basilicum*	(-) Linalool (~70%)
6.	CIM-Sharda	*Ocimum basilicum*	Methyl chavicol (89%)
7.	Kusumohak	*Ocimum basilicum*	Methyl chavicol (~37%) and linalool (~45%)
8.	CIM-Jyoti	*Ocimum africanum*	Citral (~76.6%)
9.	Vikarsudha	Hybrid	Methyl chavicol (~78%) and linalool (~24%)
10.	CIM-Snigdha	Hybrid	Methyl cinnamate (~75–80%)
11.	CIM-Shishir	Hybrid	Linalool content (~75%) and camphor (9.03%)
12.	CIM Suvaas (Paan tulsi)	Hybrid	Chavibetol (~16–25% and camphor (~6.9%)
13.	CIM-Sukhda	Hybrid	β-Linalool (~75–80%) and citral (~3.6%)
14.	CIM-Akshay	*Ocimum gratissimum*	Thymol (~50%).

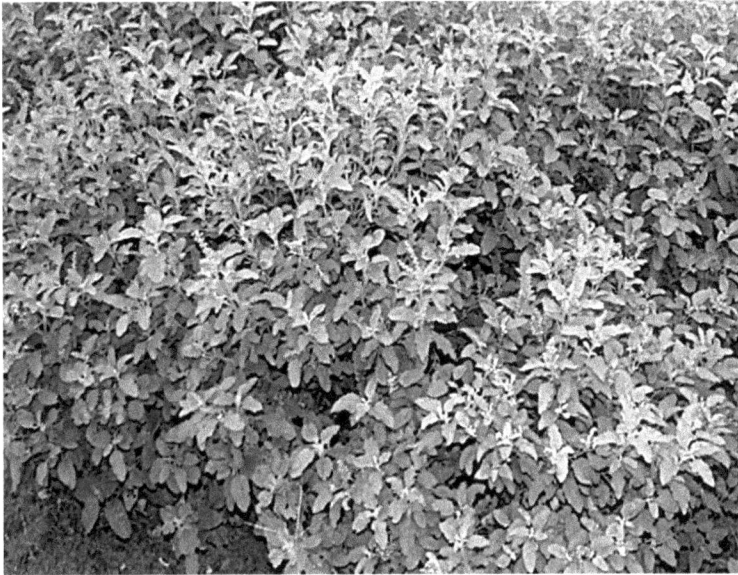

FIGURE 5.1 *Ocimum sanctum* var. CIM-Ayu.

TABLE 5.2 Genome Sequencing of Ocimum Unravels Key Genes behind its Strong Medicinal Properties (Upadhyay et al., 2015)

SL. No.	Metabolite	Disease Implication	Enzymes Involved
Flavonoids			
1.	Apigenin	Anti-cancer	Flavone synthase I [EC:1.14.20.5], Naringenin [EC:1.14.11.9], NADPH oxygen oxidoreductase [EC:1.14.13.7]
2.	Luteolin	Anti-cancer	Flavone synthase I, Naringenin, NADPH oxygen oxidoreductase Flavone 3'monooxygenase [EC:1.14.14.19 1.14.14.32], Naringenin 3' hydroxylase [EC:1.14.11.9], Eriodictyol NADPH oxygen oxidoreductase
Phenylpropanoids			
3.	Rosmarinic acid Pathway 1	Anti-cancer, anti-oxidant	4-coumaroyl-4'-hydroxyphenyllactate3-hydroxylase, Tyrosine transaminase [EC:2.6.1.5]
4.	Rosmarinic acid pathway 2	Anti-cancer, anti-oxidant	Hydroxyphenylpyruvate_reductase [EC:1.1.1.237], Tyrosine-3-monooxygenase [EC:1.14.16.2]

TABLE 5.2   *(Continued)*

SL. No.	Metabolite	Disease Implication	Enzymes Involved
5.	Eugenol	Anti-infective	Alcohol-o-acetyltransferase [EC:2.3.1.84], Eugenol synthase [EC:1.1.1.318], Isoeugenol synthase [EC:1.1.1.319]
6.	Methyl chavicol	Anti-fungal, antiparasitic, antioxidant	Eugenol-o-methyltransferase [EC:2.1.1.146]
Terpenes			
7.	Citral	Antiseptic	Geraniol synthase [EC:4.2.3.27], Geraniol dehydrogenase [EC:1.1.1.347]
8.	Linalool	Anti-infective	Farnesyl-pyrophosphate synthase [EC:2.5.1.1 2.5.1.10] r-linool synthase s-linool synthase
Sesquiterpenes			
9.	Caryophyllene	Anti-inflammatory	Alpha humulene synthase [EC:4.2.3.104 4.2.3.57] Beta-caryophyllene synthase [EC:4.2.3.104 4.2.3.57]
10.	Selinene	Anti-oxidant	Alpha selinene synthase [EC:4.2.3.198] Beta selinene synthase
11.	Taxol	Anti-cancer	Taxadiene synthase [EC:4.2.3.17] Taxadiene 5-alpha hydroxylase Taxadien-5-alpha-ol O-acetyltransferase Taxane 10-beta-hydroxylase Taxoid 14-beta-hydroxylase 2-alpha-hydroxytaxane 2-O-benzoyltransferase 10-deacetylbaccatin III 10-O-acetyltransferase 3'-N-debenzoyl-2'-deoxytaxol Nbenzoyltransferase
12.	Ursolic acid	Anti-cancer	Cytochrome P450 monooxygenase
13.	Oleanolic acid	Anti-cancer	Beta-amyrin synthase Cytochrome P450 monooxygenase [EC:2.1.1.214]
Sterols			
14.	Sitosterol	Anti-cancer	24C methyltransferase [EC:2.1.1.214]

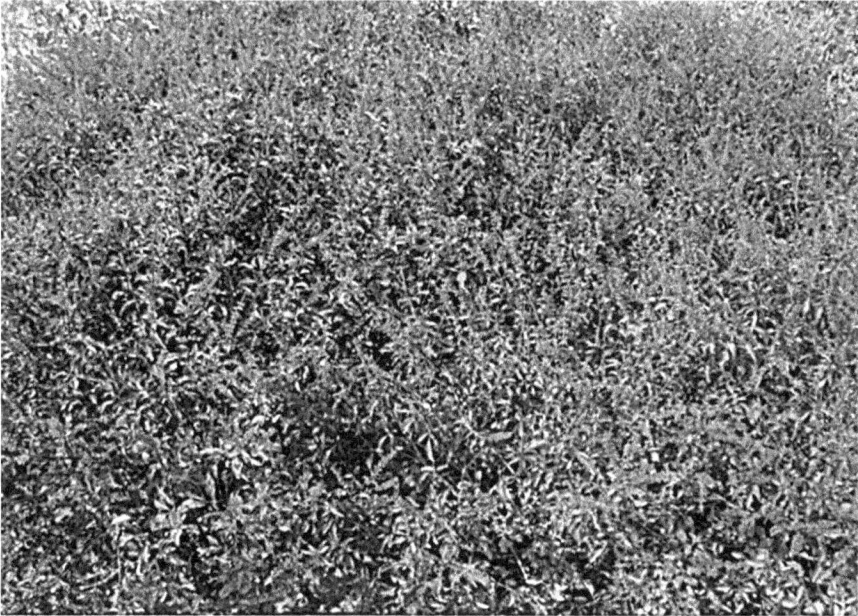

FIGURE 5.2   *Ocimum sanctum* var. CIM-Angna.

5.2.2   *KRISHNA TULSI*

➤ Common name: Dark holy basil;
➤ Scientific name: *Ocimum tenuiflorum*
    Krishna Tulsi is used to cure malaria fever, bronchitis, asthma, urogenital disorder, vomiting, Earache, antibacterial, anti-tuberculosis, leucoderma, etc. It has a strong aroma of dark purple leaves; dark stems and leaves are much smaller than Rama Tulsi:

1. **CIM Kanchan:** CIMAP developed a new chemotype Kanchan of *O. tenuiflorum* containing methyl eugenol as the dominant constituent (> 70%) in its essential oil. The chemotype Kanchan is perennial in nature and has high essential oil yield potential also (Figure 5.3). The chemotype Kanchan is a selection from extensive evaluation of the germplasm collections of *O. tenuiflorum* from different locations of South and peninsular India (Kothari et al., 2004).

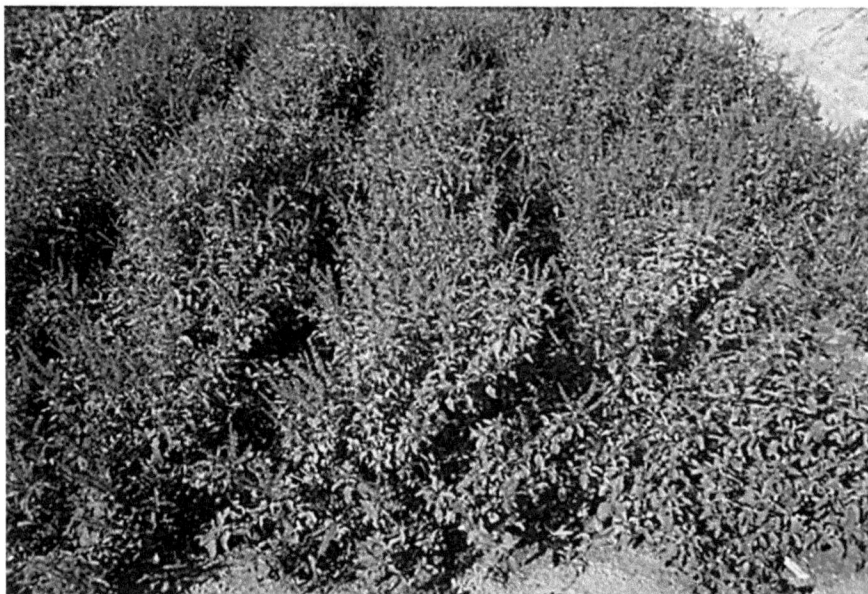

FIGURE 5.3 *Ocimum sanctum* var. CIM Kanchan.

5.2.3 SWEET BASIL

➤ Scientific name: *Ocimum basilicum*;
➤ Common name: Indian/French basil).

Sweet basil or *Ocimum basilicum* is used for many years as a medicinal herb and for cooking purposes. It acts basically on the nervous and digestive systems. Antispasmodic, aromatic, carminative, digestive, galactagogue, and stomachic properties are present in its flowers and leaves. They are taken internally in the treatment of especially fever, influenza, cough, and colds, poor digestion, depression, nausea, abdominal cramps, gastroenteritis, migraine, insomnia, and exhaustion. They are used externally to cure acne, smell loss, stings of insects, snake bites and infections of the skin. It can be cultivated in subtropical and tropical climates. This crop is not suitable for temperate climates.

CIM-Saumya and CIM-Surabhi are two varieties developed by CSIR-CIMAP:

1. **CIM-Saumya:** It was developed by selecting the progeny raised by seed. It is a short duration crop of 3 months (Figure 5.4) and essential oil yield is about 85 to 110 kg per ha. Methyl chavicol content is high with 62% and linalool with 25%. CIM-Saumya is an early, short duration, dwarf, and high essential oil yield. Rastogi et al. (2014) reported transcription factors identification and pathway genes in biosynthesis pathway of phenylpropanoids/terpenoids in CIM Saumya, a methyl-chavicol rich variety of *O. basilicum* (Lal et al., 2004).

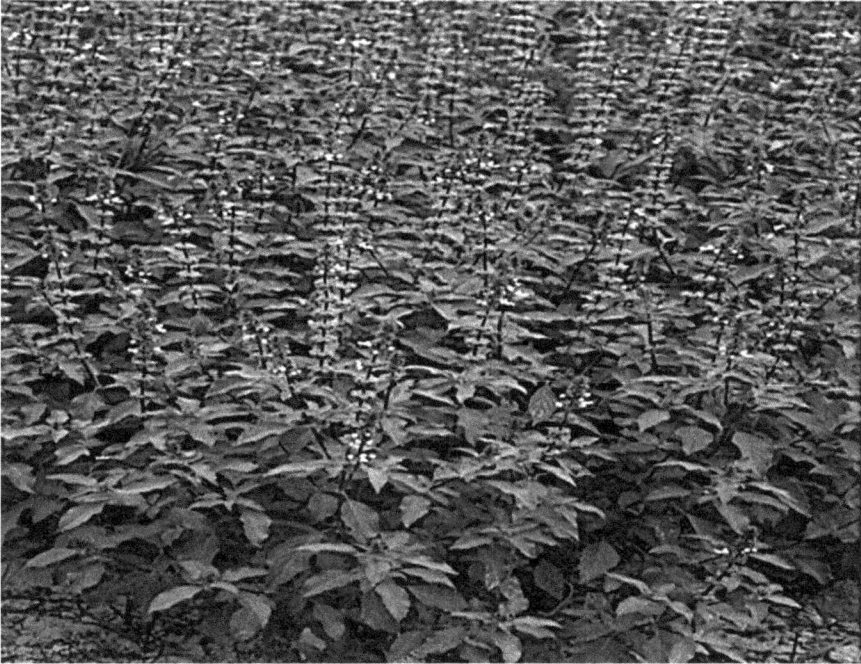

FIGURE 5.4   *Ocimum basilicum* var. CIM-Saumya.

2. **CIM-Surabhi:** This variety was developed through breeding method and by processes of selection (Figure 5.5). It is high essential oil-producing variety 100–120 kg/ha with 70–75% (-) linalool. Besides being a high linalool containing genotype. The new cultivar also fits in crop rotation/intercropping between wheat and paddy and with other vegetables crops (Lal et al., 2017b).

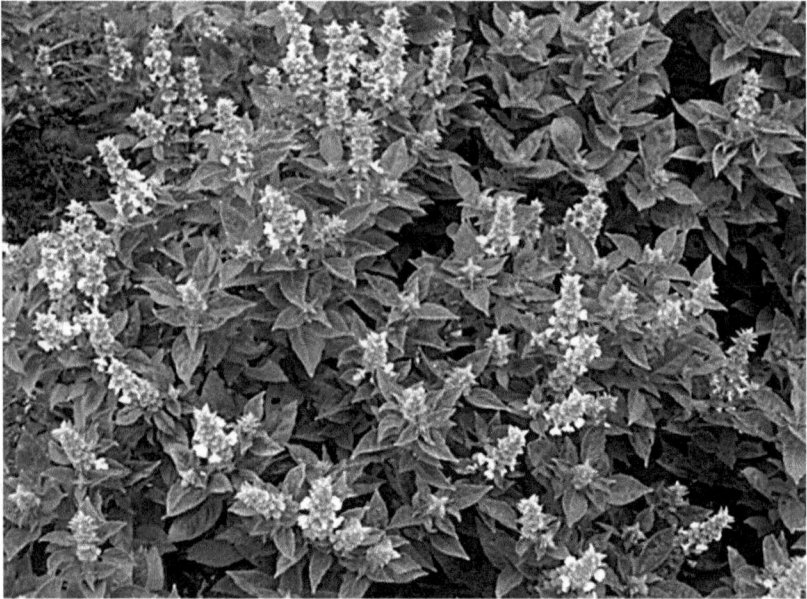

FIGURE 5.5   *Ocimum basilicum* var. CIM-Surabhi.

3. **CIM-Sharda:** Developed through intensive breeding approach and
    this variety is early maturing and high essential oil yielding, short
    duration, suitable for rainfed conditions. Herb yield: 280–290 q/ha,
    essential oil yield: 190–200 kg/ha and high Methyl Chavicol 85–89%
    (Lal et al., 2015). CIM-Sharada has been developed by CSIR-CIMAP
    through intensive breeding efforts for improved herb. The variety has
    consistently recorded a higher biomass and oil yield with high methyl
    chavicol content in the field evaluation trials. Development of new
    methyl chavicol-rich variety was utmost required to formulate value
    added industrial products. This variety matures in a short duration of
    80–90 days and hence, fits very well into crop rotation/intercropping
    cycle between wheat and paddy along with other vegetables crops of
    small farmers. It is ideally suited for rain fed cultivation. The unique
    leaf morphology and high survival in the winter season are the two
    main distinctive features of this variety as depicted in Figure 5.6. The
    newly developed variety CIM-Sharada was released at CSIR-CIMAP
    in 2015 towards its commercial cultivation by Indian farmers (Lal et
    al., 2018).

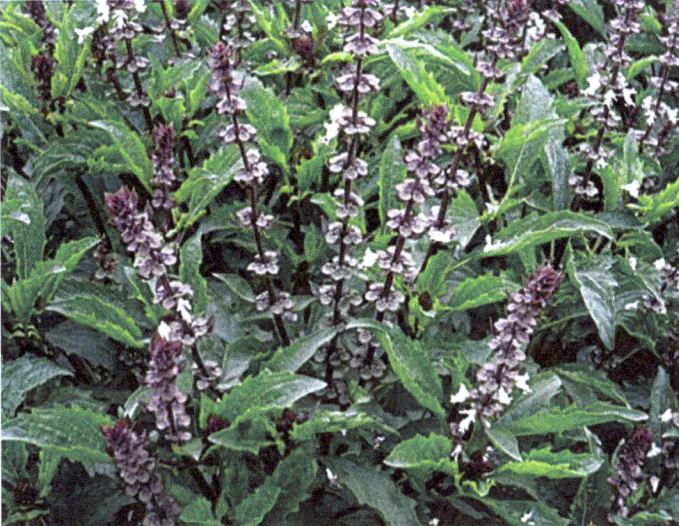

FIGURE 5.6 *Ocimum basilicum* var. CIM-Sharda.

4. **Kusumohak**: It is developed through seed raised progeny selection introduced by strain from Argentina. It has high oil yielding suitable for perfumery, cosmetic, and related industries. Yield parameters of this variety for herb is 391 q/ha, essential oil-134 kg/ha and essential oil composition shows methyl chavicol-37% and linalool 45% (Figure 5.7).

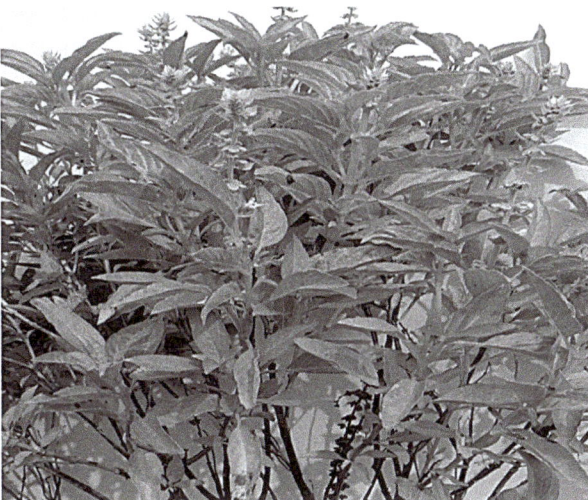

FIGURE 5.7 *Ocimum basilicum* var. Kusumohak.

5.2.4 LEMON BASIL/TULSI

➢ Scientific name: *Ocimum africanum*;
➢ Common name: citral/lemon tulsi.
➢ The plant has property of carminative, diaphoretic, and stimulant. Leaf extract is used in flue, dysentery, bronchitis, and in mouth wash for relieving toothache. It is also a good source of Vitamin A.
1. CIM-Jyoti: It is high citral rich essential oil yielding variety of *Ocimum africanum* Lemon-scented Ocimum (*Ocimum africanum*) belongs to the family Lamiaceae. The cultivar CIM Jyoti of *Ocimum africanum* has been developed by CSIR-CIMAP through intensive breeding efforts containing desirable content of citral (76.05%). The average essential oil and herb yield of this variety is 200 q/ha and 150 kg/ha, respectively. The citral (Neral+Geranial) content in its essential oil ranged from 68–76%. CIM-Jyoti which is a short duration (70–80 days) variety fits very well in crop rotation/ intercropping between wheat and paddy and with other vegetables crops. Leaves of this variety can also be used in lemon teas (Lal et al., 2017c). It also fits in crop rotation/intercropping between wheat and paddy and with other vegetables crops of small farmers. Leaves of this variety can be used in lemon tea. The new developed variety CIM-Sharada was released at CSIR-CIMAP in 2014 on the occasion of CSIR Foundation Day (Figure 5.8).

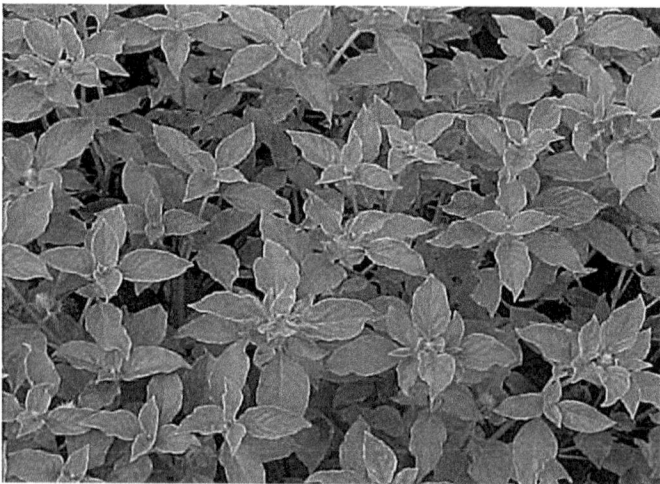

FIGURE 5.8 *Ocimum africanum* var. CIM-Jyoti.

5.2.5   INTRASPECIFIC/INTERSPECIFIC HYBRID OF OCIMUM SPECIES

1. **Vikarsudha:** It is developed through intraspecific hybridization between basil and local strain (Figure 5.9). It has long late maturity, herb yield is 335 q/ha, essential oil yield is 167.50 kg/ha, essential oil content is 0.5% and contains methyl chavicol 78% and linalool 0.16% (http://intranet.cimap.res.in/cimvariety/showvariety) (Dwivedi et al., 1999).

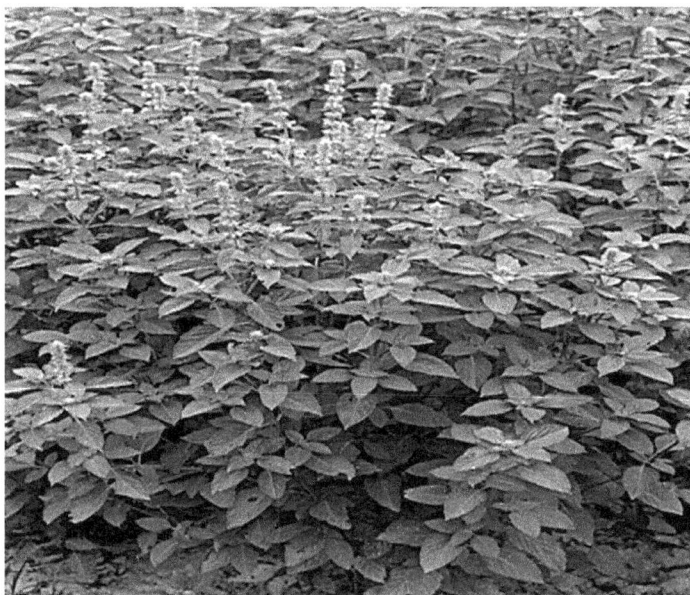

FIGURE 5.9   Intraspecific hybrid of *Ocimum basilicum* var. Vikarsudha.

2. **CIM-Snigdha:** This variety is an intraspecific hybrid of *Ocimum basilicum* developed by CSIR-CIMAP as shown in Figure 5.10. It has a unique aroma with different types of leaf morphology. It has methyl cinnamate content with 78% and this variety maturity time is from 80–90 days (Lal et al., 2017a). CIM-Snigdha has been developed by CSIR-CIMAP through intensive breeding efforts for improved herb and essential oil yield. The variety has consistently recorded a higher biomass and oil yield with high methyl cinnamate content in the field evaluation trials. The potential average herb and oil yield of this new variety is 221 q/ha and 190 kg/ha, respectively. The variety matures

within a short duration of 80–90 days and hence fits very well into crop rotation/intercropping cycle between wheat and paddy along with other vegetable crops. The distinct leaf morphology and high tolerance to cold conditions are the two important economic features of this variety. The new developed variety CIM-Snigdha was released at CSIR-CIMAP in 2017 on the occasion of Kisan Mela.

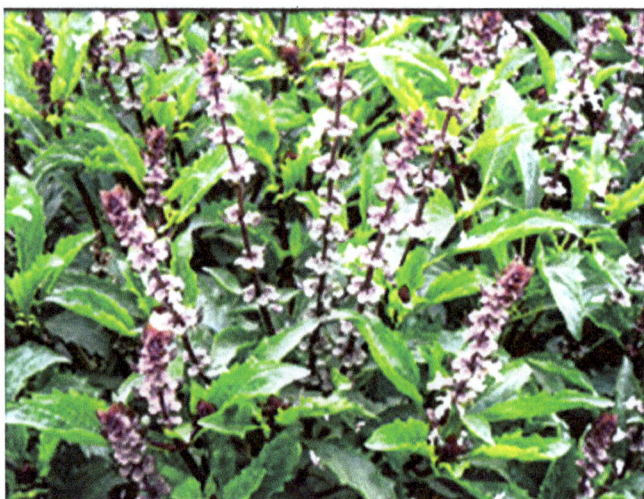

FIGURE 5.10   Intraspecific hybrid of *Ocimum basilicum* var. CIM-Snigdha.

3. **CIM-Shishir:** This variety is a multicut, lodging resistant, cold tolerant, high essential oil yielding with linalool rich strain from interspecific hybrid of *Ocimum* (Figure 5.11). It is morphologically distinct from other *Ocimum basilicum* varieties and clearly identifiable by its very tall, very broad, long, undulated surface, medium-dark green with robust growth. It has purple-green stem and has a unique feature and advantage of better survival in winter season in comparison to other *O. basilicum* varieties. Essential oil extracted from this hybrid strain contain higher amount of linalool content (70–75%) with a low amount of camphor (9.03%) (Dhawan et al., 2018). It is also suitable for cultivating in whole year with multicutting up to three harvests including rain-fed conditions. It is an interspecific hybrid between *Ocimum basilicum* and *Ocimum kilimandscharicum* (Dhawan et al., 2016). The essential oil of interspecific hybrid of *Ocimum* with linalool and camphor in desired

combinations is used in various innovative cosmetic and perfumery products. Besides the premium price of linalool, this variety will also provide additional income to farmers as it is a high herb (600 q/ha) and essential oil yielding (250 kg/ha) variety with 70–75% (-) linalool. Intensive breeding techniques like inter specific hybridization and selection process were undertaken at CSIR-CIMAP, Lucknow to develop such a variety of *Ocimum*. This linalool rich genotype will be a cheap source of linalool for the perfumery and flavor industry. Therefore, production of a variety with high essential oil having high linalool content with multi cutting without much effects of environment/temperature would be helpful to overcome low essential oil. The need of winter tolerant high yielding genotype is utmost important for the future as this will add to the income of farmers as well as various industries which are dependent upon the bioactive constituents like high linalool of *Ocimum*. The new developed variety CIM-Shishir was released at CSIR-CIMAP in 2018 on the occasion of CSIR-CIMAP Diamond Jubilee for commercial cultivation by Padma Vibhushan Dr. Ragunath Anant Mashelkar.

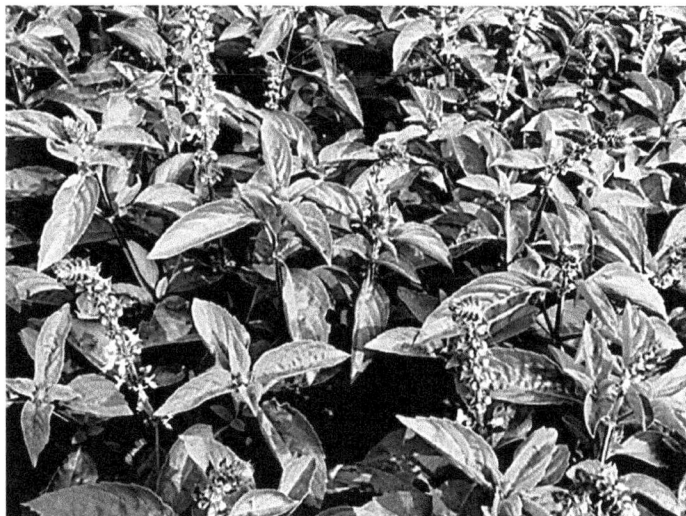

FIGURE 5.11   Interspecific hybrid of *Ocimum basilicum* and *Ocimum kilimandscharicum* var. CIM-Shishir.

4. **CIM Suvaas:** Based on the importance of chavibetol from a new source of basil, there is a need to develop a better plant type having

high essential oil yielding traits with better chavibetol content. Previously, CSIR-CIMAP developed a number of varieties but none of them having chavibetol rich essential oil and production of essential oil yield is not able to fulfill the high demand of chavibetol rich essential oil. Therefore, production of a variety with high essential oil having high chavibetol content with multi-cutting without effects of environment/temperature would be helpful to overcome low essential oil. The need of high yielding chavibetol rich genotype is utmost important for the future as this will add to the income of farmers as well as many industries. Essential oil with a new aroma like chavibetol with high essential oil is suitable for various innovative cosmetic products/ perfumery industries are required. It is also used in chewing gum, mouth wash, mouth freshener and aromatherapy traditional and therapeutic purposes. Chavibetol rich chemotypes will provide additional income to farmers. High essential oil having high chavibetol content would also be helpful to formulate value added industrial products. *Piper betel* is the main source of unique aroma chemical chavibetol, but the cultivation of betel crop is very difficult on a large scale. Therefore, the new basil chavibetol rich essential oil 'CIM-Suvaas' variety will be a new cheaper source of important aroma compound chavibetol. This is also the first world report that shows the presence of chavibetol in basil oil (Figure 5.12). The new developed variety CIM-Suvaas was released at CSIR-CIMAP in 2019 on the occasion of CSIR Kisan Mela.

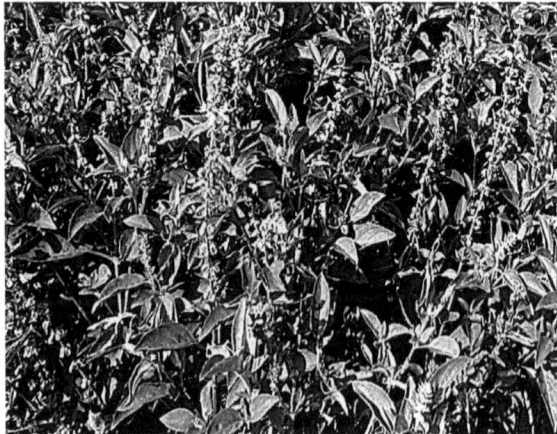

FIGURE 5.12   Interspecific hybrid of *Ocimum basilicum* and *Ocimum kilimandscharicum* var. CIM-Suvaas (Paan tulsi).

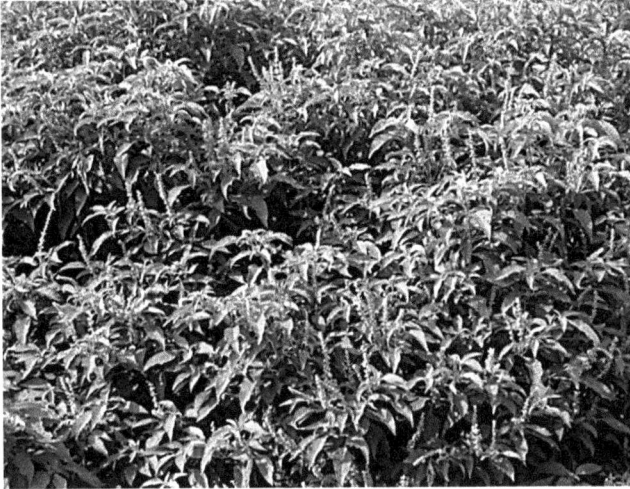

FIGURE 5.13 *Ocimum gratissimum* var. CIM-Akshay.

5.2.6 VANA TULSI

➤ Common name: Wild leaf holy basil;

➤ Scientific name: *Ocimum gratissimum*.

Vana Tulsi is used for the treatment of malaria, tuberculosis, diabetes, asthma, urinary disease, etc. Wild leaf Tulsi looks like Rama Tulsi, but has a white flower, a stronger flavor and is taller than other tulsi genotypes.

1. **CIM-Akshay:** CIM-Akshay of *Ocimum gratissimum* is yielding variety released for cultivation from CSIR-CIMAP. The only source of Thymol to meet the demand is *Thymus* and *Tachyspermum ammi*. It is perennial nature. It is high Thymol rich essential oil yielding variety of *Ocimum gratissimum* belongs to the family "Lamiaceae." The cultivar CIM Jyoti of *Ocimum africanum* has been developed by CSIR-CIMAP through breeding efforts for higher herb and essential oil containing desirable content of Thymol (50.70%). The average herb and essential oil yield of this variety is 300–320 q/ha and 100–120 kg/ha, respectively. Leaves of this variety are broad, inflorescence is small. The new developed variety CIM-Akshay was released at CSIR-CIMAP in 2019 on the occasion of CSIR Kisan Mela.

5.2.7 KAPOOR TULSI

> Common name: Camphor basil
> Scientific name: *Ocimum kilimandscharicum*.
> Kapoor Tulsi is used to cure Anti-fungal, cold, and cough, flu, Dysentery, Chronic Diarrhea, Indigestion, Eczema, Snakebite, etc. Kapoor Tulsi is commonly originated in the USA as it can be cultivated in temperate regions. It attracts many bees because of its strong aroma (Dhawan et al., 2016). *Ocimum kilimandscharicum* (Figure 5.14) is perennial and an economically important herb used for various purposes like in agriculture, medicine, and ornamental industrial. The leaves of *O. kilimandscharicum* are acrid, spasmolytic, thermogenic, aromatic, insecticidal, antibacterial, antiviral, appetizing, antioxidant, ophthalmic, and deodorant. It is useful in cough, bronchitis, catarrh, foul ulcers and wounds, anorexia, and vitiated conditions (Misra and Das, 2016).

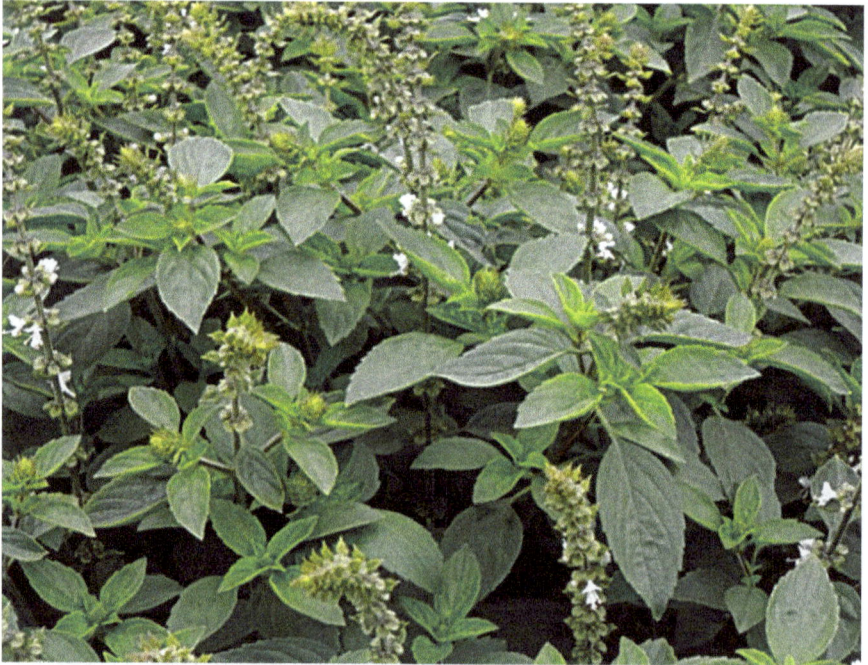

FIGURE 5.14 *Ocimum kilimandscharicum.*

5.3 GENE EXPRESSION AND TRANSCRIPTOME ANALYSIS OF *OCIMUM* SPECIES

The genome of sweet basil *O. basilicum* L. (var: CIM Saumya) was deciphered in CSIR CIMAP first time. Chromosome number of *O. basilicum* is 2n=48. The analysis of KEGG has identified 952 transcripts of *O. basilicum* for secondary metabolism with a higher percentage of transcripts for Phenylpropanoid biosynthesis. This is the first report of a comparative transcriptome analysis of *Ocimum* species and can be used to characterize genes related to secondary metabolism, its regulation and the breeding of special chemotypes with an essential oil constituent's composition. The sequence assembly resulted in an average length of 1363 ± 1139.3 bp for *O. basilicum* 130,043 transcripts. Of the total transcripts, 105,470 (81.10%) by *O. basilicum* was reported. The total number of transcripts recorded in all databases was 105,470 (81.10%) (Rastogi et al., 2014; Rastogi and Shasany, 2018; Shah et al., 2018).

In Ayurveda (Indian system of medicine), many diseases including bronchitis can be treated from the essential oils (EOs) metabolites of *Ocimum* as it has antioxidant and antifungal properties. Plants produce specific metabolites which protect from biotic and abiotic stress, and these metabolites have many medicinal properties that can treat many types of diseases caused in human beings. They are extracted from different plant parts that include flowers, leaves, roots, bark, stems, and seeds. The studies and research on chemical constituents and pharmacological screening of plant metabolites make available to develop new medicines (Khair-ul-Bariyah et al., 2012). Geraniol, linalool, citral, eugenol, camphor, methyl chavicol, ursolic acid, etc., are some of the major secondary metabolites reported in *Ocimum* species. In pharmaceutical, perfume, and cosmetic industries, these metabolites have tremendous value (Lal et al., 2018). Metabolites produce from *Ocimum* species contain many medicinally important properties like anti-inflammatory and antifungal, anti-cancer, antioxidant, malaria treatment, bronchitis, diarrhea, dysentery, etc. Specialized metabolites synthesis in *Ocimum* seeds, leaves, roots, and flowers used in pharmaceuticals and many traditional Indian medicine systems. Transcriptome and genome sequencing of medicinal plants is an important technique for drug and biochemical discovery of major secondary metabolites (Lal et al., 2017).

5.4   TRICHOME ANALYSIS IN *OCIMUM* SPECIES

Ocimum basilicum species produces EOs whose chemical constituents are widely used in cosmetics for fragrances, food as flavorings, and medicine for the treatment of many diseases (Burt, 2004). Ocimum EOs are secreted, stored, and synthesized from different types of secretory cells and structures from glandular secretory trichomes. Two types of glandular secretory trichomes that are usually present on the abaxial and adaxial surface of leaves that include large peltate and small capitate (Maurya et al., 2019). Peltate trichome head is consisting of 4 large head cells. The Capitate trichome head is consisting of 2 wide head cells type I in one layer or type II a single oval head cell. Naidoo et al. (2013) reported that the secretory cells of trichomes (glandular) are usually consists of aromatic oils, polysaccharides, and substances of lipophilic and chemical composition of secretions in glandular trichomes was reported by histochemical analysis to know its medicinal values and its role in during secretion formed by *Ocimum* species (Dhawan et al., 2016).

Peltate and capitate glandular trichomes are present in various *Ocimum* species. Capitate trichomes in *O. basilicum* consisting of one stalk cell, one basal cell and head of either elongated, two cells broad or oval cell (Werker, 2000). In *O. gratissimum*, the peltate and capitate glandular trichomes on the leaves are similar to those found on the leaves of *O. selloi*. The existence of terpenes in the EOs of the glandular trichomes of *O. obovatum* leaves has many medicinal properties. These compounds reveal antifeedant activity, mammal toxicity, antibiotics, and molluscicidal (Harborne, 1996; Nishida, 2002).

5.5   COMPOSITION OF ESSENTIAL OIL OF *OCIMUM BASILICUM*

In *O. basilicum* species qualitative analyzes of essential oil by GC/MS, it was reported that the major compounds are mono, sesquiterpenes, and Phenylpropanoids. In *O. basilicum* from Bangladesh, linalool, and geraniol are reported as the major constituents (Dev et al., 2010). In Colombia and Bulgaria essential oil produce from this species has linalool and methyl cinnamate as main compound respectively (Viña and Murillo, 2003). Linalool and methyl eugenol were also reported in these species from Mali and Guinea (Moussa et al., 2000). The differences observed may be due to different genetic and environmental factors, different chemotypes and plant nutritional status, as well as other factors that may affect the different compositions of the essential oil. Padalia and Verma (2011) also reported the major constituents identified in both cultivars *O. basilicum* (Vikarsudha and

CIM-Saumya) of northern plains of India were methyl chavicol and linalool, both belong to phenolic chemotypes as the marker constituents.

5.6 OTHER USES OF *OCIMUM BASILICUM*

The essential oil produced by *Ocimum basilicum* species are used as flavoring in cooking, in cosmetic, perfumery, dental treatment, etc. An average yield of 1.5% essential oil is produced from leaves and flowering tops. It is also used as mosquito repellent. It is an effective insect repellent also when growing or dried plant is used. It repels flies when it is growing in the home or in the greenhouse where it can keep all types of pests, insects, mosquitoes, etc., away from nearby areas.

5.7 POTENTIAL HEALTH BENEFITS OF *OCIMUM BASILICUM* SEED

Seeds of *Ocimum basilicum* are have anticancer antioxidant, antiviral, antibacterial, antifungal, and antispasmodic properties. In patients with type 2 diabetes, its seeds are helping in controlling blood sugar level. When *O. basilicum* seeds soaked in water, the outer seed coat becomes mucus-like and they are very fibrous which in helps indigestion. There is also little research suggested that this fiber has a laxative effect. Basil seeds are also helpful in relieve of stomach ache, constipation, flatulence, and indigestion. The fibers in the soaked seeds help to reduce appetite and assist with weight loss. Traditionally, its seeds are used to cure coughs and colds, flu, and asthma. Utilization of basil seeds help to reduce many types of stress, uplifting your mood, migraine headaches and depression. Basil seeds can be crushed into oil and its paste is used for skin treatment for wounds, any types of injuries and cuts or skin fungal infections. Sweet basil seeds could be used to reduce cholesterol levels in patients. It has antibacterial properties also therefore, basil seeds are also helpful in the treatment of bladder infections and vaginal infections. It is also very helpful in nutritional breakdown as basil seeds contains all the concentrated nutrients and building blocks needed to grow. There is no toxicity or any harmful effects have ever been found for basil seeds and therefore it is very safe to consume (https://www.care2.com/greenliving/are-basil-seeds-a-new-superfood.html).

5.8   CONCLUSION

The importance of medicinal plants has increased over time, as there are a number of side effects in synthetic medicines in addition to many advantages. These plants have identified and known for pharmacological uses that we have acquired. The purpose of this review is to describe the importance of *Ocimum basilicum* in a holistic view. The large range of studies on these herbal plants indicated that it is very useful for the improvement of existing drugs molecules and more efforts and improvement can be done to exploit the possible remedial properties of this plant. The *Ocimum* genotypes are potential hub or could be utilized as biofactories for the production of specific chemicals and genetic manipulation for producing various industrially important molecules. The genome analysis of this plant provides a basic model for understanding of biosynthesis and gene regulation of other aromatic plant species. Therefore, this plant is providing a model plant system for medicinal as well as for aromatic plant species.

5.9   FUTURE PROSPECTS

Plants have been used to treat enormous numbers of diseases worldwide. *Ocimum* is used in both the Ayurvedic and Unani medicine systems as well as in culinary and ornamental applications. From a medicinal point of view, the extensive literature survey showed that *O. basilicum* has a wide range of pharmacological work. The essential oil and extract produced from *Ocimum* used for their antibacterial, anticancer, anticonvulsant, antidiabetic, antihyperlipidemic, anti-inflammatory, antioxidant, antistress, hepatoprotective, and immunomodulatory properties. Sweet basil with various biological potential has a great potential for further research related to pharmaceutical industries and drug formulations. Therefore, this crop would become a designer cash crop for providing specific molecules as well as a hub for basic understanding of biosynthesis of various chemical moieties and the gene regulation involved in this complex cross-linking. Thus, catering the need on the one hand for pharma sector and on the other hand providing support to farmers. Future research should focus on *Ocimum* species for the evaluation of its pharmacological properties and for the control of various diseases, in particular cancer, cardiac, neuropsychological disorders for human welfare.

KEYWORDS

- **next-generation sequencing (NGS)**
- *Ocimum kilimandscharicum*
- *Ocimum spp.*
- **phenylpropenes**
- **terpenes**
- **transcriptome analysis**

REFERENCES

Bahl, J. R., Singh, A. K., Lal, R. K., & Gupta, A. K., (2018). High-yielding improved varieties of medicinal and aromatic crops for enhanced income. In: Singh, B., & Peter, K. V., (eds.), *New Age Herbals: Resource, Quality and Pharmacognosy* (pp. 247–265). Springer Singapore, Singapore. https://doi.org/10.1007/978-981-10-8291-7_12.

Burt, S., (2004). Essential oils: Their antibacterial properties and potential applications in foods—a review. *Int. J. Food Microbiol., 94*, 223–253. https://doi.org/10.1016/j.ijfoodmicro.2004.03.022.

Cohen, M. M., (2014). Tulsi - *Ocimum* sanctum: A herb for all reasons. *J. Ayurveda Integr. Med., 5*, 251–259. https://doi.org/10.4103/0975-9476.146554.

Dev, N., Das, A. K., Hossain, M. A., & Rahman, S. M. M., (2010). chemical compositions of different extracts of *Ocimum basilicum* leaves. *J. Sci. Res., 3*. https://doi.org/10.3329/jsr.v3i1.5409.

Dhawan, S. S., Shukla, P., Gupta, P., & Lal, R. K., (2016). A cold-tolerant evergreen interspecific hybrid of *Ocimum kilimandscharicum* and *Ocimum basilicum*: Analyzing trichomes and molecular variations. *Protoplasma, 253*, 845–855. https://doi.org/10.1007/s00709-015-0847-9.

Dwivedi, S., Tajuddin, Yaseen, M., Singh, K., Naqvi, A. A., Singh, A. P., & Kumar, S., (1999). Registration of a new variety "vikarsudha" of *Ocimum basilicum. J. Med. Arom. Pl. Sci., 21*, 373–374.

Dzoyem, J. P., McGaw, L. J., Kuete, V., & Bakowsky, U., (2017). Chapter 9 - anti-inflammatory and anti-nociceptive activities of African medicinal spices and vegetables. In: Kuete, V., (ed.), *Medicinal Spices and Vegetables from Africa* (pp. 239–270). Academic Press. https://doi.org/10.1016/B978-0-12-809286-6.00009-1.

Harborne, J. B., (1996). Plant secondary metabolism. In: Crawley, M. J., (ed.), *Plant Ecology* (pp. 132–155). Blackwell Publishing Ltd., Oxford, UK. https://doi.org/10.1002/9781444313642.ch5.

Jamshidi, N., & Cohen, M. M., (2017). The clinical efficacy and safety of tulsi in humans: A systematic review of the literature [WWW Document]. *Evid. Based Complement. Alternat. Med.* https://doi.org/10.1155/2017/9217567.

Khair-ul-Bariyah, S., Ahmed, D., & Ikram, M., (2012). *Ocimum basilicum*: A review on phytochemical and pharmacological studies. *Pak. J. Chem., 2*, 78–85. https://doi.org/10.15228/2012.v02.i02.p05.

Kothari, S. K., Bhattacharya, A. K., Singh, C. P., Singh, K., Rao, B. R. R., Shyamasundar, K. V., Ramesh, S., et al., (2004). Registration of a new chemotype "Kanchan" of sacred basil/ holy basil, *Ocimum tenuiflorum* (syn. *O. sanctum*) rich in methyl eugenol. *J. Med. Arom. Pl. Sci., 26*, 336–340.

Kumar, S., Bahl, J. R., Bansal, R. P., Khanuja, S. P. S., Darokar, M. P., Shasany, A. K., Garg, S. N., et al., (1999). Registration of a new variety "Kusumohak" of *Ocimum basilicum. J. Med. Arom. Pl. Sci., 21*, 46.

Lal, R. K., Chanotiya, C., Gupta, A., Singh, V., Shasany, A., Singh, S., Maurya, R., et al., (2017a). *Registration of Variety: CIM-Snigddha: A Methyl Cinnamate Rich and High Essential oil Yielding Variety of French Basil (Ocimum basilicum)*, 6.

Lal, R. K., Gupta, P., Chanotiya, C. S., & Sarkar, S., (2018). Traditional plant breeding in *Ocimum*, In: Shasany, A. K., & Kole, C., (eds.), *The Ocimum Genome* (pp. 89–98). Springer International Publishing, Cham. https://doi.org/10.1007/978-3-319-97430-9_7.

Lal, R. K., Khanuja, S. P. S., Agnihotri, A. K., Misra, H. O., Shasany, A. K., Naqvi, A. A., Dhawan, O. P., et al., (2003). High yielding eugenol rich oil-producing variety of *Ocimum sanctum*- 'CIM-Ayu.' *J. Med. Arom. Plant Sci., 25*, 746–747.

Lal, R. K., Khanuja, S. P. S., Agnihotri, A. K., Shasany, A. K., Naqvi, A. A., Dwivedi, S., Misra, H. O., et al., (2004). An early, short duration, high essential oil, methyl chavicol, and linalool yielding variety of Indian Basil (*Ocimum basilcum*) 'CIM- Saumya.' *J. Med. Arom. Plant Sci., 26*, 77, 78.

Lal, R. K., Khanuja, S. P. S., Rizavi, H., Shasany, A. K., Ahmad, R., Chandra, R., Naqvi, A. A., et al., (2008). Registration of high yielding dark purple pigmented variety "CIM-angana" of shyamaa tulsi (*Ocimum sanctum* L.). *J. Med. Arom. Pl. Sci., 30*(1), 92–94.

Lal, R. K., Shasany, A., Singh, S., Sarkar, S., Singh, V. R., Chanotiya, C., Yadav, R., et al., (2017b). *Registration of Variety: CIM-Surabhi: A Linalool Rich, High Essential Oil Yielding Variety of Sweet Basil (Ocimum basilicum)*, 6.

Lal, R. K., Shasany, A., Singh, V., Gupta, A., Singh, S., Sarkar, S., Chanotiya, C., et al., (2017c). *Registration of High Citral Rich Essential Oil Yielding Variety-CIM Jyoti of Ocimum africanum*, 5.

Lal, R. K., Singh, S., Gupta, P., Dhawan, S. S., Sarkar, S., & Verma, K., (2017). *Quantification of Ursolic Acid, Correlations and Contribution by Other Traits Towards Accumulation of Ursolic Acid in Six Ocimum Species*, 8.

Maurya, S., Chandra, M., Yadav, R. K., Narnoliya, L. K., Sangwan, R. S., Bansal, S., Sandhu, P., et al., (2019). Interspecies comparative features of trichomes in *Ocimum* reveal insights for biosynthesis of specialized essential oil metabolites. *Protoplasma, 256*, 893–907. https://doi.org/10.1007/s00709-018-01338-y.

Misra, R. C., & Das, G., (2016). *Ocimum* kilimandscharicum guerke (Lamiaceae): A new distributional record for peninsular India with Focus on its Economic Potential. *Proc. Natl. Acad. Sci. India Sect. B Biol. Sci., 86*, 795–803. https://doi.org/10.1007/s40011-015-0526-9.

Moussa, K. S., Vincent, C., & Bélanger, A., (2000). Essential oil composition of *Ocimum basilicum* L., *O. gratissimum* L., and *O. suave* L. in the republic of guinea. *Flavor Fragr. J., 15*, 339–341. https://doi.org/10.1002/1099-026(200009/10)15:53.3.CO;2-8.

Naidoo, Y., Kasim, N., Heneidak, S., Nicholas, A., & Naidoo, G., (2013). Foliar secretory trichomes of *Ocimum obovatum* (Lamiaceae): Micromorphological structure and histochemistry. *Plant Syst. Evol., 299*, 873–885. https://doi.org/10.1007/s00606-13-0770-5.

Nishida, R., (2002). Sequestration of defensive substances from plants by lepidoptera. *Annu. Rev. Entomol., 47*, 57–92. https://doi.org/10.1146/annurev.ento.47.091201.145121.

Padalia, R. C., & Verma, R. S., (2011). Comparative volatile oil composition of four *Ocimum* species from northern India. *Nat. Prod. Res., 25*, 569–575. https://doi.org/10.1080/147864 19.2010.482936.

Rastogi, S., & Shasany, A. K., (2018). *Ocimum* genome sequencing—A futuristic therapeutic mine. In: Shasany, A. K., & Kole, C., (eds.), *The Ocimum Genome* (pp. 127–148). Springer International Publishing, Cham. https://doi.org/10.1007/978-3-319-97430-9_10.

Rastogi, S., Meena, S., Bhattacharya, A., Ghosh, S., Shukla, R., Sangwan, N., Lal, R., et al., (2014). De novo sequencing and comparative analysis of holy and sweet basil transcriptomes. *BMC Genomics, 15*, 588. https://doi.org/10.1186/1471-2164-15-588.

Shah, S., Rastogi, S., & Shasany, A. K., (2018). Genomic resources of *Ocimum*. In: Shasany, A. K., & Kole, C., (eds.), *The Ocimum Genome* (pp. 99–110). Springer International Publishing, Cham. https://doi.org/10.1007/978-3-319-97430-9_8.

Upadhyay, A. K., Chacko, A. R., Gandhimathi, A., Ghosh, P., Harini, K., Joseph, A. P., Joshi, A. G., et al., (2015). Genome sequencing of herb tulsi (*Ocimum tenuiflorum*) unravels key genes behind its strong medicinal properties. *BMC Plant Biol., 15*, 212. https://doi.org/10.1186/s12870-015-0562-x.

Upadhyay, R. K., (2017). Tulsi: A holy plant with high medicinal and therapeutic value. *Int. J. Green Pharm. IJGP, 11*. https://doi.org/10.22377/ijgp.v11i01.869.

Viña, A., & Murillo, E., (2003). Essential oil composition from twelve varieties of basil (*Ocimum* sp.) grown in Colombia. *J. Braz. Chem. Soc., 14*, 744–749. https://doi.org/10.1590/S0103-50532003000500008.

Werker, E., (2000). Trichome diversity and development. In: *Advances in Botanical Research* (pp. 1–35). Elsevier. https://doi.org/10.1016/S0065-2296 (00)31005-9.

CHAPTER 6

SYZYGIUM AROMATICUM, CURCUMA LONGA, AND *LAVANDULA*: VOLATILE COMPONENTS AND ANTIOXIDANT ACTIVITIES

HIROKO F. KASAI

Faculty of Pharmaceutical Sciences, Hoshi University, Ebara 2-4-41, Tokyo – 142-8501, Japan, E-mail: kasai@hoshi.ac.jp

ABSTRACT

Smelling fragrances of plants directly is believed to deliver not only pleasure but also beneficial therapeutic properties for people. The volatile components originating from three plants: *Syzygium aromaticum, Curcuma longa,* and *Lavandula*, cultivated in a medicinal plant garden of Hoshi University in Tokyo, were investigated. Sampling of volatile components was performed using polydimethylsiloxane-coated bars and fibers and then analyzed using thermal desorption-gas chromatography-mass spectrometry (TD-GC-MS). The analysis of volatile components, rather than essential oils (EOs), of plants was a special feature of this study, and effects of different growth phases, parts, and solution for extract were investigated. Investigation of antioxidant activity of plant extracts was carried out using the electron spin resonance (ESR) spin-trapping method. The plants cultivated in the medicinal plant garden were extracted with either water solution or methanol, and then potent scavenging activity against superoxide anion radical (O_2^{-}) was measured.

6.1 INTRODUCTION

Information technology development has brought greater convenience to modern society. Amounts of obtainable information increase and numerous communication methods are available. People need time alone to stand still and think because this can also be stressful. Circumstances and human relationships have a great influence on mental and physical fatigue. Many are affected by allergies, e.g., asthma, and atopy, mental conditions like depression and feelings of anxiety, hypertension, heart disease, digestive problems, and lower back pain. Advances in medical science and healthy living environments lengthen life spans, and in superannuated societies, the quality of life is particularly important for maintaining health. Lowering stress levels is required. Plant-based materials such as herbs, flowers, buds, and rhizomes have been used in aromatherapy. A walk-in forest is useful for relieving us from stress. Plants release various volatile compounds, e.g., terpenes, and aromatic compounds, into the atmosphere. The compounds are useful as air fresheners and induce relaxation (Yatagai, 2000).

The medicinal plant garden of Hoshi University, located in southern Tokyo has many plant varieties. Fragrances originating from plants can affect the sense of well-being and stress relief. Increasing applications of volatile compounds to improve human health requires additional information on the fragrances of plants cultivated in the garden. Odor profiles of the plants in the garden are necessary because fragrance consists of several volatile compounds which are influenced by surrounding conditions (Letchamo, Ward, and Heard, 2004). Thermal desorption-gas chromatography-mass spectrometry (TD-GC-MS) was carried out for analyzes of volatile components.

Cloves are commonly known as *choji* in Japan and is a natural medicine originating from the flower buds of *Syzygium aromaticum* in the family Myrtaceae. Clove essential oil obtained from the buds is effective to toothache and is used as a sterilizer (Clove/Crude Drugs and Related Drugs, 2016). The color of flower buds changes with ripening, and the fragrance also changes. Sampling of volatile compounds from buds were performed at three development stages, i.e., phase I (green), phase II (pink), and phase III (bright red). The characteristic attractive fragrance of buds is the strongest at phase III. We analyzed changes in volatile compounds originating from living clove buds through growth phases (Kasai, Shirao, and Ikegami-Kawai, 2016) (Figure 6.1).

Curcuma longa is the family of Zingiberaceae, and is known as *ukon* in Japan (Turmeric/crude drugs and related drugs, 2016). The color of turmeric, i.e., the rhizomes located underground, is yellow, and has been used as a dye and a spice in curry. It is also used for medicinal purposes (Singh, Singh, and Maurya, 2002). In the medicinal plant garden, *C. longa* plant is cultivated. Seed rhizomes harvested in the previous November are planted in the ground in May, young, and white rhizomes emerge in July, and the white turmeric flowers bloom in September. At last thick rhizomes in yellow color are harvested in late November. As the volatile compounds originating from rhizomes at three different development stages, i.e., July, September, and November, assumed to be different, the analyzes were carried out (Kasai, Ishii, and Yaoita, 2017). Although there were previous reports relating to essential oils (EOs) obtained from *C. longa* plants (McCarron, Mills, and Whittaker, 1995), we investigated the fragrances produced by fresh plants (Figure 6.2).

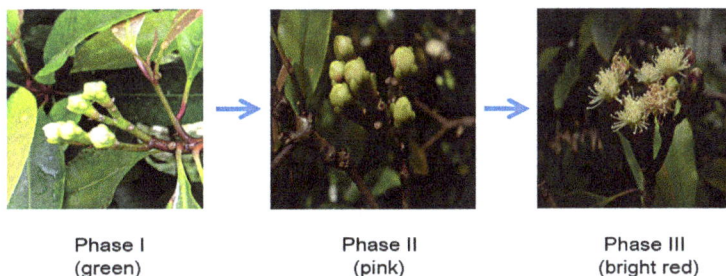

Phase I
(green)

Phase II
(pink)

Phase III
(bright red)

FIGURE 6.1   The flower buds of *S. aromaticum* are at first pale in color and gradually become green (phase I), then pink (phase II), and finally bright red (phase III).

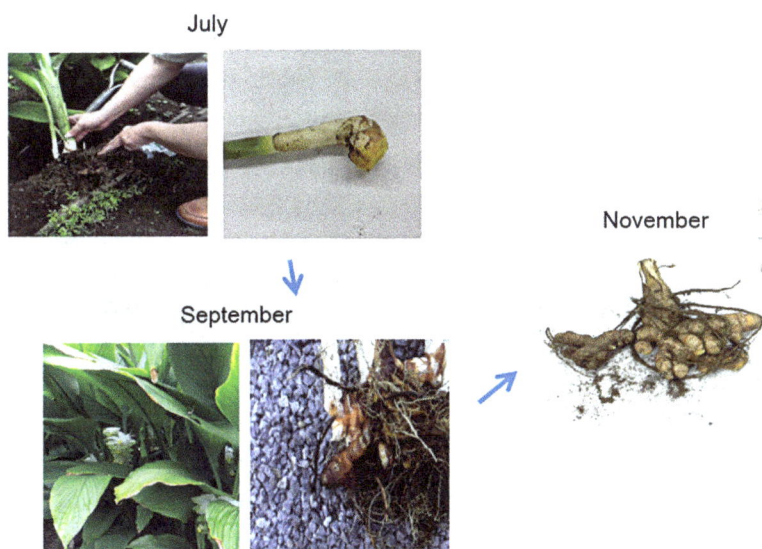

July

September

November

FIGURE 6.2   *C. longa* rhizomes at three different development stages, i.e., in July (young), September (flowering time), and November (harvest time).

Lavandula is a plant in the family Lamiaceae, and the dried flowers are familiar fragrant elements of potpourri, sachets, and pillows to promote relaxation. Lavender has been used not only in perfumery, cosmetics, food processing, and insect repellent but also in traditional medicine (TM), e.g., epilepsy, and migraine. Lavender essential oil is very popular and has been used for aromatherapy for effective relief of antianxiety, depression, and sleeplessness. The antimicrobial effect and antioxidant activity of lavender are also known (Lis-Balchin, 2011; Kunicka-Styczyńska, Śmigielski, and Prusinowska, 2015; Won, Cha, and Yoon, 2009; Adaszyńska, Swarcewicz, and Dzięcioł, 2013; Tomi, Fushiki, and Murakami, 2011; Yakuso Guide Book, 2006; Gülçin, Şat, and Beydemir, 2004).

Although the medicinal plant garden of Hoshi University contains several lavender species, we analyzed volatile components obtained from both true lavenders, i.e., *Lavandula angustifolia* Miller Hidcote (*LA*) and lavandin, i.e., *L. x intermedia* Emeric ex Loiseleur Grosso (*LX*) (Lis-Balchin, 2004). At different developmental stages (summer, autumn, and winter) sampling of the *LA* and *LX* flowers and herbs was performed, and the volatile compounds from fresh and dried herbs were also compared (Kasai and Kubota, 2018) (Figure 6.3).

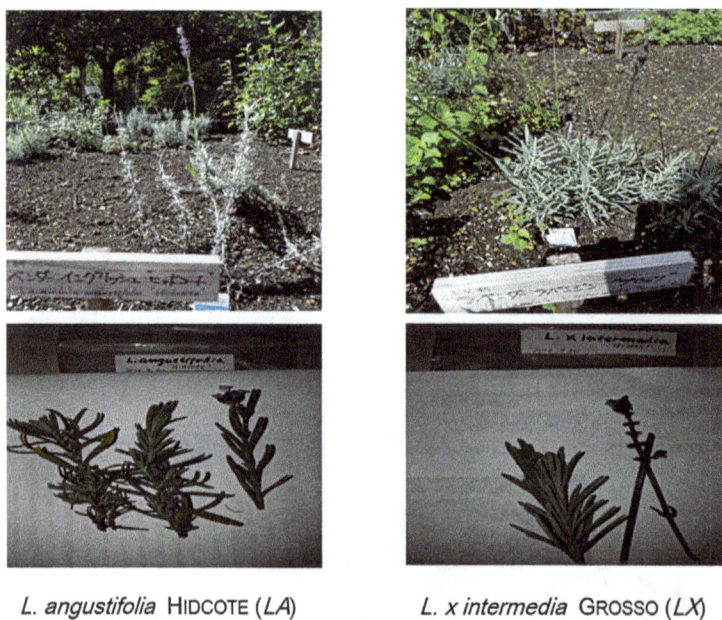

L. angustifolia HIDCOTE (*LA*)   L. x intermedia GROSSO (*LX*)

FIGURE 6.3   *L. angustifolia* Hidcote (*LA*) and *L. x intermedia* Grosso (*LX*).

Reactive oxygen species (ROS), e.g., the superoxide anion radical ($O_2^{\cdot-}$), hydrogen peroxide, and hydroxyl radical ($\cdot OH$), are known to be harmful to surrounding tissues and may affect sickness and aging. As eliminating ROS is one of the most effective defenses against oxidative stress, several antioxidants (Gülçin, Şat, and Beydemir, 2004; Kramer, 1985) and various assays (Politeo, Jukic, and Milos, 2010; Lee and Shibamoto, 2001) were reported.

The antioxidant activity of clove and turmeric in the medicinal plant garden was investigated using the electron spin resonance (ESR) spin-trapping method (Kasai, Ishii, and Yaoita, 2017; Kasai and Kubota, 2018).

6.2 TD-GC-MS METHOD

Sampling of the volatile compounds originating from each plant was performed using two kinds of adsorption devices, i.e., a solid-phase microextraction (SPME) fiber and a bar coated with polydimethylsiloxane (PDMS) (Ochiai, Tsunokawa, and Sasamoto, 2014; Ochiai, Sasamoto, and Ieda, 2013). The harvested plant material was cut into small pieces and then headspace sorptive extraction was carried out in a 40-mL vial equipped with a clean pinhole septum fixed with adsorption device. The TD-GC-MS procedure was immediately performed (see the Methodology in Kasai, Shirao, and Ikegami-Kawai, 2016; Kasai, Ishii, and Yaoita, 2017).

In order to identify compounds their retention indices (RIs) (Aroma Office 2D. Version 3.00.01, 2014) and their mass spectra were compared with those in the National Institute of Standards and Technology library (NIST) (Gaithersburg, MD, USA). When authentic standard was available, further confirmation was performed.

6.3 ESR SPIN-TRAPPING METHOD

ESR spectrometry was carried out using JES-RE1X ESR spectrometer (JEOL, Tokyo, Japan). $O_2^{\cdot-}$ was generated from the hypoxanthine (HPX)-xanthine oxidase (XOD) reaction and then was trapped by 5,5-dimethyl-1-pyrroline-N-oxide (DMPO) as a spin-trapping agent, and was added to the reaction system (see methodology in Kasai, Shirao, and Ikegami-Kawai, 2016; Kasai, Ishii, and Yaoita, 2017). When a plant extract exhibited anti-oxidant activity, decrease in the ESR signal intensity of DMPO-OO$^-$ was observed. The signal intensity was normalized using the manganese oxide marker.

6.4   VOLATILE COMPONENTS

6.4.1   *SYZYGIUM AROMATICUM* (CLOVE)

6.4.1.1   PLANT MATERIAL

Clove buds and leaves were harvested from the plant cultivated in the medicinal garden, and volatile compounds were adsorbed to a bar or to a SPME fiber coated with PDMS as a device.

6.4.1.2   BUDS AND LEAVES IN DIFFERENT GROWTH PHASES

The volatile compounds were adsorbed to the bar for 60 min and then TD-GC-MS procedure was performed. The number of volatile compounds originating from clove buds was influenced by growth phases. In phase III (bright red) it was greater compared with that in phase II (pink) as shown in Table 6.1. Although β-caryophyllene, eugenol, eugenol acetate, α-farnesene, α-humulene, and γ-murolene were identified in all growth phases, α-copaene, ethyl hexanoate, methyl salicylate, 2-nonanone, and β-ocimene were newly present in phase II and phase III. In phase III acetophenone, ethyl benzoate, ethyl octanoate, and methyl benzoate, were identified. It is assumed that characteristic fragrance originating from ripened buds is influenced from the increased compounds. From clove leaves 3-hexen-1-ol and hexyl acetate were identified as compounds characteristic of leaves (Table 6.1).

TABLE 6.1   Volatile Components of *S. aromaticum* in Different Growth Phases Identified by TD-GC-MS Using PDMS-Coated Bars (Kasai, Shirao, and Ikegami-Kawai, 2016)

Component[a]	RI[b]	RI lit[c]	Bud			Leaf	ID[e]
			Phase I	Phase II	Phase III		
3-Hexen-1-ol	[d]	–	–	–	–	–	MS, Std
Ethyl hexanoate	1000	1000	–	○	○	–	MS, RI, Std
3-Hexen-1-yl acetate	1004	1004	–	○	–	○	MS, RI, Std
Hexyl acetate	1017	1017	–	–	–	○	MS, RI, Std

TABLE 6.1   *(Continued)*

Component[a]	RI[b]	RI lit[c]	Bud			Leaf	ID[e]
			Phase I	Phase II	Phase III		
Benzyl alcohol	1031	1031	–	○	–	–	MS, RI, Std
β-Ocimene	1053	1051	–	○	○	–	MS, RI, Std
Acetophenone	1072	1071	–	–	○	–	MS, RI, Std
2-Nonanone	1098	1093	–	○	○	–	MS, RI, Std
Methyl benzoate	1100	1102	–	–	○	–	MS, RI, Std
Ethyl benzoate	1172	1168	–	–	○	–	MS, RI, Std
Methyl salicylate	1196	1193	–	○	○	–	MS, RI, Std
Ethyl octanoate	1201	1200	–	–	○	–	MS, RI
Eugenol	1373	1373	○	○	○	○	MS, RI, Std
α-Copaene	1379	1379	–	○	○	–	MS, RI, Std
β-Caryophyllene	1424	1423	○	○	○	○	MS, RI, Std
α-Humulene	1456	1456	○	○	○	○	MS, RI, Std
γ-Muurolene	1487	1490	○	○	○	–	MS, RI
α-Farnesene	1503	1502	○	○	○	–	MS, RI, Std
Eugenol acetate	1526	1512	○	○	○	–	MS, Std

[a]Compounds are listed in order of their elution from a DB-5 column.

[b]Linear retention index on DB-5 column, experimentally determined using homologous series of C_9-C_{33} *n*-alkanes.

[c]Relative retention index taken from previously analyzed compounds in Aroma Office database.[20]

[d]Retention time is outside of retention times of homologous series of C_9-C_{33} *n*-alkanes.

[e]Identification methods: MS, by comparing their mass spectra with those in the NIST library; RI, by comparing RIs with those reported in the literature recorded in Aroma Office database; Std, by comparing retention time and mass spectrum with those available authentic standard.

Note: ○: identified; –: not identified.

6.4.1.3   *FRAGRANCE OF LIVING CLOVE BUDS STILL ON THE BRANCH*

The volatile compounds originating from living clove buds still on the branch were analyzed. Adsorption was performed using a PDMS-coated SPME fiber for 3 h. As shown in Table 6.2, an increase in the number of volatile compounds was observed upon ripening as mentioned before.

Although α-humulene was not detected in growth phase I (green), it was detected upon ripening, i.e., in phase II (pink) and in phase III (bright red). And benzyl alcohol was detected in phase III.

TABLE 6.2 Volatile Components of *S. aromaticum* in Different Growth Phases Identified by GC-MS Using PDMS Fibers (Kasai, Shirao, and Ikegami-Kawai, 2016)

Component[a]	Bud			ID[b]
	Phase I	**Phase II**	**Phase III**	
β-Ocimene	○	○	○	MS, Std
α-Copaene	○	○	○	MS, Std
β-Caryophyllene	○	○	○	MS, Std
Methyl benzoate	○	○	○	MS, Std
α-Humulene	–	○	○	MS, Std
α-Farnesene	○	○	○	MS, Std
Methyl salicylate	○	○	○	MS, Std
Benzyl alcohol	–	–	○	MS, Std
Eugenol	○	○	○	MS, Std
Eugenol acetate	○	○	○	MS, Std

[a]Compounds are listed in order of their elution from an inert cap pure WAX column.

[b]Identification methods: MS, by comparing their mass spectra with those in the NIST library; Std., by comparing retention time and mass spectrum with those of available authentic standard.

Note: ○: identified; –: not identified.

6.4.2 CURCUMA LONGA (TURMERIC)

6.4.2.1 PLANT MATERIAL

C. longa obtained from a domestic market in Japan was cultivated in the medicinal plant garden. The rhizomes, roots, and leaves collected from the plants were cleaned, washed, and cut into small pieces. Adsorption was carried out using three SPME fibers, i.e., PDMS, PDMS/carboxene (CAR), and PDMS/CAR/divinylbenzene (DVB). As a device the PDMS-coated bar was also used.

6.4.2.2 LEAVES AND RHIZOMES IN DIFFERENT GROWTH PHASES

Odor compositions were adsorbed using the PDMS-coated bar as a device. The volatile compounds at different developmental stages are shown in Table 6.3. Although β-caryophyllene, 1,8-cineol, ar-curcumene, and α-terpinolene, were the predominant constituents in most cases, changes in volatile components with development stages were observed. ar-Turmerone was found in ripened rhizomes and it possesses antifungal, mosquitocidal, and anticancer activities (Dhingra, Jham, and Barcelos, 2007; Roth, Chandra, and Nair, 1998; Orellana-Paucar, Afrikanova, and De Witte, 2013; Oh, Baik, and Jung, 1992). From older rhizomes which had been harvested the previous November, additional compounds, i.e., β-bisabolene, β-elemene, and β-myrcene, were identified. Storage in soil over winter was assumed to be effective for producing additional compounds. 3-Hexen-1-ol was found as a characteristic compound from fresh leaves (Table 6.3).

TABLE 6.3 Volatile Components of *C. longa* Rhizomes and Leaves Identified by TD-GC-MS Using PDMS-Coated Bars (Kasai, Ishii, and Yaoita, 2017)

Compound[a]	RI[b]	RI lit[c]	Leaf	Rhizome July	Rhizome September	Rhizome November	ID[e]
3-hexen-1-ol	*d*	–	○	–	–	–	MS, Std
β-Myrcene	982	982	–	–	○	–	MS, RI, Std
1,8-Cineole	1026	1026	○	○	○	○	MS, RI, Std
a-Terpinolene	1085	1085	○	○	○	○	MS, RI, Std
β-Elemene	1390	1390	○	○	○	–	MS, RI
β-Caryophyllene	1420	1420	○	○	○	○	MS, RI, Std
ar-Curcumene-	1482	1482	○	○	○	○	MS, RI
β-Bisabolene	1508	1508	–	–	○	–	MS, RI
ar-Turmerone	1663	1664	–	–	○	○	MS, RI

[a]Compounds are listed in order of their elution from a DB-5 column.
[b]RI on DB-5 column, experimentally determined using homologous series of C_9-C_{33} *n*-alkanes.
[c]RI taken from previously analyzed compounds in Aroma Office data base, 2014.
[d]Retention time is outside of retention times of homologous series of C_9-C_{33} *n*-alkanes.
[e]Identification methods: MS, by comparing their mass spectra with those in the NIST library; RI, by comparing RIs with those reported in the literature recorded in Aroma Office database; Std, by comparing retention time and mass spectrum with those available authentic standard.

Note: ○: identified; –: not identified.

6.4.2.3   EFFECTS OF SPME FIBER SPECIES

The effectiveness of SPME fiber species was investigated. As adsorption devices PDMS-coated, PDMS/CAR-coated, and PDMS/CAR/DVB-coated fibers were used. When the CAR- and DVB-coated devices were used, additional volatile compounds were detected. p-Cymene, β-myrcene, α-terpinene. ar-Turmerone was detected additionally when the PDMS/CAR/DVB-coated fiber was used. They were not detected when the PDMS-coated fiber was used (Table 6.4).

TABLE 6.4   Effects of Material Used to Coat SPME Fibers on the Detection of Volatile Components Originating from *C. longa* Rhizomes Harvested in November (Kasai, Ishii, and Yaoita, 2017)

Compound	RI	RI lit	SPME Fiber			ID
			PDMS	PDMS/ CAR	PDMS/ CAR/DVB	
β-Myrcene	992	992	–	–	○	MS, RI, Std
α-Terpinene	1016	1016	–	–	○	MS, RI, Std
p-Cymene	1024	1024	–	○	○	MS, RI, Std
1,8-Cineole	1031	1031	○	○	○	MS, RI, Std
α-Terpinolene	1091	1091	○	○	○	MS, RI, Std
β-Elemene	1395	1394	○	○	○	MS, RI
β-Caryophyllene	1424	1423	○	○	○	MS, RI, Std
E-β-Farnesene	1458	1458	○	○	○	MS, RI, Std
ar-Curcumene	1485	1485	○	○	○	MS, RI
β-Bisabolene	1512	1512	○	○	○	MS, RI
β-Seesquiphellandrene	1529	1531	○	–	○	MS, RI
ar-Turmerone	1663	1664	–	–	○	MS, RI

6.4.3   LAVANDULA (LAVENDER)

6.4.3.1   PLANT MATERIAL

In the medicinal garden, the flowers and herbs of *LA* and *LX* were collected. Adsorption of volatile compounds was performed at 26°C for 60 min using the PDMS/CAR-coated SPME fiber.

6.4.3.2   FLOWERS AND HERBS IN DIFFERENT GROWTH PHASES

6.4.3.2.1   Flowers

Odor components of *LA* and *LX* flowers in summer and autumn were identified by TD-GC-MS using PDMS/CAR-coated fiber. Linalool, terpinen-4-ol, β-caryophyllene, β-myrcene, β-ocimene, and α-ocimene were predominant components of *LA* and *LX* in both summer and autumn. α-Humulene was obtained from *LA*, and eucalyptol, camphor, borneol, and γ-cadinene were detected from *LX*. Limonene, cryptone, and bornyl acetate were obtained from *LA* in summer; hexyl acetate and α-terpinolen were obtained from *LX* in summer; and α-terpineol was obtained from *LX* in autumn. Lavandulyl acetate and *trans*-α-bergamotene were obtained in summer from both *LA* and *LX* (Table 6.5).

TABLE 6.5   Volatile Components of *LA* and *LX* Flowers in Summer and Autumn Identified by TD-GC-MS Using PDMS/CAR-Coated SPME Fibers (Kasai and Kubota, 2018)

Component[a]	RI[b]	RI[lite]	LA Summer	LA Autumn	LX Summer	LX Autumn	ID[d]
β-Myrcene	990	992	○	○	○	○	MS, RI
Hexyl acetate	1015	1015	–	–	○	–	MS, RI
p-Cymene	1023	1024	○	○	–	○	MS, RI, Std
Limonene	1029	1029	○	–	–	–	MS, RI, Std
Eucalyptol	1030	1030	–	–	○	○	MS, RI
β-Ocimene	1038	1038	○	○	○	○	MS, RI
α-Ocimene	1049	1049	○	○	○	○	MS, RI
trans-Sabinenehydrate	1066	1066	–	–	○	○	MS, RI
α-Terpinolene	1089	1089	–	–	○	–	MS, RI, Std
Linalool	1100	1100	○	○	○	○	MS, RI
allo-Ocimene	1129	1127	○	○	○	–	MS, RI
Camphor	1145	1145	–	–	○	○	MS, RI, Std
Borneol	1166	1166	–	–	○	○	MS, RI, Std

TABLE 6.5   *(Continued)*

Component[a]	RI[b]	RI[litc]	*LA* Summer	*LA* Autumn	*LX* Summer	*LX* Autumn	ID[d]
Terpinen-4-ol	1177	1177	○	○	○	○	MS, RI, Std
Cryptone	1184	1184	○	-	–	–	MS, RI
α-Terpineol	1190	1191	–	–	–	○	MS, RI, Std
Linalyl acetate	1257	1257	○	○	○	–	MS, RI, Std
Bornyl acetate	1290	1290	○	–	–	–	MS, RI
Lavandulyl acetate	1296	–	○	–	○	–	MS
α-Humulene	1382	1382	○	○	–	–	MS, RI
β-Caryophyllene	1424	1425	○	○	○	○	MS, RI, Std
trans-α-Bergamotene	1440	1439	○	–	○	–	MS, RI
β-Farnesene	1458	1458	–	○	–	○	MS, RI
ar-Curcumene	1485	1485	–	○	–	○	MS, RI
γ-Cadinene	1520	1520	–	–	○	○	MS, RI

[a]Components are listed in order of their elution from a DB-5 column;

[b]RI on DB-5 column;

[c]RI taken from previously analyzed compounds in Aroma office database;

[d]Identification methods: MS, by comparing the MS with that in the NIST library; RI, by comparing RI with that reported in the literature recorded in Aroma Office database; Std, by comparing time and MS with those of available authentic standard.

Note: ○: identified; –: not identified.

6.4.3.2.2   Herbs

The odor components of *LA* and *LX* herbs in summer, autumn, and winter identified by TD-GC-MS using PDMS/CAR-coated fiber are shown in Table 6.6. Borneol and camphor were identified from both *LA* and *LX* in all three seasons. β-Caryophyllene in summer and autumn, limonene, and β-myrcene in summer, and 3-carene and eucalyptol in autumn were obtained from both *LA* and *LX*. Linalool was obtained from *LA* herbs in summer and from *LX* herbs in autumn. 3-Hexen-1-ol, *p*-cymene, β-ocimene, *trans*-sabinene hydrate, linalool, *p*-cymen-8-ol, and γ-cadinene were identified from both *LA* and *LX* (Table 6.6).

6.4.3.3   EFFECTS OF OTHER FACTORS

6.4.3.3.1   Cultivar Type

Linalyl acetate, cryptone, verbenone, cumin aldehyde, carvone, *trans*-α-bergamotene, and aromadendrene were obtained from *LA* alone, and α-phellandrene, α-terpinolene, α-terpineol, lavandulyl acetate, α-gurjunene, α-farnesene, ar-curcumene, and *trans*-calamenene were obtained from *LX* alone.

6.4.3.3.2   Season

Verbenone, linalyl acetate, and aromadendrene were obtained from *LA* in summer alone, and lavandulyl acetate was detected from *LX*. In autumn alone, α-phellandrene, α-terpinolene, α-gurjunene, β-farmasene, and ar-curcumene were identified. Compound obtained in winter alone was not existent.

6.4.3.3.3   Plant Parts

In both *LA* and *LX* species α- and allo-ocimene, and terpinen-4-ol were detected from flowers, and 3-hexen-1-ol, 3-carene, and *p*-cymen-8-ol were obtained from herbs. These are characteristic components specific to plant parts.

Characteristic volatile components were obtained not only from flowers but also from herbs, and they were affected by cultivar type, plant part, and growth season. Camphor, which activates sympathetic nerves, was identified from *LX* flowers in the plant garden. In both species, the number of volatile components from flowers in summer was greater than that in autumn. In summer, plants produce more volatile components to attract the insects essential for pollination. The number of volatile compounds originating from herbs varies with the growth season, with the fewest produced in winter.

TABLE 6.6 Volatile Components of *LA* and *LX* Herbs in Summer, Autumn, and Winter Identified by TD-GC-MS Using PDMS/CAR-Coated SPME Fibers (Kasai and Kubota, 2018)

Component	RI	RI^{lit}	LA Summer	LA Autumn	LA Winter	LX Summer	LX Autumn	LX Winter	ID
3-Hexen-1-ol	–	–	○	○	–	○	–	–	MS
β-Myrcene	990	992	○	–	–	○	○	–	MS, RI
α-Phellandrene	1003	1004	–	–	–	–	○	–	MS, RI
3-Carene	1009	1009	–	○	–	–	○	–	MS, RI, Std
p-Cymene	1023	1024	○	○	○	–	○	○	MS, RI, Std
Limonene	1029	1029	○	–	–	○	–	–	MS, RI, Std
Eucalyptol	1030	1030	○	○	–	–	○	○	MS, RI
β-Ocimene	1038	1038	○	–	–	–	○	–	MS, RI
trans-Sabinenehydrate	1066	1066	○	–	–	–	○	–	MS, RI
α-Terpinolene	1089	1089	–	–	–	–	○	–	MS, RI
Linalool	1100	1100	○	–	–	–	○	–	MS, RI
Camphor	1145	1145	○	○	○	○	○	○	MS, RI, Std
Borneol	1166	1166	○	○	○	○	○	○	MS, RI, Std
p-Cymen-8-ol	1181	1181	–	○	–	–	–	○	MS, RI
Cryptone	1184	1184	○	–	○	–	–	–	MS, RI
α-Terpineol	1190	1191	–	–	–	○	○	–	MS, RI
Verbenone	1222	1221	○	–	–	–	–	–	MS, RI
Cumin aldehyde	1238	1239	○	–	○	–	–	–	MS, RI
Carvone	1242	1242	○	–	○	–	–	–	MS, RI
Linalyl acetate	1257	1257	○	–	–	–	–	–	MS, RI, Std

TABLE 6.6 *(Continued)*

Component	RI	RI^{lit}	LA Summer	LA Autumn	LA Winter	LX Summer	LX Autumn	LX Winter	ID
Lavandulyl acetate	1296	–	–	–	–	○	–	–	MS
α-Gurjunene	1414	1413	–	–	–	–	○	–	MS, RI
β-Caryophyllene	1424	1425	○	○	–	○	○	–	MS, RI, Std
trans-α-Bergamotene	1440	1439	○	–	–	–	–	–	MS, RI
Aromadendrene	1449	1449	○	–	–	–	–	–	MS, RI
β-Farnesene	1458	1458	–	–	–	–	○	–	MS, RI
Ar-Curcumene	1485	1485	–	–	–	–	○	–	MS, RI
γ-Cadinene	1520	1520	–	–	–	–	○	–	MS, RI
trans-Calamenene	1528	1529	–	–	–	○	○	–	MS, RI

6.4.3.4   *DIFFERENCES BETWEEN DRIED AND FRESH LAVENDER*

The differences between the odors of dried lavender and fresh lavender were compared. Volatile compounds originating from the fresh plants that people who visit the garden can easily smell were compared with those of dried herbs. The volatile components from fresh *LA* and *LX* herbs in summer and autumn were compared with those from dried ones.

6.4.3.4.1   **Dried Plant Materials**

LA and *LX* herbs (0.1 g) were harvested in summer and autumn and then dried at 26°C for 1 month. Extraction of volatile compounds was carried out at 26°C for 60 min.

6.4.3.4.2   **LA Herbs**

As shown in Table 6.7, the 12 components: 3-hexen-1-ol, β-ocimene, *trans*-sabinene hydrate, linalool, camphor, borneol, cryptone, verbenone, linalyl acetate, β-caryophyllene, *trans*-α-bergamotene, and aromadendrene, present in fresh herbs in summer and the five components: 3-carene, camphor, borneol, *p*-cymen-8-ol, and β-caryophyllene, present in fresh herbs in autumn were not found in dried herbs. Camphor, borneol, and β-caryophyllene were not detected in dried herbs in both seasons (Table 6.7).

TABLE 6.7   Comparison of Volatile Components of Dried *LA* Herbs with Those of Fresh *LA* Herbs in Summer and Autumn Identified by TD-GC-MS Using PDMS/CAR-Coated SPME Fibers (Kasai and Kubota, 2018)

Component	RI	RI[lite]	Summer Fresh	Autumn Fresh	Summer Dried	Autumn Dried	ID
3-Hexen-1-ol	–	–	○	○	–	○	MS
β-Myrcene	990	992	○	–	○	○	MS, RI
α-Phellandrene	1003	1004	–	–	–	–	MS, RI
3-Carene	1009	1009	–	○	–	–	MS, RI, Std
p-Cymene	1023	1024	○	○	○	○	MS, RI, Std
Limonene	1029	1029	○	–	○	–	MS, RI, Std
Eucalyptol	1030	1030	–	○	–	○	MS, RI
β-Ocimene	1038	1038	○	–	–	–	MS, RI

TABLE 6.7 *(Continued)*

Component	RI	RI[lite]	Summer Fresh	Autumn Fresh	Summer Dried	Autumn Dried	ID
trans-Sabinenehydrate	1066	1066	○	–	–	–	MS, RI
α-Terpinolene	1089	1089	–	–	–	○	MS, RI
Linalool	1100	1100	○	–	–	–	MS, RI
Camphor	1145	1145	○	○	–	–	MS, RI, Std
Borneol	1166	1166	○	○	–	–	MS, RI, Std
p-Cymen-8-ol	1181	1181	–	○	–	–	MS, RI
Cryptone	1184	1184	○	–	–	–	MS, RI
α-Terpineol	1190	1191	–	–	–	–	MS, RI, Std
Verbenone	1222	1221	○	–	–	–	MS, RI
Cumin aldehyde	1238	1239	○	–	○	–	MS, RI
Carvone	1242	1242	○	–	○	–	MS, RI
Linalyl acetate	1257	1257	○	–	–	–	MS, RI, Std
Lavandulyl acetate	1296	–	–	–	–	–	MS
α-Gurjunene	1414	1413	–	–	–	–	MS, RI
β-Caryophyllene	1424	1425	○	○	–	–	MS, RI, Std
trans-α-Bergamotene	1440	1439	○	–	–	–	MS, RI
Coumarin	1432	1432	–	–	○	–	MS, RI
Aromadendrene	1449	1449	○	–	–	–	MS, RI
β-Farnesene	1458	1458	–	–	–	–	MS, RI
Ar-Curcumene	1485	1485	–	–	–	○	MS, RI
γ-Cadinene	1520	1520	○	–	○	–	MS, RI
trans-Calamenene	1528	1529	–	–	–	–	MS, RI

6.4.3.4.3 LX Herbs

As presented in Table 6.8, in summer the seven components: 3-hexen-1-ol, camphor, borneol, α-terpineol, lavandulyl acetate, β-caryophyllene, and trans-calamenene, and in autumn the nine components: α-phellandrene, 3-carene, β-ocimene, *trans*-sabinene hydrate, camphor, α-terpineol, α-gurjunene, β-caryophyllene, and β-farnesene, were not detected in dried herbs. Camphor, β-caryophyllene, and β-ocimene were absent in herbs dried for 1 month. β-Myrcene was still present after drying (Table 6.8).

TABLE 6.8 Comparison of Volatile Components of Dried *LX* Herbs with Those of Fresh *LX* Herbs in Summer and Autumn Identified by TD-GC-MS Using PDMS/CAR-Coated SPME Fibers (Kasai and Kubota, 2018)

Component	RI	RI[lite]	Summer Fresh	Autumn Fresh	Summer Dried	Autumn Dried	ID
3-Hexen-1-ol	–	–	○	–	–	○	MS
β-Myrcene	990	992	○	○	○	○	MS, RI
α-Phellandrene	1003	1004	–	○	–	–	MS, RI
3-Carene	1009	1009	–	○	–	–	MS, RI, Std
p-Cymene	1023	1024	–	○	○	○	MS, RI, Std
Limonene	1029	1029	○	–	○	–	MS, RI, Std
Eucalyptol	1030	1030	–	○	–	○	MS, RI
β-Ocimene	1038	1038	–	○	–	–	MS, RI
trans-Sabinenehydrate	1066	1066	–	○	–	–	MS, RI
α-Terpinolene	1089	1089	–	○	–	○	MS, RI
Linalool	1100	1100	–	○	–	○	MS, RI
Camphor	1145	1145	○	○	–	–	MS, RI, Std
Borneol	1166	1166	○	○	–	○	MS, RI, Std
p-Cymen-8-ol	1182	1181	–	–	–	–	MS, RI
Cryptone	1184	1184	–	–	–	–	MS, RI
α-Terpineol	1190	1191	○	○	–	–	MS, RI, Std
Verbenone	1222	1221	–	–	–	–	MS, RI
Cumin aldehyde	1238	1239	–	–	–	–	MS, RI
Carvone	1242	1242	–	–	–	–	MS, RI
Linalyl acetate	1257	1257	–	–	–	–	MS, RI, Std
Lavandulyl acetate	1296	–	○	–	–	–	MS
α-Gurjunene	1414	1413	–	○	–	–	MS, RI

TABLE 6.8 *(Continued)*

Component	RI	RI^lite	Summer Fresh	Autumn Fresh	Summer Dried	Autumn Dried	ID
β-Caryophyllene	1424	1425	○	○	–	–	MS, RI, Std
trans-α-Bergamotene	1440	1439	–	–	–	–	MS, RI
Coumarin	1432	1432	–	–	○	–	MS, RI
Aromadendrene	1449	1449	–	–	–	–	MS, RI
β-Farnesene	1458	1458	–	○	–	–	MS, RI
Ar-Curcumene	1485	1485	–	○	–	○	MS, RI
γ-Cadinene	1520	1520	–	○	–	○	MS, RI
trans-Calamenene	1528	1529	○	○	–	○	MS, RI

6.5 ANTIOXIDANT ACTIVITY

6.5.1 *SYZYGIUM AROMATICUM* (CLOVE)

6.5.1.1 *SAMPLE PREPARATION*

Each extract from 0.2 g of clove buds or leaves was prepared prior to ESR analyzes. Either 1 mL of sodium phosphate buffer water solution (PB; pH 7.8) or 1 mL of methanol (MeOH) was used as solution (see the Methodology in Kasai, Shirao, and Ikegami-Kawai, 2016).

6.5.1.2 *SUPEROXIDE DISMUTASE (SOD) AS A STANDARD*

In order to compare the superoxide scavenging activity (SOSA) of each extract the superoxide dismutase (SOD) equivalent (U/mg) of extract was calculated using SOD as a standard (Al-Mamun, Yamaki, and Masumizu, 2007; Saito, Kohno, and Yoshizaki, 2008; Mitsuta, Mizuta, and Kohno, 1990).

The relative inhibitory effect on DMPO-OO⁻ formation and various concentrations of SOD is shown in Figure 6.4. The median inhibitory concentration (IC_{50}) values of SOD were calculated graphically (Figure 6.4).

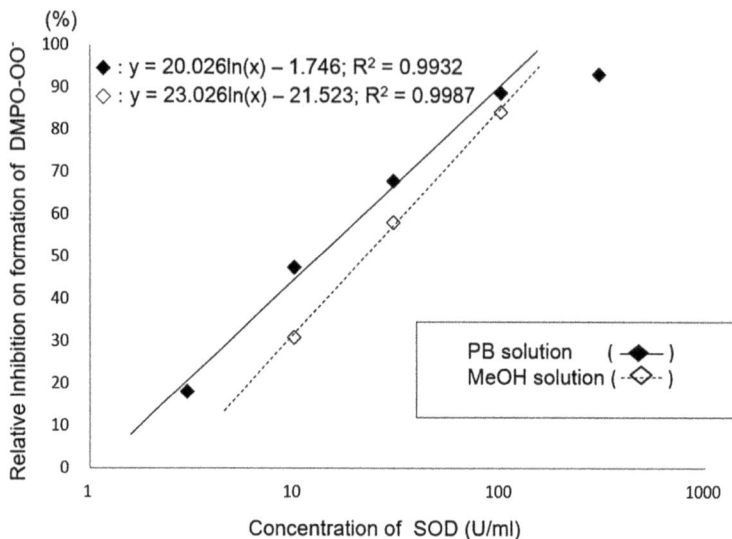

FIGURE 6.4 Relationship between the concentration of standard SOD and the relative inhibition of the formation on DMPO-OO⁻.

6.5.1.3 EFFECTS OF PLANT PARTS: BUD VS. LEAF

Each extract from clove buds and leaves functioned as an $O_2^{·-}$ scavenger. As shown in ESR spectra in Figure 6.5(a) reduction in the signal intensity was observed when the extract was added to the HPX-XOD reaction system. The reduction was dependent upon the increase in the concentration of extract (Figure 6.5).

The relative inhibition of the formation of DMPO-OO⁻ increased with the increasing concentration of clove extracts from both buds and leaves as shown in Figure 6.6.

6.5.1.4 EFFECTS OF EXTRACT SOLUTION: WATER VS. METHANOL

Effect of extract solution, i.e., PB, and MeOH, were investigated. Clove buds and leaves were extracted using PB and MeOH, and the IC_{50} values and the antioxidant unit were compared. The IC_{50} values were obtained from the linearity between relative inhibitory effects and the logarithm of concentrations. As shown in Table 6.9 each antioxidant unit of the MeOH extracts from leaves and buds was higher than that of the PB extracts. Because the amount of total phenolic compounds exhibiting antioxidant activity, i.e., eugenol, eugenol acetate, and gallic acid (Lee and Shibamoto, 2001), in MeOH extract was greater than that in water extract, the antioxidant activity of the MeOH extract assumed to be greater than that of the PB extract (Table 6.9).

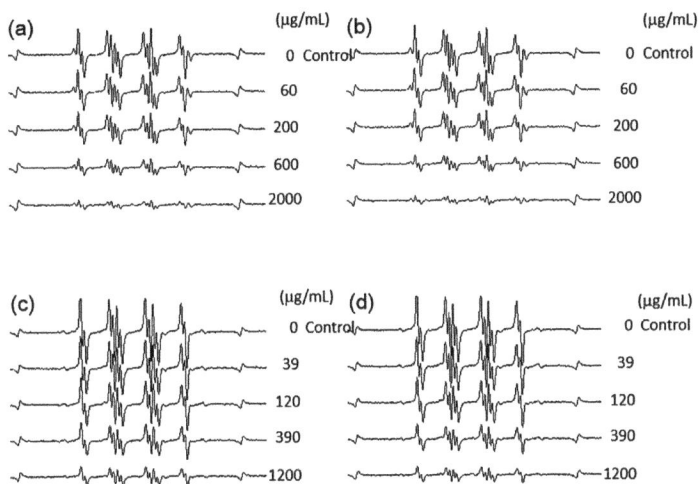

FIGURE 6.5 ESR spectra of DMPO-OO⁻ observed upon the addition of various concentrations of extract from clove buds and leaves. (a) PB extract from buds; (b) PB extract from leaves; (c) MeOH extract from buds; (d) MeOH extract from leaves.

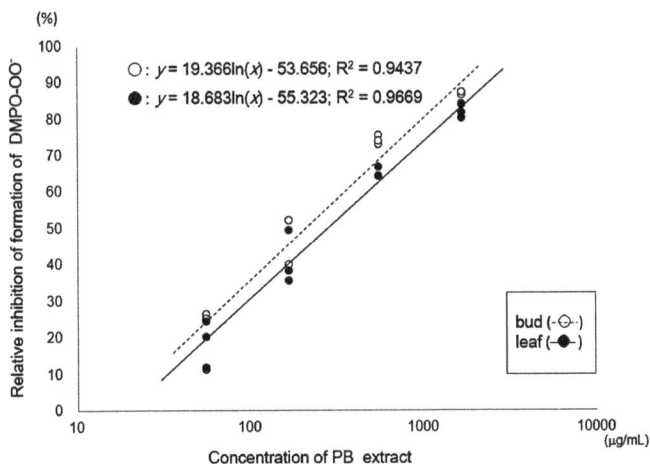

FIGURE 6.6 Inhibitory effects of various concentrations of PB extracts from clove buds and leaves on the formation of DMPO-OO⁻.

TABLE 6.9 IC_{50} Values and SOD Equivalent Values of *S. aromaticum* Extracts on Superoxide Anion Radical (O_2^{-})-Scavenging Activity (Kasai, Shirao, and Ikegami-Kawai, 2016)

	IC_{50} (µg/mL) of Extract	IC_{50} (U/mL) of SOD	Antioxidant Unit of Extract (U/mg)
PB extract of bud	211	12.8	60.7
PB extract of leaf	281	12.8	45.6
MeOH extract of bud	357	22.3	62.5
MeOH extract of leaf	250	22.3	89.2

6.5.2 *CURCUMA LONGA* (TURMERIC)

6.5.2.1 *SAMPLE PREPARATION*

Each extraction from 0.1 g of *C. longa* rhizomes was carried out using either 1 mL of PB or 1 mL of MeOH. Subsequent centrifugation gave a "supernatant of extract." Further filtration of a supernatant through a filter gave a "filtrated extract."

6.5.2.2 *COMPARISON OF SOSA OF THE SUPERNATANT OF PB EXTRACT AND FILTRATED PB EXTRACT*

The antioxidant activities of the "supernatant of PB extract" and the "filtrated PB extract" were evaluated. Both extracts exhibited antioxidant activity. The relative inhibitory effect on DMPO-OO⁻ formation increased with the increase of concentration of each PB extract, and the "supernatant of PB extract" tended to exhibit greater activity as shown in Figure 6.7. Suspension in the PB solution was assumed to exert effective antioxidant activity. From the linearity of graphs, the IC_{50} values of the "supernatant of PB extract" and the "filtrated PB extract" were 6.3 mg/mL and 8.2 mg/mL, respectively (Figure 6.7).

6.5.2.3 *EFFECTS OF HARVEST SEASON: JULY VS. NOVEMBER*

ESR spectra of DMPO-OO⁻ observed upon the addition of extracts from *C. longa* rhizomes were shown in Figure 6.8. As a reduction in the signal intensity dependent upon the increase in the concentration was observed, antioxidant activity of the extract was confirmed (Figure 6.8).

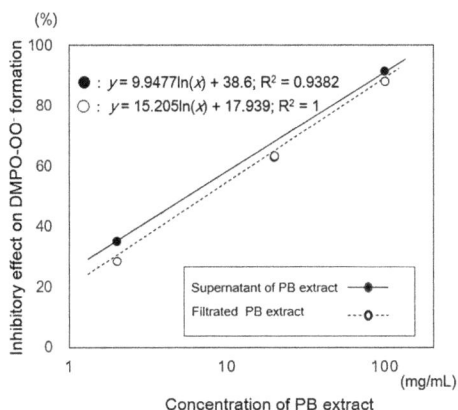

FIGURE 6.7 Inhibitory effects of various concentrations of supernatants of PB extracts and filtrated PB extracts from *C. longa* rhizomes on the formation of DMPO-OO⁻.

Relationship between the relative inhibitory effect on DMPO-OO⁻ formation and various concentrations of the PB extracts are shown in Figure 6.9. From each linearity the IC_{50} values were obtained (Figure 6.9).

MeOH extracts exhibited the same tendency. Every extract present antioxidant activity. The linearity was observed in each extract as shown in Figure 6.10. The IC_{50} values were obtained (Figure 6.10).

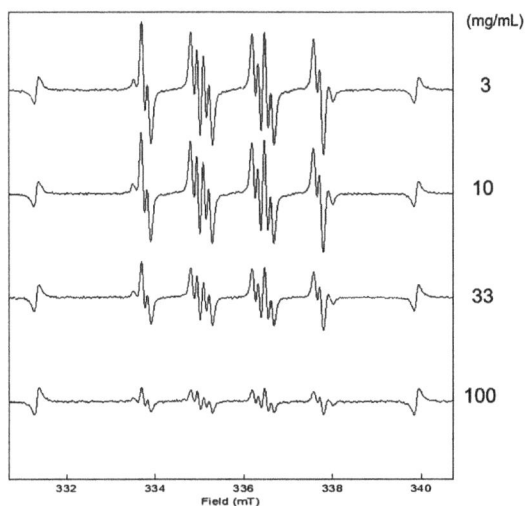

FIGURE 6.8 ESR spectra of DMPO-OO⁻ observed upon the addition of various concentrations of PB extracts from *C. longa* rhizomes harvested in November.

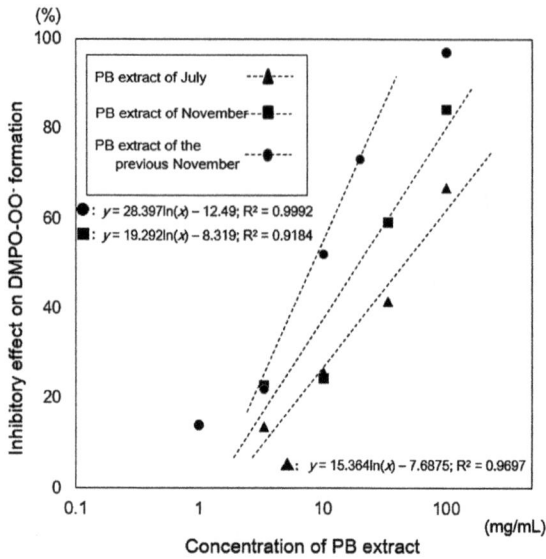

FIGURE 6.9 Inhibitory effects of various concentrations of PB extracts from *C. longa* rhizomes harvested in July, November, and the previous November on the formation of DMPO-OO⁻.

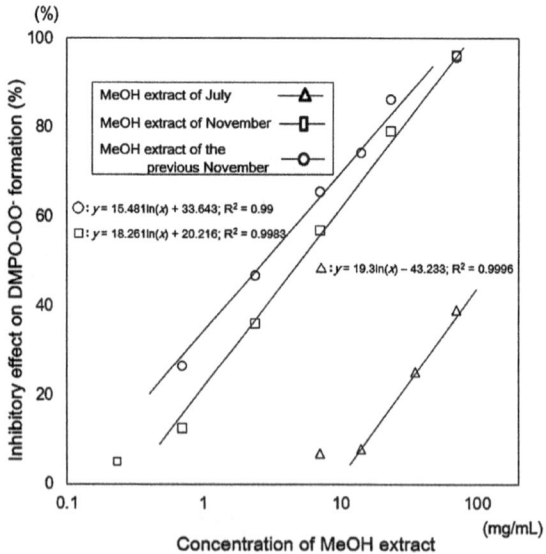

FIGURE 6.10 Inhibitory effects of various concentrations of MeOH extracts from *C. longa* rhizomes harvested in July, November, and the previous November on the formation of DMPO-OO⁻.

6.5.2.4   EFFECTS OF EXTRACT SOLUTION: WATER VS. METHANOL

The values of the IC_{50} and antioxidant unit of each sample obtained from Figures 6.9 and 6.10 are presented in Table 6.10.

In both PB and MeOH solution, order of antioxidant unit of the extracts exhibits the same tendency. The values of rhizomes harvested the previous November and then stored over the winter indicated the greatest activity. And the values of the current November were greater than those of July. During storage in soil over the winter, greater activity was assumed to be accumulated.

The antioxidant units of MeOH extracts were higher than those of the PB extracts because MeOH extracts contained higher levels of phenolic compounds such as tetrahydro curcuminoids (Table 6.10).

TABLE 6.10 IC_{50} Values and SOD Equivalent Values of *C. longa* Rhizome Extracts on Superoxide Anion Radical (O_2^{-})-Scavenging Activity (Kasai, Ishii, and Yaoita, 2017)

	IC_{50} of Extract (mg/mL)	IC_{50} of SOD (U/mL)	Antioxidant Unit of Extract (U/mg)
PB extract of July	42.7	16.7	0.39
PB extract of November	20.5	12.1	0.59
PB extract of the previous November	9.0	16.7	1.86
MeOH extract of July	125.3	19.2	0.15
MeOH extract of November	5.1	18.9	3.71
MeOH extract of the previous November	2.9	19.2	6.62

6.6   CONCLUSION

The volatile components and antioxidant activity of the plants cultivated in a medicinal plant garden located in Tokyo were investigated. Analyzes of volatile components originating from clove, turmeric, and lavender were carried out using TD-GC-MS, and qualitative differences in different growth phases were observed. Measurement of antioxidant activity of the plants was performed using ESR. The extracts from clove and turmeric exhibited effective antioxidant activity. Changes in volatile components and antioxidant activity as affected by the growth phase were identified. It is useful for profiling the medicinal plant garden and may contribute to knowledge of the therapeutic effects of the plants.

KEYWORDS

- antioxidant activity
- *Curcuma longa*
- electron spin-resonance
- *Lavandula*
- *Syzygium aromaticum*
- thermal desorption-GC-MS
- volatile component

REFERENCES

Adaszyńska, M., Swarcewicz, M., & Dzięcioł, M., (2013). Comparison of chemical composition and antibacterial activity of lavender varieties from Poland. *Nat. Prod. Res., 27*, 1497–1501.

Al-Mamun, M., Yamaki, K., & Masumizu, T., (2007). Superpxode anion radical scavenging activities of herbs and pastures in northern Japan determined using electron spin resonance spectrometry. *Int. J. Biol. Sci., 3*, 349–355.

Turmeric/crude drugs and related drugs, (2016). *The Japanese Pharmacopoeia* (17th edn., pp. 2005–2007). (JP17); Ministry of Health and Welfare of Japan: Tokyo. https://jpdb.nihs.go.jp/jp/index.aspx (accessed on 01 November 2021).

Aroma Office 2D. Version 3.00.01, (2014). Gerstel K.K.: Tokyo.

Clove/crude drugs and related drugs, (2016). *The Japanese Pharmacopoeia* (17th edn, pp. 1833–1834). Ministry of Health and Welfare of Japan: Tokyo.

Dhingra, O. D., Jham, G. N., & Barcelos, R. C., (2007). Isolation and identification of the principal fungitoxic component of turmeric essential oil. *J. Essent. Oil Res., 19*(4), 387–391.

Gülçin, İ., Şat, İ. G., & Beydemir, Ş., (2004). Comparison of antioxidant activity of clove (*Eugenia caryophylata* Thunb.) buds and lavender (*Lavandula stoechas* L.). *Food Chem., 87*, 393–400.

Kasai, H., & Kubota, Y., (2018). Analyses of volatile components of lavender (*Lavandula angustifolia* HIDCOTE and *Lavandula x intermedia* GROSSO) as influenced by cultivar type, part, and growth season. *Yakugaku Zasshi., 138*(12), 1569–1577.

Kasai, H., Ishii, H., & Yaoita, H., (2017). Analysis of volatile compounds of *Curcuma longa* (turmeric) and investigation of the antioxidant activity of rhizome extracts. *Med. Aromat. Plants, 6*(4), 302.

Kasai, H., Shirao, M., & Ikegami-Kawai, M., (2016). Analysis of volatile compounds of clove (*Syzygium aromaticum*) buds as influenced by growth phase and investigation of antioxidant activity of clove extracts. *Flavor Fragr. J., 31*(2), 178–184. doi: 10.1002/ffj.3299.

Kramer, R. E., (1985). Antioxidants in clove. *J. Am. Oil Chem. Soc., 62*(1), 111–113.

Kunicka-Styczyńska, A., Śmigielski, K., & Prusinowska, R., (2015). Preservative activity of lavender hydrosols in moisturizing body gels. *Lett. Appl. Microbio., 60*, 27–32.

Lee, K. G., & Shibamoto, T., (2001). Antioxidant property of aroma extract isolated from clove buds [*Syzygium aromaticum* (L.) Merr. et Perry]. *Food Chem., 74*, 443–448.

Letchamo, W., Ward, W., & Heard, B., (2004). Essential oil of *Valeriana officinalis* L. cultivars and their antimicrobial activity as influenced by harvesting time under commercial organic cultivation. *J. Agric. Food Chem., 52*, 3915–3919.

Lis-Balchin, M., (2004). In: *Lavender: The Genus Lavandula, History of Nomenclature of Lavandula Species, Hybrids and Cultivars* (pp. 51–56). Taylor & Francis, London.

Lis-Balchin, M., (2011). Aromatherapy science. *Fragrance Journal*. Tokyo.

McCarron, M., Mills, A. J., & Whittaker, D., (1995). Comparison of the monoterpenes derived from green leaves and fresh rhizomes of *Curcuma longa* L. from India. *Flavor Fragr. J., 10*, 355–357.

Mitsuta, K., Mizuta, Y., & Kohno, M., (1990). The application of ESR spin-trapping technique to the evaluation of SOD-like activity of biological substances. *Bull. Chem. Soc. Jpn., 63*, 187–191.

Ochiai, N., Sasamoto, K., & Ieda, T., (2013). Multi-stir bar sorptive extraction for analysis of odor compounds in aqueous samples. *J. Chromatogr. A, 1315*, 70–79.

Ochiai, N., Tsunokawa, J., & Sasamoto, K., (2014). Multi-volatile method for aroma analysis using sequential dynamic headspace sampling with an application to brewed coffee. *J. Chromatogr. A, 1371*, 65–73.

Oh, W. G., Baik, K. U., & Jung, S. H., (1992). The role of substituents of Ar-turmerone for its anticancer activity. *Arch. Pharm. Res., 15*, 256–262.

Orellana-Paucar, A. M., Afrikanova, T., & De Witte, P. A. M., (2013). Insights from zebrafish and mouse models on the activity and safety of Ar-turmerone as a potential drug candidate for the treatment of epilepsy. *PloS One, 8*, e81634.

Politeo, O., Jukic, M., & Milos, M., (2010). Comparison of chemical composition and antioxidant activity of glycosidically bound and free volatiles from clove (*Eugenia Caryophyllata* Thumb.). *J. Food Biochem., 34*, 129–141.

Roth, G. N., Chandra, A., & Nair, M. G., (1998). Novel bioactivities of *Curcuma longa* constituents. *J. Nat. Prod., 61*(4), 542–545.

Saito, K., Kohno, M., & Yoshizaki, F., (2008). Antioxidant properties of herbal extracts selected from screening for potent scavenging activity against superoxide anions. *J. Sci. Food Agric., 88*, 2707–2712.

Singh, G., Singh, O. P., & Maurya, S., (2002). Chemical and biocidal investigations on essential oils of some Indian *Curcuma* species. *Prog. Crystal Growth Charact, 45*, 75–81.

Tomi, K., Fushiki, T., & Murakami, H., (2011). Relationships between lavender aroma component and aromachology effect. *Acta Hortic., 925*, 299–306.

Won, M. M., Cha, E. J., & Yoon, O. K., (2009). Use of head-space mulberry paper bag micro solid-phase extraction for characterization of volatile aromas of essential oils from Bulgarian rose and Provence lavender. *Anal. Chim. Acta, 631*, 54–61.

Yakuso Guide Book, (2006). *YakusoenenoIzanai* (p. 20). Nihon ShokubutsuenKyokai Dai 4 bukai, Nihon Shokubutsuen Kyokai: Tokyo.

Yatagai, M., (2000). Tree aroma and its function of relaxation and rest. *Aroma Res., 1*(1), 2–7.

CHAPTER 7

ANTI-HYPERGLYCEMIC PROPERTY OF MEDICINAL PLANTS

KARANPREET SINGH BHATIA, ARPITA ROY, and
NAVNEETA BHARDAVAJ

Department of Biotechnology, Delhi Technological University,
Shahbad Daulatpur Village, Rohini, New Delhi – 110042, India,
E-mail: navneetab@dce.ac.in (N. Bhardavaj)

ABSTRACT

Hyperglycemia is one of the chronic diseases of metabolism which is procuring around 2.8% of the world's demography. It is up surging across every continent in the world. Treatment to prevent this disease is an important challenge for researchers. Conventional drugs for treatment of this disease improve insulin sensitivity. Increase production of insulin results in a decrease blood glucose level. However, they have additional side effects and not always provide satisfactory results. Herbal or medicinal plants are paramount source for potential lead candidates' discovery, which can play an utmost role in drug discovery and drug development projects. Plants are an alternative source to overcome this problem as they contain various phytocompounds which show protective effects against hyperglycemia. Using bioactive compounds may be one of the possible ways to control this disease. Due to the availability, low production cost and least undesirable adverse effects make medicinal plants as a potential candidate of anti-hyperglycemic agents. Consumption of plants phytocompounds possess an important approach to fight against hyperglycemia and yield promising outcomes. In this respect the present chapter provides the details of 54 plants which possess anti-hyperglycemic activity. Anti-hyperglycemic potential in medicinal plants is due to the presence of terpenoids, flavonoids, coumarins, polyphenols, and other constituents which results in abatement in blood glucose levels. Also, plants elicit a more potent response in amelioration of hyperglycemia as compared to synthetic drugs like glibenclamide or metformin and production of drugs from plants can be cheaper than the existing one.

7.1 INTRODUCTION

Diabetes Mellitus or Diabetes is a metabolism malady resulting in under production or no production of insulin in our body due to which glucose metabolism in our body becomes faulty. Production of insulin occurs through the pancreatic gland in our body and responsible for glucose uptake and breakdown, thus in its absence glucose starts to build up in the body creating a metabolic disorder. Diabetes is epidemic in nature and highest prevalence of hyperglycemia has been reported among adults in North Africa and Middle East region, i.e., 10.9% whereas, highest number of adults has been diagnosed in the region of Western Pacific, i.e., 37.5% (Kharroubi and Darwish, 2015). It plays an important role as a contributor to ill health and premature death worldwide. In India, hyperglycemia was considered to be a disease of urban population as it was more common in cities due to lifestyle changes and gradual increase of junk and fast-food intake. Diabetes symptoms include increase thirst, frequent urination, fatigue, hunger, and blurred vision.

WHO has been reported that population suffering from hyperglycemia has expanded from 108 million (1980) to 22 million (2014). The global prevalence of hyperglycemia in adults (>18 years) has increased from 4.7% to 8.5% in 2014 (WHO factsheet). Prevalence of diabetes is particularly rising in low- and middle-income countries. Diabetes is majorly responsible for vision loss, renal failures, lower limb amputations, heart attack and strokes. WHO's global report stated that diabetes directly took 1.6 million lives in 2016 (WHO factsheets). WHO have estimated that out of several causes of mortality, diabetes was the seventh leading reason of mortality in 2016 and almost half of the live claimed reported hyperglycemia occur prior to the 70 years' age. In global report of diabetes 2016 by WHO it has been reported that in India mortality or number of deaths due to diabetes for men are 75,900 (age: 30–69) and 46,800 (age: 70+) whereas women are 51,700 (age: 30–69) and 45,600 (age: 70+). Major risk factors of diabetes in India are overweight, obesity, and physical inactivity. Due to poor health infrastructure in rural areas, many cases of diabetes do not get proper care and medication and thus they are also not getting reported. In primary care facilities, insulin, metformin, sulfonylurea medicines are generally available as an option for medication in case of diabetic patients. WHO also reported that number of death due to high blood glucose (hyperglycemia) in case of men are 251,300 (age: 30–69) and 135,700 (age: 70+) and in case of women are 145,700 (age: 30–69) and 139,900 (age: 70+). India will lose certain amount of human resources in future due to potential danger imposed by diabetes. In India diabetes causes due to multiple factors which includes genetic factors as well as acquired traits like obesity associated with rising living standards, lifestyle changes and urban development of cities. Various treatment methods for diabetics are available, but these methods sometimes adversely affect health of the patient.

Natural products are promising therapeutic agents and possess various remedies. The endless diversity of plants provides opportunity to develop novel anti-hyperglycemic drugs. Plants contain various compounds that perform various roles in the body. Herbal remedies are useful as it is easily available and cost effective in nature. Many of the drugs that are usually used nowadays for the management of different diseases are of herbal origin. A number of drugs are prepared from plant extracts, and others are synthesized to imitate the natural plant compound. Benefit of traditional medicine (TM) use is more sensible as it reduces the adverse effects of synthetic medicines. Major use of herbal medicines is for betterment of human health and to take care of chronic ailments. The aim of this chapter is to provide a summary of various scientific evidences that support the use of plants as an anti-hyperglycemic agent.

7.2 TYPES OF DIABETES

In 1997, American Diabetes Association (ADA) suggested classification of hyperglycemias type 1, type 2, gestational diabetes mellitus (GDM) and other types. This classification is still in adoption by ADA and is the most accepted in the current scenario (ADA, 2015).

7.2.1 TYPE 1: INSULIN DEPENDENT HYPERGLYCEMIA

Type 1 or insulin dependent hyperglycemia is a medical condition resulting in loss of pancreatic beta islet cells due to our body's own immune defense attacks (autoimmune) against our pancreatic cells responsible for production of insulin thus leading to decrease in production of insulin in the body. This type of diabetes can start from childhood thus also denoted as Juvenile onset hyperglycemia. It may be due to faulty beta cells or genetic predisposition. T-cell mediated inflammatory response or humoral response (B-cell mediated) against pancreatic cells result into wrecking of cells secreting insulin (Devendra et al., 2004). Presence of auto-antibodies against the insulin secreting cells is distinctive feature of insulin dependent hyperglycemia. Its development in the body is sudden and often shows symptoms such as excessive thirst, frequent urination, enuresis, sluggishness, excessive eating, blurred vision, slow-healing wounds, sudden weight loss and frequent infections (IDF, 2013).

➤ **Molecular Factors:** It has been reported that autoimmune hyperglycemia has some strong connections with HLA and shows linkage with DQ and DR genes. HLA-DQ/DR alleles could be likewise protective or predisposing in nature (ADA, 2015). Several viral factors have also been reported for diabetes in humans. Other factors can include vitamin D deficiency (Hyppönen et al., 2001), vulnerability to pollutants before birth, hygiene hypothesis or autoimmune infection due to non-exposure to infection inefficient nutrient delivery to infants in case of feeding cow's milk formula rather than breast feeding (Knip et al., 2014) moreover resistance against insulin can be developed in juveniles because of obesity or enhanced speed of height growth. Single nucleotide polymorphism (SNP) and single gene mutations are found to be linked with insulin dependent hyperglycemia. Initially, two gene mutations in the burgeoning of insulin dependent hyperglycemia were reported which includes mutations in AIRE (autoimmune regulator) gene which leads to auto immunity by affecting immune tolerance to self-antigens and mutations in FOXP3 gene which give rises to defective T regulatory cells (Bennett et al., 2001).

7.2.2 TYPE 2: HYPERGLYCEMIA OR INSULIN INDEPENDENT HYPERGLYCEMIA

Hyperglycemia or insulin independent hyperglycemia is relatively ubiquitous and related to obese and overweight individuals. With insulin independent hyperglycemia, pancreatic β cells usually lead to underproduction of insulin which due to which insulin is not capable to meet the body's requirement or cells in the body shows resistance against insulin. Insulin resistance, or insensitivity, occurs primarily in liver, fat, and muscle cells. Incidence of insulin independent hyperglycemia has seen a tremendous increase in youth mainly due to lifestyle changes like more sedentary life and intake of junk food. Obesity has been cited as the major responsible factor for insulin resistance in the body and thus solely a plausible reason for insulin independent hyperglycemia (Ginsberg et al., 1975).

➢ **Molecular Factors:** Demographic genome wide association studies (GWAS) in United Kingdom, United States, China, Malaysia, Asian-Indian, and Africa have provided many genetic markers linked with insulin independent hyperglycemia. These are: CDKN2A/B, CDKAL1, SLC30A8, HHEX/IDE, IGFBP2, KCNQ1, TCF7L2 and CAPN10 (Horikawa et al., 2000; Dupuis et al., 2010).

7.2.3 GESTATION DIABETES MELLITUS (GDM)

Gestation diabetes mellitus (GDM) is described as hyperglycemia or glucose sensitivity occurring first time in the body after onset of pregnancy (ADA, 2011). This description does not mean that after pregnancy, glucose level in the body would come to normal level. Dysfunctional pancreatic beta cells lead to insulin depletion during late pregnancy but it has been reported that three major mechanisms may be responsible for dysfunctionality of pancreatic cells in GDM. Firstly, in some women blood (<10% cases of GDM), it has been found that there are anti-glutamate decarboxylase 65 antibodies or antibodies against islet cells circulating in the blood. This antibody has similarly found in cases of type 1 diabetes too (Catalano et al., 1996). Secondly, some women (accounting for 1–5% of cases) have genetic variant like as in case of monogenic type of diabetes (Kousta et al., 2001). And in last the third major cause of beta cells malfunctioning in GDM is contributed by obesity and chronic insulin resistance as in case of type 2 diabetes. This observation might sound good for major scenarios of GDM, but the complete overview of Gestation diabetes also includes other possible reasons of malfunctioning of β-cell in lesser aged women (Buchanan et al., 2012).

7.2.4 MONOGENIC DIABETES

Monogenic form of diabetes is a scarce state of body which is because of transmutations in single gene of β cells and can be inherited. Insulin dependent and independent hyperglycemia has many genetic variants in contrast to monogenic hyperglycemia. Monogenic form of hyperglycemia affects mostly young population. Similar to other type of diabetes, the resulting effect is less insulin production or rarely insulin resistance in the body. Most of the times it is not diagnosed correctly as its symptoms are same as other types of diabetes and this leads to wrong medication and complications. Classification of monogenic diabetes is based on the age when onset of disease has occurred. It is characterized into neonatal diabetes (prior the 6 months age) or maturity-onset diabetes of the young (MODY) prior the 25 years of age (Schwitzgebel, 2014). Mutation in homeodomain transcription factor PDX1 lead to onset of MODY and its expression get reduced before the arrival of disorder (Kushner et al., 2002). PDX1 transcription factor has a role in beta cells differentiation.

> **Molecular Factors:** A large set of genes responsible for monogenic diabetes has been identified (Schwitzgebel, 2014). Monogenic diabetes ultimately results in reduced number of β-cell or reduction in their functionality. These molecular factors majorly encodes either transcription factors which are responsible for management of nuclear genes expression or proteins that reside on the endoplasmic reticulum, cytoplasm or plasmalemma, gene products responsible for production of insulin and its secretion, and proteins like autoimmune diabetic proteins and exocrine pancreatic proteins (Schwitzgebel, 2014). Thus, these genes overall have a crucial role to play in glucose metabolism pathway and their hierarchy determines the arrival of diabetes whether it is neonatal or expressed later. Many genes responsible for monogenic diabetes have also been cited for insulin dependent as well as independent diabetes thus have been overlooked (Table 7.1).

TABLE 7.1   Genes and Molecular Markers for Different Type of Diabetes

Genes and Molecular Markers Found to be Responsible for Type 1 Diabetes		
Genes in which Mutations have been Reported	**Functions**	**References**
SIRTI (deactylation of histone) gene in β cells	Adjusts the insulin production and bring changes in peripheral tissues such that their insulin sensitivity is increased or decreased	Bordone et al. (2006); Sun et al. (2007)

TABLE 7.1 *(Continued)*

Single nucleotide polymorphisms in the HLA-DQB1 and *CTLA-4* +49A/G and VNTR alleles in insulin gene (INS)	Responsible for differentiation of latent autoimmune insulin dependent and insulin independent hyperglycemia	Haller et al. (2007)
HLA-DR, together with HLA-DQB1 alleles and a polymorphic form in *PTPN22* gene	Responsible for age inception of late insulin dependent hyperglycemia	Okruszko et al. (2012); Ahmadi et al. (2013)
SNPs in CLEC16A gene in chromosome 16	Reduction in DEX1 expression in B lymphoblastoid cells	Tomlinson et al. (2014)

Genes and Molecular Markers Reported to be Associated with Insulin Independent Diabetes

TCF7L2	Over expression leads to lesser sensitization of β islet cells to produce insulin and majorly responsible for regulating fusion between secretory granules that contributes to a late event in insulin secretion pathway.	Da Silva et al. (2009)
Single nucleotide polymorphism in hematopoietically-expressed homeobox (HHEX) gene	–	Li et al. (2012)
Islet zinc transporter protein (SLC30A8)	Mutations may have a safeguarding role against type 2 diabetes which could be an effective approach for treatment in patients	Flannick et al. (2014)
Interleukin-6 (IL-6), IL-10, TNF-α, IL12B, IL23R and IL23A genes	–	Saxena et al. (2013); Eirís et al. (2014)
Peroxisome proliferator-activated receptor gamma (PPARG) gene	Rare variations lead to functional erosion of the gene product in adipocytes differentiation, which were remarkably found to be linked with type 2 diabetes	Majithia et al. (2014)
Single nucleotide polymorphism in the α 2A adrenergic receptor (ADRA2A) gene	Has a role in the sympathetic nervous system (SNS), management of lipolysis and insulin secretion	Långberg et al. (2013)

TABLE 7.1 *(Continued)*

Genes Found to be Responsible for Monogenic Diabetes Mellitus		
Glucokinase gene (GCK)	Responsible for pancreatic sensing of blood sugar, mutations exceeding than 70 have been identified	Osbak et al. (2009)
Two hepatocyte nuclear factor genes	One codes for HNF4A transcription factor associated with MODY1;	Lyssenko et al. (2008)
	One codes for HNF1A transcription factor associated with MODY2	

7.2.5 SYNTHETIC ANTI-DIABETIC DRUGS AND THEIR SIDE EFFECTS

Metformin is a hypoglycemic agent which has the property to reduce plasma glucose levels by inhibiting hepatic gluconeogenesis. It also able to reduce sugar absorption in intestine and LDL and VLDL level reduction with HDL level enhancement was seen in patients treated with metformin for 4–6 weeks. Side effect of this drug includes reduction in cardiovascular mortality, decreased appetite, decrease in pH of blood due to lactate build up (lactose acidosis) especially in patients suffering from congestive heart failure. Pioglitazone is another drug which binds to receptor, i.e., PPAR-γ and enhances insulin sensitivity of hepatocytes, adipocytes, and skeletal muscle cells. After administration of this drug, hyperglycemia reduction, decline-ment of HbA1c and triglycerides levels occurs with increase in HDL levels. Side effects include hepatotoxicity that may be deadly. Miglitol is another drug which helps in delaying carbohydrate metabolism in the body. It inhibits glucosidase enzyme which is present in the intestinal brush borders that mediate carbohydrates digestion. Side effects include flatulence, diarrhea, and cramps. Glimipride enhances insulin binding capacity to target cells and reduces secretion of glucagon. Side effects include hyperinsulinemia, weight gain, and hypoglycemia (Chcipa et al., 2019). Due to these problems associated with synthetic drugs an alternative to treat diabetes is required. Medicinal plants contain various phytochemical which can be utilized for the treatment of this disease.

7.3 MEDICINAL PLANTS FOR DIABETES TREATMENT

As this deadly disorder is persistently increasing, the necessity to create awareness in public and deploy methods to reduce the risk of someone being affected, diagnose, and recognizing the arrival of the disorder and determining the most applicable and easily available treatment have become today's dire need. Extract from natural herbal plants have been used from several years in Ayurvedic medicines and are proved to be effective against several diseases. Several reports have suggested that globally we have a rich diversity of medicinal plants which can eradicate many diseases. Medicinal plants like *Capparis deciduas* (Sharma et al., 2009)., *Abelmoschus esculentus* (Erfani et al., 2018), *Achillea millefolium* (Chávez-Silva et al., 2017), *Capparis deciduas* (Sharma et al., 2009)., *Cinnamom icassiae* (Kim et al., 2010), and *Silybum marianum* (Guigas et al., 2007; Pferschy-Wenzig et al., 2014), in *Capparis deciduas* (Sharma et al., 2009) *Phyllanthus amarus* (Shetti et al., 2012), *Achillea millefolium* (Chávez-Silva et al., 2017), *Andrographis paniculata* (Yu et al., 2003), *Azadirachta indica* (Satyanarayana et al., 2015), *Beta vulgaris* (UlKabir et al., 2015), *Trigonella foenumgraecum* (Kumar et al., 2012) and *Vinca rosea* (Al-Shaqha et al., 2015) are some of the medicinal plants which has shown retarding TNF alpha expression retardation or enhanced expression of PPAR-alpha and gamma, glucokinase (GK), or glucose transporter 4. Various plants are reported to have potential for diabetes treatment which will be discussed in detail.

7.3.1 ABELMOSCHUS ESCULENTUS (OKRA)

Abelmoschus esculentus commonly known as okra, belongs to family Malvaceae, is primarily from Ethiopia but now can be found in region such as West Africa, Caribbean, Asia, and United States. Ben-Chioma et al. (2013) reported that dried powdered and aqueous form of *A. esculentus* has remarkably showed an antihyperglycemic effect and lowered the blood glucose concentration in alloxan induced (AI) hyperglycemic Wister rats. Anti diabetic property of okra is found to be linked with dietary fibers and polyphenols (Gunness et al., 2010). In another study, okra extract has improved histological damages in pancreatic beta cells and have shown to reduce the expression levels of PPAR-α and γ gene which results in decrease in incidence of type 2 diabetes (Erfani et al., 2018).

7.3.2   ACACIA ARABICA (BABOOL)

Acacia arabica with a vernacular name Babool in Hindi, is a member of Leguminoseae family, has worldwide approximately 1,380 species of Arabica with 920 species of them endemic to Australia and rest to the subtropical and tropical parts of the globe (Maslin et al., 2003). In India, it has been used as a multi-purpose tree for treatment of tooth related problems, skin disorders and stomach problems. Hydro alcoholic and aqueous (cold and hot) extract of babool have been evaluated for their potential hypoglycemic activity. Oral intake of aqueous extract (cold water) at a concentration of 0.4 g/kg b.w. in hyperglycemic rats proceeded in a noteworthy decrease in blood sugar, triglycerides, and cholesterol levels. This hypoglycemic action was ascribed to phenolic compounds which were found in the extract (Yasir et al., 2010). Antioxidative, anti-hyperlipidemic, and hypoglycemic activity of *A. arabica* extract was investigated on streptozotocin induced (STZ-I) hyperglycemic rats. There were 3 groups made and the first one being untreated was taken as a control and other two were given at dosage of 0.1 g/kg and 0.2 g/kg b.w. for 3 weeks. The treated groups demonstrated a reduction in insulin resistance, serum sugar levels, cholesterol, triglycerides, etc. (Hegazy et al., 2013).

7.3.3   ACHILLEA MILLEFOLIUM (YARROW)

Achillea millefolium with a vernacular name Yarrow, is included in Asteraceae family, is endemic to mild temperature zones of Northern Hemisphere in Europe, Asia, and North America and has been brought in New Zealand and Australia as an animal feed. It has been shown to have an anti-hyperglycemic activity by down regulating IL-1β and inducible nitric oxide synthase (iNOS) gene in β cells in STZ-I hyperglycemic rats. Expression level of iNOS and IL-1β was screened and found that the expression level in diabetic rat was significantly ameliorated after treatment with *A. millefolium* extract (Zolghadri et al., 2014). Hydro alcoholic extract of *A. millefolium* was tested on normoglycemic and insulin independent diabetic mice model to analyze the anti-diabetic effect and its potential mode of action. It was reported that hydroalcoholic extract ameliorated glucose levels and promoted inhibition of alpha-glucosidase enzyme by 55% at 0.001 g/ml with respect to control, increased PPAR gamma (fivefold) and GLUT4 (two-fold) expression level and also increased secretion of insulin and Ca++ ions in comparison with control exhibits multitarget mode of action (Chávez-Silva et al., 2017).

7.3.4 AEGLE MARMELOS (BAEL OR BHEL OR BENGAL QUINCE)

Aegle marmelos commonly known as bael or Bhel or Bengal quince or wood apple, is a fellow of Rutaceae and indigenous to Indian Subcontinent and Southeast Asia. Its hypoglycemic effects in hyperglycemic rats were tested using an aqueous extract of its seeds at a dosage of 100, 250 and 500 mg/kg. It was found that 0.25 g/kg was the most potent dosage resulting in reduction of blood sugar levels by 35.1% in normal healthy rats, 33.2% in mild and 41.2% in sub hyperglycemic rats (Kesari et al., 2006). In another study it was observed that *A. marmelos* extract resisted the blood glucose increase after oral sucrose intake (250 mg/kg) and remarkably improved oral glucose tolerance in type 2 hyperglycemic rats. This extracts also demonstrated a remarkable change in secretion of insulin in interval of half an hour. This hypoglycemic activity was due to the prevention of carbohydrates digestion and assimilation (alpha-amylase inhibition), and increase insulin secretion (Ansari et al., 2017).

7.3.5 ALLIUM SATIVUM (GARLIC)

Allium sativum normally called garlic, is a fellow of Amaryllidaceae family and endemic to Northeast (NE) Iran and Central Asia. It has been used as a common seasoning worldwide since years. Garlic extract possess anti-bacterial, anti-oxidant, anti-carcinogenic, anti-mutagenic, antiasthmatic, immunomodulatory, and prebiotic effects which are proven to be beneficial for human health (Corzo-Martínez, 2007; Santhosha et al., 2013). Several research studies have proven anti-hyperglycemic activity of garlic. One research study established hypoglycemic effect of aqueous extract of *A. sativum* (0.01 l/kg/day) in rabbits eating a sucrose diet (Zacharias et al., 1980). S-allyl cysteine sulfoxide, a sulfur containing amino acid, has shown to stimulate beta cells isolated from normal rats to secrete glucose metabolizing hormone and also control lipid peroxidation better than glibenclamide (an anti-diabetic drug) and insulin (Augusti et al., 1996). In another study, ethanolic extract of garlic were fed orally to normal and STZ-I hyperglycemic rats and proven to be hypoglycemic and significant decrease in serum glucose, uric acid, triglycerides, AST (aspirate aminotransferase), total cholesterol, urea, creatinine, and ALT (alanine aminotransferase) were reported (Eidi et al., 2006).

7.3.6   ALOE BARBADENSIS (ALOE VERA)

Aloe barbadensis, vernacular name Aloe vera, is commonly grown as a household plant, is a fellow of Asphodelaceae family, has its roots in Arabian Peninsula but now has spreaded to other tropical parts of the world. It has been cultivated for its medicinal effects and is exploited in various commodities like skin lotions, toothpastes, beverages, cosmetic products and others. Five phytosterols were identified in aloe vera and their anti-hyperglycemic potential was tested on type 2 diabetic mice. These compounds were: cyclo-artanol, 24-methylene-cycloartanol, lophenol, and two variants of lophenol. These phytosterols remarkably reduced fasting blood sugar levels after being treated for 28 days (51%, 55%, 64%, 28%, and 47% respectively) (Tanaka et al., 2006). In a clinical trial with insulin independent hyperglycemic patients (40–60 age) who were not prescribed any other anti-hyperlipidemic agents and resistant to standard treatment (metmorfin and glyburide tablets) were given one 0.3 g capsule of aloe vera twice a day after interval of 12 hours for two months in combination with metformin and glyburide. This administration resulted in remarkable lowering in total cholesterol, LDL, fasting blood glucose (FBG) and HbA1c (Huseini et al., 2011). In another study, ethanolic extract of aloe leaf were tested for their anti-hyperglycemic effects in STZ-I hyperglycemic rats and resulted in amelioration in FBG at a dosage of 0.3 and 0.5 g/kg after being treated for 42 days (Shinde et al., 2014).

7.3.7   ANDROGRAPHIS PANICULATA (GREEN CHIRETA)

Andrographis paniculata, commonly known as green chireta, belongs to Acanthaceae family and endemic to Sri Lanka and India. It is an herbaceous plant and cultivated for its roots and leaves which have been used in medicinal preparations for long time. Andrographolide, an active constituent present in the green chireta leaves has been evaluated for its hypoglycemic potential in STZ-I hyperglycemic rats. Dosage of 0.15 g/kg prompted a lowering in glucose levels in plasma. This effect was due to increased expression of GLUT4 protein (Yu et al., 2003). It is hypoglycemic and anti-hyperlipidemic effect have also been tested in type 2 hyperglycemic rats which were fed on a diet containing high fructose. Treatment with pure extract of *A. paniculata* leads to a considerable amelioration in blood sugar, LDL, and triglycerides in hyperglycemic rats (Nugroho et al., 2012).

7.3.8 ANNONA SQUAMOSA (SUGAR APPLE)

Annona squamosa, with a common name sugar apple fruit, belongs to Annonaceae family and endemic to the tropical America and West Indies but now being grown in Tropical and sub-tropical environments of Thailand, Taiwan, and Indonesia for its fruit. A research study was conducted to evaluate anti-hyperglycemic activity of sugar apple extracts and histological changes in pancreas. FBG level and oral glucose tolerance test (OGTT) were conducted after oral application of glibenclamide (0.003 g/kg) and aqueous extract of sugar apple leaves at a dosage of 1,250, 2,500, and 5,000 mg/kg for 12 days. Dosage of 2.5 and 5 g/kg were found to be most potent and resulted in hypoglycemic activity and there was significant improvement in pancreatic beta Islet cells morphology (Rabintossaporn et al., 2009). Anti-hyperglycemic effects of hydroalcoholic extract of *Annona* were evaluated in STZ-I diabetic rats at a dose of 0.350 g/kg in combination with 0.005 g/kg glibenclamide for 4 weeks. Results showed a noteworthy reduction in blood sugar level, triglycerides, and LDL (Tomar et al., 2012).

7.3.9 ARECA CATECHU (INDIAN NUT OR ARECA NUT)

Areca catechu with a vernacular name Indian nut is a fellow of Arecaceae family. It is native to Philippines, but now has distributed to other countries like India, Bangladesh, Southern China, Malaysia, Taiwan, Thailand, and others. Anti-hyperglycemic potential of chloroform, petroleum ether, and methanol fraction of *Areca* leaves was analyzed in a study involving Wister rats. The streptozotocin-induced hyperglycemic rats were given 200 mg/kg extracts daily for half a month. All the extracts elicited reduction in FBG, but most effective one was found to be methanolic extract (Mondal et al., 2012). In another study, ethanolic, aqueous, and petroleum ether extract of *Areca* flowers were evaluated at a dosage of 500 mg/kg in AI hyperglycemic rats for 3 weeks. It was reported that ethanol and aqueous extract produced a noteworthy lowering in blood glucose as well as improvement of body weight and various diabetic parameters associated with the disease (Ghate et al., 2014).

7.3.10   ARGYREIA NERVOSA (ELEPHANT CREEPER) OR ARGYREIA SPECIOSA

Argyreia nervosa with a vernacular name Vidhara or Elephant creeper is a fellow of Convolvulaceae family and native to Indian Subcontinent and has spread to regions worldwide like Africa, Caribbean, and Hawaii. It has been used for its medicinal properties in Ayurvedic medicines. It has been reported that application of alcoholic extract of elephant creeper at a dosage of 250, 500, 750 mg/kg leads to amelioration in blood sugar in normal as well as AI hyperglycemic rats (HemaLatha et al., 2008). Ethanolic extract of *A. nervosa* roots (0.5 g/kg b.w.), when administrated orally, elicited a lowering effect on blood glucose levels in normoglycemic (at 6 hour) as well as in STZ-I hyperglycemic rats (after 7 days) (Kumar et al., 2010).

7.3.11   AVERRHOVA BILIMBI (BILIMBI OR CUCUMBER TREE)

Averrhova bilimbi with a vernacular name bilimbi or cucumber tree, is a fellow of Oxalidaceae. It is endemic to Indonesia but now grown in Sri Lanka, Philippines, Bangladesh, Maldives, Malaysia, Myanmar, and Southern India. Ethanolic extract of bilimbi leaves at a dosage of 0.125 g/kg was investigated for its anti-hyperglycemic and anti-hyperlipidemic effects in STZ-I hyperglycemic rats. It was observed that level of blood glucose went down by 50% and triglycerides level by 130% (Pushparaj et al., 2000). In another study, streptozotocin-induced hyperglycemic rats were given ethyl acetate extract of *A. bilimbi* fruit (0.025 g/kg b.w.) for 2 months and it was found that there was noteworthy lowering in serum glucose, glycated hemoglobin and also a considerable increase in plasma insulin. This extract also had a positive effect on hepatic antioxidant potential by increasing the activities of various peroxidase and catalase. HPLC analysis of extract demonstrated the presence of quercetin, a phenolic compound, might be responsible for hypoglycemic potential of the extract (Kurup et al., 2016).

7.3.12   AZADIRACHTA INDICA (NEEM)

Azadirachta indica, with a common name neem in India, is a fellow of Meliaceae family. It is endemic to Indian Subcontinent and is normally grown in tropical and sub-tropical regions. It is traditionally associated with Indian culture and is a prestigious part of Ayurveda. Hypoglycemic activity of aqueous extract of neem bark and root has been analyzed in diabetic rats and it was reported that 0.250 g/kg b.w. dose was effective in amelioration of serum glucose, triglycerides, urea, creatinine, and cholesterol within 24 hours after treatment (Hashmat et al., 2012). In another study with fructose-induced diabetic male rats, hypoglycemic potential of neem aqueous extract was investigated at 0.4 g/kg b.w. for 1 month. The treatment ameliorated FBG levels, serum lipids and improved serum insulin and GLUT4 protein (Satyanarayana et al., 2015).

7.3.13   *BETA VULGARIS (BEET)*

Beta vulgaris, vernacular name beet, is a member of Amaranthaceae family and widespread in Southwestern, southeastern, and northern Europe, North Africa, to western Asia. Aqueous extract of beet root has been evaluated in hyperglycemic rats. 0.05 g/kg was the most active fraction of aqueous beet extract. It was reported that administration of aqueous fraction resulted in anti-hyperglycemic activity which were attributed to enhancement in insulin production due to GLP-1 and acetylcholine and also glucose uptake was increased due to more number of membranes bound GLUT-4 transporters (UlKabir et al., 2015). In another study, ethanolic extract of beet root was given to STZ-I hyperglycemic rats at a dosage of 0.4 g/kg and glibenclamide (0.005 g/kg). It was reported that glucose levels were drop down from 280.6 to 118.2 mg/dl in case of ethanolic extract as compare to glibenclamide in which the result was 116.6 from 282.2 mg/dl (Sravan et al., 2016).

7.3.14   *BIOPHYTUM SENSITIVUM (LITTLE TREE PLANT)*

Biophytum sensitivum with a common name little tree plant, is a fellow of Oxalidaceae family. It is native to tropical India, wet lands of Nepal and other Southeast Asian countries. For its medicinal properties, it has been used since long times in India and Nepal. In a study involving aqueous and methanolic extract of *B. sensitivum* it was found that 0.2 g/kg was ideal dosage for hypoglycemic activity of methanolic extract in AI Wister hyperglycemic rats (Mishra et al., 2007). It has been reported that *B. sensitivum* leaf extract exerts hypoglycemic potential by stimulating β cells to secrete insulin in hyperglycemic male rabbits (Ayodhya et al., 2010). In another study, it was shown that oral treatment with little tree plant extract at a dose of 0.2 g/kg for 4 weeks in STNZ-I hyperglycemic rabbits produced a significant decrease in blood glucose, glycosylated hemoglobin and an increment in liver glycogen, total hemoglobin and plasma insulin (Pawar et al., 2014).

7.3.15 BOERHAVIA DIFFUSA (PUNARNAVA)

Boerhavia diffusa with a vernacular name Punarnava (in Ayurveda), is a member of Nyctaginaceae family. It is used as a leafy green vegetable which is distributed throughout India, Pacific, and Southern United States. In one study, anti-hyperglycemic, and anti-obesogenic capabilities of ethyl acetate, aqueous, and ethanol extract of *Boerhavia's* aerial parts was evaluated. It was found that ethanolic extract possesses more potent ferric reducing antioxidant power and DPPH scavenging activities in comparison with other extracts. Ethanol extract also showed anti-lipidemic and hypoglycemic activity by preventing digestion of carbohydrates, fats, and abdominal glucose uptake and also by enhancing uptake of glucose by muscle tissues (Oyebode et al., 2018). In another study, methanolic extract of roots of *B. diffusa* was tested for treatment of diabetes in STZ-I hyperglycemic rats. Intake of 100 and 200 mg/kg body weight resulted in remarkable amelioration in blood glucose, plasma enzymes and other diabetes associated complications. It also showed DPPH, NO_2 and H_2O_2 radical scavenging and restored antioxidant enzymes activity (Alam et al., 2018).

7.3.16 BOMBAX CEIBA (COTTON TREE OR SEMAL)

Bombax ceiba with a common name cotton tree or semal is a fellow of the Malvaceae family It is a deciduous tree widely grown in Southeast Asia, India, and Pakistan. One study investigated hypoglycemic and hypolipidemic potential of bark extract of *Bombax* in STZ-I hyperglycemic rats indicated that 0.6 g/kg body weight dose was most effective one among 0.2, 0.4, and 0.6 g/kg dosages. It resulted in remarkable hypoglycemic and hypolipidemic effect and also reduced the total cholesterol and triglyceride levels. Triterpenoid was the major constituent present in the extract found to be responsible for anti-hyperglycemic activity (Bhavsar et al., 2013). Another study used ethanol extract of leaves of *B. ceiba*, 0.07, 0.14, and 0.28 g/kg dosages were given to the high fat diet and STZ-I diabetic rats. It was reported that extract resulted in a remarkable lowering of FBG levels, LDL, total cholesterol, glycosylated hemoglobin, triglyceride, and others. It also simulated insulin production from remaining pancreatic β cells (Xu et al., 2017).

7.3.17 BRASSICA NIGRA (BLACK MUSTARD)

Brassica nigra, with a vernacular name black mustard is a fellow of Brassicaceae family. It is a spice ornament and natively found in regions of Asia, temperate regions of Europe and tropical regions of North Africa. In a study with different types of seed extracts (aqueous, acetone, chloroform, and ethanol), glucose tolerance test was conducted and increase in serum glucose was measured between 0 and 1 hours and it was observed that aqueous extract was the most effective one in resisting increase in serum glucose and optimum concentration for its hypoglycemic activity was found to be 200 mg/kg (Anand et al., 2007). In another study, involving STZ-I insulin independent hyperglycemic rats, hypoglycemic, and antioxidant potential of *B. nigra* seeds oil was evaluated and it was reported that dosage of 0.5 and 1 g/kg b.w. effectively reduce blood glucose level from 335 to 280 mg/dl and 330 to 265 mg/dl in 4 hours respectively. Rats were treated for 28 days and in vivo studies on diabetic rats maintain that antioxidant activity is due to increased glutathione and decreased malondialdehyde (Kumar et al., 2013).

7.3.18 BRYONIA LACINIOSA (SHIVLINGI)

Bryonia laciniosa with a vernacular name shivlingi in India, is belongs to Cucurbitaceae family and native to Western Eurasia, North Africa, South Asia and the Canary Islands. In a study, ethanolic extract of shivlingi seeds were prepared and its saponin fraction was investigated for anti-hyperglycemic and anti-hyperlipidemic effect in STZ-I hyperglycemic rats. It was observed that oral intake of ethanolic extract (0.25 and 0.5 g/kg) and saponin fraction (0.1 and 0.200 g/kg) for 4 weeks resulted in amelioration in blood sugar levels and an improvement in insulin level (Patel et al., 2012). In streptozotocin-induced hyperglycemic Wister rats, it has been reported that treatment with ethanolic extract of *B. laciniosa* at a dosage of 0.25 and 0.5 g/kg resulted in lowering of MDA values and effectively reversed the diabetic nephropathic changes in induced diabetic rats (Bhide et al., 2017).

7.3.19 CAESALPINIA BONDUCELLA (GREY NICKER)

Caesalpinia bonducella commonly known as Grey Nicker or Nicker bean, is a fellow of Fabaceae family, and found in Tropical regions in India, Andaman, and Nicobar Islands and Sri Lanka. Hypoglycemic and antioxidant potential of hydromethanolic extract of *C. bonducella* seeds was investigated in STZ-I hyperglycemic male albino rats. It was reported that dosage of 0.250 g/kg b.w. effectively corrected with FBG levels and glycogen levels in treated rats and also enzymatic activities of catalase and superoxide dismutase (SOD) were improved (Jana et al., 2012). An aqueous extract of *C. bonducella* containing seed and shell was analyzed for various chemical constituents and its anti-hyperglycemic activity was evaluated. The study reported that flavonoids, saponins, and alkaloids were present in the extract and effective dosage for anti-hyperglycemic activity was 1,000 microgram/ml (Subbiah et al., 2019).

7.3.20   CAJANUS CAJAN (PIGEON PEA)

Cajanus cajan commonly known as pigeon pea, is included in Fabaceae family Itis a perennial legume plant with its center of origin in peninsular India but now consumed as a food in Asia, Africa, and Latin America as well. Oral administration of methanolic and ethyl acetate extract of *C. cajan* in diabetic mice proven to be the most effective extract by lowering the glucose levels and increasing insulin activity at 0.25 g/kg in 10 days (Dolui et al., 2012). In another study, methanolic extract of *C. cajan* was evaluated for its anti-oxidant and hypoglycemic potential in AI hyperglycemic rats. They reported that at a dosage of 0.2 and 0.4 g/kg b.w., there were remarkable reduction in FBG, decrease in blood glucose levels in 5 days (Nahar et al., 2014). In a recent study, it was documented that ethanolic extract of leaves of *C. cajan* at dosage of 400 and 800 mg/kg body weight produced hypoglycemic effect in ICR mice and have improved blood sugar levels (Manzo et al., 2017).

7.3.21   CAPPARIS DECIDUAS (KARIRA)

Capparis deciduas with a vernacular name karira, is a fellow of Capparaceae family and found in deserted regions in Southern Asia, Africa, and Middle East. To investigate upon antihyperglycemic potential of aqueous and ethanolic extract of *C. deciduas*, an investigation was conducted on albino rats. Extracts (at a dosage of 0.25 and 0.5 g/kg b.w.) were fed orally to diabetic rats for 21 days and after 21 days a quite noticeable decrease in FBG levels was observed (58.5, 83.6% for aqueous extract and 60.2, 98.5% for ethanolic extract) (Rathee et al., 2010). In another study, alkaloid rich fraction of karira was given to STZ-induced hyperglycemic rats for 28 days. It was found that alkaloid rich fraction prevented acute increase in sugar levels during OGT test and also lowered triglyceride and total cholesterol. There was impairment in glucose-6-phosphatase activity by 44%, and also glycogen content in muscle and liver were significantly improved. Gene expression of phosphoenolpyruvate carboxykinase (PEPCK), G6Pase, tumor necrosis factor-alpha (TNF-alpha) and aldose reductase were significantly decreased on other hand expression of GLUT-4, PPAR-gamma, and GK improved significantly (Sharma et al., 2009).

7.3.22   CAPSICUM ANNUUM (CAYENNE PEPPER)

Capsicum annuum, common name cayenne pepper or bell pepper, is included in Solanaceae family and endemic to Northern South America and Southern North America. It is a spicing agent due to the compound capsaicin which creates a burning sensation. *C. annuum* has been reported to possess anti-hyperglycemic activity by mechanisms like inhibition of alpha amylase, inhibition of alpha glucosidase, antioxidant activity, insulin mimetic, activation of TRPV-1 resulting in improvement of insulin resistance, by increasing insulin sensitivity of peripheral tissues and others (Watcharachaisoponsiri et al., 2016; Earnest et al., 2013). A four-week study on AI hyperglycemic rats showed that a diet rich with high fat after treatment with 0.015% capsaicin significantly shows anti-hyperglycemic effects by reversing the serum level of glucose, cholesterol, and total glycerides (TG) (Magied et al., 2014).

7.3.23   CARUM CARVI (CARAWAY)

Carum carvi with a common name caraway or meridian fennel, is a member of Apiaceae family. It is endemic to Western Asia, Europe, and North Africa. Aqueous extract of caraway when administrated to STZ-I hyperglycemic rats at a dosage of 0.03 and 0.06 g/kg b.w. for 2 months resulted in a decrease in serum sugar levels, creatinine, total urinary protein and thus demonstrated anti-hyperglycemic as well as reno-protective ability. These properties were due to flavonoids and carvones present in caraway extract (Sadiq et al., 2010). Oral administration of *C. carvi* at a dosage of 1 g/kg b.w. daily in hyperglycemic male Wistar rats resulted in a remarkable lowering of blood glucose levels, alleviation of their loss in body weight and reduction in total cholesterol and LDL levels (Haidari et al., 2011).

7.3.24   CICHORIUM INTYBUS (COMMON CHICORY)

Cichorium intybus, commonly known as common chicory, is a member of Asteraceae family, indigenous to Europe now commonly found in North America, China, and Australia. Pushparaj et al. (2006) reported the anti-hyperglycemic and anti-hyperlipidemic ability of ethanolic extract of chicory. STZ-I hyperglycemic male Sprague-Dawley rats were administered with this extract and most potent dose was found to be 125 mg/kg body weight in oral glucose tolerant test. There was remarkable decrease in total cholesterol (19%), serum glucose (20%) and triglycerides (91%) (Pushparaj et al., 2006). In another study, natural chicoric acid extract (NCRAE) from chicory roots was shown to improve insulin secretion and glucose uptake by muscle cells in Wistar rats (Azay-Milhau et al., 2013). In a recent study, LC-MS analysis of NCRAE was done and it was found that 83.8% of this extract is chicoric acid and chlorogenic acid. A comparative study between NCRAE and SCCAM (Chicoric acid and chlorogenic acid) was done for their anti-hyperglycemic action in STZ-I hyperglycemic rats and in L6 muscle cell line. It was reported that NCRAE as well as SCCAM were able to improve glucose tolerance but only NCRAE showed a significant reduction in basal hyperglycemia after treatment of six days (Ferrare et al., 2018).

7.3.25   CINNAMOM ICASSIAE (CINNAMON)

Cinnamom icassiae, commonly known as cinnamon, is a fellow of Lauraceae family, an evergreen tree from southern China and now widely grown in Southern and Eastern Asia too. Cinnamon is used as a spicing agent in various cuisines worldwide. Anti-diabetic property of cinnamon has been observed in insulin independent hyperglycemic animal model (C57BIKsj db/db) at a dosage of 0.2 g/kg. This study shows that cinnamon extract has a regulatory role in blood glucose and lipids (Kim et al., 2006). Increased expression of PPAR alpha and PPAR gamma have been reported in Male C57BIKs db/db mice when they were treated with cinnamon extract for a period of 12 weeks (Kim et al., 2010).

7.3.26   CITRULUS COLOCYNTHIS (COLOCYNTHIS OR BITTER APPLE)

Citrulus colocynthis with a common name colocynthis or bitter apple, is belongs to Cucurbitaceae family, and indigenous to Mediterranean Basin and

Asia, in Middle East countries like Turkey and Nubia. In a study, aqueous extract of seeds of *C. colocynthis* and hydroalcoholic extract of peel of the colocynthis fruit was investigated for hypoglycemic potential and Insulin Resistance Index. It was found that at a dosage of 0.2 g/kg b.w. seed extract induced a lowering in serum glucose and improvement in serum insulin whereas peel extract did the opposite (Ahangarpour et al., 2013). In another study, with hydro-ethanolic extract of Colocynthis seeds, it was observed that at a dosage of 0.3 g/kg body weight, it prompted a reduction in blood glucose level and promoted regeneration of B cells, increase in size of pancreatic islets and improved hepatic tissue (Oryan et al., 2014). In another study, four different extracts (aqueous, saponins, total alkaloids and glucosidic) of bitter apple seeds were prepared and evaluated for their hypoglycemic potential in normal and STZ-I hyperglycemic Wistar rats. Most effective extract was found to be aqueous extract with reduction in blood glucose (>57.6%) (Lahfa et al., 2017).

7.3.27   *CORIANDRUM SATIVUM (CHINESE PARSLEY OR CILANTRO)*

Coriandrum sativum with a common name Chinese parsley or Cilantro in North America belongs to Apiaceae family and endemic to Northern Africa, Southern Europe and Southwestern Asia. Its fresh leaves and dried seeds are used in cooking in various cuisines throughout the world. Hypoglycemic and antioxidant activity of leaf and stem extract of *C. sativum* has been investigated in AI diabetic rats by Sreelatha et al. (2012) They reported that there was significant amelioration in blood glucose levels as well as LDL, total cholesterol and triglycerides level were lowered and anti-oxidant potential was due to enhancement in activity of catalase, glutathione peroxidase, SOD, and lowering of lipid peroxidation (Sreelatha et al., 2012). In another study, ethanolic extract of *C. sativum* seeds at a dose of 125 and 250 mg/kg body weight resulted in hypoglycemic, anti-oxidant, and protection of pancreatic organ from diabetic damage (Widodo et al., 2015).

7.3.28   *DOREMA AUCHERI (BILHAR)*

Dorenma aucheri with a vernacular name Bilhar belongs to Apiaceae family and is native to Iran. Hydroalcoholic extract of leaves of *D. aucheri* has been investigated for hypoglycemic and hypolipidemic effect in STZ-I hyperglycemic rats with three different doses of 0.1, 0.2, and 0.4 g/kgb.w. It was reported that treatment with this extract induced lowering in blood glucose, significant change in lipid profiles, leptin, and insulin levels and most potent dose was discovered to be 0.2 g/kg (Ahangarpour et al., 2014). In another study, a clinical trial was conducted on human insulin independent hyperglycemic patients in which they were treated with aqueous extract of Bilhar. Results showed that there was a remarkable improvement in FBG levels, HbA1c, and lipid profile of diabetic patients who were given treatment with *D. aucheri* extract (Tavana et al., 2015).

7.3.29   ECLIPTA ALBA (FALSE DAISY OR BHRINGRAJ)

Eclipta alba, vernacular name Bhringraj or False Daisy, is a fellow of Asteraceae family and widely grown in India, Nepal, Thailand, China, and Brazil. Leaf suspension of Bhringraj at a dose of 2,000 and 4,000 mg/kg b.w. were given orally to alloxan-induced hyperglycemic rats for 60 days and it was reported that treatment prompted an amelioration in blood glucose (from 372 to 117), HbA1c, reduction in enzymatic activities of glucose-6-phosphatase and fructose-1,6-biphosphatase and improvement in liver hexokinase activity (Ananthi et al., 2003). In another study, hypoglycemic activity of ethanolic extract of *E. alba* was investigated in STZ-I hyperglycemic rats. Single dose treatment and treatment for 21 days was given and results were documented. Remarkable decrease in blood glucose levels, creatinine, HbA1c and other parameters as well as inhibition of alpha-glucosidase (noncompetitive) and aldose reductase took place (Jaiswal et al., 2012).

7.3.30   EMBLICA OFFICINALIS (INDIAN GOOSEBERRY OR AMLA)

Emblica officinalis with a vernacular name Indian Gooseberry or Amla, belongs to Phyllanthaceae family and natively from Indian Subcontinent. In one study aqueous extract of fruits of amla showed improvement in OGTT in insulin independent hyperglycemic rats after four weeks of feeding and remarkable decrease in FBG levels after 8 weeks (Ansari et al., 2014). In another study, methanolic extract of *E. officnialis* consists of quercetin and quercetin was found to be a major contributing factor in reduction of blood glucose level by 14.78% (0.075 g/kg) after one week of treatment. Quercetin extracted from methanolic extract also improved HDL, LDL, triglycerides, and total cholesterol levels at a dose of 0.05 and 0.075 g/kg body weight (Srinivasan et al., 2018).

7.3.31 *ENICOSTEMA LITTORALE (WHITE HEAD OR NAHI)*

Enicostema littorale, with a common name White head or Nahi, is a fellow of Gentianacae family and widely grown in India, South America, Africa, and other Asian countries (Saranya et al., 2013). It has been used to cure multiple disorders in ancient times. A study was conducted by Prince et al. (2005) in which they investigated anti-hyperglycemic and anti-oxidant potential of aqueous extract of whole plant in AI hyperglycemic rats. They reported that after feeding with aqueous extract for 45 days at a dose of 1,000 and 2,000 mg/kg, blood glucose levels were significantly dropped, antioxidant enzyme activities were increased, and most effective dosage was found to be 2,000 mg/kg (Prince et al., 2005). In another study, two types of aqueous extract (hot and cold) were used for treatment of STZ-I hyperglycemic rats. Hot aqueous extract (1,000 and 2,000 mg/kg) clearly lowered the serum glucose, total cholesterol, triglycerides, but hot aqueous extract at 500 mg/kg only lowered the serum glucose and triglycerides. Swertiamarin was discovered to be one of the major components of hot aqueous extract which was responsible for anti-hyperglycemic activity of hot extract (Vishwakarma et al., 2010).

7.3.32 *ERIOBOTRYA JAPONICA (LOQUAT)*

Eriobotrya japonica, with a common name loquat, is belongs to Rosaceae family. It is natively from cooler hill China to southern China but also quite common in Japan, Himachal, Korea, Potohar, and foot hill region of Pakistan. Sesquiterpene glycoside isolated from dried leaves has shown to possess anti-hyperglycemic effect in alloxan-induced mice models at a dosage of 0.025 and 0.075 g/kg b.w. (Chen et al., 2008). Anti hyperglycemic and anti-hyperlipidemic activity of ethanol extract of *E. japonica* was observed in AI albino rats with a dosage of 200 mg/kg of body weight (Shafi et al., 2013).

7.3.33 *GLYCYRRHIZA GLABRA (LIQUORICE)*

Glycyrrhiza glabra with common name liquorice, is a fellow of Fabaceae family. It is an herbaceous perennial plant, native of Middle East, southern

Europe and part of Asia such as India. Sweetness in liquorice comes from the compound glycyrrhizin present in *G. glabra*. Anti-hyperglycemic effect of liquorice is attributed to glycyrrhizic acid and glycyrrhizin present in roots. Glycyrrhizic acid has been reported to improve the insulin sensitivity, enhanced lipoprotein lipase expression in subcutaneous and visceral adipose tissue, kidney, and heart, it also shows reduction in serum levels of fatty acid, LDL, total cholesterol and lipid deposition in insulin independent hyperglycemic rat tissue (Eu et al., 2010). In another study, glycyrrhizin has been shown to possess anti-hyperglycemic activity by enhancing serum insulin level, reinforcing antioxidant function in diabetic rats and by improving pancreatic and kidney tissue in STZ-I hyperglycemic rats (Sen et al., 2011). Rani et al. (2017) used nanoformulations or nanoparticles loaded with glycyrrhizin or metaformin and tested in vivo for their anti-hyperglycemic activity against type-II diabetes in rats and results proved a significant decrease in serum blood glucose levels (Rani et al., 2017).

7.3.34   HYPOXIS HEMEROCALLIDEA (AFRICAN POTATO)

Hypoxis hemerocallidea, with a vernacular name African potato, is a fellow of Hypoxidaceae family, and indigenous to South Africa, Zimbabwe, and Mozambique. African potato aqueous extract has been investigated for antinociceptive, anti-inflammatory, and anti-hyperglycemic activity in rats and mice. This extract at a dose of 0.050–0.8 g/kg b.w. produced significant hypoglycemia in normal as well as glycemic rats (John, 2006). In another study, aqueous extract of *H. hemerocallidea* at a dose of 0.2 and 0.8 g/kg body weight was used for treatment of STZ hyperglycemic rats. It was observed that both dosages resulted in decrease blood glucose but 0.8 g/kg dose resulted in rectification of liver enzymes activity and elevation in FRAP and catalase activities in kidney thus showing anti-hyperglycemic, antioxidative, and reduction in oxidative stress (Oguntibeju et al., 2016).

7.3.35   JUNIPERUS COMMUNIS (JUNIPER BERRY)

Juniperus communis, commonly known as juniper berry, is a member of Cupressaceae family, and widely grown in North America, Asia, and Europe. It is a small coniferous plant or shrub and has anti-hyperglycemic and anti-hyperlipidemic potential. Sánchez de Medina et al. (1994) reported that juniper decoction at a dosage of 0.25 g/kg, significantly decreased glucose levels in normoglycemic rats and a dosage of 125 mg/kg was efficient for STZ-I hyperglycemic rats. They suggested that the hypoglycemic effect of juniper can be due to either an increase in peripheral glucose consumption or a potentiation of glucose-induced insulin secretion (Sánchez et al., 1994). Methanolic extract of juniper has been evaluated against type 2 diabetes in streptozotocin nicotinamide induced (STZN-I) hyperglycemic rats. A significant reduction in blood glucose level along with different lipid profile parameters was reported (Banerjee et al., 2013).

7.3.36   *LEPIDIUM SATIVUM (GARDEN CRESS)*

Lepidium sativum, with common name garden cress, belongs to Brassicaceae family and normally grown in France, England, Scandinavia, and Netherlands. Methanolic extract of *L. sativum* 20% (w/w) was shown to be able to induce hypoglycemia in STZ-I hyperglycemic rats and also it was observed that various parameters associated with diabetes like high lipid peroxidation, serum uric acid, creatinine, LDL, etc., were reversed and brought to normal levels (Qusti et al., 2016). In another study, methanolic extract of garden cress seeds, treatment was given to AI hyperglycemic rats for four weeks and it was found that restoration of several parameters like triglycerides levels, HbA1c, LDL, and many others. It also ameliorated lipid profile and increased antioxidants concentrations (Attia et al., 2017).

7.3.37   *MANGIFERA INDICA (MANGO)*

Mangifera indica with a common name mango is included in Anacardiaceae family and indigenous to Indian Subcontinent. Ethanolic extract of leaves of *M. indica* has shown to possess anti-hyperglycemic potential in AI hyperglycemic rats as it is intake in diabetic rat's led to reduction in blood glucose, triglycerides, total cholesterol, creatinine, and other diabetic associated parameters (Kemasari et al., 2011). Aqueous and methanolic extract of seed kernels of mango also possesses anti-hyperglycemic activity as shown by Rajesh et al. (2014). They reported that 0.2 g/kg b.w. of these extracts effectively decreased FBG levels and thus can be used for diabetic treatment (Rajesh et al., 2014). Mango peel extract at 5 and 10% concentration in basal diet in hyperglycemic rats have shown to exert not only hypoglycemic activity in diabetic rats but also increased antioxidant enzyme activities and reduction of lipid peroxidation in serum, kidney, and liver (Gondi et al., 2014).

7.3.38   MOMORDICA CHARANTIA (BITTER GOURD)

Momordica charantia, with common name bitter gourd, is a member of Cucurbitaceae family and grown in Asia, Africa, and the Caribbean for its edible fruit. It is a tropical and subtropical vine and has been used as an herbal medicine in Asian and African countries from a long time. Triterpene, protein, steroid, alkaloids, lipids, and phenolic compounds present in bitter gourd are responsible for its anti-diabetic potential (Saeed et al., 2010). *M. charantia* has been shown to possess anti-hyperglycemic and anti-oxidant activity in AI hyperglycemic rats. Treatment of diabetic rats for 30 days with aqueous extract of bitter gourd and seed powder of *T. foenum-graecum* showed significant reduction in FBG level (p<0.001) (Tripathi et al., 2010). Ahmed et al. (2004) have investigated role of bitter gourd which showed improved insulin secretion in STZ-I hyperglycemic rats. They confirmed the secretion of insulin through beta cells after administration of bitter gourd orally by using immunohistochemical methods (Ahmed et al., 2004). Potential of bitter gourd as an anti-hyperglycemic agent in type 1 Diabetes male Wister rats was investigated using plasmatic cytokine quantification. It was shown that by decreasing high blood glucose, bitter gourd juice prompted a favorable phenotypic shift from proinflammatory Th1 towards an anti-inflammatory Th2 status in T1D rats as it consists of anti-oxidant components in its juice (Fachinan et al., 2017).

7.3.39   NIGELLA SATIVA (BLACK CARAWAY)

Nigella sativa, commonly known as black caraway or kalonji, is included in Ranunculaceae family and indigenous to South and Southwest Asia. Its seeds are being used as a spicing agent in Indian cuisine. Long term anti-hyperglycemic effect of *N. sativa* was investigated in insulin independent hyperglycemic patients by Kaatabi et al. (2015). Treatment with *N. sativa* was given orally at a dosage of 2 g daily for 1 year in addition to the standard medications. FBG levels, HbA1c, anti-oxidative enzyme activities were measured at the baseline and every 3 months for comparison. It was reported that hypoglycemic effect was seen in the patients and insulin resistance were too lowered in treated patients and also anti-oxidant defense mechanism as well as beta cell activity was enhanced (Kaatabi et al., 2015). In another study on STZ-I diabetic rats, 20% (w/w) methanolic extract of *N. sativa* resulted in significant reduction in several parameters associated with diabetes like blood glucose levels, lipid peroxidation, and others and improved anti-oxidant defense mechanism (El Rabey et al., 2017). *N. sativa* oil contains thymoquinone and has shown to exert positive effects in STZ-I hyperglycemic rats by ameliorating FBG levels and improving insulin secretion (Heba et al., 2018).

7.3.40   OCIMUM SANCTUM (HOLY BASIL OR TULSI)

Ocimum sanctum or Ocimum tenuiflorum with a vernacular name Holy Basil or Tulsi, is a fellow of Lamiaceae family. It is indigenous to Indian Subcontinent and is cultivated throughout the Southeast Asian tropics. Aqueous extract of *O. sanctum* at a dosage of 0.3 g/kg body weight has been investigated for its anti-hyperglycemic potential in AI hyperglycemic rats and it was found that treatment resulted in significant lowering in blood glucose levels from 345 to 263 mg/dL and it also exerted insulin sensitization (Raja et al., 2015). In another study, five different extracts (hexane, water, methanol, ethyl acetate and chloroform) were prepared and their anti-hyperglycemic potential was tested in STZ-I hyperglycemic rats. It was found that methanolic extract (acute dosage of 1 g/kg) resulted in 31% reduction in FBG levels, methanol, and hexane extracts shown similarity with metformin in sub-cutaneous glucose tolerance test and after 2 weeks, both of these extracts resulted in 63.33% FBG reduction (Mousavi et al., 2016).

7.3.41   ORIGANIUM VULGARE (OREGANO)

Origanium vulgare, commonly known as Oregano, is included in Lamiaceae family, and indigenous to Southwestern Eurasia, temperate Western and the Mediterranean region. In STZ-I hyperglycemic rats, an aqueous extract of *O. vulgare* leaves (20 mg/kg) leads to significant decrease in blood sugar, glycosylated hemoglobin, and pancreatic amylase as compare with treatment with standard drug glibenclamide (Mohamed et al., 2013). In another study, potential of aqueous as well as methanolic extract of oregano leaves was determined against type 1 diabetes. Methanolic extract as compare to aqueous extract resulted in reduction of diabetic incidence and preservation of normal insulin secretion in the body in C57BL/6 mice. Methanolic extract reduced the requirement of up-regulation of antioxidant enzymes, prevented beta cells to undergo apoptosis via blocking caspase 3 and a compound rosmarinic acid in methanolic extract resulted in partial protection from diabetes (Vujicic et al., 2015).

7.3.42   PHYLLANTHU SAMARAS (JANGLI AMLA)

Phyllanthus amarus, commonly known as jangli amla in Hindi has many vernacular names in other countries. Itis a member of Euphorbiacea family and native to Caribbean area and has been distributed to tropical as well as subtropical region in the world (Webster, 1957). It has been reported that 0.2 g/kg b.w. dosage of aqueous extract of *P. amarus* resulted in anti-hypergly-cemic, anti-hyperlipidemic, and antioxidant activity in STZ-I hyperglycemic rats. It also ameliorated renal problems associated with diabetes as well as helped in body weight correction in diabetic rats (Karuna et al., 2011). Ethanolic extract of *P. amarus,* when fed orally to AI hyperglycemic rats for 45 days at a dosage of 0.4 g/kg/body weight, resulted in amelioration of blood glucose levels and improvement in the body weight of rats. Activities of phosphatases (glucose-6, and fructose-1,6) was found to be lowered while GK activity was observed to be increased in the treated rats (Shetti et al., 2012).

7.3.43   PRANGOS FERULACEA (COMMON BASILISK)

Prangos ferulacea with a common name common basilisk is a fellow of Apiaceae family, and a perennial herbaceous plant mainly found in Italy and Mediterranean basin. It is used in TMs to cure inflammation and diabetes as its extracts consist of monoterpenes compounds like sesquiterpenes, flavo-noids, coumarins, saponins, tannins, alkaloids, terpenoids, etc. When 0.1 g/kg dosage of hydro-alcoholic extract of *Pragnos* root was given to hypergly-cemic rats, it was observed that extract resulted in lowering of blood glucose, LDL, total cholesterol and an improvement in HDL levels. It also reversed liver and kidney damages in diabetic rats as well as adjusted the white blood cells (WBCs) number to normal (Kafash-Farkhad et al., 2013). In another study with hydro-alcoholic extract (0.3 and 0.5 g/kg), it was shown that there was remarkable decrease in blood glucose levels, LDL, total cholesterol, triglycerides, and improvement in lipid profile and body weight in STZ-I hyperglycemic rats (Mohammadi et al., 2013).

7.3.44 *PTEROCARPUS MARSUPIUM (INDIAN KINO TREE)*

Pterocarpus marsupium with a vernacular name Indian kino tree or vijayasar, is a fellow of Fabaceae family, and a deciduous tree endemic to India in Western Ghats in Karnataka-Kerala region and the central India, Nepal, and Sri Lanka. Manickam et al. (1997) reported that phenolic constituents present in the heartwood of *P. marsupium* was responsible for anti-hyperglycemic activity. These major constituents are marsupsin, pterosupin, and pterostilbene. They reported that marsupsin and pterosupin were majorly responsible for hypoglycemic action and sufficiently reduce glucose levels in STZ-I hyperglycemic rats and anti-hypercholestrolemic effect was comparable to metformin, a conventional diabetic drug (Manickam et al., 1997). A study investigated ethanol and aqueous extracts of *P. marsupium* which were prepared by conventional and non-conventional extraction methods. They concluded that ultrasound assisted extraction (UAE) derived extract was more consistent in producing hypoglycemic results in diabetic rats as compared to conventional methods (Devgan et al., 2013).

7.3.45 *PUNICA GRANATUM (POMEGRANATE)*

Punica granatum, commonly known as pomegranate, is a member of Lythraceae family. It is indigenous to Iran and Northern India and widely harvested in Middle East and Caucasus region, Southern, and Central Asia, Northern Africa and many others. Khalil et al. (2004) treated hyperglycemic rats with aqueous peel extract of pomegranate (430 mg/kg body weight) for 4 weeks and found that blood glucose level of diabetic rats considerably reduced and number of beta islet cells were increase due to which it ultimately helps in more insulin secretion. In another study, ethanolic extract of pomegranate leaves at a dose of 0.5 g/kg were given to diabetic rats for 7 days. It was reported that ethanolic extract considerably reduced the blood glucose levels, total cholesterol, triglycerides, LDL, and increased serum HDL (Das et al., 2012). Other studies have been conducted to isolate the phenolic constituents in the peel (Kulkarni et al., 2004; Gil et al., 2000), phytochemical constituents in the fruit rinds (Jain et al., 2012) to decipher the chemical constituent responsible for anti-hyperglycemic activity.

7.3.46 RHUS CORIARIA (SICILIAN OR TANEER'S OR ELMLEAVED SUMAC)

Rhus coriaria, commonly known as sicilian or taneer's or elmleaved sumac, belongs to Anacardiaceae family and endemic to Southern Europe. In a study ethanolic extract of sumac fruit was used and it was observed that single dose resulted in lowering of PBG by 24% and during long run (21 days), 26% reduction in PBG was observed. HDL was raised by 34%, LDL was observed to be lowered by 32% and a significant antioxidant effect was observed (Mohammadi et al., 2010). In another study, a clinical trial was done on 41 insulin independent hyperglycemic volunteers to assess the anti-diabetic potential of sumac powder. A dose of 3 g/day was given to the volunteers for 3 months. A considerable reduction in serum glucose, HbA1c, apoB levels and an increase in apoA-I and total antioxidant activity was reported (Shidfar et al., 2014).

7.3.47 SALACIA RETICULATE (KOTHALAHIMBUTU)

Salacia reticulata, vernaluclar name kothalahimbutu in Sinhalese, belongs to Celastraceae family. It is widely distributed in Asian countries like Sri Lanka, China, Indonesia, India, Vietnam, and others (Anurakumara, 2010). Various constituents responsible for anti-hyperglycemic effect of *Salacia* have been reported which include ponkorinol, salacinol, salaprinol, kotalanol, and their respective de-0-sulphonated compounds (Stohs and Ray, 2015). A study has been conducted on 30 insulin independent hyperglycemic in which 2 g *Salacia* bark powder was given in capsule form for 3 months. A remarkable reduction in FBG, HbA1c and lipid was observed in the patients (Radha et al., 2009). In another randomized, double blind, placebo-controlled study, 29 prehyperglycemic and mildly hyperlipidemic human patients were given leaf or bark aqueous extract (0.5 g/day) for 6 weeks. It was reported that in patients who were given bark extract, blood glucose levels and lipid profiles were lowered in 21 and 42 days and patients who received leaf extract showed lower blood glucose levels only at 42 days (Shivaprasad et al., 2013).

7.3.48 SCOPARIA DULCIS (LICORICE WEED)

Scoparia dulcis, with a common name licorice weed, is a fellow of Plantaginaceae family. It is indigenous to Neotropics but distributed throughout the tropical and subtropical countries. Das and Chakraborty (2011) used aqueous extract of *S. dulcis* in treatment of STZ-I hyperglycemic rats. They administered two dosages 0.125 demonstrated better hypoglycemic activity by decreasing the level of urine sugar and FBG and also improved body weight of rats. In another study with methanolic extract, antidiabetic as well as antioxidant activity of S. *dulcus* was evaluated. In vitro analysis demonstrated that methanolic extract was potent enough to limit the postprandial glucose level and in vivo analysis on STZ-I hyperglycemic rats demonstrated remarkable decrease in blood glucose level against the control as well as glibenclamide (Mishra et al., 2013). A clinical trial with type 2 diabetic patients was performed to evaluate the *S. dulcis* porridge (commercially available) for its hypoglycemic potential. Two groups were made (test and control) and cross overed after first three months to randomize the trial. Test group was given the porridge 3 days/week and control group was let to take any other food. The results showed that in both test groups there was reduction in HbA1c (glycosylated hemoglobin), FBG but no change in cholesterol and insulin (Senadheera et al., 2015).

7.3.49   SILYBUM MARIANUM (MILK THISTLE)

Silybum marianum, with a common name milk thistle is a fellow of Asteraceae family. It is natively from coast of South England has been widely introduced to other parts like North America, Iran, New Zealand and Australia. Milk Thistle got its name because of milky sap released when its leaves are squeezed. Silimarin (flavanoligans), a dried mixture of compounds which consists of silibins (A, B), isosilibins (A, B), taxifolin, silichristin A, silidianin, and other compounds in lesser concentrations, is present in Milk Thistle (Shojaii et al., 2011). Silibin has been shown to act as anti-hyperglycemic and anti-obesitic in SY5Y neuroblastoma cells (acting as an inhibitor of aldose reductase), in dihydroxyacetone perfused rats (by decreasing DHA gluconeogenesis and glucolysis) and recently Isosilibin A was identified as the first PPARγ flavonoglycan agonist (Guigas et al., 2007; Pferschy-Wenzig et al., 2014).

7.3.50   SWERTIA CHIRAYITA (CHIRETTA)

Swertia chirayita with a vernacular name chirettais belongs to Gentianaceae family, and native plant of temperate Himalayas and naturally grown in

India (Himachal Pradesh, Uttarakhand, Sikkim, Sheilong), Nepal, Bhutan, and Myanmar (Kumar et al., 2016). Phoboo et al. (2013) investigated anti-hyperglycemic activity of crude aqueous and 12% ethanol fraction of chiretta collected from nine districts of Nepal. They reported that crude extract not only contains swerchirin but also mangiferin, swertiamarin, and amaro-gentin which were responsible for anti-hyperglycemic potential of chiretta (Phoboo et al., 2012). In another study, effect of *S. chirayita* aqueous bark extract on insulin secretion capability of BRIN-DB11 cell line and protein glycation (using model peptide) was analyzed. It was found that there was concentration dependent stimulation of BRIN-DB11 cells to secrete insulin and also there was inhibition of protein glycation (dose-dependent), thus demonstrating the antidiabetic potential of *S. chirayita* by increasing insulin secretion, enhancing insulin action and preventing protein glycation to counter diabetic complications (Heather-Anne et al., 2014).

7.3.51   TERMINALIA CHEBULA (HIRDA)

Terminalia chebula, with a common name hirda belongs to Combretaceae family. It is indigenous to South Asia (India and Nepal), southwest China, Sri Lanka, Vietnam, and Malaysia. In one study *Terminalia* fruit was used and observed that 80% ethanolic extract was more effective against maltase activity than 50 and 100% ethanol extract. The active constituent found in these extracts was chebulagic acid and it was later observed that the chebulagic acid was responsible for downregulation of maltase activity and when orally given to maltose-loaded Sprague-Dawley rats, it resulted in lowering of postprandial blood glucose by 11.1% (Huang et al., 2012). In another study, methanolic extract of *T. chebula* leaves was investigated for anti-hyperglycemic effect *in vitro* as well as in vivo. It was found that crude extract showed 100% inhibition of alpha glucosidase and when given orally to diabetic rats, resulted in an appreciable decrease in postprandial hyperglycemia as compared to acarbose (standard drug used for diabetes treatment) (Dutta et al., 2018).

7.3.52   TRIGONELLA FOENUM-GRAECUM (FENUGREEK)

Trigonella foenum-graceum commonly known as fenugreek belongs to Fabaceae family and indigenous to Western Asia, Turkey, and Egypt. India is one of the major producers of fenugreek and it is widely used in Indian,

Egyptian, and Turkish cuisine. Ethanol extract of fenugreek at dosage of 1,000 mg/kg in AI hyperglycemic rats has shown hypoglycemic effect (Mowla et al., 2009). Treatment of STZ-I hyperglycemic rats with fenugreek extracts for 6 weeks at middle dose (0.87 g/kg.d) and high dose (1.74 g/kg.d) as compared with Metformin HCL (0.175 g/kg.d) were proven to be beneficial and showed hypoglycemic effect by decreasing glucose levels, triglycerides, plasma viscosity, and cholesterol (Xue et al., 2007). Oral administration of fenugreek seed powder for 21 days at 5% concentration in the diet with 2IU insulin in alloxan-induced diabetic rat were shown to reverse the monoamine oxidase activity and showed neuroprotective effects and increased GLUT4 expression (Kumar et al., 2012).

7.3.53   VINCA ROSEA (MADAGASCAR PERIWINKLE OR SADABAHAR)

Vinca rosea or *Catharanthus roseus,* common name Madagascar periwinkle, is a fellow of Apocynaceae family, and indigenous to Madagascar and widely grown in India, Pakistan, Australia, Malaysia, and Bangladesh. In an *in vivo* study, aqueous extract of *V. rosea* was orally given to AI hyperglycemic rats for one week at a dosage of 0.4 g/kg. It was observed that the extract resulted in a noteworthy lowering in blood glucose level and the results were in par with glibenclamide, 0.01 g/kg (Raja et al., 2008). In another study, methanolic extract was fed to AI hyperglycemic rats for 14 days. It was observed that 0.5 g/kg dose was more efficient than 0.3 g/kg dose in hypoglycemic activity. This extract also ameliorated lipid profile, body weight and regeneration of β islet cells (Ahmed et al., 2010). To explore and elucidate the mechanism of action of anti-hyperglycemic activity, a study with ethanolic extract of Madagascar periwinkle was conducted. It was found that anti hyperglycemic effect was due to the complex mechanism of GLUT gene mRNA expression or amplification (Al-Shaqha et al., 2015).

7.3.54   WITHANIA SOMNIFERA (ASHWAGANDHA OR INDIAN GINSENG)

Withania somnifera with a vernacular name Ashwagandha or Indian Ginseng, belongs to Solanaceae family, and widely grown in dry regions in India, Nepal, China, and Yemen. To investigate the hypoglycemic and hypolipid-emic potential of ashwagandha, Udayakumar et al. (2009) tested roots and leaves extract against glibenclamide in diabetic rats for 8 weeks. After eight weeks of treatment with these two extracts, lowering of urine sugar, blood glucose, HbA1c, transaminases (aspartate, alanine), phosphatases (acid and alkaline), Glucose-6-P and serum lipids and significant increase in HDL (Udayakumar et al., 2009) was found. In another study, 0.0625 g/kg per diet *W. somnifera* were fed to hyperglycemic rats for 8 weeks and glucose, insulin, interleukin-6 and TNF-alpha was measured in blood samples after 56 days. It was reported that ashwagandha ameliorated the glucose, interleukin-6, TNF-alpha, insulin, and homeostasis model assessment for insulin resistance by reducing inflammatory markers and improving insulin sensitivity (Samadi et al., 2015).

7.4   ANTI-HYPERGLYCEMIC PLANTS IN CLINICAL TRAILS

There are many problems and undesirable effects associated with conventional drugs used in the treatment of hyperglycemia such as in case of sulfonylureas (Glibenclamide) weight gain, stomach problems, skin irritations and severe hypoglycemia has been reported (Derosa et al., 2014), biguanides (Metformin) has been associated with renal failures, parageusia, stomach problems and lethargy (Scheen et al., 2013), thus a hyperglycemic treatment with lesser or nil side effects is desired. As medicinal plants do not have such undesirable effects, drug formulations from these plants can be a major game changer in diabetes treatment. Some plants which are in clinical trials include *Nigella sativa* (Oil at 2 gm daily dosage), *Cichorium intybus* (with other plants formulations as herbal tea), *Balanites aegyptiaca, Melissa officinalis,* etc. In Ghana, bark, and root of *Momordica charantia* (Ooi et al., 2012), *Cinnamomum zeylanicum* (Altschuler et al., 2007) aqueous extract of *Allium sepa, Allium sativum, Guiera senegalensis* (Gaber et al., 2013) *Zingiber officinale* (Hass, 2015), bulb, and, capsule extract of *Allium sativum* (Shoshi and Akter, 2017) are some medicinal plants which are in clinical trials against hyperglycemia. Goh et al. (2014) used resveratrol from *Polygonum cuspidatum,* in patients having type 2 diabetes mellitus. They found that resveratrol increased skeletal muscle SIRT1 and AMPK expression and prevents diabetes. Rahimi et al. (2016) performed a clinical trial in T2DM patients for a period of 3 months where they evaluated curcumin nanomicelles (80 mg/ day) for anti-hyperglycemic activity and found significant reduction in HbA1c level as well as TAG, TC, and BMI. Giuseppe et al. (2017) evaluates efficacy and safety of *Berberis aristata* and *Silybum marianum* against 143 patients for 3 months and found reduction of lipid profile, decrease of triglycerides, total cholesterol and low-density lipoprotein. Rashad et al. (2017) used *Balanites aegyptiaca,* which was incorporated in hard gelatin capsules (400 mg/day) and given to 30 type 2 diabetes patients (Egyptian) for 8 weeks. It was found that there was considerable reduction in total cholesterol, plasma triglyceride, and LDL and enhancement in HDL. Asadi et al. (2018) did clinical assessment of hydroalcoholic extract of *M. officinalis* in type 2 diabetic patient for its potential antidiabetic properties.

7.5 CONCLUSION AND FUTURE PERSPECTIVES

Diabetes or hyperglycemia is a multifaceted metabolic disorder which affects kidney (renal failure), heart, lipid peroxidation and eyes (blindness) and it is a dreadful disorder which is detrimental to human health. The major causes of various types of diabetes include lifestyle changes, molecular genetic factors, etc. There are many undesirable effects associated with standard drug used in the treatment of diabetes like nausea, diarrhea, stomach upset or weight gain. Glibenclamide and metformin solely or in combination can cause many side effects in the body. Thus, there is a need of a treatment which is more beneficial or as par beneficial to the standard drugs and produce less side effects and should be less toxic to the body.

Herbal plants which have been studied so far for anti-hyperglycemic potential have mostly the same mechanism to ameliorate diabetics malfunctioning. They might act by improving histology of pancreas and thus improve insulin secretion in the body, they might relieve oxidative stress occurred due to diabetes by enhancing anti-oxidant enzyme activities, they might lead to upregulating or down regulating some molecular factors associated with diabetes, they may act on alpha-glucosidase or lead to renal correction. The majority of plants studied so far have led to the amelioration of diabetic symptoms and if prolonged treatment is given, it would be safer than the standard drugs and results would also be more beneficial. There is no requirement of the whole plant for the production of potential drugs as the main compound associated with anti-diabetic factors are present in specific parts of the plants like seeds, oils, leaves, roots or fruits and in some cases peel too. Many of these plants consist of flavonoids, tannins, phenolic, and alkaloids fractions which are majorly responsible for their anti-hyperglycemic, anti-oxidative, anti-hyperlipidemic, anti-hypercholestrolimic, and nephron healing action. Thus, the main task for researchers is to make a potential drug from these herbal plants. Two approaches can be taken, first is to use tissue culture and culture the plant specific parts for the compound isolation and second is to chemically synthesize the compound responsible for anti-diabetic property which would be similar in structure as well as function to the natural herbal product.

KEYWORDS

- **fasting blood glucose**
- **gestational diabetes mellitus**
- **hyperglycemic**
- **maturity-onset diabetes of the young**
- **oral glucose tolerance test**
- **phytocompounds**

REFERENCES

Abdelrazek, H., Kilany, O. E., Muhammad, M. A., Tag, H. M., & Abdelazim, A. M., (2018). Black seed thymoquinone improved insulin secretion, hepatic glycogen storage, and oxidative stress in streptozotocin-induced diabetic male Wistar rats. *Oxid. Med. Cell Longev.*

Ahangarpour, A., & Oroojan, A. A., (2013). Effect of crust and seed hydro-alcoholic and aqueous extracts and pulp hydro-alcoholic extract of *Citrullus colocynthis* on glucose, insulin and FIRI level in insulin resistant male rat's. *Horizon Med. Sci., 19*(3), 149–154.

Ahangarpour, A., Zamaneh, H. T., Jabari, A., Nia, H. M., & Heidari, H., (2014). Antidiabetic and hypolipidemic effects of doremaaucherihydroalcoholic leave extract in streptozotocin-nicotinamide induced type 2 diabetes in male rats. *Iran J. Basic Med. Sci., 17*(10), 808–814.

Ahmadi, S., Rostamzadeh, J., Khosravi, D., Shariati, P., & Shakiba, N., (2013). Association of CTLA-4 gene 49A/G polymorphism with the incidence of type 1 diabetes mellitus in the Iranian Kurdish population. *Pak. J. Biol. Sci., 16*, 1929–1935.

Ahmed, I., Cummings, E., Sharma, A. K., Adeghate, E., & Singh, J., (2004). Beneficial effects and mechanism of action of *Momordica charantia* fruit juice in the treatment of streptozotocin-induced diabetes mellitus in rats. *Mol. Cell Biochem., 261*, 63–70.

Ahmed, M. F., Kazim, S. M., Ghori, S. S., Mehjabeen, S. S., Ahmed, S. R., Ali, S. M., & Ibrahim, M., (2010). Antidiabetic activity of vincarosea extracts in alloxan-induced diabetic rats. *Int. J. Endocrinol.*, 1–6.

Alam, P., Shahzad, N., Gupta, A. K., Mahfoz, A. M., Bamagous, G. A., Al-Ghamdi, S. S., & Siddiqui, N. A., (2018). Anti-diabetic effect of *Boerhavia diffusa* L. root extract via free radical scavenging and antioxidant mechanism. *Toxicol. Environ. Health Sci., 10*(3), 220–227.

Al-Shaqha, W. M., Khan, M., Salam, N., Azzi, A., & Chaudhary, A. A., (2015). Anti-diabetic potential of *Catharanthus roseus* Linn. and its effect on the glucose transport gene (GLUT-2 and GLUT-4) in streptozotocin induced diabetic Wistar rats. *BMC complementary and Alternative Medicine, 15*, 379.

American Diabetes Association, (2014). Diagnosis and classification of diabetes mellitus. *Diabetes Care, 37*(1), S81–S90.

Anand, P., Murali, K. Y., Tandon, V., Chandra, R., & Murthy, P. S., (2007). Preliminary studies on antihyperglycemic effect of aqueous extract of *Brassica nigra* (L.) Koch in streptozotocin induced diabetic rats. *Indian J. Exp. Biol., 45*, 696–701.

Ananthi, J., Prakasam, A., & Pugalendi, K. V., (2003). Antihyperglycemic activity of *Eclipta alba* leaf on alloxan-induced diabetic rats. *Yale J. Biol. Med., 76*(3), 97–102.

Ansari, A., Shahriar, M. S. Z., Hassan, M. M., Das, S. R., Rokeya, B., Haque, M. A., Haque, M. E., Biswas, N., & Sarkar, T., (2014). *Emblica officinalis* improves glycemic status and oxidative stress in STZ induced type 2 diabetic model rats. *Asian Pac. J. Trop. Med., 7*(1), 21–25.

Ansari, P., Afroz, N., Jalil, S., Azad, S. B., Mustakim, M. G., Anwar, S., Haque, S. M. N., et al., (2017). Anti-hyperglycemic activity of *Aegle marmelos* (L.) corr. is partly mediated by increased insulin secretion, α-amylase inhibition, and retardation of glucose absorption. *J. Pediatr. Endocrinol. Metab., 30*(1), 37–47.

Attia, E. S., Amer, A. H., & Hasanein, M. A., (2017). The hypoglycemic and antioxidant activities of garden cress (Lepidiumsativum L.) seed on alloxan-induced diabetic male rats. *Nat Prod Res., 1–5*.

Augusti, K. T., & Shella, C. G., (1996). Antiperoxide effect of s-allylcysteine sulfoxide, an insulin secretagogue in diabetic rats. *Experientia, 52*, 115–120.

Ayodhya, S., Kusum, S., & Anjali, S., (2010). Hypoglycaemic activity of different extracts of various herbal plants Singh. *Int J Ayurveda Res Pharm., 1*(1), 212–224.

Azay-Milhau, J., Ferrare, K., Leroy, J., Aubaterre, J., Tournier, M., Lajoix, A. D., & Tousch, D., (2013). Antihyperglycemic effect of a natural chicoric acid extract of chicory (Cichoriumintybus L.): A comparative in vitro study with the effects of caffeic and ferulic acids. *J Ethnopharmacol., 150*(2), 755–760.

Banerjee, S., Singh, H., & Chatterjee, T. K., (2013). Evaluation of anti-diabetic and anti-hyperlipidemic potential of methanolic extract of *Juniperus communis* (L.) in streptozotocin-nicotinamide induced diabetic rats. *International Journal of Pharma and Bio Sciences, 4*(3), 10–17.

Ben-Chioma, A. E., Tamuno-Emine, D. G., & Dan, D. B., (2015). The effect of Abelmoschus esculentus in alloxan-induced diabetic Wistar rat. *International Journal of Science and Research, 4*(11), 540–543.

Bennett, C. L., Christie, J., Ramsdell, F., Brunkow, M. E., Ferguson, P. J., Whitesell, L., Kelly, T. E., et al., (2001). The immune dysregulation, polyendocrinopathy, enteropathy, X-linked syndrome (IPEX) is caused by mutations of FOXP3. *Nat. Genet., 27*, 20, 21.

Bhavsar, C., & Talele, G. S., (2013). Potential anti-diabetic activity of Bombax ceiba. *Bangladesh J. Pharmacol., 8*(2), 102–106.

Bhide, S. S., Maurya, M. R., Gajbhiye, S. V., & Tadavi, F. M., (2017). Evaluation of nephroprotective effect of *Bryonia lacinosa* on streptozotocin induced diabetic nephropathy in rats. *Int. J. Basic Clin. Pharmacol., 6*, 1193–1200.

Bordone, L., Motta, M. C., Picard, F., Robinson, A., Jhala, U. S., Apfeld, J., McDonagh, T., et al., (2006). Sirt1 regulates insulin secretion by repressing UCP2 in pancreatic beta cells. *PLoS Biol., 4*(2), e31.

Buchanan, T. A., Xiang, A. H., & Page, K. A., (2012). Gestational diabetes mellitus: Risks and management during and after pregnancy. *Nat. Rev. Endocrinol., 8*(11), 639–649.

Catalano, P. M., Tyzbir, E. D., & Sims, E. A. H., (1990). Incidence and significance of islet cell antibodies in women with previous gestational diabetes. *Diabetes Care, 13*, 478–482.

Chávez-Silva, F., Cerón-Romero, L., Arias-Durán, L., Navarrete-Vázquez, G., Almanza-Pérez, J., Román-Ramos, R., Ramírez-Ávila, G., Perea-Arango, I., Villalobos-Molina, R., & Estrada-Soto, S., (2017). Antidiabetic effect of *Achillea millefollium* through multitarget interactions: α-glucosidases inhibition, insulin sensitization and insulin secretagogue activities. *J. Ethnopharmacol., 212*, 1–7.

Chen, J., Li, W. L., Wu, J. L., Ren, B. R., & Zhang, H. Q., (2008). Hypoglycemic effects of a sesquiterpene glycoside isolated from leaves of loquat (*Eriobotrya japonica* (Thunb.) Lindl.). *Phytomedicine, 15*(1, 2), 98–102.

Corzo-Martínez, M. C. N., (2007). Biological properties of onions and garlic. *Trends Food Sci. Technol., 18*(12), 609–625.

Da Silva, X. G., Loder, M. K., McDonald, A., Tarasov, A. I., Carzaniga, R., Kronenberger, K., & Rutter, G. A., (2009). TCF7L2 regulates late events in insulin secretion from pancreatic islet β-cells. *Diabetes, 58*(4), 894–905.

Das, H., & Chakraborty, U., (2011). Anti-hyperglycemic effect of *Scoparia dulcis* in streptozotocin induced diabetes. *Res. J. Pharm. Biol. Chem. Sci., 2*, 334–342.

Das, S., & Barman, S., (2012). Antidiabetic and antihyperlipidemic effects of ethanolic extract of leaves of *Punica granatum* in alloxan-induced non-insulin-dependent diabetes mellitus albino rats. *Indian J. Pharmacol., 44*(2), 219–224.

Derosa, G., Limas, C. P., Macías, P. C., Estrella, A., & Maffioli, P., (2014). Dietary and nutraceutical approach to type 2 diabetes. *Arch. Med. Sci., 10*, 336–344.

Devendra, D., Liu, E., & Eisenbarth, G. S., (2004). Type 1 diabetes: Recent developments. *British Medical Journal-BMJ., 328*, 750–754.

Devgan, M., Nanda, A., & Ansari, S. H., (2013). Comparative evaluation of the anti-diabetic activity of *Pterocarpus marsupium* roxb. heartwood in alloxan induced diabetic rats using extracts obtained by optimized conventional and non conventional extraction methods. *Pak. J. Pharm. Sci., 26*(5), 973–976.

Dolui, A., & Segupta, R., (2012). Antihyperglycemic effect of different solvent extracts of leaves of *Cajanus cajan* HPLC profile of the active extracts. *Asian J. Pharm. Clinical Res., 5*, 116–119.

Dupuis, J., Langenberg, C., Prokopenko, I., Saxena, R., Soranzo, N., Jackson, A. U., & Lindgren, C. M., (2010). New genetic loci implicated in fasting glucose homeostasis and their impact on type 2 diabetes risk. *Nat. Genet., 42*, 105–116. https://doi.org/10.1038/ng0510-464a.

Dutta, J., & Kalita, M. C., (2018). Anti-hyperglycemic evaluation of *Terminalia chebula* leaves. *Int. J. Pharm Pharm. Sci., 10*(11), 43–48.

Earnest, E. O., Lawrence, E., & Ilevbare, F. R., (2013). The roles of capsicum in diabetes mellitus. *Wilolud J., 6*, 22–27.

Eidi, A., Eidi, M., & Esmaeili, E., (2006). Antidiabetic effect of garlic (Allium sativum L.) in normal and streptozotocin-induced diabetic rats. *Phytomed., 13*(9), 624–629.

Eirís, N., González-Lara, L., Santos-Juanes, J., Queiro, R., Coto, E., & Coto-Segura, P., (2014). Genetic variation at IL12B, IL23R and IL23A is associated with psoriasis severity, psoriatic arthritis and type 2 diabetes mellitus. *J. Dermatol. Sci., 75*, 167–172.

El Rabey, H, A., Al-Seeni, M. N., & Bakhashwain, A. S., (2017). The antidiabetic activity of *Nigella sativa* and propolis on streptozotocin-induced diabetes and diabetic nephropathy in male rats. *Evid. Based Complement. Alternat. Med.*, 5439645.

ErfaniMajd, N., Tabandeh, M. R., Shahriari, A., & Soleimani, Z., (2018). Okra (abelmoscusesculentus) improved islets structure, and down-regulated PPARs gene expression in pancreas of high-fat diet and streptozotocin-induced diabetic rats. *Cell J., 20*(1), 31–40.

Eu, C. H., Lim, W. Y., Ton, S. H., & Bin, A. K. K., (2010). Glycyrrhizic acid improved lipoprotein lipase expression, insulin sensitivity, serum lipid and lipid deposition in high-fat diet-induced obese rats. *Lipids Health Dis., 9*, 81.

Fachinan, R., Yessoufou, A., Nekoua, M. P., & Moutairou, K., (2017). Effectiveness of antihyperglycemic effect of *Momordica charantia*: Implication of t-cell cytokines. *Evid, Based Complement, Alternat. Med.*, *2017*.

Ferrare, K., Bidel, L. P., Awwad, A., Poucheret, P., Cazals, G., Lazennec, F., Azay-Milhau, J., et al., (2018). Increase in insulin sensitivity by the association of chicoric acid and chlorogenic acid contained in a natural chicoric acid extract (NCRAE) of chicory (Cichoriumintybus L.) for an antidiabetic effect. *J. Ethnopharmacol., 215*, 241–248.

Flannick, J., Thorleifsson, G., Beer, N. L., Jacobs, S. B., Grarup, N., Burtt, N. P., & Blangero, J., (2014). Loss-of-function mutations in SLC30A8 protect against type 2 diabetes. *Nat. Genet., 46*, 357–363.

Ghate, R., Patil, V. P., Hugar, S., Matha, N. H., & Kalyane, N. V., (2014). Antihyperglycemic activity of *Areca Catechu* flowers.*Asian Pac. J. Trop. Dis., 4*, S148–S152.

Ginsberg, H., Kimmerling, G., Olefsky, J. M., & Reaven, G. M., (1975). Demonstration of insulin resistance in untreated adult onset diabetic subjects with fasting hyperglycemia. *J. Clin. Invest., 55*(3), 454–461.

Giuseppe, D., Angela, D. A., Davide, R., & Pamela, M., (2017). Effects of a combination of berberis aristata, silybummarianum and monacolin on lipid profile in subjects at low cardiovascular risk; a double-blind, randomized, placebo-controlled trial. *Int. J. Mol. Sci., 18*(2), 343.

Goh, K. P., Lee, H. Y., Lau, D. P., Supaat, W., Chan, Y. H., & Koh, A. F., (2014). Effects of resveratrol in patients with type 2 diabetes mellitus on skeletal muscle SIRT1 expression and energy expenditure. *Int. J. Sport Nutr. Exerc. Metab., 24*(1), 2–13.

Gondi, M., Basha, S. A., Bhaskar, J. J., Salimath, P. V., & Rao, U. J., (2014). Anti-diabetic effect of dietary mango (Mangiferaindica L.) peel in streptozotocin-induced diabetic rats. *J. Sci. Food Agric., 95*(5), 991–999.

Guigas, B., Naboulsi, R., Villanueva, G. R., Taleux, N., Lopez-Novoa, J. M., Leverve, X. M., & El-Mir, L. Y., (2007). The flavonoid silibinin decreases glucose-6-phosphate hydrolysis in perifused rat hepatocytes by an inhibitory effect on glucose-6-phosphatase. *Cell Physiol. Biochem., 20*(6), 925–934.

Gunness, P., & Gidley, M. J., (2010). Mechanisms underlying the cholesterol lowering properties of soluble dietary fibre polysaccharides. *Food Funct., 1*(2), 149–155.

Haidari, F., Seyed-Sadjadi, N., Taha-Jalali, M., & Mohammed-Shahi, M., (2011). The effect of oral administration of *Carum carvi* on weight, serum glucose, and lipid profile in streptozotocin-induced diabetic rats. *Saudi Med. J., 32*(7), 695–700.

Haller, K., Kisand, K., Pisarev, H., Salur, L., Laisk, T., Nemvalts, V., & Uibo, R., (2007). Insulin gene VNTR, CTLA-4 +49A/G and HLA-DQB1 alleles distinguish latent autoimmune diabetes in adults from type 1 diabetes and from type 2 diabetes group. *Tissue Antigens, 69*, 121–127.

Hashmat, I., Azad, H., & Ahmed, A., (2012). Neem (*Azadirachta indica* A. Juss)-A nature's drugstore: An overview. *Int. Res. J. Biol. Sci., 1*, 76–79.

Hegazy, G. A., Alnoury, A. M., & Gad, H. G., (2013). The role of Acacia Arabica extract as an antidiabetic, antihyperlipidemic, and antioxidant in streptozotocin-induced diabetic rats. *Saudi Med. J., 34*(7), 727–733.

Hema, L. E., Satyanarayana, T., Ramesh, A., Durga, P. Y., Routhu, K., & Srinivas, R. L., (2008). Hypoglycemic and antihyperglycemic effect of *Argyreiaspeciosa* sweet in normal and in alloxan induced diabetic rats. *J. Nat. Rem., 8*, 203–208.

Horikawa, Y., Oda, N., Cox, N. J., Li, X., Orho-Melander, M., Hara, M., & Bosque-Plata, L. D, (2000). Genetic variation in the gene encoding calpain-10 is associated with type 2 diabetes mellitus. *Nat Genet., 26*, 163–175.

Huang, Y. N., Zhao, D. D., Gao, B., Zhong, K., Zhu, R. X., Zhang, Y., Xie, W. J., et al., (2012). Anti-hyperglycemic effect of chebulagic acid from the fruits of terminalia *Chebula Retz. Int. J. Mol. Sci., 13*(5), 6320–6333.

Huseini, H. F., Kianbakht, S., Hajiaghaee, R., & Dabaghian, F. H., (2011). Anti-hyperglycemic and anti-hypercholesterolemic effects of Aloe vera leaf gel in hyperlipidemic type 2 diabetic patients: A randomized double-blind placebo-controlled clinical trial. *Planta Med., 78*(4), 311–316.

Jain, V., Viswanatha, G. L., Manohar, D., & Shivaprasad, H. N., (2012). Isolation of antidiabetic principle from fruit rinds of *Punica granatum. Evid. Based Complementary Altern. Med., 2012*, 1–11.

Jaiswal, N., Bhatia, V., Srivastava, S. P., Srivastava, A. K., & Tamrakar, A. K., (2012). Antidiabetic effect of *Eclipta alba* associated with the inhibition of alpha-glucosidase and aldose reductase. *Nat. Prod. Res., 26*(24), 2363–2367.

Jana, K., Chatterjee, K., Ali, K. M., De, D., Bera, T. K., & Ghosh, D., (2012). Antihyperglycemic and antioxidative effects of the hydro-methanolic extract of the seeds of *Caesalpinia bonduc* on streptozotocin-induced diabetes in male albino rats. *Pharmacognosy Res., 4*(1), 57–62.

Kaatabi, H., Bamosa, A. O., Badar, A., Al-Elq, A., Abou-Hozaifa, B., Lebda, F., Al-Khadra, A., & Al-Almaie, S., (2015). *Nigella sativa* improves glycemic control and ameliorates oxidative stress in patients with type 2 diabetes mellitus: Placebo controlled participant blinded clinical trial. *PLoS One, 10*(2), e0113486.

Kafash-Farkhad, N., Asadi-Samani, M., & Khaledifar, B., (2013). A review on secondary metabolites and pharmacological effects of *Prangos ferulacea* (L.) Lindl. *J. Shahrekord Univ. Med. Sci., 15*(3), 98–108.

Karuna, R., Bharathi, V. G., Reddy, S. S., Ramesh, B., & Saralakumari, D., (2011). Protective effects of phyllanthusamarus aqueous extract against renal oxidative stress in Streptozotocin -induced diabetic rats. *Indian J Pharmacol., 43*(4), 414–418.

Kemasari, P., Sangeetha, S., & Venkatalakshmi, P., (2011). Antihyperglycemic activity of Mangiferaindicalinn. In alloxan induced diabetic rats. *J. Chem. Pharm. Res., 3*, 653–659.

Kesari, A. N., Gupta, R. K., Singh, S. K., Diwakar, S., & Watal, G., (2006). Hypoglycemic and antihyperglycemic activity of *Aegle marmelos* seed extract in normal and diabetic rats. *J Ethnopharmacol., 107*(3), 374–379.

Khalil, E. A. M., (2004). Antidiabetic effect of an aqueous extract of pomegranate (*Punicagranatum* L.) peels in normal and alloxan diabetic rats. *Egypt. J. Hosp. Med., 16*(1), 92–99.

Kharroubi, A. T., & Darwish, H. M., (2015). Diabetes mellitus: The epidemic of the century. *World Journal of Diabetes, 6*(6), 850–867.

Kim, S. H., & Choung, S. Y., (2010). Antihyperglycemic and antihyperlipidemic action of *Cinnamomi cassiae* (Cinnamon bark) extract in C57BL/Ks db/db mice. *Arch Pharm. Res., 33*(2), 325–333.

Kim, S. H., Hyun, S. H., & Choung, S. Y., (2006). Anti-diabetic effect of cinnamon extract on blood glucose in db/db mice. *J Ethnopharmacol., 104*(1, 2), 119–123.

Knip, M., Virtanen, S. M., Seppä, K., Ilonen, J., Savilahti, E., Vaarala, O., Reunanen, A., et al., (2010). Dietary intervention in infancy and later signs of beta-cell autoimmunity. *N. Engl. J. Med., 363*, 1900–1908.

Kousta, E., Ellard, S., Allen, L. I., Saker, P. J., Huxtable, S. J., Hattersley, A. T., & McCarthy, M. I., (2001). Glucokinase mutations in a phenotypically selected multiethnic group of women with a history of gestational diabetes. *Diabetic Med., 18*, 683–684.

Kulkarni, A. P., Aradhya, S. M., & Divakar, S., (2004). Isolation and identification of a radical scavenging antioxidant—punicalagin from pith and carpellary membrane of pomegranate fruit. *Food Chem., 87*(4), 551–557.

Kumar, M., Sharma, S., & Vasudeva, N., (2013). In vivo assessment of antihyperglycemic and antioxidant activity from oil of seeds of *Brassica nigra* in streptozotocin induced diabetic rats. *Adv. Pharm. Bull., 3*(2), 359–365.

Kumar, P., Kale, R. K., & Baquer, N. Z., (2012). Antihyperglycemic and protective effects of *Trigonella foenum-graecum* seed powder on biochemical alterations in alloxan diabetic rats. *Eur. Rev. Med. Pharmacol. Sci., 16*(3), 18–27.

Kumar, S., & Alagawadi, K. R., (2010). Hypoglycemic effect of *Argyreia nervosa* root extract in normal and streptozotocin-diabetic rats. *Der Pharm. Lett., 2*(2), 333–337.

Kumar, V., & Van, S. J., (2016). A review of *Swertia chirayita* (Gentianaceae) as a traditional medicinal plant. *Front. Pharmacol., 6*, 308.

Kurup, S. B., & Mini, S., (2016). *Averrhoa bilimbi* fruits attenuate hyperglycemia-mediated oxidative stress in streptozotocin-induced diabetic rats. *J. Food Drug Anal., 25*(2), 360–368.

Kushner, J. A., Ye, J., Schubert, M., Burks, D. J., Dow, M. A., Flint, C. L., Dutta, S., et al., (2002). Pdx1 restores beta cell function in Irs2 knockout mice. *J. Clin. Invest., 109*, 1193–1201.

Lahfa, F. B., Azzi, R., Mezouar, D., & Djaziri, R., (2017). Hypoglycemic effect of *Citrullus colocynthis* extracts. *Phytothérapie, 15*(2), 50–56.

Långberg, E. C., Seed, A. M., Efendic, S., Gu, H. F., & Östenson, C. G., (2013). Genetic association of adrenergic receptor alpha 2A with obesity and type 2 diabetes. *Obesity (Silver Spring), 21*, 1720–1725.

Li, X., Li, Y., Song, B., Guo, S., Chu, S., Jia, N., & Niu, W., (2012). Hematopoietically-expressed homeobox gene three widely-evaluated polymorphisms and risk for diabetes: A meta-analysis. *PLoS One, 7*, e49917.

Lyssenko, V., Jonsson, A., Almgren, P., Pulizzi, N., Isomaa, B., Tuomi, T., Berglund, G., Altshuler, D., Nilsson, P., & Groop, L., (2008). Clinical risk factors, DNA variants, and the development of type 2 diabetes. *N. Engl. J. Med., 359*, 2220–2232.

Magied, M. M. A., Salama, N. A. R., & Ali, M. R., (2014). Hypoglycemic and hypocholesterolemia effects of intragastric administration of dried red chili pepper (*Capsicum Annum*) in alloxan-induced diabetic male albino rats fed with high-fat-diet. *J. Food Nut. Res., 2*, 850–856.

Majithia, A. R., Flannick, J., Shahinian, P., Guo, M., Bray, M. A., Fontanillas, P., Gabriel, S. B., Rosen, E. D., & Altshuler, D., (2014). GoT2D consortium; NHGRI JHS/FHS allelic spectrum project; SIGMA T2D consortium; T2D-GENES consortium rare variants in PPARG with decreased activity in adipocyte differentiation are associated with increased risk of type 2 diabetes. *Proc. Natl. Acad. Sci. USA., 111*, 13127–13132.

Manickam, M., Ramanathan, M., FarboodniayJahromi, M. A., Chansouria, J. P. N., & Ray, A. B., (1997). Antihyperglycemic activity of phenolics from Pterocarpus marsupium. *J Nat Prod., 60*(6), 609–610.

Manzo, J. A. M., & Vitor, R. J. S., (2017). Antihyperglycemic effects of *Cajanuscajan* L. (pigeon pea) ethanolic extract on the blood glucose levels of ICR mice (Musmusculus L.). *Natl. J. Physiol. Pharm. Pharmacol., 7*(8), 860–864.

Maslin, B. R., Miller, J. T., & Seigle, D. S., (2003). Overview of the generic status of *Acacia* (Leguminosae: Mimosoideae). *Aust. Syst. Bot., 16*(1), 1–18.

Mishra, M. R., Mishra, A., Pradhan, D. K., Panda, A. K., Behera, R. K., & Jha, S., (2013). Antidiabetic and antioxidant activity of *Scoparia dulcis* Linn. *Indian J. Pharm. Sci., 75*(5), 610–614.

Mishra, M., Bandyopadhyay, D., Pramanik, K. C., & Chatterjee, T. K., (2007). Antihyperglycemic activity of *Biophytum sensitivum* (L.) DC. in alloxan diabetic rats. *Oriental Pharmacy and Experimental Medicine, 7*, 418–425.

Mohamed, N. A., & Nassier, O. A., (2013). The antihyperglycaemic effect of the aqueous extract of *Origanium vulgare* leaves in streptozotocin-induced diabetic rats. *Jordan Journal of Biological Sciences, 6*(1), 31–38.

Mohammadi, J., & Zare, T. G., (2013). Hypoglycemic action of *Prangos ferulacea* in normal and streptozotocin induced diabetic Wistar rats. *J. Am. Sci, 9*(10), 51–54.

Mohammadi, S., Kouhsari, S. M., & Feshani, A. M., (2010). Antidiabetic properties of the ethanolic extract of *Rhuscoriaria* fruits in rats. *DARU Journal of Faculty of Pharmacy, Tehran University of Medical Sciences, 18*(4), 270–275.

Mondal, S., Bhattacharya, S., & Biswas, M., (2012). Antidiabetic activity of Areca catechu leaf extracts against streptozotocin induced diabetic rats. *J. Adv. Pharm. Educ. Res., 2*(1), 10–17.

Mousavi, L., Salleh, R. M., Murugaiyah, V., & Asmawi, M. Z., (2016). Hypoglycemic and anti-hyperglycemic study of *Ocimumtenuiflorum* L. leaves extract in normal and streptozotocin-induced diabetic rats. *Asian Pac. J. Trop. Biomed., 6*(12), 1029–1036.

Mowla, A., Alauddin, M., Rahman, M. A., & Ahmed, K., (2009). Antihyperglycemic effect of *Trigonella foenum-graecum* (fenugreek) seed extract in alloxan-induced diabetic rats and its use in diabetes mellitus: A brief qualitative phytochemical and acute toxicity test on the extract. *Afr. J. Tradit. Complement. Altern. Med., 6*(3), 255–261.

Nahar, L., Nasrin, F., Zahan, R., Haque, A., Haque, E., & Mosaddik, A., (2014). Comparative study of antidiabetic activity of *Cajanus cajan* and *Tamarindus indica* in alloxan-induced diabetic mice with a reference to in vitro antioxidant activity. *Pharmacognosy Res., 6*(2), 180–187.

Nugroho, A. E., Andrie, M., Warditiani, N. K., Siswanto, E., Pramono, S., & Lukitaningsih, E., (2012). Antidiabetic and antihiperlipidemic effect of *Andrographis paniculata* (Burm. f.) nees and andrographolide in high-fructose-fat-fed rats. *Indian J. Pharmacol., 44*(3), 377–381.

Oguntibeju, O. O., Meyer, S., Aboua, Y. G., & Goboza, M., (2016). Hypoxishemerocallidea significantly reduced hyperglycaemia and hyperglycaemic-induced oxidative stress in the liver and kidney tissues of streptozotocin-induced diabetic male Wistar rats. *Evid. Based Complementary Altern. Med.*, 1–10.

Ojewole, J. A., (2006). Antinociceptive, anti-inflammatory and antidiabetic properties of *Hypoxis hemerocallidea* fisch. & C.A. Mey. (Hypoxidaceae) corm ['African Potato'] aqueous extract in mice and rats. *J. Ethnopharma.*, *103*(1), 126–134.

Okruszko, A., Szepietowska, B., Wawrusiewicz-Kurylonek, N., Górska, M., Krętowski, A., & Szelachowska, M., (2012). HLA-DR, HLA-DQB1 and PTPN22 gene polymorphism: Association with age at onset for autoimmune diabetes. *Arch Med. Sci.*, *8*, 874–878.

Oryan, A., Hashemnia, M., Hamidi, A. R., & Mohammadalipour, A., (2014). Effects of hydro-ethanol extract of *Citrulluscolocynthis* on blood glucose levels and pathology of organs in alloxan-induced diabetic rats. *Asian Pac. J. Trop. Dis.*, *4*(2), 125–130.

Osbak, K. K., Colclough, K., Saint-Martin, C., Beer, N. L., Bellanné-Chantelot, C., Ellard, S., & Gloyn, A. L., (2009). Update on mutations in glucokinase (GCK), which cause maturity-onset diabetes of the young, permanent neonatal diabetes, and hyperinsulinemic hypoglycemia. *Hum Mutat.*, *30*, 1512–1526.

Oyebode, O. A., Erukainure, O. L., Chukwuma, C. I., Ibeji, C. U., Koorbanally, N. A., & Islam, S., (2018). *Boerhaaviadiffusa* inhibits key enzymes linked to type 2 diabetes in vitro and in silico and modulates abdominal glucose absorption and muscle glucose uptake ex vivo. *Biomedicine & Pharmacotherapy*, *106*, 1116–1125.

Patel, S., Santani, D., Shah, M., & Patel, V., (2012). Anti-hyperglycemic and anti-hyperlipidemic effects of *Bryonia laciniosa* seed extract and its saponin fraction in streptozotocin-induced diabetes in rats. *J Young Pharm.*, *4*(3), 171–176.

Pawar, A., & Vyawahare, N., (2014). Phytocemical and pharmacological profile of *Biophytum sensitivum* LDC. *Int. J. Pharm. Pharm. Sci.*, *6*(11), 18–22.

Pferschy-Wenzig, E. M., Atanasov, A. G., Malainer, C., Noha, S. M., Kunert, O., Schuster, D., Heiss, E. H., et al., (2014). Identification of isosilybin A from milk thistle seeds as an agonist of peroxisome proliferator-activated receptor gamma. *J. Nat. Prod.*, *77*(4), 842–847.

Phoboo, S., Pinto, M. D. S., Barbosa, A. C. L., Sarkar, D., Bhowmik, P. C., Jha, P. K., & Shetty, K., (2012). Phenolic-linked biochemical rationale for the anti-diabetic properties of *Swertiachirayita (Roxb. ex Flem.) Karst. Phytother. Res.*, *27*(2), 227–235.

Prince, P. S. M., & Srinivasan, M., (2005). *Enicostemma littorale* Blume aqueous extract improves the antioxidant status in alloxan induced diabetic rat tissues. *Acta Pol. Pharm. Drug Res.*, *62*(5), 363–367.

Pushparaj, P. N., Low, H. K., Manikandan, J., Tan, B. K., & Tan, C. H., (2006). Anti-diabetic effects of Cichoriumintybus in streptozotocin-induced diabetic rats. *J. Ethnopharmacol.*, *111*(2), 430–434.

Pushparaj, P., Tan, C. H., & Tan, B. K. H., (2000). Effects of *Averrhoa bilimbi* leaf extract on blood glucose and lipids in streptozotocin-diabetic rats. *J Ethnopharmacol.*, *72*, 69–76.

Qusti, S., El Rabey, H. A., & Balashram, S. A., (2016). The hypoglycemic and antioxidant activity of cress seed and cinnamon on streptozotocin induced diabetes in male rats. *Evid. Based Complement. Alternat. Med.*, 5614564.

Rabintossaporn, P., Saenthaweesuk, S., Thuppia, A., Ingkaninan, K., & Sireeratawong, S., (2009). Antihyperglycemic and histological effects on the pancreas of the aqueous leaves extract of *Annona squamosa* L. in normal and diabetic rats. *Songklanakarin J. Sci. Technol.*, *31*(1), 73–78.

Radha, R., & Amrithaveni, M., (2009). Role of medicinal plant *Salacia reticulata* in the management of type II diabetic subjects. *Anc, Life Sci.*, *29*, 14–16.

Rahimi, H. R., Mohammadpour, A. H., Dastani, M., Jaafari, M. R., Abnous, K., Mobarhan, M. G., & Oskuee, R. K., (2016). The effect of nano-curcumin on HbA1c, fasting blood glucose, and lipid profile in diabetic subjects: A randomized clinical trial. *Avicenna J. Phytomedicine, 6*(5), 567.

Raja, N. R. L., Sundaranathavalli, S., Ananthi, J. J., Nirmaladevi, K. C., Kumaraguruparan, P., & Yaseen, K., (2008). Antihyperglycemic activity of aqueous extract of *Vinca rosea* Linn in alloxan induced diabetic rats. *Pharmacology Online, 3*, 354–362.

Raja, T. A. R., Reddy, R. R. N., & Buchineni, M., (2015). An evaluation of anti-hyperglycemic activity of *Ocimum sanctum* Linn (leaves) in Wistar rats. *The Pharma Innovation Journal, 5*, 1–3.

Rajesh, M. S., & Rajasekhar, J., (2014). Assesment of antidiabetic activity of *Mangiferai ndica* seed kernel extracts in streptozotocin induced diabetic rats. *Journal of Natural Remedies, 14*, 33–40.

Rani, R., Dahiya, S., Dhingra, D., Dilbaghi, N., Kim, K. H., & Kumar, S., (2017). Evaluation of anti-diabetic activity of glycyrrhizin-loaded nanoparticles in nicotinamide-streptozotocin-induced diabetic rats. *Eur. J. Pharm. Sci., 106*, 220–230.

Rashad, H., Metwally, F. M., Ezzat, S. M., Salama, M. M., Hasheesh, A., & Abdel, M. A., (2017). Randomized double-blinded pilot clinical study of the antidiabetic activity of *Balanites aegyptiaca* and UPLC-ESI-MS/MS identification of its metabolites. *Pharm. Biol., 55*(1), 1954–1961.

Rathee, S., Mogla, O. P., Sardana, S., Vats, M., & Rathee, P., (2010). Antidiabetic activity of *Capparis decidua* Forsk Edgew. *J. Pharm. Res., 3*, 231–234.

Sadiq, S., Nagi, A. H., Shahzad, M., & Zia, A., (2010). The reno-protective effect of aqueous extract of *Carum carvi* (black zeera) seeds in streptozotocin induced diabetic nephropathy in rodents. *Saudi J Kidney Dis Transpl., 21*(6), 1058–1065.

Saeed, M. K., Shahzadi, I., Ahmad, I., Ahmad, R., Shahzad, K., Ashraf, M., & Nisa, V., (2010). Nutritional analysis and antioxidant activity of bitter gourd (*Momordicacharantia*) from Pakistan. *Pharmacology Online, 1*, 252–260.

SamadiNoshahr, Z., Shahraki, M. R., Ahmadvand, H., Nourabadi, D., & Nakhaei, A., (2015). Protective effects of *Withania somnifera* root on inflammatory markers and insulin resistance in fructose-fed rats. *Reports of Biochemistry and Molecular Biology, 3*(2), 62–67.

Sánchez De, M. F., Gámez, M. J., Jiménez, I., Jiménez, J., Osuna, J. I., & Zarzuelo, A., (1994). Hypoglycemic activity of juniper "berries." *Planta Med., 60*(3), 197–200.

Santhosha, S. G., Jamuna, P., & Prabhavathi, S. N., (2013). Bioactive components of garlic and their physiological role in health maintenance: A review. *Food Biosci., 3*(2013), 59–74.

Saranya, R., Thirumalai, T., Hemalatha, M., Balaji, R., & David, E., (2013). Pharmacognosy of *Enicostemma littorale*: A review. *Asian Pac. J. Trop. Biomed., 3*(1), 79–84.

Satyanarayana, K., Sravanthi, K., Shaker, I. A., & Ponnulakshmi, R., (2015). Molecular approach to identify antidiabetic potential of *Azadirachta indica*. *J. Ayurveda Integr. Med., 6*, 165–174.

Saxena, M., Srivastava, N., & Banerjee, M., (2013). Association of IL-6, TNF-α and IL-10 gene polymorphisms with type 2 diabetes mellitus. *Mol. Biol. Rep., 40*, 6271–6279.

Scheen, A. J., & Paquot, N., (2013). Metformin revisited: A critical review of the benefit-risk balance in at-risk patients with type 2 diabetes. *Diabetes Metab., 39*, 179–190.

Schwitzgebel, V. M., (2014). Many faces of monogenic diabetes. *J. Diabetes Investig., 5*, 121–133.

Sen, S., Roy, M., & Chakraborti, A. S., (2011). Ameliorative effects of glycyrrhizin on streptozotocin-induced diabetes in rats. *J. Pharm.Pharmacol., 63,* 287–296.

Senadheera, S. P. A., Ekanayake, S., & Wanigatunge, C., (2015). Anti-hyperglycaemic effects of herbal porridge made of *Scoparia dulcis* leaf extract in diabetics - a randomized crossover clinical trial. *BMC Complementary and Alternative Medicine, 15*(1), 410.

Shafi, S., & Tabassum, N., (2013). Antihyperglycemic and lipid lowering activities of ethanolic extract of *Eriobotrya* japonica seeds in alloxan induced diabetic rats. *Eur. Sci. J., 3*(2), 398–405.

Sharma, B., Salunke, R., Balomajumder, C., Daniel, S., & Roy, P., (2010). Anti-diabetic potential of alkaloid rich fraction from *Capparis decidua* on diabetic mice. *J. Ethnopharm., 127*(2), 457–462.

Shetti, A., Sanakal, R., & Kaliwal, B., (2012). Antidiabetic effect of ethanolic leaf extract of *Phyllanthus amarus* in alloxan induced diabetic mice. *Asian J. Plant Sci. Res., 2*(1), 11–15.

Shidfar, F., Rahideh, S. T., Rajab, A., Khandozi, N., Hosseini, S., Shidfar, S., & Mojab, F., (2014). The effect of sumac (*Rhus coriaria* L.) powder on serum glycemic status, ApoB, ApoA-I and total antioxidant capacity in type 2 diabetic patients. *Iran J. Pharm. Res., 13*(4), 1249–1255.

Shinde, V., Borkar, A., & Badwaik, R., (2014). Evaluation and comparative study of hypoglycemic activity of aloe barbadensis miller with oral hypoglycemic drugs (glibenclamide and metformin) in rats. *Int. J. Med. Pharmaceut. Sci., 4*(6), 31–36.

Shivaprasad, H. N., Bhanumathy, M., Sushma, G., Midhun, T., Raveendra, K. R., Sushma, K. R., & Venkateshwarlu, K., (2013). *Salacia reticulata* improves serum lipid profiles and glycemic control in patients with pre-diabetes and mild to moderate hyperlipidemia: A double-blind, placebo-controlled, randomized trial. *J. Med. Food, 16,* 564–568.

Shojaii, A., Dabaghian, F. H., Goushegir, A., & Fard, M. A., (2011). Antidiabetic plants of Iran. *Acta Med. Iran., 49*(10), 637–642.

Sravan, K. P., Bhaumik, A., Chopra, M., & Devi, K. N., (2016). Evaluation of anti diabetic activity of ethanolic extract of beet root (EEBT- Beta vulgaris) against streptozocin induced diabetic Rats. *Journal of Drug Discovery and Therapeutics, 37*(4), 01–06.

Sreelatha, S., & Inbavalli, R., (2012). Antioxidant, antihyperglycemic, and antihyperlipidemic effects of *Coriandrum sativum* leaf and stem in alloxan-induced diabetic rats. *J. Food Sci., 77*(7), T119–T123.

Srinivasan, P., Vijayakumar, S., Kothandaraman, S., & Palani, M., (2018). Anti-diabetic activity of quercetin extracted from *Phyllanthus emblica* L. fruit: *In silico* and *in vivo* approaches. *J. Pharm. Anal., 8*(2), 109–118.

Stohs, S. J., & Ray, S., (2015). Anti-diabetic and anti-hyperlipidemic effects and safety of *Salacia reticulata* and related species. *Phytother. Res., 29*(7), 986–995.

Subbiah, V., Nagaraja, P., Narayan, P., & Nagendra, H. G., (2019). Evaluation of pharmacological properties of *Caesalpinia bonducella* seed and shell extract. *Pharmacog. J., 11*(1), 150–154.

Sun, C., Zhang, F., Ge, X., Yan, T., Chen, X., Shi, X., & Zhai, Q., (2007). SIRT1 improves insulin sensitivity under insulin-resistant conditions by repressing PTP1B. *Cell Metab., 6,* 307–319.

Tanaka, M., Misawa, E., Ito, Y., Habara, N., Nomaguchi, K., Yamada, M., Toida, T., et al., (2006). Identification of five phytosterols from *Aloe vera* gel as anti-diabetic compounds. *Biol. Pharm. Bull., 29*(7), 1418–1422.

Tavana, A., Pourrajab, F., Hekmatimoghaddam, S. H., Khalilzadeh, S. H., & Lotfi, M. H., (2015). The hypoglycemic effect of *Dorema aucheri* (Bilhar) extract in diabetic type 2 patients: A first clinical trial. *International Journal of Pharmaceutical and Clinical Research, 7,* 343–347.

Tomar, R. S., & Sisodia, S., (2012). Antidiabetic activity of *Annona squamosa* L. in experimental induced diabetic rats. *Int J Pharm Biol Arch, 3,* 1492–1495.

Tomlinson, M. J., Pitsillides, A., Pickin, R., Mika, M., Keene, K. L., Hou, X., Mychaleckyj, J., et al., (2014). Fine mapping and functional studies of risk variants for type 1 diabetes at chromosome 16p13.13. *Diabetes, 63,* 4360–4368.

Tripathi, U. N., & Chandra, D., (2010). Anti-hyperglycemic and anti-oxidative effect of aqueous extract of *Momordica charantia* pulp and *Trigonella foenum-graecum* seed in alloxan-induced diabetic rats. *Ind. J Biochem. Biophys., 47*(4), 227–233.

Udayakumar, R., Kasthurirengan, S., Mariashibu, T. S., Rajesh, M., Anbazhagan, V. R., Kim, S. C., Ganapathi, A., & Choi, C. W., (2009). Hypoglycaemic and hypolipidaemic effects of *Withania somnifera* root and leaf extracts on alloxan-induced diabetic rats. *Int. J. Mol. Sci., 10*(5), 2367–2382.

UlKabir, A., Samad, M. B., Ahmed, A., Jahan, M. R., Akhter, F., Tasnim, J., Nageeb, H. S. Met al., (2015). Aqueous fraction of beta vulgaris ameliorates hyperglycemia in diabetic mice due to enhanced glucose stimulated insulin secretion, mediated by acetylcholine and GLP-1, and elevated glucose uptake via increased membrane bound GLUT4 transporters. *PloS One, 10*(2), e0116546.

Vishwakarma, S. L., Rakesh, D., Rajani, M., & Goyal, R. K., (2010). Evaluation of effect of aqueous extract of *Enicostemma littorale* Blume in streptozotocin- induced type 1 diabetic rats. *Ind. J. Exp. Bio., 48,* 26–30.

Vujicic, M., Nikolic, I., Kontogianni, V. G., Saksida, T., Charisiadis, P., Orescanin-Dusic, Z., Blagojevic, D., et al., (2015). Methanolic extract of *Origanum vulgare* ameliorates type 1 diabetes through antioxidant, anti-inflammatory and anti-apoptotic activity. *Br. J. Nutr., 113*(5), 770–782.

Watcharachaisoponsiri, T., Sornchan, P., Charoenkiatkul, S., & Suttisansanee, U., (2016). The α-glucosidase and α-amylase inhibitory activity from different chili pepper extracts. *Int. Food Res J., 23,* 1439–1445.

Widodo, G. P., Handayani, R., & Herowati, R., (2015). Antihyperglycemic, antioxidant, and pancreas protective effects of Coriandrum Sativum seed in alloxan induced diabetic rats. *Indonesian J. Pharm., 25,* 129–133.

Xu, G. K., Qin, X. Y., Wang, G. K., Xie, G. Y., Li, X. S., Sun, C. Y., Liu, B. L., & Qin, M. J., (2017). Antihyperglycemic, antihyperlipidemic and antioxidant effects of standard ethanol extract of Bombax ceiba leaves in high-fat-diet-and streptozotocin-induced type 2 diabetic rats. *Chin. J. Nat. Med., 15*(3), 168–177.

Xue, W. L., Li, X. S., Zhang, J., Liu, Y. H., Wang, Z. L., & Zhang, R. J., (2007). Effect of *Trigonella foenum-graecum* (fenugreek) extract on blood glucose, blood lipid and hemorheological properties in streptozotocin-induced diabetic rats. *Asia Pac J Clin Nutr., 16*(Suppl 1), 422–426.

Yasir, M., Jain, P., Debajyoti, D., & Kharya, M. D., (2010). Hypoglycemic and antihyperglycemic effect of different extracts of acacia arabica LAMK bark in normal and alloxan induced diabetic rats. *International Journal of Phytomedicine, 2*(2), 133–138.

Yu, B. C., Hung, C. R., Chen, W. C., & Cheng, J. T., (2003). Antihyperglycemic effect of andrographolide in streptozotocin-induced diabetic rats. *Planta Med., 69*(12), 1075–1079.

Zacharias, N. T., Sebastian, K. L., Philip, B., & Augusti, K. T., (1980). Hypoglycemic and hypolipidaemic effects of garlic in sucrose fed rabbits. *Ind. J. Physiol. Pharmacol., 24,* 151–154.

Zolghadri, Y., Fazeli, M., Kooshki, M., Shomali, T., Karimaghayee, N., & Dehghani, M., (2014). *Achillea millefolium* L. hydro-alcoholic extract protects pancreatic cells by down regulating IL-1β and iNOS gene expression in diabetic rats. *Int. J. Mol. Cell Med.,* (4), 255–262.

CHAPTER 8

IMPROVED PRODUCTION AND POSTHARVEST TECHNOLOGIES IN ASHWAGANDHA (INDIAN GINSENG)

A. C. JNANESHA and ASHISH KUMAR

CSIR-Central Institute of Medicinal and Aromatic Plants, Research Center, Boduppal, Hyderabad, Telangana – 500092, India, E-mail: jnangowda@gmail.com (A. C. Jnanesha)

ABSTRACT

Withania somnifera is a miracle medicinal crop used traditionally in Ayurveda and Siddha for treating various diseases in South Asia. The root is the principal productive part of the Ashwagandha plant employed widely in the Indian system of medicine. The root is having potential medicinal properties and contains several alkaloids. One of the major alkaloids, Withanoloides, helps improving reproductive system in men and women, antistress, anti-oxidant, antiaging, diuretic, hypothyroid, immunomodulatory, antidementia, antihyperglycemic, anti-hypercholesterolemic, and cardiovascular activity. Leaves contain Withaferin A and B used for the treatment of thyroid and insomnia problems. It is drought tolerant cultivated mainly in Andhra Pradesh, Telangana, Karnataka, Rajasthan, Madhya Pradesh, and other states of India. Simple cultivation practices and higher root price attracting the farmer to grow *Withania somnifera* crop in large scale. The main challenges posed by farmers are interference of middlemen, lack of organized market, fluctuation in root price, demand-supply of roots, climatic variation, lower root yield, lack of availability of improved varieties, high fiber content in some location, lack of knowledge about improved post-harvest technology and problem occurrence with long term storage of roots.

8.1 INTRODUCTION

Withania somnifera (L.) Dunal is often known as Winter cherry, Indian ginseng, and Ashwagandha. It is one such traditional plant whose roots have been employed as a valuable drug for the treatment of rheumatoid arthritis, stiff joints, neurosis, and tremor. It is mainly indicated as an aphrodisiac, diuretic, restorative, and rejuvenative drug. Ashwagandha roots are compared with ginseng roots for their restorative properties and have been given the name 'Indian ginseng' besides the roots of this plant, its leave has been used as a folk remedy for all types of skin bruise, blisters, simmer, minimizing pus secretion and swelling. These medicinal properties of ashwagandha have been attributed to the chemical constituents, mainly the alkaloids in the roots and withanolides in the leaves. There is considerable documentary evidence on the successful traditional uses of ashwagandha for above mentioned kinds of medicaments. The utilization of Withania was mentioned in many literatures as tonic, astringent, heat, and stimulant and is advised in arthritic, cough, edema, consumption, and senile debility (Kumar and Jnanesha, 2019). The dried roots of ashwagandha (*Withania somnifera*, a dry land medicinal plant) are the primary economic part and the starch and fiber contents play a dominant role in determining root quality. Brittle roots having high starch and low fiber are highly-priced. In India, the major Ashwagandha producing states are Punjab, Himachal Pradesh, Jammu, Rajasthan, Madhya Pradesh, Andhra Pradesh, Karnataka, and Telangana. Approximately more than 40,000 Ha is under cultivation of Ashwagandha in Ananthpur and Kurnool district of Andhra Pradesh (Kumar and Jnanesha, 2018).

8.1.1 TAXONOMICAL POSITION

The plant Withania somnifera confined to Solanaceae family is dicotyledonous in nature. This family consists of more than 3,000 species and 90 genera materialize throughout the globe, especially in the tropics. It was Pauquy who created the genus Withania in the year 1825 and today this genus includes approximately 26 species. Among the 26 species listed worldwide, In India, the *Withania* genus consists of two species viz., *W. somnifera* and *W. coagulans*. The third species of *Withania* was reported in India from Indian germplasm using multimilitary approaches (Figure 8.1) (Mir et al., 2011; Kumar et al., 2011).

Kingdom:	Plantae	
Division:	Angiosperms	
Class:	Eudicots	
Clade:	Asterids	
Order:	Solanales	
Family:	Solanaceae	
Genus:	*Withania*	
Species:	*somnifera*	
Biological name:	*Withania somnifera*	

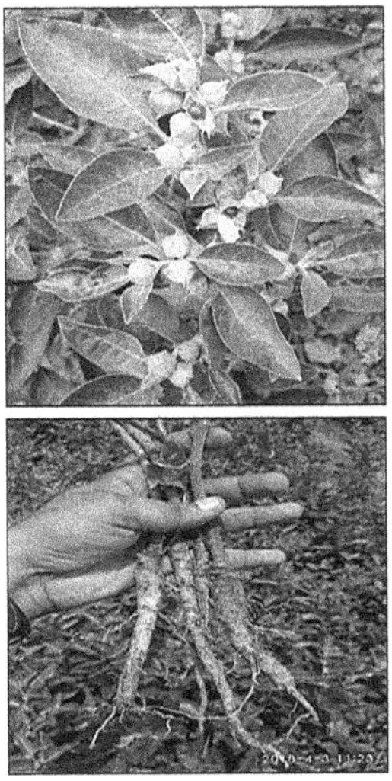

FIGURE 8.1   Ashwagandha plant and root.

8.1.2   BOTANICAL DESCRIPTION

This plant is normally shrubby, branched, unarmed, and erect in nature. It can capable to grow to a height of 1.25 m, veins on the leaf, calyx, and stellate tomentose minutely on the stem. Leaves are simple petiolate, elliptic-ovate to broadly ovate, entire, exstipulate, acute, cuneate or oblique, glabrous, and up to 10 cm long. Leaves on vegetative shoots are alternate and large; leaves on floral branches are opposite, arranged somewhat laterally in pairs of one large and one small leaf, having in their axil acymose cluster of 5–25 inconspicuous pale green flowers. Flowers shortly pedicellate, 4–6 mm in diam. Calyx gamosepalous, enlarged, and inflated in fruit; Partite 5 sepals, 5 lobed gamopetalous with 5 acute corolla, linear lobes and persistent lobes spreading or recur 5, attached near the base of the corolla; epipetalous; anthers oblong, dehiscing longitudinally; filaments linearly slender. Syncarpous gynoecium, made of small distended ovary attached by a long fragile style; stigma shortly 2-fid or 2-lobed. Berry globose enclosed in the green persistent calyx, 5 mm in diameter, green when unripe, orange-red when mature, containing numerous small smooth discrete seeds.

8.2   AREA AND PRODUCTION

Withania somnifera is a shrubby bush which grows in dry arid soils of subtropical regions. It is widespread species disseminating from the southern Mediterranean area to the Islas Canarius and to southern and eastern Africa, Congo, Madagascar; to North India, Pakistan, Baluchistan, Israel, Jordan, Egypt, Iran, and Afghanistan, representing extensive variations of soil, rainfall, temperature, and altitude (Atal et al., 1975). In India, the crop thrives better in dry region and in sub-tropical and semi temperate regions, including the states of Maharashtra, Madhya Pradesh, Gujarat, Rajasthan, Uttar Pradesh, Haryana, and Punjab extending to Himachal Pradesh, Jammu, and Kashmir from plains to the height of 1,700 meters (Figure 8.2) (Jnanesha and Kumar, 2019).

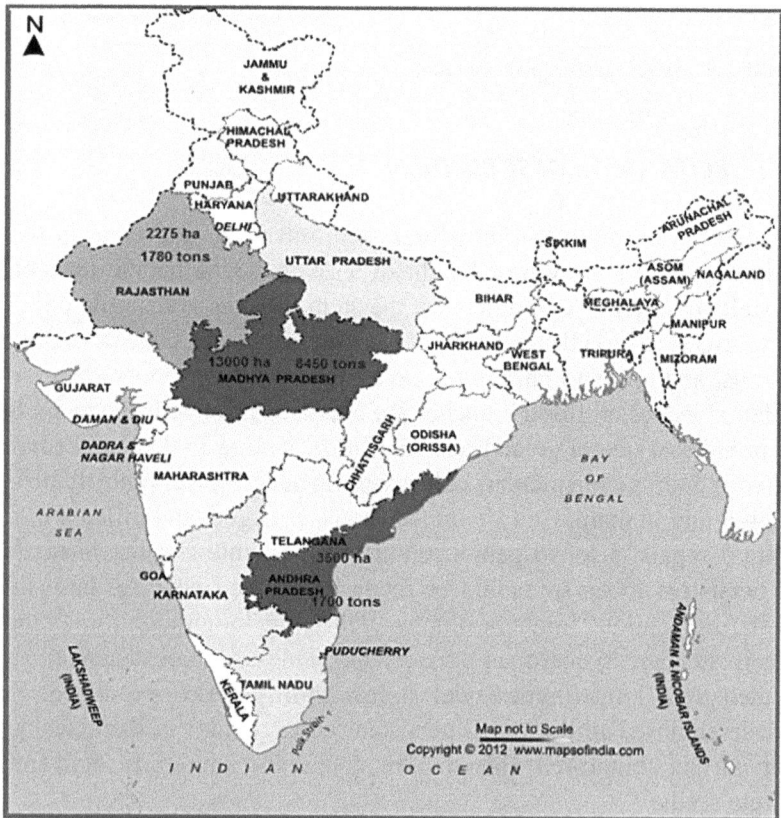

FIGURE 8.2   Area and production of Ashwagandha in India.

In South India, Anantapur, Kadapa, and Kurnool district of Andhra Pradesh owing to intervention of CSIR-Central Institute of medicinal and aromatic plants (MAPs), Research Center, Boduppal, Hyderabad, the area under cultivation of Ashwagandha was increased over the years and now the area of Ashwagandha is around 25,000 acres. Initially, the farmers of Anantapur district are cultivating cotton, chilly, maize, and pigeon pea due to climate change the rainfall received in recent years were very minimal and finally fallowing the land. CSIR-CIMAP suggested alternative crop to farmers is Ashwagandha which thrive well even under very little rainfall and getting higher income compared to traditional crop. The farmers are very happy in cultivating of ashwagandha in Southern India (Table 8.1) (Kumar et al., 2015).

TABLE 8.1 Cultivating Area of Ashwagandha in Northern Region and Southern Region of India

States	Districts	Area in ha	Production in ton
Rajasthan	Shriganganagar, Hanumangarh, Churu, Jhunjhunu, Kota, Boondi, Bara, Jhalawar, Tonk, Sawaimadhopur	2,275	1,780
Madhya Pradesh	Mandsaur District of Jawad, Neemuch, and Manasa tehsils	13,000	8,450
Andhra Pradesh and Telangana state	Anatapur, Kadapa, and Kurnool districts in Andhra Pradesh Ranga Reddy and Mahbub Nagar districts in the Telangana States	3,500	1,700
Odisha	Bhubaneswar	18.5	10

8.3 MEDICINAL PROPERTIES AND USES

W. somnifera and *W. coagulans* have delineated various biological activities viz., anti-inflammatory, cytotoxic, anti-stress, anti-aging, diuretic, immunomodulatory, diuretic, hypothyroid, antioxidant, anti-Alzheimer's disease (AD), anti-hypercholesterolemic, antimicrobial, antifeedant, radiosensitizing activity, cell-differentiation-inducing activity and cardiovascular, etc. (Maurya et al., 2008, Singh et al., 2001, Bhattacharya et al., 2001, Malhotra et al., 1965, Kaul et al., 2005). *W. somnifera* aids the whole body and mind and have wider applications. It acts as a powerful immune-regulator, cures various ailments, prevent cancer, and it also shows aphrodisiac virtues. This plant will efficaciously reduce the stress and insomnia problems. It also improves reproductive system and metabolic activity of various organs.

In Ayurveda, *W. somnifera* is widely claimed to have aphrodisiac, sedative, rejuvenate, and anti-aging properties. It is also used in preparation of Medharasayana tonic (promotes learning and memory) and in geriatric problems (Nadkarni, 1976; Kapoor, 2001). The plant has traditionally been used to promote youthful vigor, endurance, strength, health, developing growth components of the body and enhance the secretion of vital fluids, muscle growth, semen, blood, lymph, and cells (Williamson, 2002). It also helps counteract chronic fatigue, weakness, dehydration, weakness of bones and loose teeth, immature aging, appetite, infertility, anorexia, faintness, and muscles stiffness. The leaves have sour in taste and employed as an anthelmintic. The mixture is inclined in fever. Pulverized berries and leaves are locally applied to ulcers, tubercular glands, and cyst (Nadkarni, 1976; Kapoor, 2001). The berries of the Ashwagandha plant have milk solidifying property, which is used in cheese preparation (Atal and Sethi, 2015).

8.4   SPECIES AND VARIETIES

Withania somnifera is a well-known medicinal plant comprised of 23 species, spread over different parts of Northern Africa, Canary Islands, Middle East and Mediterranean region (Mirjalili et al., 2009). Among 23 species, *Withania somnifera* and *Withania coagulans* are explored well and recognized economically important species in various regions for their medicinal uses (Table 8.2) (Mirjalili et al., 2009).

TABLE 8.2   Development of Improved Varieties of *W. somnifera* from CSIR-CIMAP, Lucknow

Varieties	Herb Yield (q/ha)	Dry Root Yield (Q/ha)	Constituents	Origin/ Development
Poshita	2.83	14	Alkaloids: 1.3 kg/ha Withaferin (dry leaves): 0.53%	Half-sib selection
Pratap	5.39	34.95	Withanolide: 0.31% Withaferin A: 0.72%	Half-sib selection
Chetak	1.72	11.77	Withanolide: 0.40% Withaferin: 1.22%	Half-sib family selection

TABLE 8.2   *(Continued)*

Varieties	Herb Yield (q/ha)	Dry Root Yield (Q/ha)	Constituents	Origin/ Development
NMITLI 118	2.9	15	Withaferin A: Up to 2%, withanone in leaves	–
NMITLI 101	3.8	23	Withanolide: 0.28%	–
CIM-Pushti	–	9–10	Withanolide A:0.71 mg/g	Intraspecific hybridization

High yielding cultivars viz., NMITLI-118, NMITLI-108, Chetak Poshita, Pratap, Pushti, and Rakshita are released by CSIR-CIMAP, Lucknow (Kumar and Jnanesha, 2017). Varieties developed by other universities and institutes are Jawahar 20 grown in Madhya Pradesh. Regional Research Laboratory, Jammu released improved variety WSR.

8.4.1   *OPPORTUNITIES FOR CULTIVATION*

The ease of cultivation and high demand for its roots provide an opportunity to cultivate this plant on a commercial scale (Kattimani et al., 1999, 2001). Ashwagandha grown well in dry area and fertilizer and labor requirement is also very less. The crop can be grown as intercrop or sequential crop with existing traditional crop. Demand for seed, leaves, and stem also increasing over the year and farmer also get additional income by selling these products. Export demand for value added products like Ashwagandha powder and Ashwagandha tea is increasing and further value-added products need to be explored (Rajeswara et al., 2012).

8.4.2   *PRODUCTION TECHNOLOGY*

The estimated annual production of Ashwagandha roots in India is about 10,000 tons. The plant is cultivated mainly in the north-western region and part of Andhra Pradesh on about 40,000 ha land. It is grown marginal land in Manasa, Neemach, Jawad, Bhanpur, and nearby tehsils of Mandsaur district of Madhya Pradesh, Ananthpur, and Kurnool district of Andhra Pradesh and adjoining villages of Kota district of Rajasthan.

Generally, seed was sown late in the Kharif season around August-September and reaped in the next February/ March. The areas which receive annual rainfall of 500–750 mm rainfall having semi-tropical conditions are ideal for growing of this crop. During the growing period, it requires dry conditions and minimal winter rains are ideal for proper growth and development of roots. *Withania somnifera* thrives well in light red soil or sandy loam, having good drainage with pH 7.5–8.0. High fertile soil is not suitable for cultivation of *Withania somnifera*, However, plant grows robust and vigorously but root becomes fibrous. The crop can be sown either by broadcasting or in lines or transplanting by making nursery. It requires around 20–25 kg/ha for broadcasting method of sowing, 10–12 kg for line sowing and crop can also be raised by transplanting nursery raised (500 g/ha) in areas where irrigation facilities exist. When sown in lines the plant-to-plant distance is kept 10 cm and row to row distance 30 cm. While broadcasting, mix the seed with sand in the ratio of 1:4 to avoid thick population. A light shower after sowing ensures good germination but excessive rain affects the germination adversely. Seed should be treated with Thiram or Captan at the rate of 3 g/kg seed before sowing to protect the seedlings from seed borne diseases (Kumar and Jnanesha, 2017). The crop requires lesser inputs, In Andhra Pradesh and Madhya Pradesh, the farmers generally do not apply any fertilizer, and the crop is cultivated on the marginal, submarginal and surplus farm without applying any inputs. Application of farmyard manure and vermicompost is recommended, in some studies, the increasing levels of fertilizers (NPK) had no effect on the yield of dry roots of ashwagandha. This might be due to low fertility adoption during natural selection.

The seeds were sown by broadcasting or line sowing in furrows and maintained the optimum plant population after 25–30 days after sowing by manual thinning. Whereas, organically grown ashwagandha root fetches higher price and export demand. So, the application of farmyard manure, vermicompost, and spray of panchagavya, jeevamrutha, and waste decomposer is recommended along with biofertilizer such as phosphorous solubilizing bacteria for getting higher root yield and quality root on sustainable basis. Meanwhile, apply Nitrogen, Phosphorous, and Potash at the rate of 30 kg each, P, and K is applied as basal dose at the time of sowing at 30- and 60-days nitrogen is applied in split doses after sowing. The crop is normally cultivated as a rain-fed crop. However, where water facility is prevailed, it has to be irrigated 15–20 days for better growth. A number of pests (mites, aphids, and beetles) and diseases (Dieback, leaf blight and seedling blight, etc.), are reported on ashwagandha. Foliar spray at 15 days interval with a combination of Kelthane (0.3%) and Malathion (0.5%) will regulate the pests. Similarly spraying of copper oxychloride (COC) or Mancozeb will control the fungal diseases. Use of botanical pesticides such as cow urine, garlic, and chili extracts and custard apple leaf decoction, etc., as a prophylactic measures to protect the crop from diseases and pests. After 6–7 month of sowing, the crop has to be harvested. While, in some place, the crop is harvested within 150 days after planting. Leaves drying and red berries will indicate the maturity of the crop (Rajeswara et al., 2012). The entire plant is pulled out; Stem has to be cut 1–2 cm above the crown, segregates the roots. Clean the root and cut into 7–10 cm long pieces and shade dried under the sun. Plucked the matured berries with hand, suns dried and collect the seeds for next crop. On an average crop produces 1,000–1,200 kg/ha dried roots and 200–250 kg seeds (Farooqui and Khan, 1993; Janardhan et al., 2007).

8.5   CHEMICAL CONSTITUENTS

Withanolides, withaferins, tropine, pseudo-tropine, anferine, sitoindoside VII and VIII, ginsenosides, somniferine, somnine, withanine, somniferinine, pseudo-withanine, pseudo-tropine, 3-a-gloyloxytropane, choline, cuscohygrine, isopelletierine, anaferine, and 2 acyl sterylglucoside (Mishra et al., 2000). Withasomniferin-A and 5-dihydroxy withanolide-R are present in aerial parts of Withania somnifera (Rahman et al., 1993). It is also rich in iron. Different chemicals present in different parts of the plant are depicted in subsections.

8.5.1   ROOTS

The Ashwagandha root contain alkaloids in the range of 0.13% to 0.31%, even higher yields (up to 4.3%) have been noticed somewhere (Anonymous, 1982, 2007). Root contains alkaloids, starch, reducing sugars, glycosides, steroids, volatile oil, amino acids, hentriacontane, dulcitol, and withaniol. The other basic alkaloids present in root are, pseudo-withanine, somnine, withananinine somniferinine. somniferine, further alkaloids comprise withasomnine, tropine, withanine, cuscohygrine, anahygrine, pseudotropine, anaferine, isopelletierine, withananine, and visamine. The free amino acids found in the root include glycine, aspartic acid, proline, alanine, glutamic acid, and cystine (Khare, 2007).

8.5.2 LEAF

Withaferin A, a steroidal lactone is the most important alkaloid segregated from the leaves and dried roots extractants of *Withania somnifera*. The leaves contain 12 withanolides, 5 unidentified alkaloids, free amino acids, chlorogenic acids, glucose, tannins, and flavonoids (Khare, 2007).

8.5.3 FRUIT

The fruit contains free amino acids such as proline, glutamic acid, alanine, glycine, cystine hydroxyproline, tyrosine, aspartic acid and cysteine. The green berries also contain amino acids, proteolytic enzyme, condensed tannins, and flavonoids. The existence of chamase a proteolytic enzyme, in the berries may be culpable for the more content of the amino acid (Khare, 2007).

8.5.4 OTHER PARTS

The stem of the plant contains flavonoids and condensed tannins. The bark contains a number of free amino acids and the rich in phosphorous, calcium, and protein in tender shoots and also reported to contain scopoletin (Figure 8.3) (Anonymous, 1982).

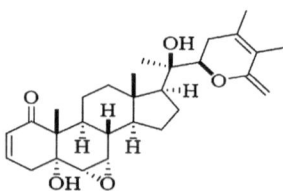

Withanolide A

FIGURE 8.3   Chemical structure of Withanolide A.

8.6 BIOACTIVITY

Withaferin A shows anti-inflammatory and anti-arthritic activities. Anti-stress agents present in Ashwagandha are Acylsteryl glucosides and sitoindosides.

The active principles present in Ashwagandha viz., Withaferin-A, and sitoindoside show eloquent results against acute models on stress (Bhattacharaya et al., 1987). Many of its chemical constituent's support immunoregulatory actions (Ghosal et al., 1989).

8.7 POST-HARVEST MANAGEMENT

After 160 to 180 days after sowing, the entire plant was uprooted and roots are separated from the plants and shade dried for one week. Cut the dried root transversely into small and finally washed, cleaned, trimmed, and graded.

8.7.1 GRADING OF ROOTS

The entire roots are then carefully sorted into four grades based on the thickness and uniformity of the piece:

1. **A-Grade:** Length of the root pieces up to 7 cm in length, with 1.0–1.5 cm diameter; solid; they should be brittle and inside is pure white.
2. **B Grade:** Length of the root pieces up to 5 cm with less than 1 cm diameter, they should be brittle and inside is white.
3. **C-Grade:** Length of the root pieces is 3–4 cm with 1 cm or less in diameter, side branches are solid.
4. **Lower Grade:** Root pieces are small, semi-solid, very thick or very thin, chopped, and yellowish on the side.

8.7.2 PACKING AND STORAGE

Ashwagandha root must be packed in nylon or poly bags to prevent the entry of moisture. Roots can be hoarded in warm condition.

8.7.3 VALUE ADDITIONS AND PATENTS

The main products derived from *Withania somnifera* are root extract, tonic, tablets, and root powder along with these, energy drinks, herbal tea, nutritious food, and superfood are some improved products on which small and medium ventures can establish. Different organizations from India and

Japan filed 8 patents with regard to value added products and extractants. Due to potential medicinal quality, many companies show interest to develop product out from this plant.

8.8 AGRO-ECONOMICS

One-hectare plantation of Ashwagandha yields on an average 6–8 q of dried roots which are sold at about Rs 15,000 per quintal giving a gross income of Rs. 75,000 to 1,05,000 having net return of Rs 40,000–60,000 from a 6- to 8-month crop. CSIR-Central Institute of MAPs, Lucknow, and its Hyderabad Research Center initiatives in popularizing this important crop in Anantapur, Kadapa, and Kurnool districts of Andhra Pradesh have shown an improvement in socio-economic status. Demand for Ashwagandha root is 7,000 tons annually, whereas 1,500 tons are being produced in India are exported to other countries.

8.9 THE MAJOR CONSTRAINTS FACED BY THE GROWERS

8.9.1 LACK OF KNOWLEDGE WITH REGARD PRODUCTION TECHNOLOGY

Transfer of technology from lab to land is meager. The improved practices like, variety, recommended dose of fertilizer, method of sowing, time of sowing, irrigation, plant protection measures, harvesting, grading processing, etc., are not available to the farmer. Another problem faced by the growers are if they apply more fertilizer, i.e., urea or giving more irrigation, the plants grow luxuriantly. However, the root becomes starchier (Fibrous) and fetches lower price in the market. Experiment was conducted by many scientists in order to address this problem and develop a package of practice for high quality root production but still the farmers are not aware about improved management practices for high quality root production.

8.9.2 LACK OF AVAILABILITY OF GOOD QUALITY PLANTING MATERIAL AND HIGH COST OF SEED MATERIAL

The farmers are not aware of improved cultivars of Ashwagandha released by CSIR-Central Institute of MAPs Lucknow, The Indian Council of

Agricultural Research (ICAR) and state universities owing to lack of transfer of technology and still farmers are using local cultivar yielding very less and getting lower income. Ashwagandha is commercially propagated through seeds. With different methods of planting seed requirement may vary transplanting method (750 g/acre), line sowing (5 kg/acre) and broadcasting (7–8 kg/acre). The existing cost of seed material will be sold at the rate of Rs. 500 per kg. Increase seed cost discouraged the many small and marginal to cultivate Ashwagandha crop.

8.9.3 INCIDENCE OF PEST AND DISEASE

There is no major pest and disease for this crop. However, *Spodoptera litura* were noticed in winter (Rabi) season and the occurrence was below Economic threshold level so it can be considered negligible. The major disease observed in Ashwagandha crops are seed rotting, seedling blight, leaf blight and powdery mildew. Some farmers are using captan (3 g/kg of seed) during seed treatment and followed to spray with Dithane M-45 at the rate of 3 g per liter of water to fungal diseases (Seedling rot and powdery mildew). Ashwagandha crop is highly sensitive to waterlogging condition and susceptible to root rot, when the conditions of high temperature and humidity prevail, this becomes serious concern to farmer. No awareness was given to farmers in order to control seedling rot diseases However, it can be controlled by effective seed treatment or application of Trichoderma before sowing will reduce the incidence. Recently, incidence of cuscuta parasitic weed is a major threat in Ashwagandha crop. Due to this nearly 50–60% of the yield will be declined. Owing to monocropping of Ashwagandha crop rather rotation with another crop will enhance the occurrence of this infestation. By giving training and creating awareness on incidence and control measures, the farmers will overcome from above problems.

8.9.4 HARVESTING AND GRADING

Harvesting of Ashwagandha starts after 160–175 days after sowing and has to be done manually. There is a machine to harvest or dig the roots and fetches higher price for labor to harvest the plant. Drying of leaves and berries indicate the maturity of the crop and alkaloid content decrease in the roots is due to source-sink relationship. Anyway, crop has to be harvested before seed maturity owing to reduction in alkaloid content in the root. For the sake of seed, many farmers go for harvesting of the crop after seed formation, by creating awareness on quality of alkaloid content in the root, we can address the issue. After the harvest of the crop, the roots are just dried under open sun and packed in gunny bags without grading the produce will affect the price drastically. Thus, technical knowledge and training has to be given with regarding grading of produce to get good price in the market.

8.9.5   MARKETING PROBLEMS

There is no organized market for selling of the produce locally. Market is at Neemuch place of Madhya Pradesh and middleman problem is more during sale of produce and many of the farmer's do not know where to sell their produce. Due to this, many farmers are selling their produce at a cheaper rate. Owing to variation in market price and lack of information about market and price will affect the income of the Ashwagandha grower and finally dependent on the middlemen or village traders and lack of knowledge with regard to standardization and consistency in quality for international marketing and another major constraint is Financial and logistic constraints make it difficult for growers to interact more closely with prospective clients. High cost of cultivation and poor market facility will affect the farmer to take up Ashwagandha cultivation in larger area.

8.10   FUTURE PROSPECTS

- Conducting training program frequently in collaboration with SAU's, KVK, and Agriculture and Horticulture department to create awareness on improved production technologies in Ashwagandha.
- Government has to create an organized market for sale of produce without interference of middlemen.
- Development of suitable cultivars of Ashwagandha with high yield and alkaloid content.
- Developing need-based package of practice in Ashwagandha crop.
- Training to the Ashwagandha farmer regarding value addition in Ashwagandha crop to increase income of the farmer.
- Identification of suitable crop to intercropping with Ashwagandha under rainfed situation in order to increase remuneration from dual crop.

- Distribution of planting material in time at subsidized rate in order to increase the area under cultivation of Ashwagandha crop.
- Reducing/minimizing the gap between grower and buyer.

KEYWORDS

- **anti-inflammatory**
- **chemical constituents**
- **cultivation**
- **Indian council of agricultural research**
- **medicinal uses**
- ***Withania somnifera***

REFERENCES

Anonymous, (1982). *The Wealth of India* (Vol. X (Sp-W), pp. 580–585). Publications and Information Directorate, Council of Scientific and Industrial Research (CSIR), New Delhi.

Anonymous, (2007). *The Unani Pharmacopoeia of India: Part I* (Vol. I, pp. 7, 8). Depart. of AYUSH, Ministry of Health & Family Welfare, Govt. of India, New Delhi.

Ashish, K., & Jnanesha, A. C., (2017). Cultivation, utilization and role of medicinal plants in traditional medicine in Deccan eco-climate. *Int. J. Agric Sci., 8*(1), 98–103.

Ashish, K., & Jnanesha, A. C., (2017). Medicinal and Aromatic plants agro technologies developed by CSIR-Central institute of medicinal and aromatic plants. *J. Pharmacognosy and Phytochem., 6*(3), 173–175.

Ashish, K., & Jnanesha, A. C., (2018). Role and cultivation of important medicinal plants. In: Manzoor, H., (eds.), *Research Trends in Medicinal Plant Sciences* (Vol. 1, pp. 65–86). AkiNik Publications, Delhi, India.

Ashish, K., & Jnanesha, A. C., (2019). *Medicinal Herbs for Home Gardens and their Uses* (Vol. 17, No. 11, pp. 68, 69). Agrobios Newsletter.

Ashish, K., Rajput, D. K., Dayal, S. Y., Nagaraju, S., & Pandu, S. K. (2015). Introduction of CSIR-CIMAP improved varieties and promotion of cultivation of Ashwagandha (*Withania somnifera*) for improving the economy of small and marginal farmers in semi-arid tropical (SAT) regions of Deccan plateau. *International Conference on Medicinal Plants: Resource for Affordable New Generation Healthcare (ICOMP) at CSIR-CIMAP*, Lucknow. Abstract page No: 18.

Atal, C. K., & Sethi, P. D. A., (2015). Preliminary chemical examination of *Withania coagulans*. *Indian J. Pharm, 25,* 163, 164.

Atal, C. K., Gupta, O. P., & Afaq, H., (1975). *Commiphor amukul*: Source of guggal in Indian systems of medicine. *Economic Botany, 29,* 208–218.

Bhattacharya, A., Ghosal, S., & Bhattacharya, S. K., (2001). Antioxidant effect of *Withania somnifera* glycowithanolides in chronic footshock stress-induced perturbations of oxidative free radical scavenging enzymes and lipid peroxidation in rat frontal cortex and striatum. *J. Ethnopharmacol., 74*, 1–6.

Bhattacharya, S. K., Goel, R. K., Kaur, R., & Ghosal, S., (1987). Anti-stress activity of sitoindosides VII and VIII. New Acylsterylglucosides from *Withania somnifera. Phytother Res., 1*, 32–37.

Chen, L. X., He, H., & Qiu, F., (2011). Natural withanolides: An overview. *Nat. Prod. Rep., 28*, 705–740.

Farooqui, A. A., & Khan, M. M., (1993). *Production Technology of Medicinal and Aromatic Crops*. Indian Herbs Res and Supply Co., Bangalore.

Ghosal, S., Srivastava, R. S., Bhattacharya, S. K., Upadhyay, S. N., Jaiswal, A. K., & Chattopadhyay, U., (1989). Immunomodulatory and CNS effects of sitoindosides IX and X, two new glycol withanolides form *Withania somnifera. Phytother Res., 2*, 201–206.

Hepper, F. N., (1991). Old world Withania (Solanaceae): A taxonomic review and key to the species. In Hawkes, Lester, Nee & Estrada, (eds.): *Solanaceae III: Taxonomy, Chemistry, Evolution*. Royal Botanic Gardens Kew and Linnean Society of London.

Hunziker, A. T., (2001). *Genera Solanacearum: The Genera of Solanaceae Illustrated, Arranged According to a New System* (p. 500). A.R.G. Gantner, Germany: Koeltz Scientific Books. ISBN:3-904144-77-4.

Janardhan, R. K., Bahadur, B., Bhadraiah, B., & Rao, M. L. N., (2007). *Advances in Medicinal Plants* (pp. 112–122). Universities Press Private Limited, Hyderabad, India.

Jnanesha, A. C., & Ashish, K., (2018). Nutritional value of medicinal plants and their cultivation. In: Hemlata, P., Srivastava, D. K., Preeti, S., Devendra, S., & Kamlesh, S., (eds.), *New Approaches in Agricultural, Environmental and Nutritional Technology* (Vol. 1, pp. 124–131). Society of biological sciences and rural development, Allahabad, India.

Jnanesha, A. C., & Ashish, K., (2019). Agro-technology and Bio-prospecting in important medicinal plants. In: Akhil, B., (ed.), *Medicinal, Aromatic & Spice Plants* (Vol. 1, pp. 65–86). Eastern Book House Publication, Guwahati, India.

Kapoor, L. D., (2001). *Handbook of Ayurvedic Medicinal Plants* (pp. 337, 338). CRC Press: London, UK.

Kattimani, K. N., Reddy, Y. N., & Rajeshwara, R. B. R., (2001). Influence of pre-sowing seed treatment on seedling vigor, root length, and dry root yield of ashwagandha (*Withania somnifera* (L.) Dunal) under semi-arid climate of Hyderabad. *J. Med. Arom. Pl. Sci., 22(4A) and 23(1A)*, 221–223.

Kattimani, K. N., Reddy, Y. N., & Rajeswara, R. B. R., (1999). Effect of pre-sowing seed treatment on germination, seedling emergence, seedling vigor and root yield of Ashwagandha (*Withania somnifera* Dunal.). *Seed Sci. Technol., 27*(2), 483–488.

Kaul, M. K., Kumar, A., & Sharma, A., (2005). Reproductive biology of *Withania somnifera* (L.) dunal. *Curr. Sci., 88*(9), 1375–1377.

Kaur, N., Niazi, J., & Bains, R., (2013). A Review on Pharmacological Profile of *Withania somnifera* (Ashwagandha). *Res. Rev. J. Bot. Sci., 2*(4), 6–14.

Khare, C. P., (2007). *Indian Medicinal Plants-an Illustrated Dictionary* (pp. 717, 718). First Indian Reprint, Springer (India) Pvt. Ltd., New Delhi.

Khodaei, M., Jafari, M., & Noori, M., (2012). Remedial use of withanoloides from *Withania coagulans* (Stocks) Dunal. *Adv. in Life Sci., 2*(1), 6–19.

Kumar, A., Mir, B. A., Sehgal, D., Koul, S., Dar, T. H., Maharaj, K. K., Soom, N. R., & Qazi, G. N., (2011). Utility of multidisciplinary approach for genome diagnostics of cultivated and wild germplasm resources of medicinal *Withania somnifera*, and status of new species, W. ashwagandha, in the cultivated taxon. *Plant Sys. Evol., 291*, 141–151.

Malhotra, C. L., Mehta, V. L., Das, P. K., & Dhalla, N. S., (1965). Studies on *Withania-ashwagandha*, Kaul. V. The effect of total alkaloids (ashwagandholine) on the central nervous system. *Ind. J. Physiol. Pharmacol., 9*, 127–136.

Maurya, R., & Akanksha, J., (2010). Chemistry and pharmacology of *Withania coagulans*: An Ayurvedic remedy. *J. Pharm. Pharmacol., 62*, 153–160.

Maurya, R., Akanksha, J., Singh, A. B., & Srivastava, A. K., (2008). Coagulanolide, a withanolide from *Withania coagulans* fruits and antihyperglycemic activity. *Bioorg Med. Chem. Lett., 18*, 6534–6537.

Mir, B. A., Koul, S., Kumar, A., Kaul, M. K., Soodan, A. S., & Raina, S. N., (2011). Assessment and characterization of genetic variability in *Withania somnifera* (L.) dunal using biochemical and molecular markers. *African J. Biotech., 10*(66), 14746–14756.

Mirjalili, M. H., Moyano, E., Bonfill, M., Cusido, R. M., & Palazón, J., (2009). Steroidal lactones from *Withania somnifera*, an ancient plant for novel medicine. *Molecules, 14*(7), 2373–2393.

Mishra, L. C., Singh, B. B., & Dagenais, S., (2000). Review scientific basis for the therapeutic use of *Withania somnifera* (ashwagandha): A review. *Altern Med Rev., 5*(4), 334–346.

Muthu, C., Muniappan, A., Nagappan, R., & Savarimuthu, I., (2006). Medicinal plants used by traditional healers in Kancheepuram District of Tamil Nadu, India. *J. Ethnobiol Ethnomed., 2*, 43.

Nadkarni, K. M., (1976). *Indian Materia Medica* (3rd edn., p. 1074). Popular Prakashan, Bombay, India.

Oliver, E., & Williamson, (2002). The theory of the firm as governance structure: From choice to contract. *J. of Economic Perspectives, 16*(3), 171–195.

Rahman, A. U., Abbas, S., Dur-e-Shahwar, & Choudhary, M. I., (1993). New withanolides from *Withania* spp. *J. Nat. Prod., 56*, 1000–1006.

Rajeswara, R. B. R., Rajput, D. K., Nagaraju, G., & Adinarayana, G., (2012). Opportunities and Challenges in the Cultivation of Ashwagandha (*Withania somnifera* [L.] dunal). *J. Pharmacogn., 3*(2), 88–91.

Singh, B., Saxena, A. K., Chandan, B. K., Gupta, D. K., Bhutani, K. K., & Anand, K. K., (2001). Adaptogenic activity of a novel, withanolide-free aqueous fraction from the roots of *Withania somnifera* Dun. *Phytother. Res., 15*(4), 311–318.

Singh, G., Sharma, P. K., Dudhe, R., & Singh, S., (2010). Biological activities of *Withania somnifera*. *Annals of Biol. Res., 1*(3), 56–63.

Williamson, E. M., (2002). *Major Herbs of Ayurveda* (pp. 322, 323). Churchill Livingstone: London, UK.

CHAPTER 9

ENDANGERED MEDICINAL PLANTS OF TEMPERATE REGIONS: CONSERVATION AND MAINTENANCE

DHIMAN MUKHERJEE

Directorate of Research, Bidhan Chandra Krishi Viswavidayalaya, Kalyani – 741235, West Bengal, India, E-mail: dhiman_mukherjee@yahoo.co.in

ABSTRACT

The temperate Himalaya zone is amongst the most vulnerable and hazardous environments in the world, which is a rich repository of biodiversity of the valuable medicinal plant such as *Swertia chirayita, Valeriana jatamansi, Bergenia ciliata, Coptis teeta, Acorus calamus*, etc. The nature of these plants are very fragile and its conservation becomes very difficult because lack of suitable seed germination technique, cultivars, and improved cultivation practice. Under the influence of climate change, mountains are likely to experience wide-ranging effects on the environment, natural resources including biodiversity of medicinal plants, and socioeconomic conditions. Very little is known about the vulnerability of mountain ecosystems to climate change and its impact on high-value medicinal plant and its biodiversity pattern. Observations revealed that a good number of known and unknown medicinal plants are found in the forests of northeastern Himalayan (NEH) region in a temperate zone, and they are wiped out by miscreants or smugglers. Local inhabitants use some of these plants as herbal medicine, which is highly effective against some dreaded diseases. The unscientific, over-, and irregular exploitation of medicinal plants from their natural habitat has resulted in very fast depletion as well as the extinction of some important plant species due to shifting climate patterns. The threat of extinction can be reduced by developing in-situ and ex-situ conservation by adopting suitable agronomic management. Seed germination to crop harvesting becomes very challenging for growers as well as for research workers. An investigation was undertaken under Regional Research Station (Hill zone), Kalimpong, Uttar Banga Krishi Viswavidayalaya from 2005 to 2014, in consultation with local growers and scientists regarding various aspects of the cultivation of high altitude endangered medicinal plant species. The main objective was to generate some field-level preliminary data or observations on crop husbandry aspects for the welfare of the local community and future research program. Further, these plants have curative properties due to the presence of various complex chemical substances in different compositions, which are found as secondary plant metabolites in one or more parts of these plants. Exploitation of *Swertia chirayita* and *Valeriana jatamansi* mainly from wild sources, results in depletion of resource bases and ultimately endangering the species. Realizing the importance, it has been felt necessary to undertake both in-situ, as well as ex-situ conservation. Ex-situ conservation may be done in the form of depositing the live materials in the gene bank, establishing field gene banks and also promoting the cultivation of medicinal plants. Marketing of valuable medicinal herbs becomes a very challenging aspect especially for *Coptis teeta, Swertia chirayita,* etc., and this needs to be channelized with proper trade and marketing forum aided through various new schemes from state or central government.

9.1   INTRODUCTION

Human beings have depended on nature in general and plants in particular for their simple needs as being the sources for medicines, shelters, food-stuffs, fragrances, clothing, flavors, nutrients, and means of transportation throughout the ages. For the large proportions of the world's population, medicinal plants continue to show a dominant role in the healthcare system and this is mainly true in developing world, where herbal medicine, particularly high-altitude medicinal plants of North Eastern Himalaya, has a continuous history of long usage (Fakim, 2006). The foundations of archetypal traditional systems of medicine that have been in existence for thousands of years have formed from these plants.

Medicinal plant treatment is based on the experimental outcome of hundreds to thousands of years. The earliest information imprinted on clay tablets in cuneiform date since 2600 BC is from Mesopotamia; among the materials that were used were oils of *Commiphora* species (Myrrh), *Cedrus* species (Cedar), *Glycyrrhiza glabra* (Licorice), *Papaver somniferum* (Poppy juice), *Swertia chirayita* (chirota), *Valeriana jatamansi* and *Coptis teeta* (mismi teta) are still used today for the cure of diseases extending from colds and coughs to inflammation and parasitic infections (Jones, 1998; Mukherjee, 2018a). The traditional medicine (TM) practice is widespread in China, India, Japan, Pakistan, Sri Lanka, and Thailand. About 30% of the total medicinal consumption is attributed to traditional tribal medicines alone by China. In diversified industries, the contribution of plants is remarkable such as fine chemicals, cosmetics, pharmaceuticals drugs, and industrial raw materials, etc. For the development of new drug discovery, medicinal plants perform a dynamic part. Medicinal plants have proved their sole role in coping with several deadly diseases, including cancer and the diseases associated with viral onslaught viz. Hepatitis, AIDS, etc. Recently in the drug market, more than 100 plants as sources of new drugs are presented which mainly include vincristine, reseinnamine, vinblastin, deseridine, and reserpine from different plants. Fresh medicines chiefly in use are artemisinin, guggulsterone, ginkgolides, lectinam, E-guggulsterone, teniposide, etoposide, plaunotol, and nabilone appeared all around the world (Harrison, 1998; Pradhan and Lama, 2012). Indian indigenous tree of *Nothapodytes nimmoniana* (*Mappia faetida*) is frequently used in Japan for the cure of cervical cancer. Some of the most important medicinal plants in the Indian Himalayan range are *Swertia chirayita, Valeriana jatamansi, Coptis teeta Dioscorea deltoidea, Rheum emodi, Arnebia benthamii, Inula racemosa, Datura stramonium Aconitum heterophyllum, Artemisia spp., Podophyllum hexandrum, Juniperus macropoda, Hypericum perforatum, Hyoscyamus niger, Saussurea spp., Picrorhiza kurroa*, etc. Amongst all these plants, the first three are highly endangered and available to a limited area in the world. They are mostly confined to North Eastern Himalaya zone (Mukherjee, 2008). Importance of medicinal plant cultivation is:

- To ease pressure on natural resources;
- To make the available fresh, genuine, and quality raw material for manufacturing of standardized and efficacious drugs;
- To evolve better strains and high yielding crops through improvement programs such as tissue culture, etc.;
  To standardize the collection, storage, and post-harvest technology;
- To provide the regular and alternative source of income to the farmers for the amelioration of their economic conditions;

To conserve the biological and genetic diversity in medicinal plants for posterity.

9.2 CONSERVATION AND UTILIZATION

Plant genetic resources have made substantial contributions to the domestication, utilization, and improvement of all kinds of crops, including medicinal plants with high soil microbial activity (Mukherjee, 2019). Collection, characterization, and their efficient utilization are keys to the efficient management of any kind of genetic resource (Uniyal et al., 2006). Domestication and cultivation of valuable medicinal plants have become a very challenging task for the grower, stakeholder, and concerned department. Several researchers studied on high altitudinal medicinal plants and observed that they were highly potent and required widespread cultivation. This would help to ease pressure on natural resources, and make available fresh, genuine, and quality raw material for the manufacturing of standardized and efficacious drugs (Prakash et al., 2011). Further, the introduction and domestication of useful, exotic drug plants would help to minimize import and maximize the export of valuable herbal medicine. Few plant species such as *Coptis teeta, Swertia chirata, Picrorrhiza kurooa,* and *Taxus baccata* need intensive care so that we can protect earth's treasure. The major objectives of conservation programs are to provide safety against loss of genetic resources and to make these resources available for crop improvement at present and in the future. Each strategy for conservation has to offer relatively greater safety and cost-effectiveness (Bharat et al., 2012; Mukherjee, 2018d). Any useful plant can be considered for conservation but medicinal plants with known biological activities and chemical constituents responsible for such activities, if influenced by agro-ecological situations, need to be conserved in ideal situations to avoid loss of essential compounds responsible for biological actions. However, prioritization of species is essential to make full use of any particular strategy with justification. Most of the valuable plant species are confined to various forest ecosystems. Many of the plants in developing countries being extracted from the wild, there is a fair chance of genetic diversity loss leading to the rapid depletion of several valuable plant species from their natural habitats (Mukherjee et al., 2013). Conservation of most plant species is under severe threat due to shifting in climate patterns as well as global warming trends in the recent past (Mani and Mukherjee, 2016). The prosperity of most of the valuable plant species is confined to various forest zone under different ecosystems. They should be protected under the natural conditions for optimum biological activity (Purohit et al., 2013). These are mainly categorized as:

1. **Tropical:** *Andrographis paniculata, Ocimum basilicum, Withania somnifera, Vitex negundo, Plantago erosa, Dioscorea alata, Cryptolepis buchanani, Acorus calamus, Adhatoda vasica, Aquillaria agallocha; Centella asiatica,* and *Paedaria faetida.*
2. **Subtropical:** *Artemisia maritime, Lavendula vera, Litsea cubeba, Mucuna pruriens, Pogostemon calelin, Curcuma caesia,* and *Zanthoxylum armatum.*
3. **Temperate:** *Geranium nepalensis, Panax pseudoginseng, Swertia chirata, Picrorrhiza kurooa, Satyrium nepalensis, Taxus baccata, Orchis latifolia,* and *Rubia cordifolia.*
4. **Alpine:** *A. heterophyllum, Podophyllum hexandrum, Rheum emodi, Coptis teeta, Aconitum ferox,* and *Delphinium subulatum.*

Conservation of these valuable plants, germplasm is possible either through in-situ and ex-situ mode based on topography and environmental condition.

9.2.1   IN-SITU CONSERVATION

The parks and department should prepare a policy at the national level on the conservation and utilization of medicinal plants in protected areas (WHO, 1993). The policy should include:

- Identifying which of the protected areas are most important for medicinal plants;
- Techniques and procedures for the collection of medicinal plants within protected areas;
- The Parks division should assess the extent to which the protected areas system covers the medicinal vegetation of the country. Through this new protected area create and help to conserve genetic resources;
- Governing body of protected zone, should ensure that the preservation and utilization of medicinal plants are included into site management plans;

- Species that are deeply exhausted by over-collection should be re-introduced into locality where they once grew natural (Mukherjee, 2008a).

9.2.2 EX-SITU CONSERVATION

Protection of medicinal plants can be made by the ex-situ, i.e., outside from the natural habitat by cultivating and maintaining vegetation in botanic gardens, parks, other suitable sites, and through long term protection of plant propagules in gene banks (seed bank, pollen bank, DNA libraries, etc.), and plant tissue culture repositories and by cryopreservation). Botanical gardens can play a key role in ex-situ conservation of plants, especially those facing imminent threat of extinction (Bhardwaj et al., 2011). Species conserved ex situ can also suffer genetic erosion and depend on continued human care (Mukherjee et al., 2015). The disadvantage of ex-situ protection is that the plant sample of various species conserved ex-situ (e.g., *Swertia chirayita*) might signify a thin array of heritable difference than that which occurs in the wild (Mukherjee and Chakrabarty, 2010). North Eastern Himalaya range of India is the native place of three high value endangered medicinal plants viz. *Coptis teeta, Swertia chirayita,* and *Valeriana jatamansi.* Cultivation and conservation aspects of these plants are discussed here in detail as per research findings from 2005 to 2014 in Eastern Himalaya in Darjeeling subdivision of West Bengal, India (Figure 9.1).

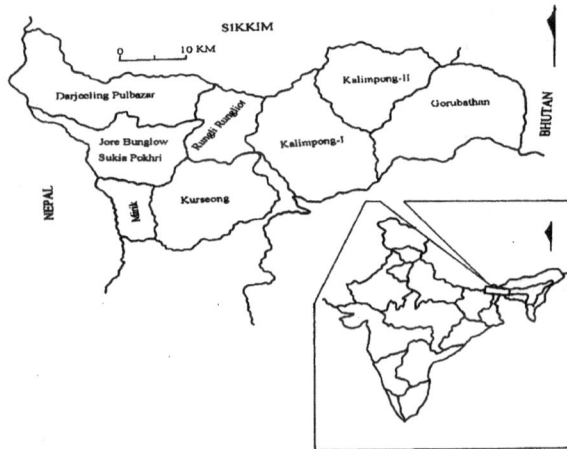

FIGURE 9.1   Study area of Eastern Himalaya range of threatened medicinal plant species.

9.3   IMPROVED CULTIVATION ASPECTS OF FEW ENDANGERED MEDICINAL PLANT OF TEMPERATE ZONE

9.3.1   COPTIS TEETA

> ➢ **Kingdom**: Plantae;
> ➢ **Division**: Magnoliophyta;
> ➢ **Class:** Magnoliopsida;
> ➢ **Order**: Ranunculales;
> ➢ **Family:** Ranunculaceae;
> ➢ **Genus**: Coptis;
> ➢ **Species:** Teeta.

Coptis teeta is a small perennial herb with the height of 20–25 cm. It is popularly known as Coptis or Mishmi tita and is an important medicinal plant used against various diseases. The explicit nomenclature 'Tita' has been come out for its bitterness. Its tenuous rhizome, known as "Yunnan goldthread" in the traditional Chinese medicine (TCM) system, has been used as an antibacterial and as an anti-inflammatory medicine for a long time (Mukherjee and Chakraborty, 2019). This has a compound leaf, serrated into three parts; the leaf blade is ovate, triangular in shape. Length of the leaf varies from 5–13 cm and breadth 4–9 cm. Leaf is papery in nature. Lateral segment subsessile to petiolate, shorter than the central, serrated leaf, unequally parted. Central segment is petiolate, pinnately divided. Leaf margin is acute, apex attenuate, scales 15–26 cm tall, glabrous. Base of the leaf is cordate. Root is fibrous with small yellow-colored. The color of the rhizome is golden yellow. Inflorescence is cymose, and root is a pungent, very bitter, cooling herb that controls bacterial and viral infections, relaxes spasms, lowers fevers and stimulates the circulation (Mukherjee, 2018b). The root contains several compounds that are effective in inhibiting various soil-inhabiting microbes, mainly bacteria and are a safe and effective treatment for many ailments, such as some forms of dysentery that are caused by bacteria (http://en.wikipedia.org/wiki/Coptis_teeta).

Several factors contribute to its endangerment. It is endemic to a very small area, where its habitat is rapidly declining due in part to deforestation, partly for over-collection, for medicinal use, and partly due to its low reproductive success (Pandit and Babu, 1998; Mukherjee, 2009). This is mainly used in Ayurveda, Unani, and Siddha system of medical prescriptions. The world distribution ranges from East Asia, particularly in the north part of China to the temperate regions of Eastern Himalayas. Few species are endemic to India, recorded only in the Himalayan region across Darjeeling in the West Bengal, Sikkim, and Arunachal Pradesh in an altitude range of 2,300–3,200 m (Pandit and Babu, 1998; Mukherjee, 2016). These are found mainly in Dibang Valley, part of Lohit and upper Subansiri districts of Arunachal Pradesh. The plant prefers light sandy, loamy, moist soils with a pH range of 4.6 to 5.4. It can grow in light shade to no shade mainly on woodland.

Because of high demand, plant population is diminishing day by day and deforestation leads to the risk of extinction. Desiccated root and rhizomes have tremendous demand in the market (Huang and Chunlin, 2007). To date, very little work has been conducted on this plant, particularly in crop production aspects. A few notable research works have been conducted from 2009 to 2014 in Darjeeling hill, under the aegis of Uttar Banga Krishi Viswavidyalaya, at Lava (2,040 m AMSL) on plant morphology and influence of various method of planting along with organic nutrient management on growth and yield of *Coptis teeta*. The study was mainly confined to the yield of rhizome weight because it is the main source of alkaloid berberine having excellent therapeutic values to fight malaria, indigestion, liver diseases, etc. Various composition of berberine will differ according to the rhizome weight, girth, and length. An exploration program was conducted during November 2009 in Arunachal Pradesh for the collection of *Coptis teeta* in Dibang Valley at an altitude of 3,000 m AMSL (Figures 9.2–9.5). The plant is locally called Mismi teeta because local primitive inhabitants (Mismi tribes) called this

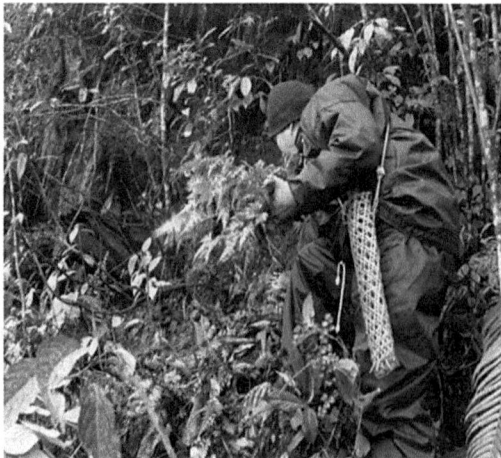

FIGURE 9.2   Collection of *Coptis teeta* plant by local growers.

medicinal plant as such from time immemorial. According to Mismi tribes and information collected from the forest department, Govt. of Arunachal Pradesh, this plant is categorically enlisted as critically endangered plant as per International Union for Conservation of Nature and Natural resources (IUCN) list of endangered species (Mukherjee and Sharma, 2014). In Myodia of Dibang valley, seedlings were collected with the help of one mismi tribe person who was a forest ranger in the Forest Department, Govt. of Arunachal Pradesh (Table 9.1).

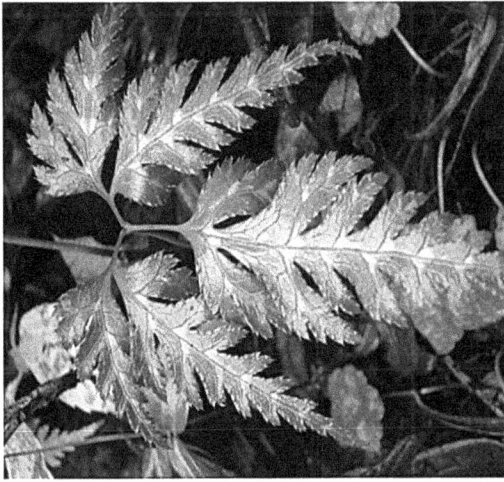

FIGURE 9.3   *Coptis teeta plant.*

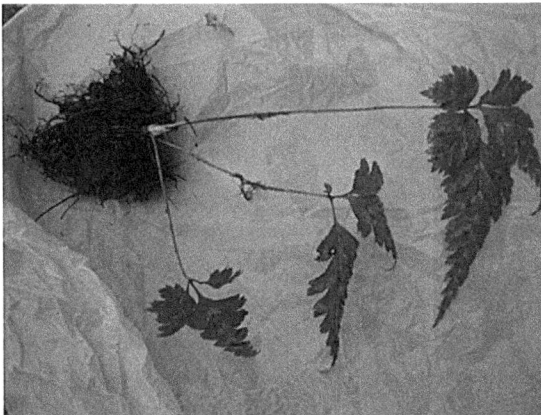

FIGURE 9.4   Plant with roots.

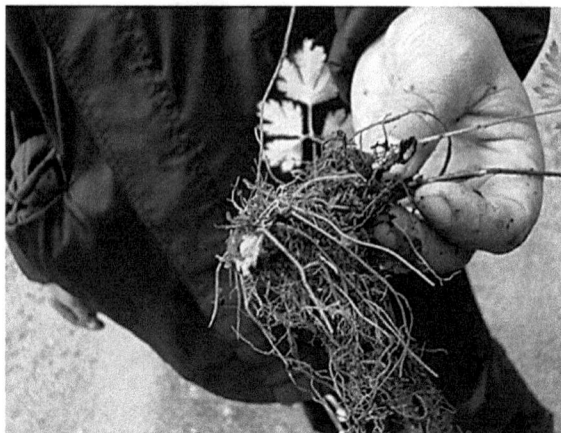

FIGURE 9.5   Plant with rhizome.

TABLE 9.1   Physicochemical Status of Soil Sample of Experimental Site (Lava, Kalimpong Block II)

pH	ECE (inch/cm)	Available (kg/ha)			Total N (%)	Organic C (%)	Organic Matter (%)	C/N Ratio
		N	P_2O_5	K_2O				
4.9	0.32	345	22.1	379	15.15	3.54	2.87	12.25

Growth of *Coptis teeta* was considerably influenced by various land configurations (Table 9.2). Studies revealed that superior plant height was registered with the sloppy terraced land sowing at eight months after sowing. It was at par with the ridge sowing, and statistically better to other methods of plantings. Leaf length was more with sloppy land sowing and significantly better for other options. A number of leaves per plant was recorded highest with sloppy land sowing and showed parity with the ridge sowing. Further, observation from Table 9.1 revealed that petiole length was more with furrow method and showed parity with ridge sowing only, and statistically better to rest of cultivation options. The greater number of flowers and fruits were observed with ridge planting. Better rhizome girth was observed with ridge methods and showed parity with all other options except the plain bed and undulated land sowing method. Better rhizome length was found with the sloppy land sowing closely followed by ridge and undulated land sowing methods. Better rhizome weight was found with sloppy land cultivation (3.01 g) and was at par with the undulated method of planting (2.55 g), and statistically better to rest of the imposed options. Root length was also found better with the sloppy land situation and comparatively superior to all other practices.

Various treatments on nutrient use aspect revealed that plant height, leaf length was more with vermicompost (@0.50 t/ha), and statistically better to rest of the nutrient doses (Table 9.3). Leaf breadth was more with leaf manure (@ 0.50 t/ha), and gave notable reply compare to other application of organic nutrient supply except vermicompost (@0.50 t/ha). The number of leaves/plant record with vermicompost (@ 0.50 t/ha), was statistically better than others (Table 9.3). The highest petiole length was observed with leaf manure (@ 0.50 t/ha) and was at par with vermicompost (@0.50 t/ha). The number of flowers/plants was more with the FYM (@0 50 t/ha), and similar to the vermicompost used field. The number of follicles and rhizome girth, more observed with the vermicompost (@0 50 t/ha), and significantly better to other options. Rhizome length was found superior with leaf manure (@0 50 t/ha). Rhizome weight was more with vermicompost (@0.50 t/ha) and was at par with leaf manure (@ 0.50 t/ha). This treatment gave 96.6 and 79.6%, more rhizomes compared to control, respectively. Root length was better with the vermicompost (@0.50 t/ha) and showed parity with the leaf manure (@0 50 t/ha) treated plots. From this finding, it revealed that, use of vermicompost and leaf manure application (@0.50 t/ha) was very effective for higher productivity of *Coptis teeta*.

9.3.2 VALERIANA JATAMANSI

> **Kingdom:** Plantae;
> **Family:** Valerianaceae;
> **Sub-family:** Valerianoideae;
> **Genus:** *Valeriana;*
> **Species:** *jatamansi;*
> **Common name:** Indian valerian;
> **Latin name:** *Valeriana jatamansi.*

V. jatamansi is an endangered medicinal herb grown wildly as under story vegetation in temperate forests. Like many other non-timber forest products, this is considered as forest gift and hence there is neither any control system in its harvest nor is its domestication started for ensuring sustainable regeneration (Chakraborty et al., 2015). This is a perennial plant growing to 0.45 to 0.65 m (approximately 1 ft 8 inch), velvet-hairy. The flowers are

TABLE 9.2 Effect of Various Planting Methods on Growth and Yield Characters of *Coptis teeta* in Darjeeling Hills

Treatments	Plant height (cm)	Leaf length (cm) (compound leaf)	Leaf breadth (cm)	No of leaves/plant	Petiole length (cm)	No. of flowers/plant	No of fruits/plant (follicle)	Rhizome girth (cm)	Rhizome length (cm)	Rhizome weight (g)	Root length (Fibrous root) (cm)
Plain bed sowing	9.11	6.21	4.22	5.33	7.01	4.03	3.11	1.39	2.11	1.83	4.11
Sloppy land sowing	13.01	8.55	5.19	7.21	7.89	3.18	3.31	2.03	3.71	3.01	7.77
Furrow sowing	11.21	5.79	4.66	6.56	9.04	2.09	3.91	1.33	3.32	2.14	5.16
Ridge sowing	13.10	5.31	5.93	6.88	10.01	5.86	4.36	2.14	3.13	2.36	6.32
Undulated land	8.01	6.08	4.11	6.12	7.11	4.93	3.78	2.04	2.71	2.55	5.11
LSD ($P=0.05$)	2.01	1.61	0.46	0.88	1.73	0.29	0.63	0.70	NS	0.60	0.91

TABLE 9.3 Effect of Various Nutrient Treatments on Plant Growth and Yield Characters of *Coptis teeta*

Treatments	Plant height (cm)	Leaf length (cm) (compound leaf)	Leaf breadth (cm)	No of leaves/plant	Petiole length (cm)	No. of flowers/plant	No of fruits/plant (follicle)	Rhizome girth (cm)	Rhizome length (cm)	Rhizome weight (g)	Root length (Fibrous root) (cm)
Control	8.02	6.55	3.11	7.33	8.31	3.25	2.82	1.41	1.11	2.41	4.21
Vermicompost (@0.50t/ha)	19.31	8.05	4.25	15.11	12.11	3.51	5.91	3.81	2.33	4.74	7.55
FYM (@0 50 t/ha)	13.33	6.11	3.10	11.35	10.12	3.92	3.25	2.36	2.04	2.23	5.18
Leaf manure (@ 0.50 t/ha)	17.05	7.30	4.34	12.56	11.01	1.51	4.85	3.04	2.64	4.33	7.36
LSD ($P=0.05$)	0.78	0.89	0.57	1.16	1.79	1.41	0.90	0.41	0.51	0.87	1.44

dioecious (individual flowers are either male or female, but only one sex is found on one plant. So, both male and female plants must be grown if seed is required) and are pollinated by insects. Rhizomes are elongate, with fibrous roots. Stems are 3–6 in number. Leaves at the base are heart-shaped or ovate, 2–10 cm x 1.5–8 cm, toothed or wavy-toothed. Stem leaves are stalkless, smaller, and uppermost often cut (Chakraborty et al., 2015a). Snow-white flowers are borne in flat-topped clusters on top of the stems. Upper bracts are linear-lance shaped, about 3 mm long. Seed-pods are velvety, shorter than the upper bracts. This plant prefers light (sand) to medium (loamy) soils with suitable pH acidic to neutral soils. Also prefers to grow in an upland sloppy situation where water stagnates rarely or under a good drainage facility. Common in forests, shrubberies, and on open slopes of the hills at a temperature ranging between 14–18°C. Valerian is a shade loving plant preferring moist soil. Its flowering time is mostly confined to March-May (Mukherjee and Chkraborty, 2014).

The plant can be grown in sandy loam soil, rich in carbon and humus. Sandy soils, containing concrete or coarse sand are favorable for its cultivation. Similarly steep land is more suitable than the plain land for its growth. Plants also grow better in the fire burnt forest and high hill areas where other wild plants grow. The growth is reported to be better in slightly acidic soil (pH 4.9–5.7). Jatamansi is found throughout the Himalayas, from Afghanistan to SW China, at altitudes of 1,500–3,600 m AMSL (Chakraborty et al., 2015c). It requires a temperate wet climate, moderate sunshine and foggy weather condition in the evening time, high relative humidity and open space. It can tolerate drought and frost for a long time. During favorable growth periods, roots of the damaged plants bear new buds. Frost can harm the plant if it occurs before the flowering stage resulting in the production of immature seeds. As the altitude and coldness increases, the plant takes more time to grow and mature (Table 9.4).

TABLE 9.4 Physicochemical Status of Soil Sample Suitable for Cultivation of *Valeriana jatamansi*

pH	ECE (mho/cm)	Available (kg/ha)			Total N (%)	Organic C (%)	Organic Matter (%)	C/N Ratio
		N	P$_2$O$_5$	K$_2$O				
4.5–5.7	0.21–026	240–319	20.3–26.71	244–280	10.25–15.02	1.44–2.89	2.31–4.09	10.11–14.34

Although the economic value of this herb is reportedly unknown to the local people until the recent past, the herb has now been widely known for its market potential. Thus, the exploitation of this valuable plant is in increasing trend leading to its rapid decline from its natural habitat, without knowing the better agronomic and cultivation aspects. The collection and, more recently, marketing of these plants has provided an important source of income for communities living in mountain areas (Mukherjee et al., 2009). Valerian is a well-known and frequently used medicinal herb that has a long and proven history of efficacy (Mukherjee et al., 2015). It is employed as a nervine and sedative. In high mountain range of Himalaya, it is used to treat insomnia and hysteria along with nausea, pimples, and rheumatism. It is noted especially for its effect as a tranquilizer and nervine, particularly for those people suffering from nervous overstrain (Singh et al., 2006). The root is antispasmodic, carminative, diuretic, hypnotic, powerfully nervine, sedative, and stimulant (Prakash, 1999). The roots of 2-year-old plants are harvested in the autumn once the leaves have died down and are used fresh or dried (Mukherjee et al., 2014). A dried rhizome is used as incense. This plant is relatively new to researchers and local people as well as far as the cultivation aspects are concerned. Because of scanty literature and limited extension programs, most of the hill people are unaware of these valuable treasures.

9.3.2.1 PROPAGATION

Major means of propagation is by seeds. Fully mature seeds fall on the ground of a mature fruit, but only a few germinate to grow into new plants. Seeds are sown in a cold frame by just covering them with soil because they require light for germination. The seedlings are picked out from different pots when they are 3–7 cm in height, and placed in the main field with the advent of summer season (April-May) or the following rainy season. Natural regeneration of this plant takes place by seeds, but it can also be propagated through vegetative means by cutting method. Seed germination study revealed that this can be increased significantly by the use of Kinetin 200 ppm (91.66 ± 5.21) and GA_3 200 ppm (Mukherjee, 2016a). Seed germination drastically enhanced with a growth regulator compared to control plots (Figures 9.6–9.9).

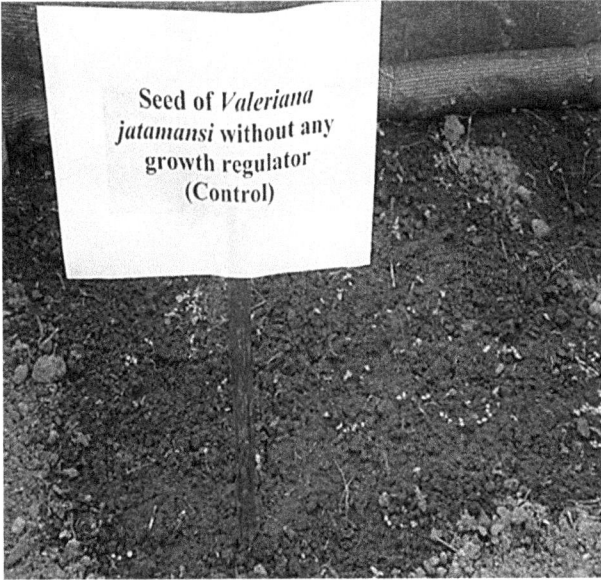

FIGURE 9.6 Seeds pretreated with distilled water (control).

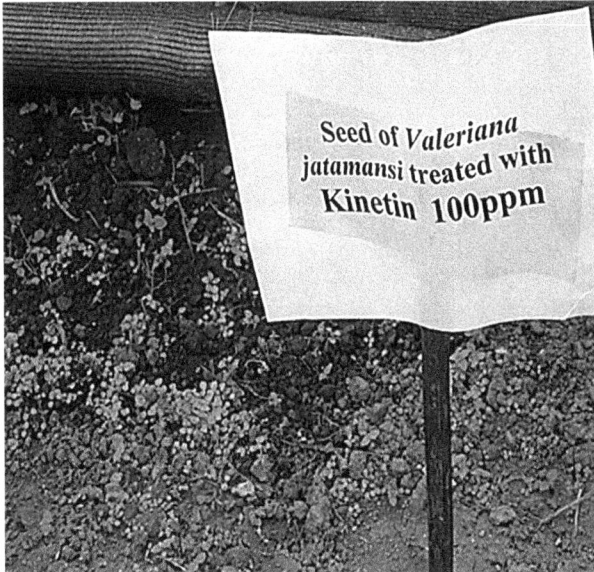

FIGURE 9.7 Seeds pretreated with Kinetin 100 ppm.

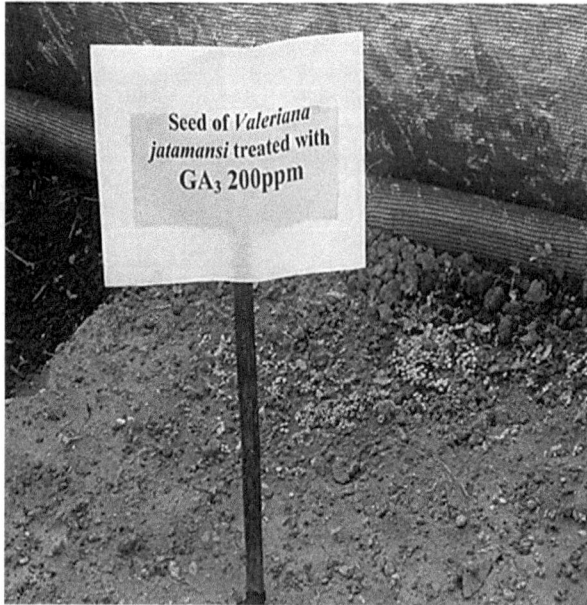

FIGURE 9.8   Seeds pretreated with GA$_3$ 100 ppm.

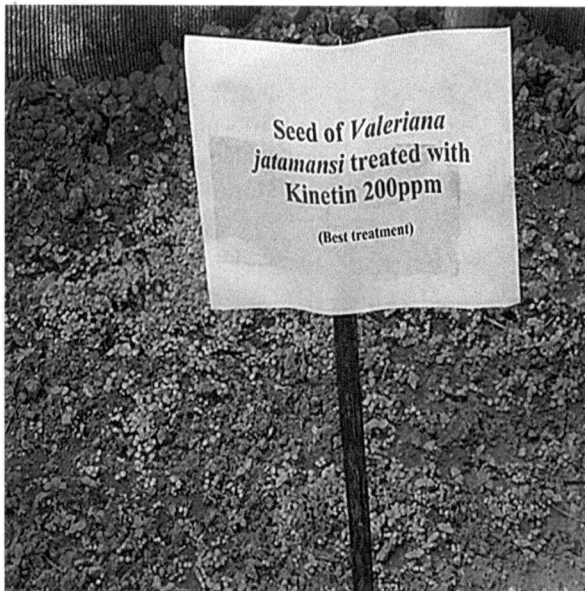

FIGURE 9.9   Seeds pretreated with Kinetin 200 ppm.

9.3.2.2   NURSERY RAISING AND PLANTING

The nursery should be maintained in a raised bed with good and healthy seeds. Following factors should be taken into account during seed germination:

- The feathery seeds must be healthy and should be used within 6 months of harvesting;
- Seeds should be freshly collected from fully mature plants and sown under shade (polyhouse);
- Nursery bed must contain one part of sand, two-parts forest soil and three-parts compost manure (w/v) (1:2:3). These should be properly mixed and sieved. The bed should be raised into 10–20 cm;
- To control harmful insects found in the soil, Malathion powder must be mixed with the soil at the rate of 3 g/sq m;
- Seeds must be sown, after mixing with sieved sand or soil, at the rate of 5 g/sq m, uniformly on the upper layer of the bed;
- After the seeds were sown, it should be covered either with light soil, straw or coirpit to conserve soil moisture for proper germination of seed;
- Water should be applied as per need; excessive watering reduces seed viability;
- The shade must be removed after one and a half months. All the weeds must be uprooted in the beginning otherwise the weeds can be harmful to the plants.

Attention must be paid to the preparation of nursery bed, method, and time of sowing and watering the plant, etc. Beds must be fully protected from trespassing animals. Seeds are sown during April-June. When the seeds germination starts, various mulching materials used should be removed. The seedling can be transferred to the perforated plastic bags 3 to 4 months after sowing. Seed Invigoration is an effective tool for the conservation of endangered or valuable medicinal plants such as *Bergia ciliate* (Mukherjee, 2019a).

9.3.2.3   SEED INVIGORATIONS

Seed germination is a very challenging task and various growth regulators can be used for effective seed emergence. An experiment was conducted on a randomized block design with 15 pre-treatment seeds of *V. jatamansi* in

TABLE 9.5　Effect of Different Treatments on Seed Germination of *Valeriana jatamansi* (Pooled Value of Two Year Data)

Treatments	Germination (%)	Days required for onset of germination (days)	Days required for completion of Germination (days)	Mean germination time (days)	Seedling vigour		Seedling Vigour Index I	Seedling Vigour Index II
					Fresh biomass (g)	Dry biomass (g)		
Control	51.33±6.16	29.33	36.33	33.03	2.03* (3.64)	1.02 (0.54)**	51.87	41.11
IBA 50	54.00±2.12	26.00	39.00	31.59	2.22 (4.43)	1.24 (1.03)	76.22	53.66
IBA 100	79.33±1.33	23.33	33.33	27.83	2.37 (5.12)	1.35 (1.32)	173.08	104.21
IBA 150	85.66±4.13	20.66	44.66	30.56	2.85 (7.65)	1.43 (1.54)	260.83	133.92
IBA 200	70.00±3.11	20.00	34.33	25.15	2.13 (4.02)	1.27 (1.11)	153.52	72.71
IBA 250	63.66±3.92	22.66	30.66	25.66	1.81 (2.79)	0.93 (0.36)	121.66	36.65
GA₃50	61.66±3.21	27.33	32.00	29.05	2.05 (3.69)	1.07 (0.65)	91.19	43.07
GA₃100	72.66±3.91	27.33	30.66	27.91	2.27 (4.67)	1.22 (0.98)	161.33	71.07
GA₃150	80.15±3.12	27.66	31.33	28.35	2.49 (5.69)	1.26 (1.09)	156.31	86.36
GA₃200	86.66±5.60	24.00	28.33	25.16	2.61 (6.32)	1.47 (1.65)	202.45	137.99
GA₃250	80.15±2.66	22.33	25.66	22.95	2.51 (5.77)	1.39 (1.44)	196.66	112.42
Kinetin 50	50.21±8.62	25.33	36.33	31.93	2.03 (3.61)	1.13 (0.77)	74.81	33.66
Kinetin 100	58.98±7.32	25.00	36.00	31.15	2.41 (5.32)	1.22 (0.98)	101.83	56.81
Kinetin 150	72.36±3.63	23.33	30.33	25.33	2.78 (7.25)	1.48 (1.69)	220.95	121.24
Kinetin 200	94.66±10.66	20.33	24.33	23.33	2.94 (8.15)	1.59 (2.03)	303.33	190.06
Kinein 250	81.33±5.33	20.00	23.33	23.65	2.71 (6.87)	1.32 (1.23)	201.66	100.66
LSD (P=0.05)	7.21	1.98	2.05	2.11	NS	0.08	8.98	9.11

N.S = Non-significant.

*Values marked are square root transformed values.

**Original values.

(*Source*: Mukherjee, 2018).

four different replications. Work was carried out in the field condition from November 2011 to November 2014. *V. jatamansi* seed osmo-priming with IBA 50, 100, 150, 200, 250 ppm; GA_3 50, 100, 150, 200, 250 ppm, kinetin 50, 100, 150, 200, 250 ppm and hydro-priming (control with distilled water). The highest seed germination percentage of *V. jatamansi* was observed with the kinetin-treated seeds @ 200 ppm and significantly better to all other treatments (Table 9.5). Days required for the onset of germination was lesser in IBA 200 and kinetin 250 ppm. Mean germination time was 32.11 days in untreated (control) seeds which was significantly reduced to 22.95 days with GA_3 250 ppm. It was 32.01% lower than the control and was at par with kinetin 200, kinetin 250 and IBA 200 ppm primed seeds. Kinetin 100 ppm showed maximum seedling vigor index I (303.33), which was 484.15% higher than the control and was significantly better than all other 14 seed priming treatments. The highest seedling vigor index II of 190.06 was registered with kinetin 200 ppm, which was 362.32% higher than the control and was statistically better than other treatments. The maximum emergence index (EI) and germination energy (GE) were exhibited by kinetin 200 ppm.

Maximum seedling length of *V. jatamansi* (3.11 cm) was registered with kinetin 200 ppm and was at par with the kinetin 200 and IBA 150 ppm pretreated seeds (Table 9.6). However, the lowest seedling length was obtained with the control (1.03 cm). EI is a parameter that reflects the seed vigor and recorded highest with kinetin 200 ppm. The lowest value of the EI was found with control followed by kinetin 50 ppm. The effect of seed invigoration treatments on GE reveals that the maximum value of 3.89 was observed with kinetin 200 ppm, which was statistically at par with kinetin 250 ppm and GA_3 200 ppm.

TABLE 9.6 Influence of Different Seed Invigoration Treatments on Seedling Length, Emergence Index, and Germination Energy of Seeds of *Valeriana jatamansi* (Pooled Value of Two-Year Data)

Treatments	Seedling Length (cm)	Emergence Index	Germination Energy
Control	1.03	1.75	1.41
IBA 50	1.43	2.08	1.38
IBA 100	2.27	3.40	2.38
IBA 150	3.08	4.15	1.92
IBA 200	2.25	3.51	2.04
IBA 250	1.90	2.81	2.08
$GA_3$50	1.44	2.26	1.93

TABLE 9.6   *(Continued)*

Treatments	Seedling Length (cm)	Emergence Index	Germination Energy
GA$_3$100	2.37	2.66	2.37
GA$_3$150	2.00	2.92	2.56
GA$_3$200	2.31	3.61	3.06
GA$_3$250	2.49	3.59	3.12
Kinetin 50	1.51	1.98	1.38
Kinetin 100	1.76	2.36	1.64
Kinetin 150	3.11	3.10	2.38
Kinetin 200	3.31	4.65	3.89
Kinein 250	2.46	4.07	3.49
LSD (P=0.05)	0.26	0.58	0.77

9.3.2.4   LAND SELECTION AND SHADING

V. jatamansi can be grown on steep barren land with no waterlogging. In the plains, there should be a proper drainage system (Chakraborty et al., 2015b). According to the necessity, weeding should be done and the land should be plowed 2–3 times. Well friable bed is more productive compared to clotted soil. Soil should be treated with carbofuran (2.5 kg/ha) for control of various nematodes and pests. Well pulverized soil for seed germination and sandy-loam soil with good water holding capacity for transplanting is advocated. Shading on cultivation land becomes very remunerative for its cultivation up to a certain extent (Chakraborty et al., 2015d). Work conducted under various shading option during 2010 to 2013 at Sukhiapokhri (Darjeeling) revealed that maximum rhizome yield, leaf yield, total crop yield was registered with the 40% shading (Table 9.7).

TABLE 9.7   Influence of Shading on Fresh Yield of *V. jatamansi*

Shade	Yield (q/ha)			
	Rhizome	Root	Leaf	Total Biomass
Open	16.33	9.66	34.11	60.1
20% shad	15.36	14.47	44.23	74.06
40% shade	25.91	21.63	48.12	95.66
60% shade	20.65	20.98	40.65	82.28
80% shade	17.32	20.33	29.05	66.7
LSD (P=0.05)	2.33	2.45	4.11	22.47

9.3.2.5   NUTRIENTS AND PESTICIDES MANAGEMENT

Use of various organic manures mainly FYM, vermicompost, green manure, etc., may be used as per the requirement of the plant (Table 9.8). The research conducted in Kalimpong (Darjeeling) revealed that use of vermicompost @ 0.50 t/ha and forest litter @ 3 t/ha was the best in producing good economic yield. To prevent diseases, bio-pesticides could be prepared (either single or mixture) from neem (kernel, seeds, and leaves), chitrakmool, dhatura, cow's urine, etc. The disease can be prevented with the help of various bio-pesticides either in a single or mixture of neem (i.e., kernel, seed, and leaves), powder, dhatura, chitrakmool, cow's urine, etc. Observation revealed that under field conditions, the plant is mostly attacked by ant and termite. To overcome this problem, Phorate should be applied as per the need and necessity.

TABLE 9.8   Organic Inputs Recommendation on Observation Basis at Field Level

Input	Quantity Required (t/ ha)	Remarks
Neem/Pongamia cake	1–2.5	Protection against termite and other soil borne pests and pathogens.
FYM	2–5	There is the possibility of weed infestation and poor establishment of the crop.
Forest litter	3–6	Act as a growth enhancer for *V. jatamansi*.
Compost	5–8	Possibility of weed and pathogen infestation and poor establishment of the crop.
Vermicompost	0.50	This source is weed-free and helps in better performance of the crop.

9.3.2.6   WEEDING

Periodical weeding and hoeing are required both in the nursery and main field. Since the crop is grown around the rainy season and since it remains in the field for a longer duration, it gets invaded by different types of weeds, viz. *Oxalis corniculata, Echinochloa colon, Eleusine indica, Digitaria sanguinalis, Cynodon dactylon, Panicum repens*, sedges viz., *Cyperus rotundus, Cyperus iria, Fimbristylis miliacea* and broad-leaved weeds viz., *Chenopodium album, Caesulia axillaris, Phyllanthus sp., Ammania baccifera, Commelina benghalensis, Fragaris indica, Artemesia vulgaris, Desmodium oxyphyllum,* etc. This plant is mostly associated with few valuable medicinal herbs, *Heracleum candicans, Bidens bipinnata, Taraxacum officinale, Cuscuta reflexa, Trifolium repens, Fumaria parviflora, Loranthus longiflorus, Plantago major, Rumex nepalensis,* and *Urtica dioica* (Mukherjee, 2013).

9.3.2.7   IRRIGATION AND DRAINAGE

The actual requirement of irrigation depends upon the climatic conditions. Even though this can tolerate dryness, but its growth gets affected when the moisture goes down the optimal level (i.e., field capacity) for the plant. It should be watered intermittently from November to April, to avoid any water stress to the crop. Regular watering at fortnight intervals should be a must during the dry period. Regular irrigation during the lean period found to be good for proper growth and flowering. The crop requires approximately 10 irrigations during in its whole cycle. The maximum vegetative growth phase (15-to-18-month stage) and pre-flowering is the most critical time for irrigation, and other irrigation applies as per need-based. Restricted or no irrigation after flowering is found to be good for remunerative rhizome and seed harvest.

Drainage is one of the key factors for good seed germination and proper growth in the field. The crop should not be over irrigated and there must be proper arrangement of drainage as excess water in the field affects crop growth adversely. In the case of improper drainage, roots of the plant get rotten which ultimately affects the plant growth and finally to the economics as a whole. As per different work, only two days of stagnation reduce 40 to 53% yield of rhizome (Mukherjee, 2016b).

9.3.2.8   ECONOMICS

Improved agronomic measures along with suitable crop husbandry practices fetch better economic yield (rhizome and root) and higher B: C ratio (Tables 9.9 and 9.10) to growers.

TABLE 9.9 Detailed Expenditure Incurred During Cultivations of *Valeriana jatamansi*

SL. No.	Particulars	Amount	Man Power Required	Rate (Rs.)	Total Cost Incurred (ha)
I.	Land rent	2 yr.	–	8,000/yr.	16000.00
II	Working capital	–	–	–	–
1.	Land preparation	–	22	178	3916.00
2.	Nursery	–	–	–	–
	(a) Seed	2.0 kg	–	1,300	2600.00
	(b) For preparation and observation	–	10	178	1780.00
3.	Manure	20 ton	–	4,500	4500.00
4.	Pit for compost and FYM	–	20	178	3560.00
5.	Biopesticide for pathogen and insect.	–	–	1,200	1200.00
6.	Biopesticide application	–	10	178	1780.00
7.	Seedlings transplanting	–	40	178	7120.00
8.	For drainage and irrigation	–	20	178	3560.00
9.	Pesticide and manure application in next season	–	10	178	1780.00
10.	Collection of plant	–	12	178	2136.00
11.	Drying place and storage	–	10	178	1780.00
III.	Total working capital (1 to 11)				35,712
IV.	Interest on total working capital @ 12% /annum				4,286
V.	Total variable cost (III+IV)				39,998
VI.	Total cost of production (I+V)				55,998
VII.	Gross returns (as per Table 9.4)				136,000
VIII.	Net returns (VII-VI)				80,002
IX.	Benefit: cost ratio (VII/VI)				2.42

Note: Cost calculation based on market value 2014–2015.

TABLE 9.10 Income Incurred from Cultivation of *V. jatamansi (per ha)*

Production (Total Biomass)	Rate/kg	Gross Return (Rs.)
1800.00 kg	76.00	1,36,000.00

9.3.2.9   HARVESTING AND MARKETING

Harvesting is done from September to November after completion of two-year life cycle. *Valeriana jatamansi* contain the valepotriates, mostly from its underground parts which possess tranquilizing property. Work conducted by Singh et al. (2010) in Palampur, Himachal Pradesh revealed that fresh weight of underground parts and length of root were significantly higher during July and August, the time of maximum rains. An enriched fraction of valepotriates was significantly lower from February to June (2.4–3.6%), the time of flowering and fruiting in the crop, and was significantly higher during January, October, and November (5.4, 4.7 and 4.9%, respectively). The essential oil in the underground parts ranged from 0.1 to 0.5% and was significantly higher from March to June (0.3–0.4%) attaining its peak in June (0.4%). An estimate of the yield of the enriched fraction of valepotriates indicates that November or January is the optimum time to harvest for enriched fraction of valepotriates production, while May is appropriate to harvest time for the production of essential oil. The whole plant is pulled out and leaves, stem, root, and rhizome are separated and sorted out for its marketing. Rhizome and root are the parts used for trading. From commercial cultivation, 1,800 to 2,000 kg of biomass are collected from well managed field. Approximately 2,500 kg of dry rhizome can be collected from one hectare of land. The collected rhizomes are cleaned or washed in water. Then each rhizome is cut into 2–4 cm long pieces. The rhizomes are dried in the sun on mats or sometimes by spreading them in trays, supported over a wood fire. Dried rhizomes are then stored. The product is sold mainly to big traders or wholesalers for pharmaceutical industries.

9.3.3   SWERTIA CHIRAYITA

- ➢ **Kingdom:** Plantae;
- ➢ **Family:** Gentianaceae;
- ➢ **Genus:** *Swertia;*
- ➢ **Species:** *chirayita;*
- ➢ **Local name:** Chiraita, Tite, or Lektite or Khalu, Pothe, Chirota;
- ➢ **English name:** Chiretta.

Swertia chirayita (Robex. ex Flem) Karsten is an essential medicinal plant endemic to the Himalayan regions (Balaraju et al., 2009) and registered in the category of the highly endangered plant (IUCN, 2009). This plant grows in the damped hillside of temperate to alpine forest between the altitudes of 1,400–3,150 m AMSL and is irrationally collected from its wild for selling and local medicinal use. Darjeeling range of Himalaya is one of the native places of different Swertia species. It is situated between the 87°59'–88°53'E and 28°31'–27°13' N in the Eastern Himalayan region of India (Yonzone et al., 1981). Swertia species contain many primary and secondary compounds that are responsible for its beneficial value such as flavonoids, terpenoids, iridoids, xanthones, and secoiridoid glycosides (Pant et al., 2000; Mukherjee, 2018c). Swertia chirayita has just been brought into farming with partial success (Mukhrjee, 2008b). The survey revealed that medicinal plants viz. *Panax pseudo-ginseng Picrorhiza kurrooa, Podophyllum hexandrum* prefer to grow with *Swertia chirata*.

9.3.3.1 MEDICINAL USES

This plant is extensively utilized in TM mainly in Unani and Siddha, also gaining importance in traditional Chinese and Tibetan medicine. Its medicinal usage is reported in the Indian pharmaceutical codex, the British and the American pharmacopeia. This species was first introduced in the Edinburgh Pharmacopoeia in 1839 and is reported in British and American Pharmacopeia to be used as an infusion or a tincture (Niiho, 2005). It becomes very helpful for indigestion, bloating, nausea, and also used as a laxative and an appetizer in addition to various liver and bile problem (Roy et al., 2008). In Ayurveda, *S. chirayita* is described as bitter (*tikta*) in taste and its thermal action defined as cooling (*shita*), easily digestible (*laghu*) and dry (*ruksha*) (Joshi and Dhawan 2005; Chakraborty et al., 2016). Owing to its medicinal importance, the plant has been harvested from the wild for a long time and is now considered endangered in its natural habitats. It requires immediate attention for conservation and sustainable management. In order to devise pragmatic conservation strategies for *S. chirayita,* identification of intra-population and inter-population diversity is a preliminary step. Further, as for most *chirayita*, authentic material is not cultivated and collected, leading to substitution. This is due to sheer ignorance on the part of the collector or unavailability of the genuine germplasm (Mukherjee et al., 2013). In such cases, diagnostic tools become essential for proper identification of authentic samples. Enormous variations at morphological and biochemical levels have been observed among different species of *Swertia*.

9.3.3.2   PLANT AND SOIL

This plant is chiefly found in India (Darjeeling hill, Kashmir, Meghalaya, and Khasi hills), Nepal, and Bhutan. It is a biennial or perennial herb of seasonal growth (Mukherjee, 2014). The plant is found at an altitude of 1,300–2,800 m AMSL, from Kashmir to Bhutan, and in the Khasi hills at 1,300–1,700 m AMSL. Usually it has a single, stout, elongated stem, about 2–5 ft long stem, the middle portion is round, while the upper is four-angled, with a prominent decurrent line at each angle. The stems are light brown to purplish in color. The stem is cylindrical in the lower side and is quadrangular upper side (Chandra et al., 2009). Ovate or lanceolate leaves with entire margin curly in nature (Bhardwaj et al., 2011). The root is simple, tapering, and stout, short, almost 8 cm long (Rai et al., 2000). Flowers are small, stalked, green-yellow, tinged with purple color. The whole inflorescence is 2 ft long (Figures 9.10 and 9.11; Table 9.11) (Chakraborty et al., 2008).

TABLE 9.11   Soil Environment Suitable for *Swertia chirayita Cultivation*

SL. No.	Particulars	Values
1.	pH	4.8–5.6 (acidic)
2.	E.C.E. (inch/cm)	0.09-.13 (neutral)
3.	Organic carbon (%)	0.93–1.62 (high)
4.	Available N (Kg/ha)	250–321 (medium)
5.	Available P_2O_5 (Kg/ha)	70–90 (high)
6.	Available K_2O (Kg/ha)	125–260 (medium)

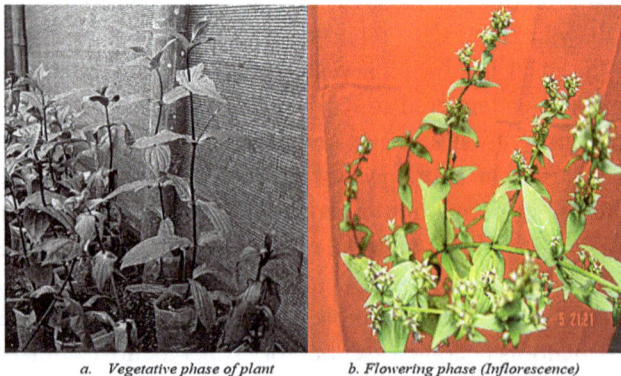

a.   *Vegetative phase of plant*   b. *Flowering phase (Inflorescence)*

FIGURE 9.10   *Swertia chirayita* plant. *(a) Vegetative phase of plant. (b) Flowering phase (inflorescence).*

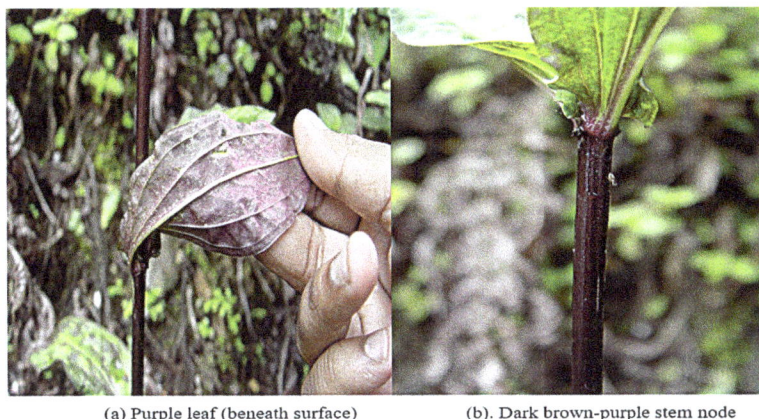

(a) Purple leaf (beneath surface)   (b). Dark brown-purple stem node

FIGURE 9.11   Purple tinge below leaf surface and on stem node. *(a) Purple leaf (beneath surface). (b) Dark brown-purple stem node.*

9.3.3.3   PRINCIPLE CONSTITUENT

Swertia chirayita contains two bitter glycosides chiratin (not a pure substance) and amarogentin. This plant is chemically characterized by the presence of taxonomically important groups of secondary metabolites such as xanthones, iridoids, mangiferin, and C-lucoflavones (Khan et al., 2014). This herb is an excellent drug for strengthening the stomach and promoting its action. It is used in the treatment of dyspepsia and diarrhea (Mukherjee, 2016c). This plant possesses anthelmintic that is, worms destroying properties and is used in killing intestinal worms, and beneficial to infants. The herb, as well as its extracts, are used as a bitter stimulant to treat fever as well as curing several skin problems (Mukherjee, 2009a). It is much employed in urinary complaints with uneasiness in the region of the kidneys, frequent urging to urinate, which is accomplished with difficulty, and in cases of uric acid deposits. It is also a remedy for convalescence from exhausting sickness, and dyspepsia. Observation revealed that amarogentin content of *S. chirayita* was quite higher in the true type of chirota. The study conducted in RRS, Kalimpong (2006–2008) revealed that concentration of amarogentin in leaf vary from 0.238 to 0.391% and in stem from 0.077 to 0.096% (Plant sample analysis was done by Directorate of Medicinal and Aromatic Plant, Gujrat, Anand) (Figure 9.12 and Table 9.12).

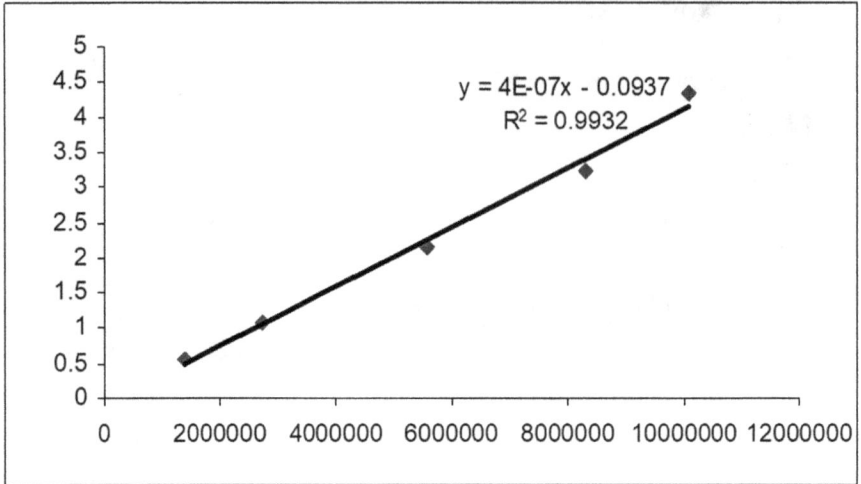

FIGURE 9.12   Calibration curve of *S. chirayita* sample analysis.

TABLE 9.12   Analysis Report of *Swertia chirayita* Plant (Sample from Darjeeling Hill)

Plant Sample Parts	Sample wt.(g)	Dissolve (ml)	Area	µg/20 µl	mg/g	Percentage (%)	Mean	St. Dev.
Leaf-1	0.5008	10	6201,894	2.3805	2.3767	0.238		
	0.5008	10	6259,112	2.4033	2.3995	0.240	0.238	0.0013
	0.5008	10	6201,894	2.3805	2.3767	0.238		
Stem-1	0.5008	10	2192,533	0.7767	0.7755	0.078		
	0.5008	10	2171,521	0.7683	0.7671	0.077	0.077	0.0005
	0.5008	10	2170,223	0.7678	0.7666	0.077		
Leaf-2	0.5000	10	10012,093	3.9045	3.9045	0.390		
	0.5000	10	10057,640	3.9228	3.9228	0.392	0.391	0.0010
	0.5000	10	10016,740	3.9064	3.9064	0.391		
Stem-2	0.5006	10	2640,542	0.9559	0.9548	0.095		
	0.5006	10	2654,262	0.9614	0.9603	0.096	0.096	0.0003
	0.5006	10	2654,282	0.9614	0.9603	0.096		

9.3.3.4   SEED TREATMENTS

Gentianaceae have mostly the physiological dormancy problem (Nikole-aeva, 1977). Proper seed germination of chirota plant is very difficult and challenging to the scientific community since long back. Due to this problem, its conservation either in-situ or ex-situ becomes difficult. Because of high demand in the pharmaceutical market and poor seed germination, the herb becomes extinct day by day from forest microhabitats and comes in the category of critically endangered. As per various reports concerned, the germination of this plant was only 12–20% (Mukherjee and Chakraborty, 2008). Understanding seed germination is a pre-requisite to ensure species conservation, viable seeds collected from six microhabitats were studied at 20°C, 25°C, and 30°C, both under a 14/10 h light/dark photoperiod and in continuous darkness. Crop micro-habitat and temperature notably influence seed germination, growth rate, and germination recovery (GR) rate. Overall, the seeds collected from under canopy showed a significantly ($p < 0.05$) higher germination than those from open habitats, at 20°C, 25°C, and 30°C (14/10 h light/dark photoperiod) (Pradhan and Badola, 2012). Observation revealed that seed germination was low in incessant darkness but after transfer to a 14/10 h light/dark photoperiod, the seeds from under canopy notably improved at 20°C and at 25°C ($p < 0.05$), and showed the maximum germination percentage compared to seeds collected from tree base, shrub-beries or grassy slope. Seeds are positively photoblastic in nature (Pradhan and Badola, 2012).

An experiment was conducted in randomized block design under the aegis of UBKV, Kalimpong (Lava) with 15 pre-treatments of *S. chirayita* seeds replicated thrice during November, 2011 to November, 2014 (Figures 9.12–9.16). The pre-treatments include osmo-priming with various concentration of GA_3 (50, 100, 200, 400 and 800 ppm), IAA (50 100 200 400 800 ppm), KNO_3 (1,2,3, and 4%) and hydro-priming (control with distilled water) for *S. chirayita*. The maximum seed germination was observed with GA_3 400 ppm and was at par with the GA_3 200 ppm (Table 9.14). Onset of germination was the earliest, i.e., 19.00 days after sowing in treatment GA_3 800 ppm for 12 hrs, which was statistically at par with IAA 200 ppm (20.33 days) and IAA 50 ppm (22 days). Mean germination time (44.11 days) in untreated (control) seeds was comparable to 27.34 days in seeds pretreated with IAA 400 ppm, which was 38.01% lower than the control. Seeds treated with GA_3 400 ppm for 24 hrs show maximum SV-I (71.11), which was 207.71% more than the control. The highest SV-II of 54.18 was registered by KNO_3 (2%), which was 67.0% higher than the control. GE of 1.16 was found in seeds pretreated with GA_3 400 ppm (Table 9.13).

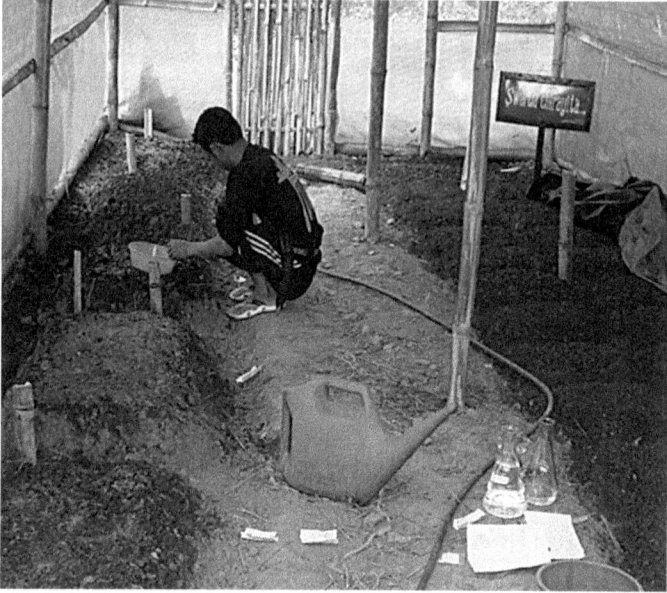

FIGURE 9.13 Layout of the experiment.

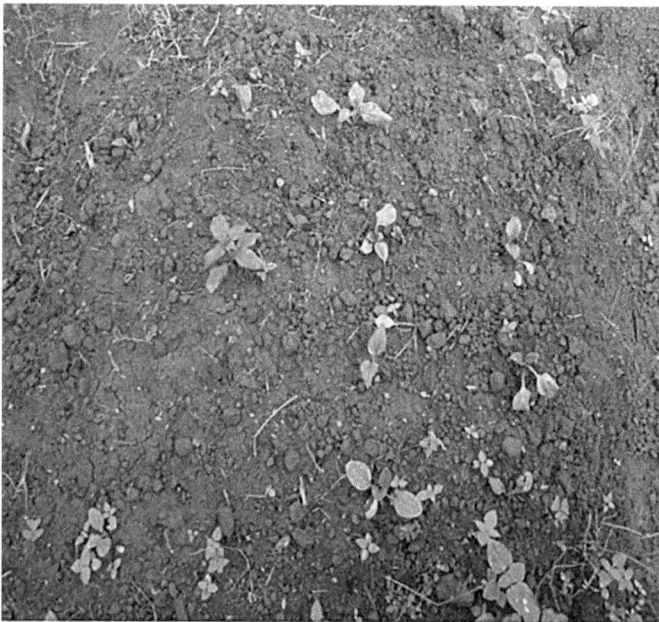

FIGURE 9.14 *Swertia chirayita* under control (untreated seed) condition.

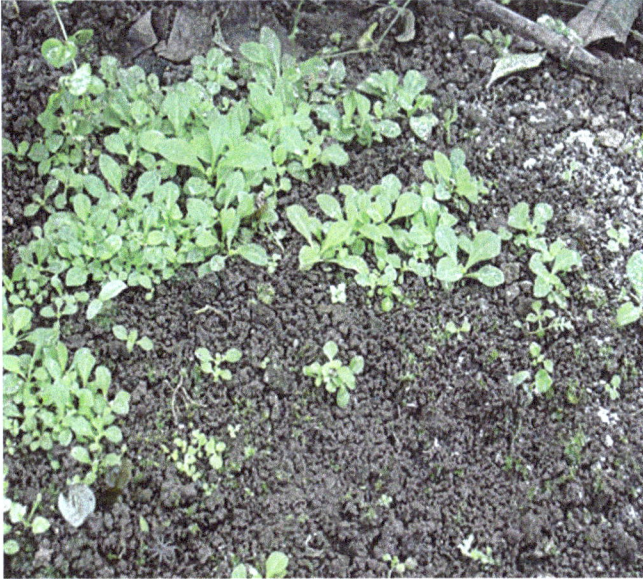

FIGURE 9.15   *Swertia chirayita* under GA$_3$400 ppm treated seeds (best treatment).

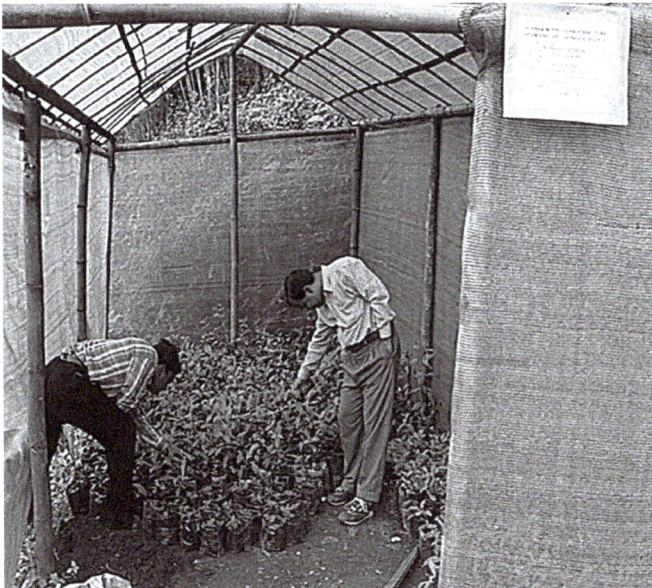

FIGURE 9.16   Conservation of *S. chirayita* at lava (2,200 m asl), Darjeeling.

TABLE 9.13　Effect of Seed Invigoration Treatments on Seed Germination Characteristics of *Swertia chirayita* (Pooled Value of Two-Year Data)

Treatments	Germination (%)	Days Require for Onset of Germination (Days)	Days Required for Completion Germination (Days)	Mean Germination Time (Days)	Seedling Vigor Fresh Biomass (g)	Seedling Vigor Dry Biomass (g)	Seedling Vigor Index I	Seedling Vigor Index II
Control	26.66±2.11	36.66	44.66	44.11	1.17* (0.87)	0.78 (0.11)**	23.11	2.93
GA$_3$50	36.00±1.31	27.33	47.00	36.36	1.49 (1.74)	0.95 (0.40)	35.21	13.64
GA$_3$100	40.44±2.33	30.33	50.33	39.37	1.84 (2.89)	0.94 (0.39)	35.98	15.36
GA$_3$200	55.87±3.44	28.00	50.00	37.11	2.32 (4.94)	1.22 (0.98)	64.08	53.74
GA$_3$400	64.00±5.91	27.00	55.33	29.63	2.01 (3.54)	0.95 (0.41)	71.11	26.53
GA$_3$800	33.66±1.72	19.00	30.66	31.00	1.20 (0.95)	0.79 (0.12)	34.33	4.37
IAA50	30.32±2.16	22.00	45.33	33.77	1.19 (0.92)	0.84 (0.21)	29.71	6.67
IAA100	44.11±1.56	33.66	55.66	40.34	2.03 (3.65)	1.19 (0.91)	48.96	39.63
IAA200	34.00±3.81	20.33	57.66	39.97	2.14 (4.12)	1.22 (0.98)	36.04	32.65
IAA400	30.15±5.11	24.33	40.66	27.34	1.74 (2.54)	1.04 (0.59)	29.24	17.18
IAA800	2.66±3.03	28.33	40.33	31.45	1.77 (2.66)	0.85 (0.23)	2.97	0.64
KNO$_3$ (1%)	44.11±1.16	34.00	41.33	39.32	1.92 (3.21)	0.96 (0.43)	38.88	19.86
KNO$_3$ (2%)	53.65±3.33	26.66	46.66	30.67	2.19 (4.32)	1.23 (1.01)	57.99	54.18
KNO$_3$ (3%)	23.54±2.19	36.33	54.66	34.17	2.27 (4.66)	1.17 (0.87)	24.95	20.47
KNO$_3$ (4%)	32.92±4.11	29.66	43.33	36.13	1.61 (2.11)	0.87 (0.25)	25.34	8.69
LSD (P=0.05)	9.60	3.07	N.S	3.65	0.22	0.16	4.98	5.33

*Values marked are square root transformed values.
**Original values.
Source: Mukherjee (2018).

TABLE 9.14 Effect of Seed Invigoration Treatments on Seedling Length, Emergence Index and Germination Energy of Seeds of (Pooled Value of Two-Year Data)

Treatments	Seedling Length (cm)	Emergence Index	Germination Energy
Control	0.87	0.73	0.61
$GA_3 50$	0.98	1.32	0.77
$GA_3 100$	0.89	1.33	0.81
$GA_3 200$	1.16	2.14	1.12
$GA_3 400$	1.11	2.37	1.16
$GA_3 800$	1.02	1.77	1.12
IAA50	0.98	1.38	0.67
IAA100	1.11	1.31	0.79
IAA200	1.06	1.67	0.59
IAA400	0.97	1.24	0.74
IAA800	0.86	0.09	0.07
KNO_3 (1%)	0.88	1.3	1.07
KNO_3 (2%)	1.08	2.01	1.15
KNO_3 (3%)	1.06	0.65	0.43
KNO_3 (4%)	0.77	1.11	0.76
LSD	0.16	0.14	0.14

The seedling length was maximum registered with the pre-treatment of seeds with $GA_3 200$ ppm (1.16 cm) and was at par with the $GA_3 400$ ppm, IAA 100 ppm, KNO_3 (2%) and KNO_3 (3%). Effect of seed invigoration treatments on EI in chirota plant revealed that (Table 9.15) pre-treatment with $GA_3 400$ ppm gave maximum EI (2.37) which was significantly higher than other mentioned treatments except for $GA_3 200$ ppm (2.14). Further, GE of seeds revealed that maximum GE of 1.16 was found in seeds pre-treated with $GA_3 400$ ppm.

Seed germination study revealed significant improvement in germination under GA_3 treatment compared to control (Table 9.13). Epigeal type of seed germination observed in chirota. Soil depth also influenced the plant physiological system of this endangered plant species. Sowing at 0.50 cm showed the highest germination with less time required for the onset of germination and significantly superior to higher depth (Table 9.15). With various soil compositions, germination percentage and onset of germination were almost similar in soil, sand, and FYM in 1:2:1 and 1:1:2 proportions. Amongst all soil media, maximum germination was found with compositions of 1:1:2 (soil: sand: FYM) and was followed by 1:2:1 and, significantly superior to rest of soil composition (Mukherjee, 2008a, b). The result of *Swertia* species, with improved germination under GA_3 and IAA treatments, correspond well with these generalizations, as both these substances are considered best for breaking physiological dormancy.

TABLE 9.15 Seed Germination as Influenced by Different Sowing Depth and Soil Composition

Treatments	Germination (%)	Days Require for Onset of Germination	Days Required for Maximum Germination
Depth of Soil (cm)			
0.50	56.25 ±3.9	26.31	44.39
1.00	44.41±2.33	32.66	48.66
LSD (P=0.05)	4.68	3.28	NS
Proportion of Soil: Sand: FYM			
1:1:1	40.66± 3.92	31.33	48.50
2:1:1	28.33±4.66	35.83	51.21
1:2:1	57.66±3.31	29.99	45.16
1:1:2	61.00±2.99	28.75	44.50
LSD (P=0.05)	9.54	2.07	2.02

People generally collect this plant from the high-altitude forest area of North Eastern Himalaya, however, from growers' point of view it may be a highly remunerative crop. The crop is usually ready for harvesting after 18–22 months. Optimum crop yield found in November-December harvesting. The collection is done by hand with the help of sickle without using any mechanical methods. The whole plant is pulled out and sun-dried for a few days and then wrapped by bamboo slip. Final produce such as root, straw, and seed are separated and kept in a dry place. As per study during 2010–2011, it revealed that, the benefit: cost ratio (BCR) in terms of rupees benefited rupee[-1] invested was quite high (3.64), due to its high demand in the pharmaceutical industry (Table 9.16).

TABLE 9.16 Cost of Cultivation, Economics Incurred for Cultivation of *Swertia chirayita* (per ha)

SL. No.	Particulars	Value (Rs.)*
I	Land rent	10,000.00
II	Working capital	–
1	Land preparation	4,375.00
2.	Nursery	–
(a)	Seed	2,500.00
(b)	For preparation and observation	1,562.50
3.	Manure	1,500.00
4.	Pit for compost and FYM	1,875.00
5.	Biopesticide for pathogen and insect	500.00
6.	Biopesticide application	625.00
7.	Seedlings transplanting	5,000.00
8.	For drainage and irrigation	1,250.00
9.	Pesticide and manure application in next season	625.00
10.	Collection	1,250.00
11.	Drying	625.00
III	Total working capital (1 to 11)	21,687.50
IV	Interest on total working capital @ 12% / annum	2,602.50
V	Total variable cost (III+IV)	24,290.00
VI	Total cost of production (I+V)	34,290.00
VII	Gross returns	1,25,000.00
VIII	Net returns (VII–VI)	90,710.00
IX	Benefit-cost ratio (VII ÷VI)	3.64

*Based on market price of 2010–2011.

9.4 PROBLEMS AND CONSTRAINTS OF CULTIVATION OF MEDICINAL PLANTS

Major constraints in commercial production of chirota plant are discussed here. Most people depend on collection from natural plant habitat; low harvesting (indiscriminate) and post-harvest treatment measures, domestication, indecent storage; improper marketing practices, and lack of synchronization of the plant-based drug industry. There is insufficient data on the demand and supply situation of chirota plants. Farmers have been taking initiatives to cultivate medicinal plants, but price instability affects the level of confidence of farmers necessary to take up large scale cultivation. Some of the constraints associated with the processing of chirota plants are:

- Poor agricultural practices;
- Poor harvesting (indiscriminate) and post-harvest treatment practices;
- Lack of research on development of high-yielding varieties, domestication, etc.;
- Poor propagation methods;
- Inefficient processing techniques leading to low yields and poor-quality products;
- Poor quality control procedures;
- High energy losses during processing;
- Lack of current good manufacturing practices;
- Lack of R and D on product and process development;
- Difficulties in marketing;
- Lack of local market for primary processed products;
- Lack of trained personnel and equipment;
- Lack of facilities to fabricate equipment locally;
- Lack of access to latest technological and market information.

Efficient cultivation of plants needs explicit cultural practices and agronomical requirements. Above mentioned aspects must have to be incorporated into protocols for the cultivation of these medicinal plants. Organic farming is another practice that is gaining wide acceptance as world demand, particularly in developed countries for organically grown crops is rapidly on the increase. Farmers have to be trained in all aspects of organic farming of medicinal plants and herbs, including obtaining certification from associations that do the monitoring starting from cultivation to final harvesting. Organic farming, which is labor-intensive, gives the developing countries the comparative advantage to be competitive.

9.5 TRADE AND MARKETING

Most of the medicinal raw materials produced by valuable herbs (*Centalla asiatica, Swertia chiryaita, Bergia cilliata*) in the country are used locally (Mukherjee, 2016d). Most of the local people/ middle man take out from forest microhabitat without proper knowledge of authority or scientific personals. Due to such illegal extractions' day by day, they are becoming extricated (Figure 9.17).

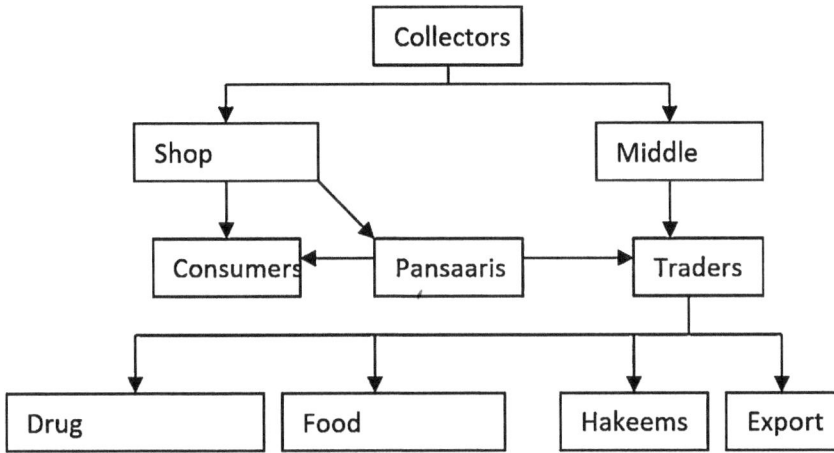

FIGURE 9.17   Chain of people involved in the medicinal plant trade in India.

However, with the introduction of cultivation of high demand plants, export is expected to rise in the coming years. India exported USD 330.18 million worth of herbs during 2017–2018 with a growth rate of 15.06% over the previous year. Also, the export of value-added extracts of medicinal herbs/herbal products during 2017–2018 stood at USD 399.12 million recording a growth rate of 12.03% over the previous year (https://pib.gov.in). India, apart from the request for temperate medicinal plant (chirota, jatamansi, etc.), for domestic use, is one of the main exporters of crude drugs, mainly to five developed countries such as Germany, Japan, France, UK, and the USA, who share 63 to 74% of the total export of crude drugs from India (Moktan and Mukherjee, 2008). In spite of the potential for producing raw material in the country, Chirayita, Jatamansi, Mismi teeta are imported from countries such as Nepal, Bhutan, Pakistan, and China. Few of the prominent medicinal plant export from are: *Glycyrrhiza glabra* L. from Afghanistan, Iran, and Pakistan; *Atropa belladonna* L. from Germany; *Hedychium spicatum* from China; *Commiphora wightii* (Arn.) Bhandari Engl. from Pakistan and *Podophyllum sp.* from Nepal (Table 9.17) (Mukherjee, 2015).

TABLE 9.17   List of Valuable Medicinal Plants Having High Export Market Demand

SL. No.	Medicinal Plants
1.	*Picrorhiza kurroa*
2.	*Nardostachys jatamansi*
3.	*Swertia chirata*
4.	*Valeriana jatamansi*
5.	*Aconitum heterophyllum*
6.	*Saussurea lappa*
7.	*Asparagus racemosa*
8.	*Rauvolfia serpentina*
9.	*Dactylorhiza hatagarea*
10.	*Withania somnifers*
11.	*Costus specious*
13.	*Bacopa monnieri*
14.	*Taxus wallichiana*
15.	*Digitalis purpurea*

All plants listed above are having high efficacy and have medicinal values, which have been widely used by the different Indian Systems of Medicines like Ayurveda, Homeopathy, Unani, Siddha, Amchi, and Allopathy. These plants have tremendous demands from pharmaceuticals and many other Herbal Based Industries.

9.6   CONCLUSION

Plant genetic resources have made substantial contributions to the domestication, utilization, and improvement of valuable temperate medicinal plants in the Himalayan region. Their adoption by farming community becomes limited due to lack of knowledge about seed germination (*Swertia chirayita, Coptis teeta, Podophyllum hexandrum*), cultivation (*Valeriana jatamansi, Bergenia ciliata*) and marketing. The practice of TM is widespread in China, India, Japan, Pakistan, Sri Lanka, and Thailand. Mostly they used products or extracts made from these endangered herbs. The protection of such plants can be made by either in-situ or ex-situ methods. However, they have a certain limit due to the narrow genetic base and lesser knowledge of seed germination and other conservation practices. Although the economic value of these herbs was reportedly unknown to the local people until the recent past, the herb has now been widely known for its market potential. Thus, the exploitation of this valuable plant is in increasing trend leading to its rapid decline from its natural habitat. Improved cultivation along with proper marketing channels becomes a valuable and economic option to the farming community in the North-Eastern Himalaya region.

KEYWORDS

- **conservation**
- **cultivation**
- **endangered**
- **marketing**
- **medicinal plant**

REFERENCES

Balaraju, K., Agastin, P., & Ignacimuthu, S., (2009). Micropropagation of *Swertia* chirata Buch- hams. Ex wall: A critically endangered medicinal herb. *Acta Physiologia Plantarum., 31*(3), 487–494.

Bharat, K., Pradhan, B. K., & Badola, H. K., (2012). Effects of microhabitat, light and temperature on seed germination of a critically endangered Himalayan medicinal herb, *Swertia chirayita*: Conservation implications. *Plant Biosystem, 146*(2), 345–351.

Bhardwaj, A., Khatri, P., & Soni, M. L., (2011). Potent herbal hepatoprotective drugs: A review. *Journal of Advanced Scientific Research, 2*(2), 15–20.

Chakraborty, S., Mukherjee, D., & Baskey, S., (2015). Indian valerian, a highly endangered medicinal plant in North Eastern Himalayan Region. *Advances in Plants and Agriculture Research, 2*(4), 1–7. (doi: 10.15406/apar.2015.02.00058).

Chakraborty, S., Mukherjee, D., & Baskey, S., (2015a). Paradigm of demographic stochasticity way to extinction of *Valeriana jatamansi* Jones, a valuable medicinal plant in North Eastern Himalaya region. *Ecology, Environment and Conservation, 21*(1), 521–528.

Chakraborty, S., Mukherjee, D., & Baskey, S., (2015b). Role of Demographic stochasticity on erosion of genetic variability of *Valeriana jatamansi* Jones, a high value introduced medicinal plant in North Eastern Himalaya region. *Journal of Agriculture and Technology, 2*(1), 44–51.

Chakraborty, S., Mukherjee, D., & Baskey, S., (2015c). Selection of lines of *Valeriana jatamansi* Jones, a high value medicinal plant in North Eastern Himalayan region. *Indian Journal of Genetics and Plant Breeding, 75*(3), 1–4.

Chakraborty, S., Mukherjee, D., & Baskey, S., (2015d). Floral homeostasis breakdown in endangered plant *Valeriana jatamansi* Jones (Valerianceae) in northeastern Himalaya. *American Journal of Plant Sciences, 6*, 3119–3138.

Chakraborty, S., Mukherjee, D., & Baskey, S., (2016). Morphological diversity and nomenclature of *Swertia chirayita* (Gentianaceae)- Recovery of endangered medicinal plant population in northeastern Himalaya. *American Journal of Plant Sciences, 7*, 741–755.

Chakraborty, S., Mukherjee, D., & Dasgupta, T., (2008). Cytological study on chromosome behavior and new report on nature of mode of pollination of *Swertia chirayita*, a high value endangered medicinal plant of North Eastern Himalayan region. *Caryologia, 62*(1), 43–52.

Chandra, S., Kumar, V., Bandopadhyay, R., & Sharma, M. M., (2009). SEM and elemental studies of *Swertia chirayita*: A critically endangered medicinal herb of temperate Himalayas. *Current Trends in Biotechnology and Pharmacy., 6*(3), 381–388.

Fakim, A. G., (2006). Medicinal plants: Traditions of yesterday and drugs of tomorrow. *Molecular Aspects of Medicine, 27*, 1–93.

Harrison, P., (1998). Herbal medicine takes roots in Germany. *Canadian Medical Association Journal, 10*, 637–639.

Huang, J., & Chunlin, L., (2007). Coptis teeta-based agroforestry system and Its conservation potential: A case study from Northwest Yunnan. *Ambio, 36*(4), 343–349. (Published by: Springer on behalf of Royal Swedish Academy of Sciences).

IUCN, (2009). *IUCN Red List of Threatened Species*.www.iucnredlist.org (accessed on 01 November 2021).

Jones, W. B., (1998). Alternative medicine-learning from the past examining the present advancing to the future. *Journal of American Medical Association, 280*, 1616–1618.

Joshi, P., & Dhawan, V., (2005). *Swertia chirayita* - an overview. *Current Science, 89*, 635–640.

Mani, J. K., & Mukherjee, D., (2016). Accuracy of weather forecast for hill zone of West Bengal for better agriculture management practices. *Indian Journal of Research, 5*(10), 325–328.

Moktan, M. W., & Mukherjee, D., (2008). Trade and marketing strategy for spice crops in Darjeeling District. *Environment and Ecology, 26*(3A), 1302–1305.

Mukherje, D., & Chakrabarty, S., (2010). Effect of hormonal treatment on seed germination of *Valeriana jatamansi*. *Journal of Medicinal and Aromatic Plant Sciences, 32*(2), 145–147.

Mukherjee, D., & Chakraborty, S., (2019). *Coptis teeta*: Conservation and cultivation practice - A rare medicinal plant on earth. *Current Investigation in Agriculture and Current Research, 6*(4), 781–787.

Mukherjee, D., & Chkraborty, S., (2014). Studies on ecology, habitats diversification and seed germination behavior of *Valeriana jatamansi* jones: A critical endangered plant. *International Journal of Agricultural Sciences, 4*(5), 203–209.

Mukherjee, D., & Sharma, B. R., (2014). Conservation and scope of medicinal plant in Eastern Himalaya. *The Himalayan Review, 1*(1), 102–110.

Mukherjee, D., (2008). Association of medicinal plants with important tree species in hills of Darjeeling. *Environment and Ecology, 26*(4A), 1697–1699.

Mukherjee, D., (2008a). Germination improvement in *Swertia chirayita*: An endangered medicinal herb. *Journal of Medicinal and Aromatic Plant Sciences, 30*(2), 136–138.

Mukherjee, D., (2008b). Cultivation of *Swertia chirayita*: A high value medicinal herb in high altitude. *Journal of Medicinal & Aromatic Plant Sciences, 30*(4), 350–355.

Mukherjee, D., (2009). In: Krishi, S., Rai, S., Mokthan, M. W., & Ali, S., (eds.), *Medicinal Plant in Darjeeling Hills* (Vol. 1, pp. 118–121). Miazik International Volunteer Center, Japan.

Mukherjee, D., (2009a). In: Krishi, S., Rai, S., Mokthan, M. W., & Ali, S., (eds.), *Swertia Chirayita an Endangered Herbs in Darjeeling Hill* (Vol. 2, pp. 122–132). Miazik International Volunteer Center, Japan.

Mukherjee, D., (2013). Improved agricultural practices for high value medicinal plants under mid to high altitude situation. *Journal of Crop and Weed, 9*(1), 201–206.

Mukherjee, D., (2014). Medicinal plant with relation to biodiversity conservation at Darjeeling hill. In: Nehra, G., & Ghosh, L., (eds.), *Biodiversity in India: Assessment, Scope and Conservation* (pp. 43–73). Lap lambert academic publishing, Deutschland, Germany.

Mukherjee, D., (2015). Studies on seed germination pattern and effect of sowing date with planting prototype on *Valeriana jatamansi* (Jones): A rare medicinal plant of Eastern Himalaya. *Journal of Crops and Weed, 11*(2), 9–13.

Mukherjee, D., (2016). Influence of various parameters on seed germination and plant growth prototype of *Swertia chirayita* (Roxb. Ex fleming): A rare plant on earth. *Indian Horticulture Journal, 6*(2), 193–197.

Mukherjee, D., (2016a). Studies on ecology and outcome of various seed and organic input treatments on yield attribute and economic yield of *Valeriana jatamansi. The Himalayan Review, 1*(2), 193–200.

Mukherjee, D., (2016b). Study the effect of various growth regulators and crop architecture on *Valeriana jatamansi* - crop raised through seed: Valuable medicinal herb of Eastern Himalaya range. *Annals of Plant Sciences, 5*(4), 1326–1329.

Mukherjee, D., (2016c). Medicinal and aromatic plants: Wealth of India. In: Hemantaranjan, A., (ed.), *Advances in Plant Physiology* (pp. 425–456). Scientific Publishers, Jodhpur, India.

Mukherjee, D., (2016d). Influence of transplanting time, plant geometry and nutrient management on growth and economics of *Centella asiatica*: Valuable NTFPs. *International Journal of Forest Usufructs Management (IJFUM), 17*(2), 37–45.

Mukherjee, D., (2018). Effect of different seed priming treatments on germination and seedling establishment of two threatened endangered medicinal plants of Darjeeling Himalaya. In: Rakshit, A., & Singh, H. B., (eds.), *Advances in Seed Priming* (pp. 241–262). Springer Publication. (doi:10.1007/978-981-13-0032-5_13.).

Mukherjee, D., (2018a). Effect cultivation aspect of endangered medicinal plant of northeastern Himalaya. *Journal of Agricultural Engineering and Food Technology, 5*(1), 5–9.

Mukherjee, D., (2018b). Challenges and opportunity of horticulture and allied sector of the farming system under Darjeeling Himalaya - a reappraisal. *Journal of Plant Biology, Chemistry and Ecophysiology, 102*(1), 1–6.

Mukherjee, D., (2018c). Improved agronomic package of practices of *Valeriana jatamansi:* An endangered valuable non timber forest product of high altitude. *Bioved., 29*(1), 17–23.

Mukherjee, D., (2018d). Conservation and utilization of high altitude valuable medicinal plant. In: Jha, S. K., (ed), *Advances in Ethnobotany* (pp. 431–468). SSPH Publishers, Delhi, India.

Mukherjee, D., (2019). Microbial intervention in soil and plant health for improving crop efficiency. In: Singh, D. P., & Prabha, R., (eds.), *Microbial Interventions in Agriculture and Environment: Soil and Crop health Management* (Vol. 3, pp. 17–47). https://doi.org/10.1007/978-981-32-9084-6_2. Springer publication.

Mukherjee, D., (2019). Seed invigoration: An effective tool for conservation of endangered and valuable medicinal plant. In: Hemantaranjan, A., (ed.), *Advances in Plant Physiology* (Vol. 28, pp. 243–272). Scientific Publishers, Jodhpur, India.

Mukherjee, D., Chakraborty, S., & Baskey, S., (2013). *Near to Extinct Medicinal Plants of Darjeeling Hills: Protect for Future, 4*(7), 17–18. Himalayan Times.

Mukherjee, D., Chakraborty, S., & Baskey, S., (2015). Threatened medicinal plants biodiversity of Eastern Himalaya and its conservation. *Journal of Agriculture and Technology, 2*(1), 101–107.

Mukherjee, D., Chakraborty, S., Baskey, S., & Ali, S., (2014). Studies on effect of time of sowing and crop geometry on growth and economic yield of *Valeriana jatamansi*. *Himalayan Research Journal, 2*(1), 80–86.

Mukherjee, D., Chakraborty, S., Roy, A., & Mokthan, M. W., (2009). Differential approach of germplasm conservation of high value of medicinal plants in north eastern Himalayan region. *International Journal of Agriculture Environment & Biotechnology, 2*(4), 332–340.

Niho, Y., (2005). Gastroprotective effects of bitter principles isolated from gentian root and *Swertia* herb on experimentally induced gastric lesions in rats. *Journal of Natural Medicine, 60*, 74–88.

Pandit, M. K., & Babu, C. R., (1998). Biology and conservation of Coptis teeta Wall. – an endemic and endangered medicinal herb of Eastern Himalaya. Environmental Conservation, 25(3), 262–272. http://www.jstor.org/stable/4315837 (accessed on 01 November 2021).

Pant, N., Jain, D. C., & Bhakuni, R. S., (2000). Phytochemicals from genus *Swertia* and their biological activities. *Indian Journal of Chemical Sciences, 39*(B), 565–586.

Pradhan, S., & Lama, P. C., (2012). Biochemical analysis during early seedling growth of *Swertia chirata* buch. ham. in Darjeeling hill of Eastern Himalayas. *Environment and Ecology, 30*(4), 1395–1398.

Prakash, V., (1999). *Indian Valerianceae: A Monograph on MEDICINALLY Important Family* (pp. 70–87). Scientific Publishers, Jodhpur, India.

Prakash, V., Bisht, H., & Prasad, P., (2011). Altitudinal variation in morpho-physiological attributes in *Plantago major*: Selection of suitable cultivation site. *Research Journal of Medicinal Plant, 5*, 302–311.

Purohit, V. K., Bahuguna, Y. M., Tiwari, D., Tiwari, A., Andola, H. C., & Negi, S. R., (2013). *Swertia chirayita* (Roxb. ex Fleming) Karsten on the verge of extinction in the Himalayan region. *Current Science, 104*(2), 161, 162.

Rai, L., Prasad, P., & Sharma, E., (2000). Conservation threats to some important medicinal plants of the Sikkim Himalaya. *Biological Conservation, 93*(1), 27–33.

Roy, K., Jash, S., Mukherjee, D., Pramanik, A., & Mukhopadhyay, A. K., (2008). A note on the incidence of *Melodogyna javanica* in *Swertia chirayita* (Family: Gentianaceae) from West Bengal. *Indian Journal of Nematology, 38*(2), 258.

Singh, N., Gupta, A. P., Singh, B., & Kaul, V. K., (2006). Quantification of valeric acid in *Valeriana jatamansi* and *Valeriana officinalis* by HPTLC. *Chromatographia, 63*, 209–213.

Singh, R. D., Gopichand, M., Sharma, R. L., Singh, B., Kaul, V. K., & Ahuja, P. S., (2010). Seasonal variation of bioactive components in *Valeriana jatamansi* from Himachal Pradesh, India. *Industrial Crops and Products, 32*(3), 292–296.

Uniyal, S. K., Kumar, A., Lal, B., & Singh, R. D., (2006). Quantitative assessment and traditional uses of high value medicinal plants in Chhota Bhangal area of Himachal Pradesh, Western Himalaya. *Current Science, 91*, 1238–1242.

WHO/IUCN/WWF, (1993). *Guidelines on Conservation of Medicinal Plants.* IUCN, Gland, Switzerland.

Yonzone, R., Mandal, S., & Chanda, S., (1981). A contribution to the ethnobotany of Darjeeling hill. *Trans. Bose Res. Inst., 44*, 75–81.

CHAPTER 10

CONSERVATION AND SUSTAINABLE UTILIZATION OF THREATENED MEDICINAL PLANTS OF NORTH EAST INDIA

KALKAME CH. MOMIN and N. SURMINA DEVI

College of Horticulture and Forestry, CAU, Pasighat, Arunachal Pradesh – 791102, India, E-mail: kalkame.momin@gmail.com (K. C. Momin)

ABSTRACT

North-East India or popularly known as the 'Seven Sister States' are among the 18 biodiversity hotspots in the world. This region is identified as the center of origin of many crop plant species and is a treasure house of traditional knowledge. The usage of locally available medicinal plants is known since time immemorial and is linked to the tradition and culture of the tribal inhabiting the NE region. The age old practice and knowledge of herbal remedies has been passed on from generation to generation. These plants are found naturally in the dense forests and they are grown domestically by the users, growers, practitioners, and marketers as well. Considering the dependence of the people on the locally available medicinal plants for their healthcare needs, cultivating and preserving the plants comes as a natural process of conservation in the region. Some of the highly valued medicinal plants found in North-Eastern region are *Acorus calamus, Aconitum heterophyllum, Aquillaria malaccensis, Bacopa monnieri, Berberis aristata, Coptis teeta, Costus speciosus, Curcuma caesia, Elaeocarpus sphericus, Embelia ribes, Gmelina arborea, Gynocordia odorata, Hydnocarpus kurzii, Homalomena aromatica, Mesua ferrea, Nardostachys jatamansi, Paris polyphylla, Picrorhiza kurroa, Rheum australe, Rubia cordifolia, Smilax China, Solanum anguivi, Swertia chirayita, Taxus wallichiana, Trichosanthis bracteata, Valeriana jatamansi, Zanthoxylum armatum,* etc. The existence of these plants is threatened by many factors and more because of population explosion leading to habitat destruction, clearing jungles for human settlements, widening of roads and so on. With the alarming decrease in forest areas and plants assuming different threat status, conservation is the need of the hour to ensure the plants survival. The farming community should be encouraged to practice the systematic cultivation of medicinal plants in order to conserve biodiversity and protect the threatened species of medicinal plants.

10.1   INTRODUCTION

The North East India covers a total area of 262,180 square kilometers accounting for about 8% of the country's total geographical area. The Northeast (NE) region boasts of having a diverse range of climate, geographical conditions and dense forest which is home to unique species of flora and fauna. Because of its vast diversity in soil, slope, altitudes, and ecological conditions, the region hosts diverse life forms including both flora and fauna. The region is a meeting ground of temperate east Himalayan flora, palaeo arctic flora of Tibetan highlands, wet evergreen flora of South East Asia and Yumnan which forms a bowl of diversity. The Brahmaputra valley includes the Eastern Himalayas, Patkai, and Nagaland, hilly areas of Meghalaya and Mikir hills. A rain forest type of climate is prevalent in the whole valley. Arunachal Pradesh is one of the largest states in terms of area, occupying nearly 83,743 sq km and hosts the maximum flora in the region. As per the latest report of the Forest Survey of India (FSI) (2018), the forest area coverage in NE region is about 65.34% of the total geographic area constituting nearly 24.2% of the country's total area. The NE India represents a region with diverse culture, ethnic tribes, food habits, rough terrain, inaccessibility, and biodiversity hotspot. Nearly 13,500 species of plants have been reported from the region and about 7,000 (52%) are reported to be endemic. Floristically, the region contributes almost 43% of the total plants' species in India. Further, the rate of endemic species percentage is also high (39%).

The use of medicinal plants in traditional health care system is an age-old practice and has been associated with all societies for centuries. There is a renewed global interest in herbal health care practices recently. This age-old practice which was believed to be no longer popular and replaced by the modern health care systems are now witnessing a comeback in the health care, despite "the traditional medicines (TMs)" attracting whole spectrum of reasons from 'uncritical enthusiasm to uninformed skepticism' on account of safety, efficacy, quality, etc. (WHO, 2002). In the NE region in particular, a very significant population still continues to rely on the medicinal plants gathered from the wild populations. The NE region is a treasure house of some of the rarest and highly valued medicinal plant which is now either threatened or endangered due to several factors, which include habitat loss, degradation as well as unscrupulous collection and over-exploitation from the wild resources. As per the reports of Karthikeyan (2000), an estimate of presence of nearly 7,500 taxa of flowering plants have been reported from the NE region, which accounts for nearly 40% of the floral diversity in the country. Owing to this reason, the entire NE region has attracted the conservation agencies in the country as well as at international level. At present, there are 16 National Parks and 55 Wildlife sanctuaries in the region. Mouling, Namdhapa, Eaglenest, Dibang, Sessa Orchid, Pakhui (Arunachal Pradesh); Manas, Kaziranga, Garampani, Nameri, DiporBil, Pobitora, Pabha, Laokhowa, Bornadi, and Oran (Assam); Balpakram, Nokrek, Baghmara Pitcher Plant WLS, Siju, and Nongkhyllem (Meghalaya); Intanki, Fakim, Puliebadze, Rangapahar (Nagaland); Keibul Lam Jao, Yangoupokpi Lokchao (Manipur); Murlen, Phawngpui Blue Mountain, Dampa, Thorangtlang, Tokalo, Khawnglung (Mizoram), Clouded leopard NP, Bison NP, Gumti, Rowa, Trishna, Sepahijala (Tripura), Kanchendzonga NP, Barsey Rhododendron WLS, Fambhong, Kyongnosla Alpine WLS, Shingba, Maenamand Kitam (Sikkim) and Jaldapara, Gorumara, Singalila, and Senchal (West Bengal) are some of the well-known national parks and wildlife sanctuaries of eastern region. The region provides an immense opportunity being a treasure house of rare and endangered flora and fauna. The forest of NE India comprises of nearly 74% gymnosperms, 49% pteridophytes, 72% orchids, 89% rhododendrons, 54.5% bamboos and 44.6% cane of the total population reported in India. The conservation efforts taken up till date is still not very strong and with the recent discoveries of many new plant species in the region, it needs further strengthening. It is possible to get different climatic zones in the entire north east region ranging from alpine type to tropical and mostly consists of acidic soils with a pH range of 4.5–5.0 (Table 10.1). The climatic zones in NE region can be classified as follows:

- Alpine Zone (> 3,500 m);
- Temperate Sub-Alpine (1,500–3,500 m);
- Sub-tropical Hill Zone (1,000–1,500 m);

- Sub-Tropical Plain Zone (800–1,000 m);
- Mild Tropical Hill Zone: (200–800 m);
- Mild Tropical Plain Zone (0–200 m).

TABLE 10.1   Biodiversity Richness in North East India

State	Species Richness (Flowering Plants)
Arunachal Pradesh	± 5,000
Sikkim	± 4,500
Meghalaya	±3,500
Assam	± 3,010
Manipur	± 2,500
Nagaland	± 2,250
Mizoram	± 2,200
Tripura	± 1,600

Source: Chatterjee et al. (2006)

10.2   MEDICINAL AND AROMATIC PLANT DIVERSITY

With its varied climatic zones, the NE region is a popular biodiversity hotspot that has been rightly termed by Takhtajan (1969) as the 'cradle of flowering plants.' The wide knowledge base on the usage of medicinal plants has been preserved and handed down over generation till today. The NE region is by far the richest area in context to floristic composition and concentration of endemic taxa contributing nearly 43% of the Indian floral diversity. The NE region is a storehouse of medicinal plants with that make their way to Indian as well as foreign markets. Reports suggests that nearly 70% of the medicinal plants are abundantly found in the forest's areas; out of which, 5% unscrupulously collected and sold in the market and 10% reported to be under threat. There is a growing demand and market for such important medicinal plants which makes it necessary to review their demand and supply in the country. There are numerous plants reported to have high medicinal importance and are found wild in the forests of North East India. This includes species like *Coptis teeta* (Mishmi teeta), *Aconitum ferox* (Indian Aconite), *Aconitum heterophyllum* (Indian Atees), *Oroxylum indicum* (Broken bones), *Illicium griffithii* (Star Anise), *Paris polyphylla* (Himalayan Paris), *Homalomena aromatica* (Scented Arum), *Swertia chiryata* (Chirayita), *Berginia ciliate* (Winter Begonia), *Garcinia spp.* (Sap tree), *Smilax glabra* (Sarsa Parilla), etc.

The ethnic communities still collect and use the medicinal plants for their healthcare needs and based upon the indigenous knowledge that they acquired, they use it for curing a simple disease as well as dreaded diseases like cancer, tumor, etc. Looking at the present scenario in the state of Assam, nearly 900 medicinal plant species have been reported, and Brahmaputra valley alone has more than 50 plant species of high commercial value. The state of Meghalaya is home to 850 medicinal plants, out of which 377 species are reported to be in use by the tribals of the state for health care needs. Sikkim, also known for its rich bio-resources, boasts of having a number of raw drugs that has been described in Ayurvedic texts. There are about 420 plants reported to be in use for the treatment of various diseases in the Sikkim Himalayan region. The tribal people of Tripura use as many as 25 of such plants for treating various ailments (De, 2016). The tribes inhabiting the state of Arunachal Pradesh use over 500 species of plants for their primary health care needs. The state is home to some of the endangered and highly valued medicinal plants *Taxus baccata, Coptis teeta, Panax pseudo-ginseng, Aconitum spp., Picrorhiza kurroa, Berberis spp.,* etc. which grow abundantly in the high altitude alpine and temperate belts in the region (Hussain and Hore, 2006). A field survey in Mizoram indicated the usage of a total of 242 plant species belonging to 86 families by different ethnic groups in the state. These plants were used for curing diseases like cancer, diabetes, tumor, epilepsy, heart related diseases, etc. (NMPB, 2006). The major tribes in Nagaland viz. Ao, Lotha, Angami, and Sema are reported to use 257 species of ethno-medicinal plants from 85 different plant families. The usage of medicinal plants reported to be used by different ethic tribes of the state are 112 species from Ao tribe, 54 species from Lotha tribe, 37 species from Angami tribe and 54 species from Sema tribe (Bhuyan et al., 2014). Another biodiversity rich state is Manipur which is bestowed with a rich and interesting floral diversity and holds an array of ethno-medicinal and aromatic plants (MAPs). A total of 456 plants having high therapeutic value and medicinal use have been reported which is being used by the various ethnic communities of the state (Das et al., 2017). Tripura has a record of over 1,500 species of plants and out of which 266 have been identified as having medicinal value. The state government has identified around 25 plants as priority species, and nearly 100 species of medicinal plants are reported to be cultivated or commercially extracted in small quantities. The setting up of Tripura State Medicinal Plants Board indicates the step towards conserving the important medicinal plants in the region (Table 10.2) (Tripura Forest Department, 2019).

TABLE 10.2   Ethno-Medicinal Diversity in NE

State	Number of Plant Species Used
Meghalaya	850
Assam	900
Arunachal Pradesh	500
Sikkim	420
Nagaland	257
Mizoram	242
Manipur	456
Tripura	266

By nature, the tribes inhabiting the NE region have a deeply rooted socio religious beliefs and have also followed a system of herbal medicines in treating their ailments. They have, by trial and error, developed their own way of diagnosing and treating diseases. They have inherited the knowledge on the identification and use of medicinal plants and have a rich experience in the field of traditional healthcare system. The rough and the rocky terrain in the North East region makes it difficult for the people to reach the nearest hospitals and health care centers. The only solution for them is to depend on the available plant resources for their primary treatment and relief. This is one way helps to explore and keep a record of the therapeutic activity of medicinal plants collected and used by them. In many of the villages throughout the region, there are one or two traditional healers who practice at home or have a separate place in the weekly markets where people come to consult him. The practice of traditional healing through plants is still prevalent in the region, which can be associated with the ethnic people's strong faith and belief in the healing properties and effectiveness over modern medicines.

Medicinal plants having high value from across the states of NE includes species like *Acorus calamus, Aconitum heterophyllum, Aquilaria malaccensis, Bacopa monnieri, Berberis aristata, Coptis teeta, Costus speciosus, Curcuma caesia, Elaeocarpus sphericus, Embelia ribes, Gmelina arborea, Gynocordia odorata, Hydnocarpus kurzii, Homalomena aromatica, Mesua ferrea, Nardostachys jatamansi, Paris polyphylla, Picrorrhiza kurrooa, Rheum australe, Rubia cordifolia, Smilax China, Solanum anguivi, Swertia chirayita, Taxus wallichiana, Trichosanthis bracteata, Valeriana jatamansi, Zanthoxylum aromaticum,* etc. (Shankar and Rawat, 2013).

10.3   THREATS TO PLANT POPULATION AND REGENERATION

With the Forest Conservation Act that came into force in the year 1980, the forest area of nearly 1.17 million hectares have been cleared for almost 23,000 developmental works in the country (MoEF, 2008). The loss of forest cover and ultimately the biodiversity in the region is driven by factors like the fast-growing human population coupled with high density, technological change-induced effects, growing economic activities and at the same time dearth of knowledge and scientific know how of the available biodiversity. Due to various anthropological factors, there has been a threat globally leading to drastic loss of habitat of flora, land fragmentation and degradation for conversion of land use for agricultural means, rapid urbanization and industrial development, invasion by alien plants, overexploitation of natural resources, etc. The manufacturing units of plant based pharmaceutical products rely on the collection and extraction of plants from the wild populations, and as a consequence of unscrupulous collection, overutilization and harvesting for production, the plants are getting endangered at an alarming rate. Plants such as *Homalomena aromatica, Coptis teeta, Thalictrum javanicum, Berberis aristata, Nardostachys jatamansi, Dipsacus inermis, Podophyllum hexandrum, Panax pseudoginseng, Picrorrhiza kurooa*, etc., are largely collected from the wild populations and are now available only in isolated pockets. For collection of such plants, the local people are mostly involved, who sell the plants at a take away price to the middlemen and later to the pharmaceutical companies at exorbitant rates. Different plant parts, be it root, leaf, stem, flower, fruit, or maybe the whole plant is collected from the jungles which in due course of time have rendered the plants rare, threatened, endangered or extinct. Some of the plants are regenerated through sexual and asexual methods. If the whole plant is uprooted, it gives a very less chance for its regeneration in the wild. Reports and studies have suggested that nearly 95% of the plants have been collected from the wild, posing a huge threat to their existence and survival in their natural habitats. The local people and the farming community needs to be educated and made aware of their cultivation practices for their preservation and future use.

The usage of over 30,000 plant species worldwide has been reported by World Health Organization (WHO). As per the latest reports of the International Union for Conservation of Nature (IUCN, (2020), nearly 40,108 plants have been listed under different threat status (Table 10.3) which poses a great concern for its conservation. Nearly 2,500 species of plants have been reported to be in use in the Indian Ayurvedic system of medicine. The threat status of plants in India numbers to 124 as endangered, 28 extinct, 81 rare and 34 insufficiently known (Akshay et al., 2014).

TABLE 10.3   IUCN Threat Status Worldwide

SL. No.	Categories	IUCN Red List Version 2020
1.	Extinct (EX)	123
2.	Extinct in the wild (EW)	37
3.	Critically endangered (CR)	3,325
4.	Endangered (EN)	6,063
5.	Vulnerable (VU)	7,072
6.	Near threatened (NT)	2,500
7.	Lower risk/conservation dependent (LR/cd)	171
8.	Data deficient (DD)	2,774
9.	Least concerned (LC)	18,043
	Total	40,108

Source: IUCN (2020).

The FSI report (2011) states that 'shifting' or 'jhum cultivation' is one of the major responsible factors for declining forest cover in NE India. The loss of forest cover as a result of shifting cultivation in the whole of NE region is estimated to be around 5,476 sq.km. This practice is still ongoing and widespread in all the states that causes a major loss to the forest wealth and disturbs the ecological balance. The age-old practice of jhumming is destructive to the surrounding environment as a whole since the forest areas are being converted to agriculture through practices, thereby diminishing the primary forest area. The fragmentation of natural habitat, destruction, and loss of native species, invasion of more exotic weeds, burning down of sun-dried vegetation pollutes the air with carbon dioxide, nitrous oxide, and many other harmful gases are some of the ill effects of shifting cultivation on the environment. This is coupled with illegal felling and poaching, diverting the forest areas for developmental projects, over-extraction of timber and non-timber forest products, particularly medicinal plants, which poses a serious threat for species for which there is high commercial demand. Further, activities like coal mining and quarrying also has a severe impact on the ecology of the biodiversity rich region as NE India. Another threat is the invasions by alien species which is a great cause of concern for the survival of the native species in their natural population and is gradually being replaced by them (Tables 10.4 and 10.5).

TABLE 10.4   Critically Endangered Medicinal Plants in India

Aconitum spp.	*Gastrochilus longiflora*
Adhatoda beddomei C. B. Clarke	*Gentiana kurrooa* Royle
Angelica glauca Edgew	*Ilex khasiana*
Aquilaria malaccensis Lam.	*Inula racemosa* Hook. f.
Arnebia benthamii (Wall. ex G. Don) Johnston	*Luvunga scandens* (Roxb.) Buch.-Ham. ex Wight
Aristolochia bracteolate Lam.	*Meconopsis aculeate* Royle
Atropa acuminate Royle ex Lindl.	*Nardostachys grandiflora* DC.
Berberis spp.	*Nepenthes khasiana* Hook. f.
Chlorophytum spp.	*Nothapodytesn immoniana* (J. Graham)
Colchicum luteum Baker	*Panax pseudoginseng* Wall.
Commiphora wightii (Arn.) Bhandari	*Przewalskia tangutica* Maxim.
Coptis teeta Wall.	*Picrorhiza kurrooa* Royle ex Benth.
Crateriostigma plantagineum Hochst.	*Podophyllum hexandrum*
Curcuma caesia Roxb.	*Rauvolfia serpentine* Benth. exKurz.
Dactylorhiza hatagirea D.Don	*Saussurea costus* (Falc.) Lipsch
Delphinium denudatum Wall.ex Hook. f. and Thomson	*Saussurea gossypiphora* D.Don
Dioscorea deltoidea Wall. ex Griseb.	*Swertia chirayita* (Roxb. ex Fleming)
Ephedra gerardiana Wall. ex Stapf	*Taxus wallichiana* Zucc.
Ferula jaeschkeana Vatke	*Valeriana jatamansi* Jones
Fritillaria roylei Hook	–

Source: Dhyani (2015); Sharma and Thokchom (2014).

TABLE 10.5   IUCN Red List Category Plants

Critically Endangered	**Endangered**	**Vulnerable**
Aconitum chasmanthum	*Cinnamomum wightii*	*Hydnocarpus pentandrus*
Chlorophytum borivilianum	*Coptis teeta*	*Magnolia nilagirica*
Gentianakurroo	*Decalepis hamiltonii*	*Malaxis muscifera*
Gymnocladus assamicus	*Dysoxylum malabaricum*	*Garcinia indica*
Lilium polyphyllum	*Gymnema khandalense*	*Nilgirianthus ciliatus*
Saussurea costus	*Illicium griffithii*	*Piper pedicellatum*

TABLE 10.5   *(Continued)*

Critically Endangered	Endangered	Vulnerable
Nardostachys jatamansi	*Humboldtia vahliana*	*Phyllanthus indofischeri*
Tribulus rajasthanensis	*Iphigenia stellata*	*Salacia oblonga*
Valeriana leschenaultia	*Lamprachaenium microcephalum*	*Terminalia pallid*
Commiphora wightii	*Nepenthes khasiana*	*Myristica dactyloides*
	Pimpinella tirupatiensis	*Aconitum violaceum*
	Piper barberi	*Boswellia ovalifoliolata*
	Syzygium alternifolium	*Calophyllum apetalum*
	Shorea tumbuggaia	*Cayratia pedata*
	Aconitum heterophyllum	*Cinnamomum macrocarpum*
	Angelica glauca	*Cinnamomum sulphuratum*
		Diospyros candolleana
		Diospyros paniculata

Source: Dhyani and Dhyani (2016).

Another big challenge for mountain and coastal eco-system is the adaptation to climate change which is slowly changing the forest patterns in such areas. The global climate change is the root cause of many disasters happening in the recent times and will continue to do so in the near future. Studies by various workers have shown that there has been an increase in global average surface temperature by 2C which is a great concern and threat to the existence and survival of the floral and faunal diversity. This rise in temperature is accompanied with the changes in species composition, productivity, and biodiversity, affecting millions of people who rely on the forest resources in their day-to-day life for their livelihood. The fragile ecosystem and biodiversity of the North-Eastern region is no exception and are very sensitive and vulnerable to sudden changes in climatic/environmental conditions. The farmers traditional crop varieties and races are now almost lost and being replaced by hybrid varieties. Further, the native forests plantations are slowly being replaced by plantation trees like rubber, eucalyptus, teak, willow, etc., which endangers the biodiversity. The popularization of medicinal plants can be only be achieved by creating awareness amongst the people in the region about its importance and need for conservation, focused survey of potential areas for species of medicinal value, documentation of the medicinal plants underuse, standardization of production technology, post-harvest, and marketing aspects, extraction of chemical compound and their application in pharmaceutical industries, DNA characterization, etc.

10.4 EXPLORATION AND CONSERVATION STRATEGIES OF UNEXPLORED MEDICINAL PLANT SPECIES UNDER NE REGION

In the NE region, exploration of herbal plant is a matter of great attraction to the researchers, scientists, traders as well as pharmaceuticals. Attempts have also been made for the acclimatization of medicinal plants by cultivating them in different zones in the NE region. It has also been reported that the crude drugs produced in North East India are highly traded in eastern (Assam, West Bengal and Bihar) and northern (Delhi) part of India (Shankar and Rawat, 2013). Further, highly valued plants having medicinal properties like the root of *Paris polyphylla* (Himalayan Paris) are collected from Arunachal Pradesh, Nagaland, Manipur, and Meghalaya and exported to Myanmar (Mao et al., 2009).

TERI (The Energy Resources Institute) NE Center has taken up the work not only to find out the rare and least explored plants of medicinal value of the region, but also on conservational aspects of the locally available plant species and providing planting material to local growers for their cultivation. This practice will help to check the destruction of the wild plant inhabitants. In NE region, following initiations were taken by TERI-NE center to explore and conserve the plants having therapeutic value (Kar, 2019). Initiatives have been taken from the central government sector for the promotion of farming of commercial medicinal plants of the region and also to explore opportunities in this sector.

- Herbal gardens were established in different school campuses to popularize and conserve local plants having medicinal value under DNA club programs.
- In Sikkim, a total of 83 accessions of sea buckthorn have been collected from the Himalayan region. Sea buckthorn's natural population is also found in Arunachal Pradesh with 37 accessions which were collected from Zimithang.
- Under a multi-institutional project, the TERI-NE Center has collected 26 species of plants having anti-ulcer property as a part of an ethnobotanical survey of locally grown plants of North East region.

- Screening of anti-ulcerogenic activity of plants surveyed will provide clues for its potential as anti-ulcer drugs.
- Good quality planting materials of Patchouli were produced at the center and evaluated for their field performance.
- Conserved seven species of *Garcinia* (Sap tree) at field level, some of which are endemic to NE India.

Raising the desire of native medicine has made alertness to the sustainability of these plants as raw drug and specially the collection of those plants which are already facing threat to their very existence. Conservation of medical and herbal plants involves two basic approaches, the *in-situ* and the *ex-situ*.

10.4.1 IN-SITU CONSERVATION

In-situ conservation involves the protecting the species in natural or semi-natural state in their dwelling environment. It has the potential to conserve wild family of crop plant species, their landraces and traditional cultivars. *In-situ* conservation can be achieved by different methods. The locally available landraces are preserved and managed in their natural area by means of *in-situ* method. Plant species and probable protected area for preserving the plants *in-situ* should be finalized based on the biodiversity map and policy of the government. An effort has been made in Garo hills district of Meghalaya, where more than 10,000 ha of land have been acknowledged as endangered reservation for different species of Citrus plants. The Ministry of Environment and Forest, Government of India, had identified 18 biosphere reserves based on survey data and four (04) of them are situated under the NE region (Table 10.6).

TABLE 10.6   Biosphere Reserves in NE Region

SL. No	Biosphere Reserve	Year	Area (sq.km)	States
1.	Nokrek	01.09.1988	820.00	Meghalaya
2.	Dihang-Dibang	02.09.1998	5,111.00	Arunachal Pradesh
3.	Manas	14.03.1989	2,837.00	Assam
4.	Khangchendzonga	02.02.2000	2,931.00	Sikkim
5.	Dibru-Saikhowa	28.07.1997	765.00	Assam

Source: Sujatha (2016). Biosphere Reserve of India. https://www.mapsofindia.com/my-india/india/biosphere-reserves-of-india.

The sacred groves are considered as the centers for conserving the native flora and fauna. The work of preserving and managing the local biodiversity is taken up by the local residents/communities in a sustainable manner who also takes the responsibility to safeguard the endemic, vulnerable, and rare plants in the sacred groves. The rare plants having medicinal value in Ayurvedic and as a general medicine which are usually not found in the wild are concentrated in sacred groves. The perceptions of sacred groves rise over the years when certain important ecological and economic species of plants and animals were protected in a grove (Deshmukh et al., 1998). Malhotra et al. (2001) stated that over 13,720 sacred groves from different parts of India. A large number of 634 sacred groves reported from different parts of Megha-laya, Manipur, and Karbi Anglong area of Assam (Tripathi, 2001). However, only a few are well preserved while many are under threat as a result of urbanization. The National Botanical Research Institute (Eco-Education Division) in Lucknow and the North Eastern Hill University (NEHU) has documented as many as 79 sacred groves in the state of Meghalaya. In Meghalaya, the sacred groves are under direct control of the headman of the village Dorbars/Syiemships/Dolloiships/Nokmaships or clan councils. The protection of the forest comes from the religious beliefs linked with the sacred groves and facts which have been followed for generations and serves as a good model for conserving the native flora and fauna in the area. In Manipur, plants used for curing and healing ailments which were reported to have disappeared earlier are now confined to the groves only. Researchers have also reported that in Manipur, 96% of the plant species that have been used for healing illnesses or sickness, content high medicinal value (Table 10.7) (Khumbongmayum et al., 2005).

TABLE 10.7   Recognized Sacred Groves in North-East India

SL. No.	State	Local Name for Sacred Groves	Total Number of Documented Sacred Groves
1.	Arunachal Pradesh	Gumpa forests (sacred groves attached to Buddhist monasteries)	65
2.	Assam	Than, Madaico	65
3.	Manipur	Umanglai, Mauhak (sacred bamboo reserves)	365
4.	Meghalaya	Ki Law Lyngdoh or Ki Law kyntang	83
5.	Sikkim	Gumpa forests	56

Source: Malhotra et al. (2001); Khumbongmayum et al. (2004).

10.4.2   EX SITU CONSERVATION

Ex-situ conservation means the safeguarding of components of biological diversity outside their environmental area (Rands et al., 2010). It involves the safeguarding of flora and fauna out of their accepted habitation by cultivation and maintaining plants in botanical gardens. The approaches of ex-situ safeguarding also involve long term preservation of flora in seed bank, *in-vitro* maintenance, DNA storage, etc.

The botanical garden plays an important role in exploration, introduction of herbal plants and plant biodiversity conservation. By embracing the ex-situ conservation method, the highly-threatened genetic materials are collected, rescued, and preserved, and at the same time, breeding of flora is carried out so as to enable them for restoration in cases where the survival in its native habitat is threatened. Further the approaches comprise the transfer of a target flora far from its natural habitat to a safer place like the plant estates and seed banks.

The practice of micro-propagation is one of the promising and quickest ways for multiplying and conserving the unexploited medicinal flora, which is otherwise difficult to propagate by conventional methods. Over the recent years, the method of tissue culture is conceived as significant means for germplasm conservation that will ensure the survival of endangered medicinal flora, their cultivation on a larger scale through tissue cultured plants and their genetic manipulation (Sharma and Thokchom, 2014). The legislative laws of Indian Government concerning to protect the natural forest reserve is one of the most operative ways of shielding biological diversity (Table 10.8).

TABLE 10.8   Laws for Conservation of Forest Framed by Government of India

SL. No.	Laws	Year
1.	Forest act	1927
2.	Wildlife (protection) act	1972
	Forest (conservation) act	1980
3.	Environment protection act	1986
4.	National forest policy	1988
5.	Wildlife (protection) amendment act	1991
6.	National biodiversity act	2002
7.	The scheduled tribes and other traditional forest dwellers act	2006

These are the laws framed by the Government of India for conservation of forest to protect the wild herbal flora (Akshay et al., 2014).

10.5   CONCLUSION

The medicinal plants are rooted with the major cultural, livelihood or economic roles amongst the tribal folk in the NE region and still continue to play a major role in their daily life. There has been a trend where too much importance has stressed on the potential for discovering new drugs, where too little attention has been given for their conservation actions and have just received a shallow treatment. The tribal people who are living close to nature and their acquired knowledge are not synergized to make them aware of the current scenario of medicinal plants and eventually empower and involve them to preserve the existing important plants of the area. This calls for an appropriate conservation measures coupled with the development and protection of the forest areas. The systematic cultivation needs to be taken up to meet the growing demands of herbal medicine, to conserve biodiversity and protect the threatened species of medicinal plants.

Diversity of medicinal plant species and the access to traditional herbal medicine is a less worked upon issue in NE region and therefore calls for serious investigation. Despite the deafening escalation of synthetic drugs in the last couple of decades, the ethnic people of NE region still depend on plants from the wild to such an extent that it is relevant to raise concerns related to the issues of their sustainability of their production and management. There is a growing concern about the risk of overexploitation to try to meet this demand without proper consideration of the proper stock for the future use. No concerted effort has been made to ensure that medicinal plants are preserved in view of their growing demand and ever-growing human population leading to extensive destruction of plant rich habitats. As a result, many medicinal plants face extinction or severe genetic loss and their detailed information is scanty. Till date, no action has been taken for the conservation of the endangered medicinal plant species. In fact, a complete database of medicinal plants is still lacking in most of the areas. Much of the knowledge of the plants and their usage is held by the traditional health practitioners which has not been properly documented and preserved. The information generated will help in linking the modern medicine with TM making it possible to complement the modern medicine and/or compliment it. At the backdrop of these facts, there is an urgent need for to bridge the gap between human and nature especially in NE region where the later has provided food, health, shelter, livelihood for generations.

KEYWORDS

- conservation
- cultivation
- medicinal value
- northeast India
- threat

REFERENCES

Akshay, K. R., Sudharani, N., Anjali, K. B., & Deepak, T. M., (2014). Biodiversity and strategies for conservation of rare, endangered and threatened medicinal plants. Research and Reviews: *Journal of Pharmacognosy and Phytochemistry, 2,* 12–20.

Anjula, P., Semwal, D. P., Ahlawat, S. P., & Sharma, S. K., (2015). Maize (*Zea mays*): Collection Status, Diversity Mapping and Gap Analysis. *National Bureau of Plant Genetic Resources: India, 34.*

Asati, B. S., & Yadav, D. S., (2004). Diversity of horticultural crops in North-Eastern region. *ENVIS Bulletin Himalayan Ecology, 12.* India.

Bhuyan, S. I., Meyiwapangla, & Laskar, I., (2014). Indigenous Knowledge and Traditional Use of Medicinal Plants by Four Major Tribes of Nagaland, North East India. *International Journal of Innovative Science, Engineering & Technology,* 1(6), 481–484.

Chatterjee, S., Saikia, A., Dutta, P., Ghosh, D., & Worah, S., (2006). *Background paper on Review of Biodiversity in North East* India. WWF, Delhi, India.

Das, A. K., Rajkumari, R., Khatoon, R., & Singh, P. K., (2017). *Glimpses of Ethnobotany and Medicinal Plants of Manipur.* N.E. India. Om Publication: India. ISBN 9789380702117.

De, L. C., (2016). Medicinal and aromatic plants of North East India. *International Journal of Development Research,* 6(11), 10104–10114.

Deshmukh, S., Gogate, M. G., & Gupta, A. K., (1998). Sacred groves and biological diversity: Providing new dimensions to conservation Issue, In: Ramakrishnan, P. S., Saxena, K. G., & Chandrashekara, U. M., (eds.), *Conserving, the Sacred for Biodiversity Management* (pp. 397–414). Oxford and IBH Publishing Co: New Delhi.

Dhyani, A., & Dhyani, S., (2016). *IUCN Red List 2015: Medicinal Plants at Risk* (pp. 12, 13). Science Reporter: India.

Dhyani, A., (2015). *Critically Endangered Indian Medicinal Plants* (pp. 42–45). Heritage Amruth.

Forest Survey of India (FSI), (2018). India State of Forest Report 2018–19, Forest Survey of India, Ministry of Environment, Forest and Climate Change, Govt. of India.

Forest Survey of India (FSI), (2011), India State of Forest Report, Dehradun: Ministry of Environment and Forest

Hussain, S., & Hore, D. K., (2006). Collection and conservation of major medicinal plants of Arunachal Pradesh. *Indian Forester*, 1663–1679.

IUCN (2020) The IUCN red list of threatened species. Version 2020–1. https://www.iucnredlist.org. Accessed on 17.11.2021

Kar, A., (2019). *Making Medicinal Plant Wealth Work for Northeast India.* https://www.teriin.org/article/making-medicinal-plant-wealth-work-northeast-india (accessed on 01 November 2021).

Karthikeyan, S., (2000). A statistical analysis of flowering plants of India; In: N. P. Singh, P. K. Singh, P. K. Hajra, and B. D. Sharma (ed.). Flora of India, Introductory volume II. Calcutta: Botanical Survey of India. pp. 201–217.

Khumbongmayum, A. D., Mohammed, L. K., & Radhey, S. T., (2005). Sacred groves of Manipur – Ideal centers for biodiversity conservation. *Current Science, 87*(4), 25.

Malhotra, K. C., Gokhle, Y., Chatterjee, S., & Srivastava, S., (2001). *Cultural and Ecological Dimensions of Sacred Groves in India.* INSA: New Delhi.

Mao, A. A., Hynniewta, T. M., & Sanjappa, M., (2009). Plant wealth of Northeast India with reference to ethnobotany. *Indian Journal of Traditional Knowledge, 8*(1), 96–103.

MOEF Forest Survey of India, (2008). *Ministry of Environment, Forest, and Climate Change.* http://www.fsi.nic.in/publications (accessed on 01 November 2021).

NMPB. (2006). *Documentation of Ethnomedicinal Plants of Mizoram.* https://www.nmpb.nic.in/content/documentation-ethno-medicinal-plants-mizoram (accessed on 01 November 2021).

Rands, M. R., Adams, W. M., Bennun, L., Butchart, S. H., Clements, A., Coomes, D., Entwistle, A., et al., (2010). Biodiversity conservation: Challenges beyond. *Science, 329*(5997), 1298–1303.

Shankar, R., & Rawat, M. S., (2013). Conservation and cultivation of threatened and high valued medicinal plants in North East India. *International Journal of Biodiversity and Conservation, 5*(9), 584–591.

Sharma, S., & Thokchom, R. V., (2014). A review on endangered medicinal plants of India and their conservation. *Journal of Crop and Weed, 10*(2), 205–218.

Singh, H., (2016). *Taxonomic Studies on Family Noctuidae Lepidoptera from North East India.* http://hdl.handle.net/10603/79515 (accessed on 01 November 2021).

Sujatha, (2016). Biosphere reserve of India. https://www.mapsofindia.com/my-india/india/biosphere-reserves-of-india.

Takhtajan, A., (1969). *Flowering Plants, Origin and Dispersal.* Tr. Jeffrey, Edinburgh.

Tripathi, R. S., (2001). Sacred groves: Community biodiversity conservation model in Northeast India. In: Ganeshaiah, K. N., Shaanker, U. R., & Bawa, K. S., (eds.), *Tropical Ecosystems Structure, Diversity and Human Welfare (Supplement)* (pp. 104–107). ATREE: Bangalore.

Tripura Forest Department, (2019). Forest Resources of Tripura, Govt. of Tripura, Tripura Forest Department. https://forest.tripura.gov.in/forest-of-tripura (accessed on 17 November 2021).

WHO (2002). *Traditional Medicine Strategy (2002–2005). WHO/EDM/TRM/2002.1.* Geneva, Switzerland: World Health Organization.

CHAPTER 11

ESSENTIAL OILS: CLINICAL PERSPECTIVES AND USES

JUGREET BIBI SHARMEEN and
MAHOMOODALLY MOHAMAD FAWZI

Department of Health Sciences, Faculty of Medicine and Health Sciences, University of Mauritius, Réduit – 80837, Mauritius E-mail: f.mahomoodally@uom.ac.mu (M. M. Fawzi)

ABSTRACT

During recent decades, the use of plant essential oils (EOs) for the procurement of health benefits has been on crescendo in the wellness and aromatherapy industries. Indeed, the scientific documentation of the therapeutic effects of EOs are diverse. They have been established as potent antimicrobial, antioxidant, immunostimulant, analgesic, anti-cancer, and anti-inflammatory agents amongst many others in numerous *in vitro* and *in vivo* investigations. Moreover, EOs has widespread applications in aromatherapy where they are either inhaled or topically applied on skin. In fact, a significant number of clinical studies have highlighted the efficacy of EOs, particularly in the context of aromatherapy, as being stress, anxiety, depression, and pain-relieving. Besides their calming and relaxing attributes, they have been shown to improve the psychological along with the biochemical and physiological parameters of individuals in clinical settings. The aromatherapeutic uses of EOs are also acknowledged to harmonize with conventional therapies, thus enhancing the treatment provided to patients. However, although EOs are generally regarded as safe and are greatly used on a daily basis in their pure form or in products containing them, they have been reported to be associated with certain adverse effects. Notably, EOs have shown to be responsible for skin allergic reactions owing to the presence of individual components that may act as sensitizing agents. Furthermore, the oxidation of EOs and their components have been documented to be more prone to cause skin irritations. Nevertheless, cases of toxicity arising from the ingestion of EOs have also been described. Hence, the present book chapter aimed to provide a broad perspective of the health benefits of EOs along with their curative uses in aromatherapy in the light of various clinical studies and highlight the possible adverse effects that may be linked to the use of EOs and their related products.

11.1 INTRODUCTION

The use of herbal products has become a significant and indispensable part of public healthcare worldwide (Lai, 2000). Numerous surveys on alternative and traditional medicine (TM) have highlighted their extensive use (Eisenberg et al., 1993; Saydah and Eberhardt, 2006; Welz et al., 2018). Nonetheless, in order to ensure their efficacy and safety, clinical studies on these herbal remedies are of utmost significance.

Essential oils (EOs) which are aromatic volatile oils, are among one of the important natural products derived from plants (Elshafie and Camele, 2017), with widespread commercial applications and a growing global market (Barbieri and Borsotto, 2018). In fact, they are acknowledged to have various traditional uses, including the treatment of ailments related to the cardiovascular, endocrine, digestive, respiratory tract, gynecological, andrological, and nervous system as well as skin infections (Firenzuoli et al., 2014). Undeniably, they are very well-known for their fragrances and are widely used in various industries such as perfumery, food and beverage and cosmetics (Irshad et al., 2019). Moreover, EOs derived from a wide range of plants have been extensively scrutinized using a number of experimental models where they have demonstrated to possess promising pharmacological potentials such as anti-cancer, anti-inflammatory, anti-diabetic, anti-allergic, analgesic, antimicrobial, and antioxidant properties amongst others (Mitoshi et al., 2014; Angelini et al., 2018; Tahir et al., 2016; Viuda-Martos et al., 2010; El Bouzidi et al., 2013; Silva et al., 2015; Sarmento-Neto et al., 2016; Kozics et al., 2017).

Besides these laboratory-based experiments, several pre-clinical and clinical studies have been undertaken to evaluate the medicinal benefits of these natural compounds on human health. For instance, aromatherapy, the use of pure EOs from aromatic plants to help alleviate health issues and improve the quality of life in general (Buckle, 2007), has demonstrated varied clinical applications. Several research conducted in this direction have shown EOs used in aromatherapy, where they are mainly absorbed via the skin or olfactory system, to be efficient as a non-pharmacological therapy or an adjunct along with conventional drug therapies, thus improving the treatment given to patients, especially those suffering from debilitating illnesses (Buckle, 1999; Martinec, 2012; Knoerr, 2018; Ganji et al., 2019). In fact, studies have also shown EOs to be useful in managing symptoms in critically ill patients (Halm, 2008).

It has also been reported that the main mechanism of aromatherapy may be associated with the brain limbic system. Aromatic components are believed to be able to activate olfactory cells for transmitting signals to the brain and therefore affect the autonomic nervous system and hormone secretion (Kagawa et al., 2003). In furtherance, aromatherapy combined with massage has been claimed to be relaxing, stress-, and pain-relieving, with the capacity to reduce blood pressure (BP) and boost the immune system (Tisserand, 1990). The use of aromatherapy massage as a complementary therapy is also increasing in popularity in palliative care owing to its positive effects on pain, psychological, and physical symptoms, and the overall quality of life (Wilkinson et al., 1999; Soden et al., 2004; Ching, 2005).

Additionally, self-medication with EOs has become a popular phenomenon eliciting substantial debate with respect to its merits. Besides, a large number of EOs' components can all together interact with many physiological target systems, thereby turning conventional pharmacological experimentations complex (Schnaubelt, 2005). Although the benefits remain controversial, many healthcare providers and patients are greatly attracted towards aromatherapy due to its low cost and minimum adverse effects. However, even though EOs are generally recognized as safe by the US Food and Drug Administration, they can cause minor skin irritation at the site of use, while ingesting them in large amounts can cause phototoxic reactions which can be lethal in rare cases (Boehm et al., 2012).

Hence, in the light of the above, the aim of the present work is to underline the different studies that have used a clinical approach to assess the healing properties of EOs in the treatment and management of several disease conditions and alongside highlight the EOs associated toxicities that have been reported.

11.2   CLINICAL STUDIES ON EOS

Clinical studies conducted on EO applications in human health and wellness are quite varied. In fact, various clinical applications of EOs in aromatherapy have gathered growing attention over the past years. Most importantly, they have been found to have emotional, psychological, as well as physiological benefits on individuals under different clinical settings. Thus, in this section, studies reporting the clinical facets of EOs will be discussed.

11.2.1   ANXIETY

Given the chronic nature of anxiety disorders, patients tend to suffer from them for a long time, sometimes even decades. Thus, long-term treatment requirements set very high safety and compliance standards for the medications bringing phytotherapy as a treatment alternative (Sarris et al., 2011). In fact, phytotherapy has been attracting momentous interest in the treatment of anxiety (Ernst, 2006; Sarris et al., 2013; Yeung et al., 2018), with many GABA-modulating medicines from herbal sources being considered for preclinical and clinical investigations (Savage et al., 2018).

Indeed, particular consideration has also been directed towards the anxiolytic-like effects of EOs, among which lavender EO has shown to possess the best profile (De Sousa et al., 2015). Accordingly, evidence pertaining to the effectiveness of the lavender EO in the pharmacotherapy of mental disorders has led to the development of silexan, a standardized preparation of the flowers of *L. angustifolia* EO obtained by steam distillation (Kasper et al., 2018). In this regard, the anxiolytic efficacy of oral administration of silexan has been evaluated in generalized anxiety disorder (GAD) and compared to paroxetine (a known anti-anxiety/anti-depressant drug) and placebo in the study of Kasper et al. (2014). Selected participants received capsules of 80 or 160 mg silexan, 20 mg paroxetine or placebo once daily for 10 weeks duration. The primary efficacy endpoint was the reduction in total score of the Hamilton anxiety scale (HAMA) from baseline to the end of treatment. Interestingly, for 80 and 160 mg/day silexan group, the HAMA total scores were 12.8 ± 8.7 and 14.1 ± 9.3 points respectively, while it was 9.5 ± 9.0 for placebo and 11.3 ± 8.0 for paroxetine. Both doses of silexan had superior effect compared to placebo in the reduction of HAMA total score, although, the difference between paroxetine and placebo was more prominent. Moreover, the incidence densities of adverse events (AEs) reported for silexan 80 and 160 mg/d were 0.008 and 0.006 AEs/day respectively. Conversely, 0.008 AEs/d for placebo and 0.011 AEs/d for paroxetine group were recorded. Silexan displayed AEs comparable to placebo but lower than that of paroxetine. Therefore, silexan was seen to be efficacious in GAD and well-tolerated even at a higher dosage of 160 mg/d. In furtherance, no withdrawal symptoms were shown following termination of the treatment after 10 weeks completion of full therapeutic dosage. Hence, silexan demonstrated convincing anxiolytic efficacy and a good safety profile.

Nevertheless, the effect of lavender EO on anxiety of dental patients was inspected by Zabirunnisa et al. (2014). A significant reduction in anxiety scores of lavender groups was observed compared to the control group. Besides, anxiety scores were seen to reduce with increase in age in the lavender group. This routine practice of EO usage can thus help to enhance the quality of dental treatments.

Moreover, a review by Mannucci et al. (2018) reported *Citrus aurantium* or *Citrus sinensis* Eos to produce anxiolytic effects in both preclinical and clinical studies. *Citrus aurantium* EO aromatherapy was observed to reduce anxiety levels in most stress conditions studied, especially in subjects affected by chronic myeloid leukemia and preoperative patients. On the other hand, *Citrus sinensis* EO exposure in clinical studies showed a positive decline in patients' anxiety level waiting to receive dental treatment and in healthy volunteers that were subjected to an anxiogenic situation. Thus, oral administration and/or inhalation of these *Citrus* EOs can be beneficial in treating anxiety (Mannucci et al., 2018).

Similarly, Lehrner et al. (2000) showed that exposure of ambient orange (*Citrus sinensis*) odor (EO) to patients waiting for dental treatment in a dental office could have a relaxant effect and help in reducing anxiety. In particular, women exposed to the orange odor displayed a lower level of state anxiety, a more positive mood, and a greater level of calmness in comparison with the control group.

Furthermore, Kim et al. (2010) investigated the effect of aroma inhalation of a mixture of orange EO along with other EOs on the level of anxiety in nursing students that were practicing their first intravenous injections. The increase in pulse rate and systolic BP was found to be inferior in the intervention group compared to the control group.

In a randomized clinical trial conducted by Rashidi-Fakari et al. (2015), the effect of aromatherapy using orange EO on women's anxiety during labor was studied. Women were exposed to 2 drops of orange peel EO in the intervention group or distilled water in the control group (placebo). Clean and non-absorbable napkins containing the EO (2%) or placebo were attached to the participants' clothes at a distance of 20 cm away from their chins. The systolic and diastolic BPs, pulse and respiration rates were the physiological parameters that were monitored in all the women before and 20 min after the intervention. The anxiety level was reduced in both intervention and control groups. However, the reduction was greater in the intervention group than in the control group based on their difference in anxiety scores before and after the intervention, although no significant change was observed in the physiological parameters of women from the intervention group.

Aromatherapy with geranium EO was also found to reduce anxiety level during first stage of labor in nulliparous women. Anxiety levels using Spielberger' questionnaire including physiological parameters before and after intervention were assessed in both experimental and control groups. The mean anxiety score as well as the diastolic BP reduced significantly after geranium EO inhalation (Fakariet al., 2015).

Aromatherapy massage is also increasingly being applied on cancer patients as a complementary therapy, particularly in palliative care setting as it is considered to improve the quality of life of patients as well as help to reduce psychological distress in patients (Fellowes et al., 2004). For instance, Corner et al. (1995) compared the effects of an 8-week course of massage, with either an EO blend or plain oil, on patients that were undertaking cancer treatment. The results from their study suggested that massage had a significant effect on patients' anxiety and was greater when EOs were used. Moreover, cancer patients receiving full body aromatherapy massage thrice over a period of 3 weeks with Roman Chamomile EO showed statistically significant improvement in post-test scores as measured by the Rotterdam Symptom Checklist physical symptom and quality of life subscales including the state anxiety scale (Wilkinson, 1995).

The anxiolytic efficacy of aromatherapy massage in breast cancer patients was also examined by Imanishi et al. (2009). Patients received a 30 min aromatherapy massage two times weekly for 4 weeks such that 8 sessions were given in total. The results during the control period, that is, one month before the aromatherapy massage were compared with those during the aromatherapy treatment and one month after completing the aromatherapy massage treatment. Interestingly, anxiety was found to reduce in one 30 min aromatherapy massage as assessed by the State-Trait Anxiety Inventory test, while it was reduced in eight sequential aromatherapy massage sessions according to the Hospital Anxiety and Depression Scale test. Concomitantly, aromatherapy massage was found to boost the immunologic state of patients.

11.2.2 HYPERTENSION

Hypertension, an irregular rise in BP, occurs when the arterioles become constricted, decreasing the capacity of blood to flow and causes the heart to work harder (Buckle, 2003). Hypertension is accountable for at least 45% of deaths due to heart disease while 51% of deaths because of stroke (WHO, 2013). Interestingly, aromatherapy has been reported to aid as an adjunctive relaxing therapy, and some EOs are believed to assist in reducing borderline hypertension (Buckle, 2003).

For instance, Li et al. (2011) investigated the effect of inhaling different concentrations of lavender EO on BP in hypertensive patients together with the possible mechanism involved. At all three different concentrations that were tested, lavender EO inhalation was found to be able to reduce high BP in patients. However, at 1% lavender EO, the decrease in BP was more significant and stayed for a longer time, with no effect on heart rate. The mechanisms accountable for the reduction of BP were by lowering plasma renin activity, angiotensin II, aldosterone, and the concentration of norepinephrine via the olfactory pathway of lavender EO.

The effects of EO inhalation on BP and salivary cortisol levels in hypertensive and pre-hypertensive subjects were also examined (Kim et al., 2012). The experimental group was asked to inhale an EO blend containing lavender, ylang-ylang, marjoram, and neroli EOs (in ratio of 20:15:10:2). The placebo group instead inhale an artificial fragrance for 24 h while no treatment was received by the control group. The daytime systolic and diastolic blood pressures (SBP and DBP) monitored throughout 24-hour ambulatory BP measurement in the experimental group were significantly decreased compared with the placebo and control groups after treatment. On the contrary, no significant difference in night-time SBP and DBP was achieved. Besides, the experimental group showed significant decrease in salivary cortisol levels compared to those in the placebo and control groups. Therefore, EO inhalation demonstrated instant and continuous effects on BP and stress reduction that can be considered as effective for controlling hypertension.

11.2.3 MIGRAINE/HEADACHES

Headaches, including migraine are prevalent and disabling disorders that can impact negatively on one's quality of life. According to WHO (2001), headache is considered as a high-priority health issue and has been ranked as

19th among the causes of years of life lived with disability in both sexes and all ages, and 12th in women.

Interestingly, a number of EOs has been positively associated with the reduction of headache/migraine occurrences in patients having these chronic disorders. Notably, in the randomized controlled clinical trial carried out by Rafie et al. (2016), the efficacy of lavender EO as a prophylactic therapy for migraine was examined. The participants selected for this study were patients that were previously being treated with propranolol and thus received lavender EO as an adjunct to that treatment. This double-blind and placebo-controlled study was performed over a period of three months. Patients involved in the study were evaluated for migraine impact at the baseline and at the end of the study using the migraine disability assessment scores (MIDAS) questionnaire. After three months of lavender therapy, a significant reduction in the MIDAS was obtained compared to the baseline as well as the control group. Furthermore, no complaints or side effects were reported by the participants during the treatment. These findings therefore indicated that the severity and frequency of migraine occurrences were reduced in patients who used the lavender EO therapy.

Similarly, Sasannejad et al. (2012) investigated the efficacy of lavender EO inhalation in the treatment of migraine in a placebo-controlled clinical trial. Around 47 patients diagnosed as having a definitive migraine headache were separated into cases and controls. Cases and controls inhaled lavender EO and liquid paraffin respectively for 15 min, following which patients recorded their headache severity and associated symptoms at 30 min intervals for a total 2 h duration. The mean reduction of headache severity obtained in cases and controls was statistically significant; with the percentage of responders in the lavender group being higher than the placebo group. Moreover, out of 129 headache attacks in cases, 92 responded partly or completely to lavender EO treatment, while 32 from 68 reporting headache attacks responded to placebo in the control group. Thus, this study demonstrated that inhalation of lavender EO could be a safe and efficient treatment modality for managing acute migraine headaches.

11.2.4 INSOMNIA/SLEEP DISORDERS

Insomnia can have devastating effects on a person's health and has been associated with the increased risk of medical conditions such as cardio-vascular diseases (CVD), weakened immune system, hypertension, and cognitive impairment (Spiegel et al., 2002; Palagini et al., 2013; Javaheri and Redline, 2017; Hamdy et al., 2018). In addition, sleep deprivation in hospitalized patients is common and can entail serious detrimental consequences on patient's convalescence (Lytle et al., 2014).

Aromatherapy, as a holistic and non-medicine therapy is considered an effective treatment for sleep disorders (Robertshawe, 2009). In this context, previous studies on aromatherapy have demonstrated to significantly improve sleep using geranium, lavender, marjoram, bergamot, citrus, and other EO mixtures through massage, inhalation, skin smear and other methods (Hwang and Shin, 2015). Moreover, lavender EO, has been particularly reported to possess sedative and hypnotic effects (Bowles, 2003) along with a safe profile (Tisserand and Young, 2014). In fact, in the study of Moeini et al. (2010), a significant improvement in sleep quality of ischemic heart disease patients was noted following aromatherapy treatment with lavender oil. Likewise, aromatherapy with lavender EO was found effective in improving sleep quality in postpartum women (Afshar et al., 2015). Lillehei et al. (2015) also studied the effect of inhaled lavender (*Lavandula angustifolia*) EO and sleep hygiene on sleep quality and quantity, which were then compared to sleep hygiene alone in college students with self-reported sleep issues. Lavender EO inhalation together with sleep hygiene displayed better sleep quality at post-intervention and two-week follow-up. Besides, a clinical effect was reported for the lavender group at post-intervention, together with a significant finding of waking feeling refreshed.

In furtherance, Lytle et al. (2014) investigated the effect of inhaling 100% pure lavender EO on the vital signs and perceived quality of sleep of patients admitted in intermediate care unit (IMCU). The treatment group was exposed to 3 ml of the lavender EO placed in a glass jar at patients' bedside from 10 pm to 6 am. Measurement of vital signs was done at intervals throughout the night, and all patients were asked to fill the Richard Campbell Sleep Questionnaire at 6 am in order to evaluate sleep quality. BP was found to be significantly inferior between midnight and 4 am in the EO group compared to the control group who received normal care. Also, based on the overall mean change score in BP between the baseline and 6 am measurements, the treatment group showed a decrease in BP, while an increase was observed in the control group. Besides, the mean overall sleep score was higher in the intervention group compared to the control group. However, the differences between the two groups were not significant.

Hence, the use of EOs can be regarded as a useful and safe treatment for treating insomnia, thereby helping to reduce the overuse of prescription drugs and the risk of sleeping disorders which affects the well-being of the body in the long or short-term (Lillehei and Halcon, 2014).

11.2.5 ARTHRITIS

The anti-inflammatory and analgesic properties of EOs are well recognized (Silva et al., 2003; Sarmento-Neto et al., 2016). Bahr et al. (2018) showed in their randomized, double-blind, placebo-controlled study that the application of aroma touch hand technique (ATHT) using EOs (Copaiba and Deep Blue oils) in patients with hand arthritis significantly increased joint flexibility. Moreover, the patients receiving the treatment (ATHT and EOs) took significantly less time to complete dexterity tasks and demonstrated around 50% reduction in pain scores, enhanced finger strength, and a notable increase in the angle of maximum flexion compared with those treated with coconut oil (placebo).

Nevertheless, Nasiri and Mahmodi (2018) evaluated the effects of aromatherapy massage with lavender EO on daily activities of patients with knee osteoarthritis. In a single-blinded, randomized clinical trial, participants were randomly assigned into three groups: intervention (massage with lavender EO), placebo (massage with almond oil) and control (without massage). The daily living activities of the patients were significantly improved immediately and one week post-intervention in the group that received massage with the EO as opposed to their initial status and that of the control group. Thus, aromatherapy massage with lavender EO can help to reduce the occurrence of daily activity disabilities in patients suffering from knee osteoarthritis.

11.2.6 DEMENTIA

Dementia is a chronic and progressive disease that causes impairment of memory, thinking, and behavior, consequently affecting the ability to take part in daily activities (Henderson and Jorm, 2002). Some of the behavioral and psychological symptoms of dementia (BPSDs) include aggression, agitation, psychotic manifestations with consequent stress, increased pain perception, and reduced quality of life (Scuteri et al., 2017).

Aromatherapy has been well-documented in the treatment and management of dementia (Scuteri et al., 2017). For instance, a placebo-controlled trial to inspect the effect of aromatherapy with *Melissa officinalis* (lemon balm) EO on agitation in people with severe dementia was conducted by Ballard et al. (2002). The active treatment or placebo oil (sunflower oil) was mixed with a base lotion and applied to patients' faces and arms two times a day. Changes in agitation was monitored using the Cohen-Mansfield agitation inventory (CMAI) and quality of life indices taking into consideration of the percentage of time spent socially withdrawn and the time engaged in constructive activities were measured using the Dementia Care Mapping. An overall improvement in agitation (mean reduction in CMAI score) of 35% in patients receiving the EO and 11% for those in the placebo group was observed. Their findings indicated that quality of life indices were improved significantly more in people receiving the EO. Importantly, no significant side effects were observed. It was therefore concluded that aromatherapy with lemon balm EO can be regarded as safe and effective for treating clinically significant agitation in people suffering from severe dementia (Ballard et al., 2002).

Likewise, Jimbo et al. (2004) studied the effect of aromatherapy on dementia patients. The therapy consisted of the use of rosemary and lemon EOs in the morning, and lavender and orange EOs in the evening. Moreover, the evaluation was done before and after the control period, after aromatherapy, and after the washout period (28 days). Patients showed significant improvement in personal orientation associated with cognitive function after the therapy. Especially, patients with Alzheimer's disease (AD) demonstrated significant progress in total Touch Panel-type Dementia Assessment Scale scores. Besides, no adverse effects associated with the use of aromatherapy was reported, suggesting that aromatherapy can be an efficacious non-pharmacological therapy with the potential of improving cognitive function in dementia as well as in AD patients.

11.2.7   DERMATOLOGICAL PROBLEMS

For instance, Kim et al. (2018) carried out clinical trials to assess the effects of myrtle EO on skin acne of Korean women. The subjects of this study, divided as the experimental group (treated with myrtle EO) and the control group (no myrtle EO applied) were provided with cosmetics for use every morning and evening for 6 weeks. Besides, the provided cosmetics are made with only a difference in the presence or absence of added myrtle substances, leaving all other substances alike in order to test the effects of the myrtle substances. Amazingly, the acne grades were significantly reduced along with a decrease in pores, erythema, sebum, desquamation including microorganism indexes in the experimental group. Thus, all evaluation indicators associated with acne improved significantly in the experimental group. Therefore, this study clinically demonstrated that myrtle EO was efficient for convergence and reduction of erythema, sebum, and dead skin cells removal, and exerted antibacterial activity on facial skin of Korean women and confirmed that myrtle EO could be regarded as a safe and skin-soothing substance for acne treatment.

Nonetheless, Malhi et al. (2017) evaluated the tolerability, efficacy, and acceptability of a tea tree oil gel and face wash in treating mild to moderate facial acne in an open-label, uncontrolled phase II pilot study. For this purpose, participants applied tea tree oil products on their face twice daily for 12 weeks and assessments were done at 4th, 8th, and 12th weeks. The total lesion counts as well as the mean investigator global assessment were found to differ significantly over time that is from baseline to 12 weeks. No serious AEs occurred and only minor local tolerability events which were restricted to dryness, peeling, and scaling, were reported to be resolved without intervention. This study thus suggested the efficacy and tolerability of these tea tree oil products in improving mild to moderate acne.

Likewise, Enshaieh and co-workers (2007) showed the efficacy of 5% topical tea tree oil gel in the treatment of mild to moderate *Acne vulgaris* in a randomized double-blind clinical trial conducted on 60 patients. The effect to the treatment was evaluated by considering the acne severity index (ASI) and total acne lesions counting (TLC) for every 15 days over a duration of 45 days. A significant difference between tea tree oil gel and placebo groups was observed in the improvement of the TLC and ASI, although they were 3.55 and 5.75 times respectively more effective in the treatment group than placebo. In contrast, side effects in both groups were relatively comparable and tolerable.

Tea tree oil has also been found to possess anti-dandruff properties. Accordingly, Satchell et al. (2002) investigated the tolerability and efficacy of 5% tea tree oil in patients with mild to moderate dandruff. Patients were randomly assigned to receive either 5% tea tree oil shampoo or placebo, which was used daily for 4 weeks. Evaluation was performed on the basis of quadrant-area-severity scale and by patient self-assessment scores of itchiness, scaliness, and greasiness. An improvement of 41% in the quadrant-area-severity score was recorded by the treatment group compared to 11% in the placebo group. Significant improvements were also observed in the total area of involvement and severity scores, including the greasiness and itchiness components, while improvement in scaliness was found not as significant according to patients' self-assessment scores.

11.2.8   PAIN

Pain can be an emotional and unpleasant experience associated with actual or potential tissue damage. In this regard, the effect of aromatherapy with orange EO on pain and vital signs of patients with fractured limbs was evaluated in a randomized clinical trial. Patients were separated into experiment and control groups. Orange EO (4 drops) was poured on a pad which was pinned to the patients' collar, about 20 cm distant from the head. The old pad was replaced by a new one every 1 h and the patients' pain and vital signs (BP, pulse rate, respiration, and body temperature) were checked every 1 h for at last 6 h. Pain scores in the intervention group showed significant differences at different times and increasing duration of pain was reduced significantly. Moreover, pain in the experiment group decreased significantly compared to the control group, although no significant effects on their vital signs was observed in both groups. Aromatherapy with orange EO can thus help to relieve pain in patients with fractured limbs and be used as a complementary medicine in such patients (Hekmatpou et al., 2017).

The efficacy of rose EO as a complementary therapy in addition to conventional therapy in the relief of renal colic was also reported by Ayan et al. (2013). Participants (n=80) were patients (19–64 years old) diagnosed with renal colic in the emergency room. Half of the patients were treated with 75 g of diclofenac sodium intramuscularly which constituted the conventional therapy together with placebo (physiological serum, 0.9% NaCl), while the other half was treated with conventional therapy along with aromatherapy with rose EO. The visual analog scale (VAS) values as measures of pain severity prior to the start of therapy, 10 and 30 minutes after therapy were obtained and compared between the two groups of participants. No significant difference between the starting VAS values of the two groups was found but 10 and 30 minutes after the initiation of therapy, the VAS values were observed to be statistically lesser in the group that were given the conventional therapy plus aromatherapy.

In another clinical situation, the effectiveness of blended EOs on pain in outpatients experiencing menstrual cramps was investigated. Patients who were diagnosed with primary dysmenorrhea were assigned randomly to an EO group against a synthetic fragrance one. Blended EOs composed of lavender, clary sage and marjoram in a ratio of 2:1:1 was diluted in an unscented cream (at 3% concentration) and given to the experimental group. This cream was daily used by outpatients to massage their lower abdomen on a regular basis from the end of their last menstruation to the commencement of their next menstruation. Verbal and numeric rating scales were used; whereby they were found to reduce significantly after one menstrual cycle intervention in both groups. However, pain duration was significantly decreased from 2.4 to 1.8 days after aromatherapy intervention in the EO group. Consequently, outpatients in the EO group experienced reduced duration of menstrual pain. Besides, the blended EO formula was reported to contain four key analgesic constituents namely linalool, linalyl acetate, β-caryophyllene and eucalyptol accounting for as much as 79.29%, indicating that it can be used as reference therapy to provide relief from primary dysmenorrhea (Ou et al., 2012).

Furthermore, eucalyptus oil has been reported to be effective in the reduction of swelling, pain, and inflammation. For instance, Jun et al. (2013) investigated the effects of eucalyptus oil inhalation on pain and inflammatory responses after total knee replacement (TKR) surgery in a randomized clinical trial. Patients inhaled eucalyptus or almond oil (intervention and control group respectively) for 30 mins in continuous passive motion for 3 successive days. Pain measurement was derived from VAS, heart rate, BP, white blood cell (WBC) count and C-reactive protein (CRP) concentration recorded before and after inhalation. Remarkably, pain on VAS on all three days as well as systolic and diastolic BPs on the second day were significantly inferior in eucalyptus EO group compared to the group inhaling almond oil, although heart rate, CRP, and WBC did not change significantly in both groups. Hence, eucalyptus oil inhalation was found effective in reducing the patient's pain and BP, suggesting that eucalyptus oil inhalation could be useful as a nursing intervention for pain relief following TKR surgery.

11.3   EOS ASSOCIATED TOXICITIES

In this section, emphasis will be laid on the different cases of human toxicities that have been reported involving the use of EOs and EOs containing products.

For instance, in a case report, a 23-months-old boy was found to ingest less than 10 ml of T36-C7@, a commercial product containing 100% melaleuca oil. While the child was in no distress, the latter appeared disoriented, with difficulty in maintaining his balance, tripping, and falling over, 30 mins later.

However, his mental status was found to improve and became asymptomatic within 5 h post-ingestion. This suggests that ingestion of a modest amount of a concentrated form of this oil could incite signs of toxicity (Jacobs and Hornfeldt, 1994). Other cases of toxicity have also been reported following tea tree oil ingestion (Morris et al., 2003).

Besides, tea tree EO, as a popular additive in cosmetics and personal hygiene products has been implicated in many allergic reactions. In fact, allergic contact dermatitis to tea tree EO is well-documented (Bruynzeel et al., 1994; Selvaag et al., 1995; Bhushan and Beck, 1997). In a related case study, a 50-year-old patient presented a 9-year history of large, red, and painful lesions on her neck and face. Despite the use of various antimicrobial agents, no effect was observed on her symptoms. The patient revealed to have been using Australian tea tree oil for skin conditions like athletes' foot and acne. Allergic contact dermatitis to tea tree oil was suspected, which was afterwards established by a usage test. At a six-month follow-up, no more lesions were demonstrated by the patient after the use of tea tree oil was stopped (Monthrope and Shaw, 2004). In this regard, effort has been made to identify the offending agents present in the tea tree EO, mostly responsible for sensitizations. For instance, limonene, eucalyptol, aromadendrene, alpha-terpinene, terpinene-4-ol, sesquiterpenoids have been detected to be among the culprits (Knight and Hausen, 1994; Southwell et al., 1997; Rubel et al., 1998). Importantly, tea tree EO that has undergone oxidization is recognized to be more prone to cause dermatitis compared to fresh tea tree oil (Khanna et al., 2000).

The major components of lavender EO, linalool and linalyl acetate have also shown to autoxidize in contact with oxygen in the air; resulting into the formation of sensitizing hydroperoxides (Sköld et al., 2004, 2008 Christensson et al., 2010; Hagvall et al., 2015). For instance, in the investigation of Hagvall and Christensson (2016), in order to inspect the frequency of contact allergy to oxidized lavender oil and the associated pattern of reactions to oxidized linalool and linalyl acetate, patients suspected to have allergic contact dermatitis were patch tested with oxidized lavender EO, linalyl acetate and linalool (tested at 6% in petroleum). Positive reactions to oxidized lavender oil were established in 2.8% of the patients. Among them, 56% reacted to oxidized linalool and/or oxidized linalyl acetate, while 52% reacted to the fragrance markers of the baseline series. Thus, oxidized lavender oil was revealed to be among the ones that caused the highest frequencies of contact allergy.

Lavender EO is also used in some topical drugs which are frequently applied for their anti-inflammatory effects (Matthieu et al., 2004); thus, giving rise to a high level of exposure to lavender oil. In this context, cases of allergic contact dermatitis arising from lavender oil present in topical medications have been described. Notably, allergic contact dermatitis to lavender oil from Difflam® gel, used against inflammation and as a topical analgesic, was reported in a 36-year-old physiotherapist having a history of episodic acute facial dermatitis. The latter was observed to react positively (2+) to the gel and lavender absolute (2% pet.) following patch-testing. She also revealed to occasionally massage her clients with the product and under one circumstance to have rubbed her face without washing her hands (Rademaker, 1994). In yet another case, photoallergic contact dermatitis was caused by lavender oil in topical ketoprofen, administered in Fastum® gel. The patient, a 45-year-old woman, presented erythematous and itching plaque, starting on her left foot and spreading onto her left leg. The patient was found to be patch positive to both 2% lavender oil and Fastum® gel, indicating that lavender oil was responsible for the photoallergic contact dermatitis and ketoprofen for contact dermatitis (Goiriz et al., 2007).

Allergic airborne contact dermatitis to EOs was also demonstrated in a 53-year-old patient with relapsing eczema resistant to therapy on several exposed skin parts, especially the hands, neck, face, and scalp. The patient revealed to use aromatherapy whereby he would utilize dressings soaked in EOs, evaporated EOs using aroma lamps or even baths. The cause of sensitization was found to be due to previous exposure to jasmine, lavender, and rosewood oils (1%). Laurel, eucalyptus, and Pomerance (2%) also produced positive reactions. Skin lesions were resolved following topical and systemic treatment with glucocorticoid. As a result of persisting presence of volatile EOs in the patient's home after a year-long employment of aroma lamps, the entire renewal of the interior of the patient's flat was considered necessary (Schaller and Korting, 1995).

Allergic contact dermatitis was also linked to *Laurus nobilis* oil used for massage as reported in a 36-year-old man presenting a generalized erythematous and edematous dermatitis being more severe at the back and dorsal parts of the legs. The latter revealed to have undergone a massage 2 weeks earlier, with a mixture of olive and *L. nobilis* oil applied to his back, thighs, and dorsal aspect of the limbs. Following exposure to the massage oils, skin dermatitis was developed three days later which progressively spread to the rest of the body. He also related to have applied once *L. nobilis* oil to his knee, under occlusion, to alleviate pain. A short course of oral steroids (40 mg/day) was started. The lesions reacted fastly to this treatment causing the erythema to fade over 2 weeks, leaving post-inflammatory pigmentation. Patch testing showed reactions to laurel oil and to the mixture of olive oil and laurel oil (Adişen and Önder, 2007).

Besides, the association of aromatherapy products and the increased risk of hand dermatitis in massage therapists were determined by Crawford et al. (2004). Among the statistically significant independent risk factors that were identified for self-reported hand dermatitis, was the usage of aromatherapy products such as massage lotions, oils or creams. Other cases of occupational contact dermatitis arising from the exposure of EOs have been described (Keane et al., 2000; Crawford et al., 2004; Boonchai et al., 2007). In addition, it is important to point out that given the multi-component nature of EOs and the variable concentrations in which they occur in EOs, it can be difficult to determine the sensitizing agent that may be responsible for the skin reactions linked to an EO (Battaglia, 1995).

Bergamot oil has also been reported to cause phototoxic reactions (Kaddu et al., 2001). The development of localized and disseminated bullous phototoxic skin reactions was observed within 48 to 72 h after being into contact with bergamot oil aromatherapy followed by ultraviolet exposure. In another circumstance, a patient with no history of direct contact with aromatherapy oil was seen to still develop bullous skin lesions after being exposed to evaporated aromatherapy oil in a sauna and subsequent UVA radiation in a tanning salon. Bergamot oil possesses melanogenic and photosensitive activities owing to the presence of furocoumarins, principally bergapten (5-methoxy psoralen [5-MOP]). The photo-mutagenic as well as toxic activities of 5-MOP are also known and hence this study highlighted the potential health hazard associated with the use of aromatherapy oils containing psoralen (Kaddu et al., 2001).

Additionally, mild to severe side effects including fatality were reported to be induced by EOs such as lavender, peppermint, ylang-ylang, and tea tree oil, greatly employed in aromatherapy. Among them, dermatitis was the most frequent adverse effect noted (Posadzki et al., 2012). Other examples of allergic reactions that have been documented in literature are associated with sensitivity development as a result of exposure to a number of oils over time as described in the study of Selvaag et al. (1995) which reported a female aromatherapist (65-year-old) to develop allergic contact dermatitis over a large part of her body. She showed sensitivity to lemongrass EO, which then developed into dermatitis upon exposure to other fragrant compounds including household cleaners. Allergy testing revealed that she reacted to 17 out of 20 EOs that she used recurrently.

Moreover, in another case of EO adverse effects, a patient was reported to have reacted to peppermint oil and menthol present in his toothpaste and throat medication and hence was found to be a case of allergic contact cheilitis. Patch testing conducted revealed patient to have positive reactions to menthol, peppermint oil and menthol-containing throat spray. Similarly, positive result was obtained with 'semi-open' testing with the patient's tooth-paste. The patient was then advised to discontinue using these products, and rather use 'homeopathic' toothpastes that were free from these substances (peppermint and menthol), following which he experienced significant improvement of his lesions (Bourgeois and Goossens, 2016).

Nevertheless, gynecomastia, a condition that causes disruption of sex-steroid signaling pathways, resulting in an increased or unopposed estrogenic action on breast tissue (Braunstein, 1993), was found to be associated with the topical application of products that contained lavender and tea tree oils in pre-pubertal boys. Interestingly, gynecomastia resolved shortly after the use of the products containing the oils was stopped in each patient. Concomitantly, studies on human cell lines demonstrated the two oils to possess estrogenic and anti-androgenic effects. Hence it was concluded that the repeated topical exposure to lavender and tea tree oils could have been responsible for pre-pubertal gynecomastia in these boys (Henley et al., 2007).

11.4   CONCLUSION AND FUTURE PERSPECTIVES

Undoubtedly, EOs have appealing therapeutic uses as demonstrated in many clinical studies elaborated in the present book chapter. For instance, they have been found to relieve pain, anxiety, migraine, arthritis, insomnia, amongst others. Moreover, they hold tremendous applications in aroma-therapy extensively employed for the promotion of health and wellness. Hence, aromatherapy as a non-pharmacological approach, low-cost, holistic, and effective treatment modality can be regarded as an alternative or comple-mentary therapy for improving the quality of life of individuals. Neverthe-less, while EOs are generally deemed as safe and are widely employed by people on a daily basis, it is significant to take into consideration of their doses to avoid toxicity. Moreover, EOs as mixtures of active compounds, may contain allergenic components, and therefore it is of great significance to perform clinical trials using EOs and their related products to minimize any possible adverse effects such as skin sensitizations and allergies. Given the increasing use of EOs in cosmetics, household and personal hygiene products, medications, and particularly aromatherapy, the establishment of standard doses and identification of sensitizing agents and awareness of their potential photoallergic nature on the basis of clinical studies are crucial and could help to alert consumers using EOs and their products; thus, helping to reduce EOs induced allergies.

KEYWORDS

- **adverse effects**
- **aromatherapy**
- **clinical studies**
- **essential oils**
- **health benefits**

REFERENCES

Adişen, E., & Önder, M., (2007). Allergic contact dermatitis from *Laurus nobilis* oil induced by massage. *Contact Derm., 56*, 360–361.

Afshar, M. K., Moghadam, Z. B., Taghizadeh, Z., Bekhradi, R., Montazeri, A., & Mokhtari, P., (2015). Lavender fragrance essential oil and the quality of sleep in postpartum women. *Iran Red Crescent Med. J.*, 17.

Angelini, P., Tirillini, B., Akhtar, M. S., Dimitriu, L., Bricchi, E., Bertuzzi, G., & Venanzoni, R., (2018). Essential oil with anticancer activity: An overview. In: *Anticancer Plants: Natural Products and Biotechnological Implements* (pp. 207–231). Springer, Singapore.

Ayan, M., Tas, U., Sogut, E., Suren, M., Gurbuzler, L., & Koyuncu, F., (2013). Investigating the effect of aromatherapy in patients with renal colic. *J. Altern. Complement. Med., 19*, 329–333.

Bahr, T., Allred, K., Martinez, D., Rodriguez, D., & Winterton, P., (2018). Effects of a massage-like essential oil application procedure using copaiba and deep blue oils in individuals with hand arthritis. *Complement Ther. Clin. Pract., 33*, 170–176.

Ballard, C. G., O'Brien, J. T., Reichelt, K., & Perry, E. K., (2002). Aromatherapy as a safe and effective treatment for the management of agitation in severe dementia: The results of a double-blind placebo-controlled trial with melissa. *J. Clin. Psychiatry*.

Barbieri, C. & Borsotto, P., (2018). Essential oils: market and legislation. *IntechOpen. Potential of Essential Oils*, 107–127.

Battaglia, S., (1995). Essential oil safety. *The Complete Guide to Aromatherapy*, pp. 123–129.

Bhushan, M., & Beck, M. H., (1997). Allergic contact dermatitis from tea tree oil in a wart paint. *Contact Dermatitis, 36*, 117–118.

Boehm, K., Büssing, A., & Ostermann, T., (2012). Aromatherapy as an adjuvant treatment in cancer care-a descriptive systematic review. *Afr. J. Tradit. Complement Altern. Med., 9,* 503–518.

Boonchai, W., Iamtharachai, P., & Sunthonpalin, P., (2007). Occupational allergic contact dermatitis from essential oils in aromatherapists. *Contact Derm., 56,* 181, 182.

Bourgeois, P., & Goossens, A., (2016). Allergic contact cheilitis caused by menthol in toothpaste and throat medication: A case report. *Contact Derm., 75,* 113–115.

Bowles, E. J., (2003). *Chemistry of Aromatherapeutic Oils.* Allen & Unwin.

Braunstein, G. D., (1993). Gynecomastia. *N. Engl. J. Med., 328,* 490–495.

Bruynzeel, D. P., Coenraads, P. J., & Weijland, J. W., (1994). Allergic contact eczema due to 'tea tree' oil. *Nederlands Tijdschrift Voor Geneeskunde, 138,* 823–825.

Buckle, J., (1999). Use of aromatherapy as a complementary treatment for chronic pain. *Alternative Therapies in Health and Medicine, 5,* 42.

Buckle, J., (2003). *Clinical Aromatherapy: Essential Oils in Practice* (2nd edn.). New York, NY, USA: Churchill Livingstone Elsevier Science.

Buckle, J., (2007). Literature review: Should nursing take aromatherapy more seriously? *British Journal of Nursing, 16,* 116–120.

Christensson, J. B., Matura, M., Gruvberger, B., Bruze, M., & Karlberg, A. T., (2010). Linalool-a significant contact sensitizer after air exposure. *Contact Derm., 62,* 32–41.

Corner, J., Cawley, N., & Hildebrand, S., (1995). An evaluation of the use of massage and essential oils on the wellbeing of cancer patients. *International Journal of Palliative Nursing, 1,* 67–73.

Crawford, G. H., Katz, K. A., Ellis, E., & James, W. D., (2004). Use of aromatherapy products and increased risk of hand dermatitis in massage therapists. *Arch. Dermatol., 140,* 991–996.

De Sousa, D. P., Hocayen, P. D. A. S., Andrade, L. N., & Andreatini, R., (2015). A systematic review of the anxiolytic-like effects of essential oils in animal models. *Molecules, 20,* 18620–18660.

Eisenberg, D. M., Kessler, R. C., Foster, C., Norlock, F. E., Calkins, D. R., & Delbanco, T. L., (1993). Unconventional medicine in the United States--prevalence, costs, and patterns of use. *N. Engl. J. Med., 328,* 246–252.

El Bouzidi, L., Jamali, C. A., Bekkouche, K., Hassani, L., Wohlmuth, H., Leach, D., & Abbad, A., (2013). Chemical composition, antioxidant and antimicrobial activities of essential oils obtained from wild and cultivated Moroccan thymus species. *Industrial Crops and Products, 43,* 450–456.

Elshafie, H. S., & Camele, I., (2017). An overview of the biological effects of some Mediterranean essential oils on human health. *Biomed Res Int., 2017,* 9268468.

Enshaieh, S., Jooya, A., Siadat, A. H., & Iraji, F., (2007). The efficacy of 5% topical tea tree oil gel in mild to moderate acne vulgaris: A randomized, double-blind placebo-controlled study. *Indian J. Dermatol. Venereol. Leprol., 73,* 22.

Ernst, E., (2006). Herbal remedies for anxiety-a systematic review of controlled clinical trials. *Phytomedicine, 13,* 205–208.

Fakari, F. R., Tabatabaeichehr, M., Kamali, H., Fakari, F. R., & Naseri, M., (2015). Effect of inhalation of aroma of geranium essence on anxiety and physiological parameters during first stage of labor in nulliparous women: A randomized clinical trial. Journal of Caring Sciences, *4,* 135.

Fellowes, D., Barnes, K., & Wilkinson, S. S., (2004). Aromatherapy and massage for symptom relief in patients with cancer. *Cochrane Database of Systematic Reviews, 3.*

Firenzuoli, F., Jaitak, V., Horvath, G., Bassolé, I. H. N., Setzer, W. N., & Gori, L., (2014). Essential oils: New perspectives in human health and wellness. *Evid. Based Complement Alternat. Med., 2014*, 467363.

Ganji, R., (2019). Aromatherapy massage: A promising non-pharmacological adjuvant treatment for osteoarthritis knee pain. *The Korean Journal of Pain, 32*, 133.

Goiriz, R., Delgado-Jiménez, Y., Sánchez-Pérez, J., & García-Diez, A., (2007). Photoallergic contact dermatitis from lavender oil in topical ketoprofen. *Contact Derm., 57*, 381–382.

Hagvall, L., & Christensson, J. B., (2016). Patch testing with main sensitizers does not detect all cases of contact allergy to oxidized lavender oil. *Actadermato-Venereologica, 96*, 679–684.

Hagvall, L., Berglund, V., & BråredChristensson, J., (2015). Air-oxidized linalyl acetate–An emerging fragrance allergen? *Contact Derm., 72*, 216–223.

Halm, M. A., (2008). Essential oils for management of symptoms in critically ill patients. *American Journal of Critical Care, 17*, 160–163.

Hamdy, R. C., Kinser, A., Dickerson, K., Kendall-Wilson, T., Depelteau, A., Copeland, R., & Whalen, K., (2018). Insomnia and mild cognitive impairment. *Gerontology and Geriatric Medicine, 4*, 2333721418778421.

Hekmatpou, D., Pourandish, Y., Farahani, P. V., & Parvizrad, R., (2017). The effect of aromatherapy with the essential oil of orange on pain and vital signs of patients with fractured limbs admitted to the emergency ward: A randomized clinical trial. *Indian J. Palliat. Care, 23*, 431.

Henderson, A. S., & Jorm, A. F., (2002). Definition and epidemiology of dementia: A review. *Dementia, 3*, 1–68.

Henley, D. V., Lipson, N., Korach, K. S., & Bloch, C. A., (2007). Prepubertal gynecomastia linked to lavender and tea tree oils. *N. Engl. J. Med., 356*, 479–485.

Hwang, E., & Shin, S., (2015). The effects of aromatherapy on sleep improvement: A systematic literature review and meta-analysis. *J. Altern. Complement Med., 21*, 61–68.

Imanishi, J., Kuriyama, H., Shigemori, I., Watanabe, S., Aihara, Y., Kita, M., Sawai, Ket al., (2009). Anxiolytic effect of aromatherapy massage in patients with breast cancer. *Evid Based Complement Alternat. Med., 6*, 123–128.

Irshad, M., Subhani, M. A., Ali, S., & Hussain, A., (2019). Biological importance of essential oils. In: *Essential Oils-Oils of Nature*. IntechOpen. doi: 10.5772/intechopen.87198.

Jacobs, M. R., & Hornfeldt, C. S., (1994). Melaleuca oil poisoning. *J. Toxicol. Clin. Toxicol., 32*, 461–464.

Javaheri, S., & Redline, S., (2017). Insomnia and risk of cardiovascular disease. *Chest, 152*, 435–444.

Jimbo, D., Kimura, Y., Taniguchi, M., Inoue, M., & Urakami, K., (2009). Effect of aromatherapy on patients with Alzheimer's disease. *Psychogeriatrics, 9*, 173–179.

Jun, Y. S., Kang, P., Min, S. S., Lee, J. M., Kim, H. K., & Seol, G. H., (2013). Effect of eucalyptus oil inhalation on pain and inflammatory responses after total knee replacement: A randomized clinical trial. *Evid. Based Complement. Alternat. Med.*, Article ID: 502727. https://doi.org/10.1155/2013/502727.

Kaddu, S., Kerl, H., & Wolf, P., (2001). Accidental bullous phototoxic reactions to bergamot aromatherapy oil. *Journal of the American Academy of Dermatology, 45*, 458–461.

Kagawa, D., Jokura, H., Ochiai, R., Tokimitsu, I., & Tsubone, H., (2003). The sedative effects and mechanism of action of cedrol inhalation with behavioral pharmacological evaluation. *Planta Med., 69*, 637–641.

Kasper, S., Gastpar, M., Müller, W. E., Volz, H. P., Möller, H. J., Schläfke, S., & Dienel, A., (2014). Lavender oil preparation silexan is effective in generalized anxiety disorder-a randomized, double-blind comparison to placebo and paroxetine. *International Journal of Neuropsychopharmacology, 17*, 859–869.

Kasper, S., Müller, W. E., Volz, H. P., Möller, H. J., Koch, E., & Dienel, A., (2018). Silexan in anxiety disorders: Clinical data and pharmacological background. *The World Journal of Biological Psychiatry, 19*, 412–420.

Keane, F. M., Smith, H. R., White, I. R., & Rycroft, R. J., (2000). Occupational allergic contact dermatitis in two aromatherapists. *Contact Derm., 43*, 49.

Khanna, M., Qasem, K., & Sasseville, D., (2000). Allergic contact dermatitis to tea tree oil with erythema multiforme [ndash] like ID reaction. *American Journal of Contact Dermatitis, 11*, 238–242.

Kim, I. H., Kim, C., Seong, K., Hur, M. H., Lim, H. M., & Lee, M. S., (2012). Essential oil inhalation on blood pressure and salivary cortisol levels in prehypertensive and hypertensive subjects. *Evid. Based Complementary Altern. Med.*, 984203. doi: 10.1155/2012/984203.

Kim, K. Y., Jang, H. H., Lee, S. N., Kim, Y. S., & An, S., (2018). Effects of the myrtle essential oil on the acne skin—Clinical trials for Korean women. *Biomedical Dermatology, 2*, 28.

Kim, M., & Kwon, Y. J., (2010). Effects of aroma inhalation on blood pressure, pulse, visual analog scale, and McNair scale in nursing students practicing intravenous injection at the first time. *International Journal of Advanced Science and Technology, 23*, 61–68.

Knight, T. E., & Hausen, B. M., (1994). Melaleuca oil (tea tree oil) dermatitis. *Journal of the American Academy of Dermatology, 30*, 423–427.

Knoerr, K., (2018). Essential oils: An adjunct to holistic nursing. *Gastroenterology Nursing, 41*, 250–254.

Kozics, K., Srancikova, A., Sedlackova, E., Horvathova, E., Melusova, M., Melus, V., Krajcovicova, Z., & Sramkova, M., (2017). Antioxidant potential of essential oil from *Lavandulaangustifolia* in *in vitro* and *ex vivo* cultured liver cells. *Neoplasma, 64*, 485–493.

Lai, S. L., (2000). *Clinical Trials of Traditional Chinese Materia Medica*. Ch. 1. Guangdong: People's Publishing House.

Lehrner, J., Eckersberger, C., Walla, P., Pötsch, G., & Deecke, L., (2000). Ambient odor of orange in a dental office reduces anxiety and improves mood in female patients. *Physiology and Behavior, 71*, 83–86.

Li, J. X., Liu, Y. F., Li, G. W., & Fu, J., (2011). Inhalation effect of different concentrations of lavender essential oil on blood pressure in hypertensive patients [J]. *Anhui Medical and Pharmaceutical Journal*, 11.

Lillehei, A. S., & Halcon, L. L., (2014). A systematic review of the effect of inhaled essential oils on sleep. *J. Altern. Complement. Med., 20*, 441–451.

Lillehei, A. S., Halcón, L. L., Savik, K., & Reis, R., (2015). Effect of inhaled lavender and sleep hygiene on self-reported sleep issues: A randomized controlled trial. *J. Altern. Complement. Med., 21*, 430–438.

Lytle, J., Mwatha, C., & Davis, K. K., (2014). Effect of lavender aromatherapy on vital signs and perceived quality of sleep in the intermediate care unit: A pilot study. *American Journal of Critical Care, 23*, 24–29.

Malhi, H. K., Tu, J., Riley, T. V., Kumarasinghe, S. P., & Hammer, K. A., (2017). Tea tree oil gel for mild to moderate acne; a 12 week uncontrolled, open-label phase II pilot study. *Australas. J. Dermatol., 58*, 205–210.

Mannucci, C., Calapai, F., Cardia, L., Inferrera, G., D'Arena, G., Di Pietro, M., Navarra, M., et al., (2018). Clinical Pharmacology of *Citrus aurantium* and *Citrus sinensis* for the Treatment of Anxiety. *Evidence-Based Complementary and Alternative Medicine*.

Martinec, R., (2012). Some implications of using aromatherapy as a complementary method in oncology setting. *Archive of Oncology, 20*, 70–74.

Matthieu, L., Meuleman, L., Van, H. E., Blondeel, A., Dezfoulian, B., Constandt, L., & Goossens, A., (2004). Contact and photocontact allergy to ketoprofen. The Belgian experience. *Contact Derm., 50*, 238–241.

Mitoshi, M., Kuriyama, I., Nakayama, H., Miyazato, H., Sugimoto, K., Kobayashi, Y., Jippo, T., et al., (2014). Suppression of allergic and inflammatory responses by essential oils derived from herbal plants and citrus fruits. *Int. J. Mol. Med., 33*, 1643–1651.

Moeini, M., Khadibi, M., Bekhradi, R., Mahmoudian, S. A., & Nazari, F., (2010). Effect of aromatherapy on the quality of sleep in ischemic heart disease patients hospitalized in intensive care units of heart hospitals of the Isfahan University of medical sciences. *Iranian Journal of Nursing and Midwifery Research, 15*, 234.

Monthrope, Y. M., & Shaw, J. C., (2004). A 'natural' dermatitis: Contact allergy to tea tree oil. Univ. *Toronto Med. J., 82*, 59–60.

Morris, M. C., Donoghue, A., Markowitz, J. A., & Osterhoudt, K. C., (2003). Ingestion of tea tree oil (Melaleuca oil) by a 4-year-old boy. *Pediatr. Emerg. Care, 19*, 169–171.

Nasiri, A., & Mahmodi, M. A., (2018). Aromatherapy massage with lavender essential oil and the prevention of disability in ADL in patients with osteoarthritis of the knee: A randomized controlled clinical trial. *Complement Ther. Clin. Pract., 30*, 116–121.

Ou, M. C., Hsu, T. F., Lai, A. C., Lin, Y. T., & Lin, C. C., (2012). Pain relief assessment by aromatic essential oil massage on outpatients with primary dysmenorrhea: A randomized, double-blind clinical trial. *J. Obstet. Gynaecol. Res., 38*, 817–822.

Palagini, L., Maria, B. R., Gemignani, A., Baglioni, C., Ghiadoni, L., & Riemann, D., (2013). Sleep loss and hypertension: A systematic review. *Curr. Pharm. Des., 19*, 2409–2419.

Posadzki, P., Alotaibi, A., & Ernst, E., (2012). Adverse effects of aromatherapy: A systematic review of case reports and case series. *International Journal of Risk and Safety in Medicine, 24*, 147–161.

Rademaker, M., (1994). Allergic contact dermatitis from lavender fragrance in Difflam® gel. *Contact Derm., 31*, 58, 59.

Rafie, S., Namjoyan, F., Golfakhrabadi, F., Yousefbeyk, F., & Hassanzadeh, A., (2016). Effect of lavender essential oil as a prophylactic therapy for migraine: A randomized controlled clinical trial. *Journal of Herbal Medicine, 6*, 18–23.

Rashidi-Fakari, F., Tabatabaeichehr, M., & Mortazavi, H., (2015). The effect of aromatherapy by essential oil of orange on anxiety during labor: A randomized clinical trial. *Iranian Journal of Nursing and Midwifery Research, 20*, 661.

Robertshawe, P., Price, S., & Price, L., (2009). Aromatherapy for Health Professionals. *Journal of the Australian Traditional-Medicine Society, 15*, 101, 102.

Rubel, D. M., Freeman, S., & Southwell, I. A., (1998). Tea tree oil allergy: What is the offending agent? Report of three cases of tea tree oil allergy and review of the literature. *Australas. J. Dermatol., 39*, 244–247.

Sarmento-Neto, J. F., Do Nascimento, L. G., Felipe, C. F. B., De Sousa, D. P., (2016). Analgesic potential of essential oils. *Molecules, 21*, 20.

Sarris, J., McIntyre, E., & Camfield, D. A., (2013). Plant-based medicines for anxiety disorders, part 2: A review of clinical studies with supporting preclinical evidence. *CNS Drugs, 27*, 301–319.

Sarris, J., Panossian, A., Schweitzer, I., Stough, C., & Scholey, A., (2001). Herbal medicine for depression, anxiety and insomnia: A review of psychopharmacology and clinical evidence. *Eur. Neuropsychopharmacol., 21*, 841–860.

Sasannejad, P., Saeedi, M., Shoeibi, A., Gorji, A., Abbasi, M., & Foroughipour, M., (2012). Lavender essential oil in the treatment of migraine headache: A placebo-controlled clinical trial. *European Neurology, 67*, 288–291.

Satchell, A. C., Saurajen, A., Bell, C., & Barnetson, R. S., (2002). Treatment of dandruff with 5% tea tree oil shampoo. *J. Am. Acad. Dermatol., 47*, 852–855.

Savage, K., Firth, J., Stough, C., & Sarris, J., (2018). GABA-modulating phytomedicines for anxiety: A systematic review of preclinical and clinical evidence. *Phytother Res., 32*, 3–18.

Saydah, S. H., & Eberhardt, M. S., (2006). Use of complementary and alternative medicine among adults with chronic diseases: United States 2002. *J. Altern. Complement. Med., 12*, 805–812.

Schaller, M., & Korting, H. C., (1995). Allergic airborne contact dermatitis from essential oils used in aromatherapy. *Clin. Exp. Dermatol., 20*, 143–145.

Schnaubelt, K., (2005). Essential oil therapy according to traditional Chinese medical concepts. *Int. J. Aromather., 15*, 98–105.

Scuteri, D., Morrone, L. A., Rombolà, L., Avato, P. R., Bilia, A. R., Corasaniti, M. T., Sakurada, S., et al., (2017). Aromatherapy and aromatic plants for the treatment of behavioral and psychological symptoms of dementia in patients with Alzheimer's disease: Clinical evidence and possible mechanisms. *Evid. Based Complement. Alternat. Med., 2017.*

Selvaag, E., Holm, J. Ø., & Thune, P., (1995). Allergic contact dermatitis in an aromatherapist with multiple sensitizations to essential oils. *Contact Derm., 33*, 354, 355.

Silva, G. L., Luft, C., Lunardelli, A., Amaral, R. H., Melo, D. A., Donadio, M. V., Nunes, F. B., et al., (2015). Antioxidant, analgesic and anti-inflammatory effects of lavender essential oil. *An. Acad. Bras. Ciênc., 87*, 1397–1408.

Silva, J., Abebe, W., Sousa, S. M., Duarte, V. G., Machado, M. I. L., & Matos, F. J. A., (2003). Analgesic and anti-inflammatory effects of essential oils of eucalyptus. *J Ethnopharmacol., 89*, 277–283.

Sköld, M., Börje, A., Harambasic, E., & Karlberg, A. T., (2004). Contact allergens formed on-air exposure of linalool. Identification and quantification of primary and secondary oxidation products and the effect on skin sensitization. *Chem. Res. Toxicol., 17*, 1697–1705.

Sköld, M., Hagvall, L., & Karlberg, A. T., (2008). Autoxidation of linalyl acetate, the main component of lavender oil, creates potent contact allergens. *Contact Derm., 58*, 9–14.

Southwell, I. A., Freeman, S., & Rubel, D., (1997). Skin irritancy of tea tree oil. *J. Essent. Oil Res., 9*, 47–52.

Spiegel, K., Sheridan, J. F., & Van, C. E., (2002). Effect of sleep deprivation on response to immunization. *JAMA, 288*, 1471–1472.

Tahir, H. U., Sarfraz, R. A., Ashraf, A., & Adil, S., (2016). Chemical composition and antidiabetic activity of essential oils obtained from two spices (*Syzygium aromaticum* and *Cuminumcyminum*). *Intl. J. Food Prop., 19*, 2156–2164.

Tisserand, R., & Young, R., (2014). *Essential Oil Safety* (2nd edn.). London: Churchill Livingstone Elsevier.

Tisserand, R., (1990). *Aromatherapy for Everyone*. London: Arkana.

Viuda-Martos, M., El Gendy, A. E. N. G., Sendra, E., Fernandez-Lopez, J., Abd El, R. K. A., Omer, E. A., & Pérez-Alvarez, J. A., (2010). Chemical composition and antioxidant and anti-listeria activities of essential oils obtained from some Egyptian plants. *J. Agri. Food Chem., 58*, 9063–9070.

Welz, A. N., Emberger-Klein, A., & Menrad, K., (2018). Why people use herbal medicine: Insights from a focus-group study in Germany. *BMC Complement. Altern. Med., 18*, 92.

WHO, (2013). *A Global Brief on Hypertension.* Silent killer, global public health crisis. World Health Organization, Geneva, Switzerland.

Wilkinson, S., (1995). Aromatherapy and massage in palliative care. *International Journal of Palliative Nursing, 1*, 21–30.

World Health Organization, (2001). *The World Health Report 2001: Mental Health: New Understanding, New Hope.* World Health Organization.

Yeung, K. S., Hernandez, M., Mao, J. J., Haviland, I., & Gubili, J., (2018). Herbal medicine for depression and anxiety: A systematic review with assessment of potential psycho-oncologic relevance. *Phytother Res., 32*, 865–891.

Zabirunnisa, M., Gadagi, J. S., Gadde, P., Myla, N., Koneru, J., & Thatimatla, C., (2014). Dental patient anxiety: Possible deal with Lavender fragrance. *Journal of Research in Pharmacy Practice, 3*, 100.

CHAPTER 12

ASPARAGUS SP.: PHYTOCHEMICALS AND MARKETED HERBAL FORMULATIONS

VIKAS BAJPAI, PRATIBHA SINGH, PREETI CHANDRA, and BRIJESH KUMAR

Sophisticated Analytical Instrument Facility, CSIR-Central Drug Research Institute, Lucknow – 226001, Uttar Pradesh, India, E-mail: gbrikum@yahoo.com (B. Kumar)

ABSTRACT

The Asparagus plants are used in the Indian traditional system of medicine, Ayurveda, Homeopathy, and Unani due to their immense medicinal properties. Asparagus species namely *Asparagus racemosus, Asparagus officinalis*, and *Asparagus adscendens* is used in treatment of various ailments such as diabetes, gonorrhea, piles, and has various biological activities such as anti-cancer, anti-diabetic, anti-diarrheal, anti-dysenteric, anti-epileptic, anti-inflammatory, anti-spasmodic, anti-tubercular, aphrodisiac, appetizer, astringent, and stomach tonic, etc. Recent studies revealed that the phytochemicals present in *A. racemosus* plants are responsible for their immune-adjuvant property and hence they can be scrutinized for use in adjuvant therapy in the management of HIV. An ultra-high performance liquid chromatography-electrospray ionization tandem mass spectrometry method has been developed and validated for simultaneous determination of 7 major bioactive compounds in plant parts of three Asparagus species namely, *A. racemosus, A. officinalis* and *A. adscendens*. The analysis was accomplished on Waters AQUITY UPLC BEH C18 column with a gradient mobile phase (A: 0.1% aqueous formic acid and B: acetonitrile) at a flow rate of 0.4 mL/min. Validation parameters were analyzed with good linear regression relationship (r^2, 0.9989–0.9999), intra-day, and inter-day precision (RSD < 1.87 and 2.03%, respectively), stability (RSD ≤ 2.39%) and recovery (RSD ≤ 3.03%) was evaluated under optimum conditions. The same method was utilized to study the content of 7 selected markers in marketed herbal formulations. These results could be used for the selection of suitable plant / phytopharmaceuticals by estimation of higher quantity of active compounds, which will be more therapeutically effective. Therefore, this strategy is rapid, simple, and feasible which may be effectively utilized for evaluating the quality of Asparagus samples and its preparations.

12.1　INTRODUCTION

12.1.1　MEDICINAL AND ANALYTICAL ASPECTS OF ASPARAGUS SPECIES

Plants are the principal component of worldwide sustainability as it provides basics to human life in the form of breath, food, shelter, medicine, fuel, condiments, aromas, perfumes, etc., (Iqbal et al., 2017). Medicinal plants are the main source of traditional medicines (TMs) and drugs and showed a significant role in modern drug discovery systems (Raskin et al., 2002). Asparagus is one of the important genuses worldwide and out of several species of Asparagus found in India, Asparagus adsendens, Asparagus officinalis and Asparagus racemosus are most commonly used as TM (Iqbal et al., 2017). Asparagus racemosus WILD (family: Asparagaceae) usually known as *Shatavari* (means "curer of hundreds of diseases") in India and it is a significant medicinal plant, inhabitant to tropical and subtropical regions in India up to the height of an altitude of 1,500 m. More than 300 species of Asparagus are recognized in the world with about 22 species are recorded in India. *A. racemosus, A. officinalis, A. adscendens, A. sprengeri, A. acutifolius, A. gonaclades* are few species which found in the European countries and eastern Asia including India, China, Korea, and Japan (Velavan et al., 2007; Hayes et al., 2008; Sharma et al., 2009). Medicinal uses of Asparagus species have been reported in the traditional systems of medicine (India) such as Ayurveda, Siddha, and Unani and as well as in the British and Indian pharmacopeia (Goyal et al., 2003; Kapoor, 2000). *Charaka Samhita* and *Susruta Samhita* have described the use of A. racemosus to cure the problems associated with the female reproductive system (Alok et al., 2013). Pharmacological activities reported are antioxidant (Visavadiya et al., 2005), immunostimulant (Gautam et al., 2009; Sharma et al., 2011; Sidiq et al.,

2011) antihepatotoxic (Muruganadan et al., 2000), antibacterial (Mandal et al., 2000; Battu et al., 2010), antiulcer (Sairam et al., 2003), antileishmanial, anticancer (Bhutani et al., 2010), hypolipidemic effects (Patel et al., 1969; Khanna et al., 1991; Vihan et al., 1998) and galactogog activity (Patel et al., 1969; Khanna et al., 1991; Vihan et al., 1998). The occurrence of steroidal saponins and sapogenins in various plant parts of Asparagus species is to be responsible for its therapeutic effectiveness. Sarsasapogenin and saponins have isolated from the aerial part, root, and fruits of plant (Manta et al., 1995).

Plant metabolomics is the most relevant and top-rated research area in the world for the study of plant systems and natural products Identification and characterization of the bioactive compounds in the polyherbal preparation by using HPLC, LC-MS. LC-NMR improves speed and sensitivity of method and found useful in the areas of plant metabolomics, pharmacokinetics, toxicity studies, drug metabolism and drug discovery process (Harvey et al., 2007; Kesting et al., 2010). Plant metabolism represents a vast range of semi-polar compounds with many important groups of secondary metabolites, which are best separated and detected only by LC-MS approaches (de Villiers et al., 2016). Liquid chromatography-mass spectrometry (LC-MS) is indicated as the technique of choice to assay polar pharmaceuticals and their metabolites, and is especially suitable for phytochemical, pharmaceutical, and environmental analysis because of the possibility for hyphenation from HPLC to UPLC with ESI and APCI in combination with more advanced mass analyzers such as ion trap, QTOF, QqQ, QTRAP, etc. (Allwood and Goodacre 2010). LC-MS has high selectivity and sensitivity for qualitative and quantitative study of bioactive compounds and their metabolites found in trace amount in plant extract (Wolfender et al., 2019). UPLC-QTRAP MS permits rapid identification of the metabolites in a very short run time with low consumption of solvents at very low sample concentration and has an increasing role in quantitation of phytochemicals in plant extract (King and Fernandez, 2006). Hence, an UPLC-MS method was developed and validated for the simultaneous quantitation of the main bioactive compounds in *Asparagus* samples.

Many analytical methods are reported in the literature for the identification and determination of phytochemical constituents of the *A. racemosus, A. officinalis* and *A. adscendens*. These literature reports reveal the use of high-performance thin-layer chromatography (HPTLC) (Satti et al., 2006; Wang et al., 2011), high-performance liquid chromatography (HPLC) (Lee et al., 2010; Negi et al., 2011), gas chromatography (GC-MS) and LC-MS (2009;

Jaiswal et al., 2014; Patil et al., 2014). These methods contributed signifi-cantly but have limitation of longer analysis time, more solvent consumption and analyzed only one or two bioactive compounds. To triumph over these restrictions, a new advanced analytical method is required. UPLC-MS/MS is a functional methodology having positive approach in separation sciences which has drawn much attention in the analysis of compounds due to its high speed, improved sensitivity and specificity (Chandra et al., 2015a; Chandra et al., 2015b, 2016a, b; Rathore et al., 2016). Till date, no analytical method is described for the simultaneous investigation of selected bioactive compounds namely saponin (shatavarin-IV), sapogenin (sarsasapogenin), flavonoids (apigenin, quercetin, and vanillin) and phenolic acids (caffeic acid and ferulic acid) in *Asparagus* species. Hence in the present study, we have developed and validated an UPLC-MS/MS method for the simultaneous quantitation of 7 bioactive phytocompounds in plant parts of three *Asparagus* species, i.e., *A. racemosus, A. officinalis* and *A. adscendens*. Authentic presence of major compounds, i.e., saponin, and sapogenin in marketed herbal formulations was also shown by applying the developed method.

12.1.2 TRADITIONAL USES AND COMMERCIAL IMPORTANCE

Selected Asparagus species *A. racemosus, A. officinalis, A. adscendens s* is used in Ayurveda for prevention and treatment of dyspepsia, gastric ulcers, inflammation, liver diseases and in infectious disease and nervous disorders. Traditionally, these plants occupy an important position in the socio-cultural, spiritual, and medicinal arena. It has anti-bacterial, antimicrobial, and immune-modulatory properties and as digestive tonic for diarrhea, dysentery, dyspepsia, and indigestion. These plants are used in the treatment of several skin diseases and hence are the best herb used in Ayurvedic medicine for the treatment of women's fertility issues like in the treatment of infertility, loss of libido, stomach ulcer, hyperacidity, vulnerable miscarriage, menopausal problems, and bronchial infection. The plants are also used in the cure of rheumatism, diabetes, and brain complaints. It is used in the management of behavioral disorder and minimal brain dysfunction. The rhizome of several Asparagus plants is used as a soothing tonic that acts mainly on the circulatory, digestive, respiratory, and female reproductive organs. The root is alterative, antispasmodic, aphrodisiac, demulcent, diuretic, and refrigerants (Hasan et al., 2016). Many plants of Asparagus species are commercially important plants and produced as food yielding crops, and used in agricultural and as horticultural plants and is a good companion plant for tomatoes, parsley, and basil, as well as it is used in preparation of herbal medicine.

12.1.3   PHYTOCHEMISTRY

Wide range of phytochemicals found in Asparagus species including poly-phones, saponins, and polysaccharides (Zhang et al., 2019). Several chemical classes, for example, acids, alcohol, aldehyde, ester, hydrocarbon, ketone, N-containing compounds were found in these plants. The flower and fruits of the plants contain hyperoside, flavonoids glycosides of quercetin and rutin. Phytochemical as shatvarins is the steroidal saponins content present in these plants. Glycosides such as Shatvarin I to VI are present in these Asparagus species. In the selected plants Shatvarin I a 3-glucose glycoside with a rhamnose moiety attached to sarsapogenin and shatavarins the glyco-side of sarsasapogenin are generally found in two types of structure such as furostanols and spirostanols rhamnose. A new isoflavone was isolated by roots of *A. racemosus* known as 8-methoxy-5,6,4'-trihydroxyisoflavone along with many bioactive compounds. Phytochemicals such as isoflavones, steroidal glycosides, polycyclic alkaloids and a dihydrophenanthrene deriva-tive were mainly obtained from roots of Asparagus plants (Chitrakar et al., 2019; Kobus et al., 2019; Okolie, 2019).

12.2   DEVELOPMENT OF UPLC-MS METHOD FOR QUANTITATION OF PHYTOCHEMICALS AND THEIR HERBAL FORMULATIONS

12.2.1   REAGENTS, CHEMICALS, AND MATERIALS

The reference standards (purity≥90%) sarsasapogenin and shatavarin-IV were purchased from Natural Remedies Pvt. Ltd. Apigenin, quercetin, vanillin, caffeic acid, and ferulic acid were purchased from Sigma Aldrich Ltd. (St. Louis, MO, USA). Five different marketed herbal formulations manufactured by a different pharmaceutical company in tablet dosage forms were purchased from local drug stores, Lucknow, UP, India. Methanol, aceto-nitrile (LC/MS grade), and formic acid (analytical grade) were purchased from Fluka, Sigma-Aldrich (St. Louis, MO, USA). Milli-Q Ultra-pure water was obtained from a Millipore water purification system (Millipore,

Milford, MA, USA). The chemical structures of seven bioactive compounds of *Asparagus* species are presented in Figure 12.1.

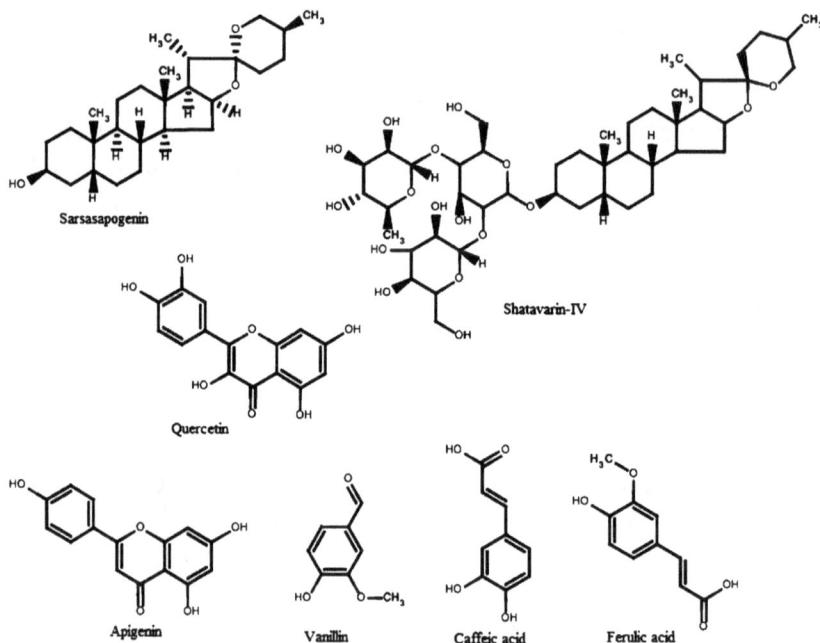

FIGURE 12.1   Structure of selected phytochemical quantified in Asparagus species.

12.2.2   PLANT MATERIAL

Plant materials of *A. racemosus* (leaf, stem, root, and twig), *A. officinalis* (twig) and *A. adscendens* (twig) were collected on 23/06/2015 from the plants grown in Jammu region, Jammu, and Kashmir. Voucher specimens of *A. racemosus* (RRLH-52911), *A. officinalis* (RRLH-52916) and *A. adsendens* (RRLH-52917) were deposited in the Janaki Ammal Herbarium.

12.2.3   EXTRACTION PROCESS AND SAMPLE PREPARATION OF PLANT MATERIAL

The dry plant parts of selected *Asparagus* species were powdered to a homogeneous size by a pulverizer and sieved through a 40-mesh sieve, respectively. The dried powder of each part (10 g) was weighed precisely and sonicated with 200 mL of 100% methanol for 30 min at room temperature using an ultrasonic water bath (53 kHz) and left for 24 hours at room temperature. Three replicates of the extraction process were carried out on each individual sample. The solution was filtered through Whatman filter paper and evaporated to dryness under reduced pressure using a rotatory evaporator (Buchi Rotavapor-R2, Flawil, Switzerland) at 40°C. Dried residue (1 mg) was weighed accurately and dissolved in 1 mL of methanol using an ultrasonicator (Bandelin SONOREX, Berlin). The solutions were filtered through 0.22 μm syringe filter (Millex-GV, PVDF, Merck Millipore, and Darmstadt, Germany). The filtrates were diluted with methanol to final working concentration and injected into the UPLC-MS/MS system for analysis.

12.2.4   EXTRACTION PROCESS AND SAMPLE PREPARATION OF HERBAL FORMULATION

The coating of each tablet was removed completely, and the remains were smashed into powder. Pulverized sample (0.5 g) was weighed precisely, and sonicated by ultrasonicator (53 kHz, Bandelin SONOREX, Berlin) using 50 ml 100% methanol at room temperature for 30 min. The extracted solution was centrifuged at 15,000 rpm for 10 min, and the supernatant was filtered through a 0.22 μm syringe filter to obtain 10,000 μg/mL. The filtrates were diluted with methanol to final working solutions and analyzed directly by injecting 5 μL aliquot in UPLC-MS/MS system.

12.2.5   PREPARATION OF STANDARD SOLUTIONS AND SAMPLES

A stock solution containing seven standards, i.e., sarsasapogenin, shatavarin-IV, apigenin, quercetin, vanillin, caffeic acid and ferulic acid were weighed accurately and dissolved in pure methanol. The standard solutions were prepared by diluting the mixed standard solution with methanol to a series of 10 concentrations that is used for plotting the calibration curves within the ranges from 0.5 to 1,500 ng/mL. All solutions were stored at 20°C until use and sonicated prior to injection.

12.2.6 INSTRUMENTATION AND ANALYTICAL CONDITIONS

The UPLC-MS analysis were carried out on an UPLC system (Waters USA) connected with linear ion trap tqd mass spectrometer (API 4000 QTRAP system, AB Sciex, Canada) with electrospray ionization source. The UPLC was contained with a solvent manager (binary), sample manager, column oven, and PDA detector. Analyst software version 1.5.1 control the LC-MS/MS system and used for data acquisition and processing. All the statistical calculations related to quantitative analysis were done on Graph Pad Prism version 5.

12.2.6.1 UPLC CONDITIONS

Chromatographic analysis was performed on a Waters Acquity BEH C_{18} column (2.1 mm× 50 mm, 1.7 μm) by using gradient mobile phase: 0.1% formic acid in water (A) and acetonitrile (B). Gradient elution was as follows: 0–3.3 min, 10–90% B; 3.3–5.5 min, 90–90% B; then from 5.5 up to 7 min returned to initial condition. The flow rate was 0.4 mL/min and the sample injection volume was 5 μL.

12.2.6.2 MS CONDITIONS

For precursor ion scan mass spectra were recorded for full ESI-MS scanning in the range of m/z 100–1,000. Nitrogen was used as the nebulizer, heater, and curtain gas as well as the collision-activated dissociation (CAD) gas. The optimized parameters for positive mode were as follows: the ion spray voltage was set to 5,500 V; the turbo spray temperature, 550°C; nebulizer gas (gas 1), 50 psi; heater gas (gas 2), 50 psi; collision gas, medium; the curtain gas (CUR) was kept at 20 psi. Optimized parameter for negative mode were as follows: the ion spray voltage was set to –4,200 V, the turbo spray temperature, 450C; nebulizer gas (gas 1), 20 psi; heater gas (gas 2), 20 psi; collision gas, medium; the curtain gas (CUR) was kept at 20 psi. The CAD gas was set at medium and the interface heater was on. Quantitative analysis was performed using MRM acquisition mode and its conditions were optimized for each compound during infusion. The optimized compound dependent MRM parameters are: declustering potential (DP), entrance potential (EP), collision energy (CE) and cell exit potential (CXP).

12.2.7   METHOD VALIDATION

The method was validated for many parameters such as linearity, limit of detection (LOD), limit of quantitation (LOQ), precision, stability, and recovery. The linearity of the calibration curve was tested by analysis of reference compound at six different concentrations. The LOD and LOQ were determined by the calibration curve method by the following equations: LOD= $3.3 \times Sy.x/S$; LOQ= $10 \times Sy.x/S$, where Sy.x is the standard deviation of residuals from line and S is the slope of the calibration curve. Intra- and inter-day precision and accuracy were determined from six replicates of samples at three concentrations on five different days. The stability experiment for the compounds was tested by replicate assays of sample solution at 0, 2, 4, 6, 8, 12 and 24 h at room temperature. Recovery was further performed to evaluate the accuracy of the method. Identified amounts of standard solutions were mixed with fixed amounts of samples. Then, the subsequent samples were extracted and analyzed by the established method, and triplicate experiments were run for each sample. The average recoveries were estimated by the formula: recovery (%) = (amount found − original amount)/ amount spiked × 100%, and RSD (%) = (SD/mean) × 100%.

12.3   APPLICATION OF UPLC-MS METHOD FOR QUANTITATION OF PHYTOCHEMICALS AND THEIR HERBAL FORMULATIONS

12.3.1   OPTIMIZATION OF UPLC-MS/MS CONDITIONS

Complete separation of adjoining reference analytes is certainly not required in MS/MS detection. Normally, a suitable chromatographic column, mobile phase, and elution mode are critically important for good separation. To obtain better resolution, various compositions of solvents were tried to get a suitable mobile phase. Acetonitrile possesses stronger elution capability over methanol, which made it more suitable for the final selection in this method. Similarly, as compared to other tested columns, an Acquity UPLC BEH C_{18} (2.1 × 50 mm, 1.7 μm; Waters, Milford, MA) column was found more suitable for acidic mobile phase with smoother baseline. After testing various concentrations (0.1%, 0.2% and 0.3%) of formic acid, 0.1% formic acid concentration was finally selected. Formic acid was found more effective for ionization of compounds detected in positive and negative ESI mode. A gradient elution with 0.1% formic acid in water and acetonitrile at a flow rate of 0.4 mL/min with a column temperature of 30°C was resulted in separation of the 7 analytes in less than 5.5 min chromatographic run time. Figure 12.2 shows the typical MRM chromatograms of reference analytes under the above optimized conditions.

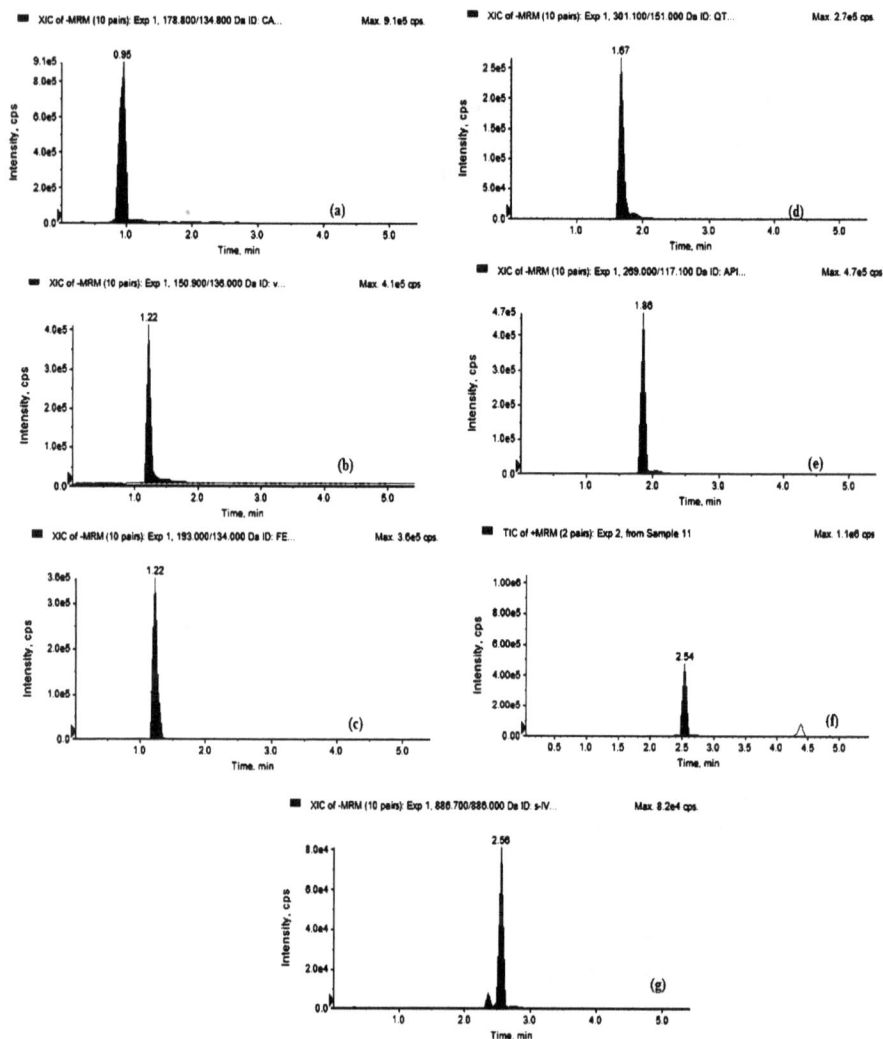

FIGURE 12.2 UPLC-MRM extracted ion chromatogram of reference analytes: (a) caffeic acid; (b) vanillic acid; (c) ferulic acid; (d) quercetin; (e) apigenin; (f) sarsasapogenin; (g) shatavarin-IV in Asparagus species.

The seven analytes were characterized according to their mass spectra which were performed by flow injection analysis (FIA) of the individual standard solution into the mass spectrometer to ascertain their precursor ions and select productions for MRM, respectively. The electrospray interface was used which provided good sensitivity and fragmentation. In this study, the mass spectral conditions were optimized in both positive and negative-ion with continuous polarity switching mode. On the basis of sensitivity and reproducibility of dominant ions in full-scan mass spectra, positive mode was selected for the detection of sapogenin, whereas negative mode was selected for saponin, flavonoids, and phenolic acids. DP is one of the most important mass spectrometer parameters which impact ion response. Therefore, DP was optimized in order to obtain the maximum sensitivity of $[M + H]^+$ and $[M - H]^-$. The most suitable CE was also determined by observing the maximal response for MS/MS monitoring of fragment ions. The ions used for quantitative analysis were selected on the basis of highest peak intensity and lowest interference. All MRM parameters were optimized to achieve the most abundant, specific, and stable MRM transitions for each compound were listed in Table 12.1.

12.3.2 ANALYTICAL METHOD VALIDATION

The linearity, regression, and linear ranges of 7 analytes were determined using the developed UPLC-MS/MS method. The results for each compound are listed in Table 12.2. The good correlation coefficient values ($r^2 > 0.9989$) indicated appropriate correlations between their peak areas and investigated compound concentration within the test ranges. The LODs and LOQs for each investigated compounds were < 4.84 and 5.19 ng/mL, which showed a high sensitivity under these chromatographic conditions. The overall intra-day and inter-day variations (RSD) of the 7 analytes were < 1.87 and 2.03%, respectively. Stability of the analytes is ≤ 2.39%. The average recovery was in the range of 98.2–102.3% with RSD ranging from 0.94 to 3.03%. The results indicate that the method was accurate and reproducible.

12.3.3 UPLC-MS BASED QUANTITATION OF PHYTOCHEMICALS

The developed UPLC-MS/MS method was applied for the quantitative analysis of 7 major active compounds in twig of *A. racemosus, A. officinalis* and *A. adscendens* and other plant parts of *A. racemosus*, i.e., leaf, stem, and root also. The contents were calculated with external standard methods based on the respective calibration curve. The results demonstrated a successful

TABLE 12.1 MRM Parameters, Retention Time (Rt), Declustering Potential (DP), Entrance Potential (EP), Collision Energy (CE) and Cell Exit Potential (CXP) for Each Analyte

Compounds	Retention Time (min)	Precursor (Q1) Mass (Da)	Product (Q3) Mass (Da)	Declustering Potential (eV)	Entrance Potential (eV)	Collision Energy (eV)	Cell Exit Potential (eV)
Caffeic acid	0.95	179.0	135.0	−48	−8	−21	−11
Vanillin	1.22	150.9	136.0	−45	−9	−21	−12
Ferulic acid	1.22	193.0	134.0	−58	−5	−23	−9
Quercetin	1.67	301.0	151.0	−107	−9	−31	−12
Apigenin	1.86	269.0	117.0	−71	−5	−45	−9
Sarsasapogenin	2.54	417.6	273.4	24	7	27	13
Shatavarin–IV	2.56	886.7	886.0	−92	−9	−13	−15

TABLE 12.2 Validation Parameters of Seven Reference Analytes

Reference Standards	Linearity		Regression Equation	LOD (ng)	LOQ (ng)	Precision (%RSD)		Stability % RSD (n = 5)	Recovery % RSD (n = 3)
	Linear Range (ng/mL)	R^2				Intra-Day (n = 6)	Inter-Day (n = 6)		
Caffeic acid	0.5–100	0.9998	y = 7416.6x + 26233	0.11	0.48	0.94	1.27	1.77	1.29
Vanillin	10–250	0.9998	y = 1084.2x − 7909.4	2.06	6.31	1.87	2.03	2.11	1.34
Ferulic acid	0.5–100	0.9995	y = 726.74x + 3027.2	0.19	0.54	1.44	0.67	0.81	1.28
Quercetin	10–500	0.9989	y = 2250x − 198.56	4.84	5.19	1.37	0.47	1.02	2.05
Apigenin	1–100	0.9999	y = 2906.5x − 601.72	0.12	0.47	0.74	1.38	2.39	1.37
Sarsasapogenin	10–500	0.9998	y = 925.8x − 6718.4	3.03	3.39	1.29	1.03	2.34	3.03
Shatavarin-IV	1–100	0.9993	y = 222.63x + 637.31	0.28	0.52	1.09	0.87	0.55	0.94

application of the developed method for the quantitation of the major saponins, sapogenins, flavonoids, and phenolic acid in different samples of *Asparagus* species. Furthermore, developed technique was applied to evaluate different marketed formulations of *Asparagus* species.

12.3.4   SAMPLE ANALYSIS

The quantitation of the major bioactive compounds in different samples of *Asparagus* species are summarized in Table 12.3. Significant differences in total contents of saponin, sapogenin, flavonoids, and phenolic acids were observed in the three species of *Asparagus* samples. Saponin, shatavarin-IV was detected highest (12.40 mg/g) in twig of *A. adscendens*. While sapogenin, sarsasapogenin was found second highest (6.55 mg/g) in roots of *A. racemosus*. Flavonoids (quercetin, apigenin) raise up to 0.75 mg/g and 0.02 mg/g, respectively. Similarly, among phenolic acids, caffeic acid (3.05 mg/g) was the highest in *A. adscendens* twig in comparison to ferulic acid (0.67 mg/g) and vanillin (0.30 mg/g), which were analyzed highest in *A. racemosus* twig. Stem and leaf of *A. racemosus* were having relatively lower content of bioactive compounds (caffeic acid, 0.24 and 0.03 mg/g; vanillin, 0.17 and 0.12 mg/g, respectively) while some of these compounds were not able to detected in *Asparagus* species samples.

TABLE 12.3   Content (mg/g) of Reference Analytes in *Asparagus* Species Samples

Sample	Caffeic Acid	Ferulic Acid	Sarsasapo-genin	Vanillin	Shatavarin-IV	Quercetin	Apigenin
A. officinalis twig	0.11	0.17	nd	0.12	0.09	0.06	nd
A. adsendens twig	3.05	0.09	5.30	0.28	12.40	0.71	0.02
A. racemosus twig	0.25	0.67	1.11	0.30	3.11	0.75	0.01
A. racemosus root	1.68	0.08	6.55	0.10	0.07	nd	nd
A. racemosus stem	0.24	nd*	nd	0.17	nd	nd	nd
A. racemosus leaf	0.03	nd	nd	0.12	0.03	0.02	nd

12.3.5 ANALYSIS OF MARKETED FORMULATION

The application of developed UPLC-MS/MS method was performed by quantitative analysis of major two marker components, i.e., sarsasapogenin, and shatavarin-IV in different marketed herbal formulations of *Asparagus* species as summarized in Table 12.4. The result clearly demonstrated that among all the selected formulations, sample F-4 was having the dominant compounds with the highest yield (%), i.e., shatavarin-IV (3.54 mg/g) and sarsasapogenin (1.18 mg/g). On the other hand, the contents of both markers were relatively low or below detection limit in other samples. Due to the number of reasons such as growth conditions, collecting time, drying process, and storage condition, might contribute to the significant differences in the content of active constituents among various samples.

However, multiple active components were considered to be responsible for the therapeutic effects of the herbal formulations, and thus the quantitative determination of multiple components is more reasonable for quality control of raw material/ products of *Asparagus* species.

12.3.6 SCIENTIFIC INTERVENTION WITH FUTURE PERSPECTIVES

An efficient, rapid, and sensitive UPLC-MS/MS method operating in positive and negative scanning modes was first established for the simultaneous quantitation of saponin (shatavarin-IV), sapogenin (sarsasapogenin), flavonoids (apigenin, quercetin, and vanillin) and phenolic acids (caffeic acid and ferulic acid) in *Asparagus* species. The results clearly demonstrated that the developed analytical method could quantitatively determine the content of major components in various *Asparagus* species, as well as in marketed herbal formulation. Validation statistics indicated the sensitivity and specificity of the accuracy and precision. Our results also demonstrated that the developed UPLC-MS/MS quantitative fingerprint worked as a reliable and practical approach for comprehensive quality evaluation of *Asparagus* species. Significant variations in the content of the detected compounds were observed. Moreover, two chemical markers, i.e., sarsasapogenin, and shatavarin-IV were proven to be outstanding distinguishable variables and could be used for the accurate discrimination and QC of *Asparagus* species and herbal formulations. These phytochemicals can also be served as bioactive markers. However, there is need of more work for identification and quantitation of other known and unknown compounds present in these medicinal plants. Dereplication and chemical profiling is also the main demand for the

TABLE 12.4 Content (mg/g) of Reference Analytes in Marketed Herbal Formulations

Sample Code	Composition	Yield % (mg/g)		Brand Name	Batch	Manufacturing Date (month/year)	Supplier
		Sarsasapogenin	Shatavarin-IV				
F-1	4.27 g	nd*	0.01	Count Plus	0I1Q	Sep-14	Nagarjuna Herbal Conc. Ltd.
F-2	165 mg	0.28	0.97	Vigoroyal-F	VFMT002	Sep-13	Maharishi Products
F-3	190 mg	0.13	0.33	Vigoroyal-M	VMMT002	Nov-13	Maharishi products
F-4	20 mg	1.18	3.54	Gariforte	37500375	Feb-15	Himalaya Drug Co.
F-5	10 mg	nd	0.13	Abana	37400156B	Jan-14	Himalaya Drug Co.

standardization and quality control of these plants. The biological activity assessment according to bioactive compounds present in them can be further explored.

KEYWORDS

- analytical method
- *Asparagus* species
- phytopharmaceuticals
- quantitation
- UPLC-MS
- validation

REFERENCES

Allwood, J. W., & Goodacre, R., (2010). An introduction to liquid chromatography-mass spectrometry instrumentation applied in plant metabolomic analyses. *Phytochemical Analysis, 21*(1), 33–47.

Alok, S., Jain, S. K., Verma, A., Kumar, M., Mahor, A., & Sabharwal, M., (2013). Plant profile, phytochemistry and pharmacology of *Asparagus racemosus* (Shatavari): A review. *Asian Pacific Journal of Tropical Disease, 3*(3), 242–251.

Battu, G. R., & Kumar, B. M., (2010). Phytochemical and antimicrobial activity of leaf extract of *Asparagus racemosus* Willd. *Pharmacognosy Journal, 2*(12), 456–463.

Bhutani, K. K., Paul, A. T., Fayad, W., & Linder, S., (2010). Apoptosis-inducing activity of steroidal constituents from *Solanum anthocarpum* and *Asparagus racemosus*. *Phytomedicine, 17*(10), 789–793.

Chandra, P., Kannujia, R., Pandey, R., Shukla, S., Bahadur, L., Pal, M., & Kumar, B., (2016a) Rapid quantitative analysis of multi-components in *Andrographis paniculata* using UPLC-QqQLIT-MS/MS: Application to soil sodicity and organic farming. *Industrial Crops and Products, 83*, 423–430.

Chandra, P., Kannujia, R., Saxena, A., Srivastava, M., Bahadur, L., Pal, M., Singh, B. P., Ojha, S. K., & Kumar, B., (2016b). Quantitative determination of multi markers in five varieties of *Withania somnifera* using ultra-high-performance liquid chromatography with hybrid triple quadrupole linear ion trap mass spectrometer combined with multivariate analysis: Application to pharmaceutical dosage forms. *Journal of Pharmaceutical and Biomedical Analysis, 129*, 419–426.

Chandra, P., Pandey, R., Kumar, B., Srivastva, M., Pandey, P., Sarkar, J., & Singh, B. P., (2015b). Quantification of multianalyte by UPLC–QqQLIT–MS/MS and in-vitro anti-proliferative screening in Cassia species. *Industrial Crops and Products, 76*, 1133–1141.

Chandra, P., Pandey, R., Srivastva, M., & Kumar, B., (2015). Quality control assessment of polyherbal formulation based on a quantitative determination multimarker approach by ultra-high performance liquid chromatography with tandem mass spectrometry using polarity switching combined with multivariate analysis. *Journal of Separation Science, 38*(18), 3183–3191.

Chitrakar, B., Zhang, M., & Adhikari, B., (2019). Asparagus (*Asparagus officinalis*): Processing effect on nutritional and phytochemical composition of spear and hard-stem byproducts. *Trends in Food Science & Technology.* 10.1016/j.tifs.2019.08.020.

De Villiers, A., Venter, P., & Pasch, H., (2016). Recent advances and trends in the liquid-chromatography-mass spectrometry analysis of flavonoids. *Journal of Chromatography A,* 16–78.

Gautam, M., Saha, S., Bani, S., Kaul, A., Mishra, S., Patil, D., Satti, N. K., Suri, K. A., Gairola, S., Suresh, K., & Jadhav, S., (2019). Immunomodulatory activity of *Asparagus racemosus* on systemic Th1/Th2 immunity: Implications for immunoadjuvant potential. *Journal of Ethnopharmacology, 121*(2), 241–247.

Goyal, R. K., Singh, J., & Lal, H., (2003). *Asparagus racemosus*-An update. *Indian Journal of Medical Sciences, 57*(9), 408–414.

Harvey, A. L., (2007). Natural products as a screening resource. *Curr Opin Chem Biol, 11,* 480–484.

Hasan, N., Ahmad, N., Zohrameena, S., Khalid, M., & Akhtar, J., (2016). *Asparagus racemosus*: For medicinal uses & pharmacological actions. *International Journal of Advanced Research, 4*(3), 259–267.

Hayes, P. Y., Jahidin, A. H., Lehmann, R., Penman, K., Kitching, W., De Voss, J. J., (2008). Steroidal saponins from the roots of *Asparagus racemosus*. *Phytochemistry, 69*(3), 796–804.

Iqbal, M., Bibi, Y., Raja, N. I., Ejaz, M., Hussain, M., Yasmeen, F., Saira, H., & Imran, M., (2017). Review on therapeutic and pharmaceutically important medicinal plant *Asparagus officinalis* L. *J. Plant Biochem. Physiol, 5*(180), 2.

Jaiswal, Y., Liang, Z., Ho, A., Chen, H., & Zhao, Z., (2014). A Comparative tissue-specific metabolite analysis and determination of protodioscin content in asparagus species used in traditional Chinese medicine and Ayurveda by use of laser microdissection, UHPLC–QTOF/MS and LC–MS/MS. *Phytochemical Analysis, 25*(6), 514–528.

Kapoor, L. D., (2000). *Handbook of Ayurvedic Medicinal Plants: Herbal Reference Library.* CRC press.

Kesting, J. R., Huang, J., & Sorensen, D., (2010). Identification of adulterants in a Chinese herbal medicine by LC–HRMS and LC–MS–SPE/NMR and comparative in vivo study with standards in a hypertensive rat model. *Journal of Pharmaceutical and Biomedical Analysis, 51,* 705–711.

Khanna, A. K., Chander, R., & Kapoor, N. K., (1991). Hypolipidemic activity of Abana in rats. *Fitoterapia, 62*(3), 271–275.

King, R., & Fernandez, M., (2006). The use of Qtrap technology in drug metabolism. *Curr. Drug Metab., 7*(5), 541–545.

Kobus-Cisowska, J., Szymanowska, D., Szczepaniak, O. M., Gramza-Michałowska, A., Kmiecik, D., Kulczyński, B., Szulc, P., & Górnaś, P., (2019). Composition of polyphenols of asparagus spears (Asparagus officinalis) and their antioxidant potential. *Ciência Rural, 49*(4), 1–8. http://dx.doi.org/10. 1590/0103-8478cr20180863.

Lee, E. J., Yoo, K. S., & Patil, B. S., (2010). Development of a rapid HPLC-UV method for simultaneous quantification of protodioscin and rutin in white and green asparagus spears. *Journal of Food Science, 75*(9), 703–709.

Mandal, S. C., Nandy, A., Pal, M., & Saha, B. P., (2000). Evaluation of antibacterial activity of *Asparagus racemosus* willd. root. *Phytotherapy Research: An International Journal Devoted to Pharmacological and Toxicological Evaluation of Natural Product Derivatives, 14*(2), 118–119.

Manta, T., Shukla, Y. N., & Tandon, M., (1995). Phytoconstituents of *Asparagus adscendens, Chlorophytum arundinaceum* and *Curculigo orchioides*: A review. *Current Research on Medicinal and Aromatic Plants, 17*, 202–210.

Muruganadan, S., Garg, H., Lal, J., Chandra, S., & Kumar, D., (2000). Studies on the immunostimulant and antihepatotoxic activities of *Asparagus racemosus* root extract. *J. Med. Arom. Pl Sci., 22*, 49–52.

Negi, J. S., Singh, P., Joshi, (nee Pant) G., & Rawat, M. S. M., (2011). High performance liquid chromatographic analysis of derivatized sapogenin of Asparagus (RP-HPLC analysis of derivatized sapogenin of Asparagus). *Journal of Medicinal Plants Research, 5*(10), 1900–1904.

Okolie, O. D., Manduna, I., & Mashele, S., (2019). Phytochemical analysis of *Asparagus africanus* root extracts. *Journal of Pharmacy and Pharmacology, 7*, 351–354.

Patel, A. B., & Kanitkar, U. K., (1969). *Asparagus racemosus* willd--form bordi, as a galactagogue, in buffaloes. *The Indian Veterinary Journal, 46*(8), 718–721.

Patil, D., Gautam, M., Gairola, S., Jadhav, S., & Patwardhan, B., (2014). HPLC/tandem mass spectrometric studies on steroidal saponins: An example of quantitative determination of Shatavari IV from dietary supplements containing *Asparagus racemosus*. *Journal of AOAC International, 97*(6), 1497–1502.

Raskin, I., Ribnicky, D. M., Komarnytsky, S., Ilic, N., Poulev, A., Borisjuk, N., Brinker, A., et al., (2002). Plants and human health in the twenty-first century. *TRENDS in Biotechnology, 20*(12), 522–531.

Rathore, A. S., Sathiyanarayanan, L., Deshpande, S., & Mahadik, K. R., (2016). Rapid and sensitive determination of major polyphenolic components in *Euphoria longan* Lam. seeds using matrix solid-phase dispersion extraction and UHPLC with hybrid linear ion trap triple quadrupole mass spectrometry. *Journal of Separation Science, 39*(22), 4335–4343.

Sairam, K., Priyambada, S., Aryya, N. C., & Goel, R. K., (2003). Gastroduodenal ulcer protective activity of *Asparagus racemosus*: An experimental, biochemical and histological study. *Journal of Ethnopharmacology, 86*(1), 1–10.

Satti, N. K., Suri, K. A., Dutt, P., Suri, O. P., Amina, M., Qazi, G. N., & Rauf, A., (2006). Evaluation of *Asparagus racemosus* on the basis of immunomodulating sarsasapogenin glycosides by HPTLC. *Journal of Liquid Chromatography and Related Technologies, 29*(2), 219–227.

Sharma, P., Chauhan, P. S., Dutt, P., Amina, M., Suri, K. A., Gupta, B. D., Suri, O. P., et al., (2011). A unique immuno-stimulant steroidal sapogenin acid from the roots of *Asparagus racemosus*. *Steroids, 76*(4), 358–364.

Sharma, U., Saini, R., Kumar, N., & Singh, B., (2009). Steroidal saponins from *Asparagus racemosus*. *Chemical and Pharmaceutical Bulletin, 57*(8), 890–893.

Sidiq, T., Khajuria, A., Suden, P., Singh, S., Satti, N. K., Suri, K. A., Srinivas, V. K., Krishna, E., & Johri, R. K., (2011). A novel sarsasapogenin glycoside from *Asparagus racemosus* elicits protective immune responses against HBsAg. *Immunology Letters, 135*(1, 2), 129–135.

Velavan, S., Nagulendran, K. R., Mahesh, R., & Begum, V. H., (2007). The chemistry, pharmacological and therapeutic applications of *Asparagus racemosus*: A review. *Pharmacognosy Reviews, 1*(2), 350–360.

Vihan, V. S., & Panwar, H. S., (1988). A note on galactogogue activity of *Asparagus racemosus* in lactating goats. *Indian J. Animal Health, 27*, 177–178.

Visavadiya, N. P., & Narasimhacharya, A. R., (2005). Hypolipidemic and antioxidant activities of *Asparagus racemosus* in hypercholesteremic rats. *Indian Journal of Pharmacology, 37*(6), 376.

Wang, L., Wang, X., Yuan, X., & Zhao, B., (2011). Simultaneous analysis of diosgenin and sarsasapogenin in Asparagus officinalis byproduct by thin-layer chromatography. *Phytochemical Analysis, 22*(1), 14–17.

Wolfender, J. L., Allard, P. M., Kubo, M., & Ferreira, E., (2019). Metabolomics strategies for the dereplication of polyphenols and other metabolites in complex natural extracts. *Recent Advances in Polyphenol Research, 6*, 183–205.

Zhang, H., Birch, J., Pei, J., Ma, Z. F., & Bekhit, A. E. D., (2019). Phytochemical compounds and biological activity in Asparagus roots: A review. *International Journal of Food Science and Technology, 54*(4), 966–977.

CHAPTER 13

PHYTOSOMES: PREPARATIONS, CHARACTERIZATION, AND FUTURE USES

PALAKDEEP KAUR and UTTAM KUMAR MANDAL

Department of Pharmaceutical Sciences and Technology,
Maharaja Ranjit Singh Punjab Technical University (MRSPTU),
Bathinda, Punjab – 151001, India,
E-mail: mandalju2007@gmail.com (U. K. Mandal)

ABSTRACT

Phytosomes are little cell-like structures. They are advanced vesicular structures like liposomes where active phytoconstituents are enclosed within a lipid core. Most of the phytoconstituents like glycosides, flavonoids, etc., are hydrophilic in nature and cannot penetrate lipid-based biological membrane. Enclosure of lipid core makes the phytosomes permeable through the biological membrane, thereby increasing the bioavailability and desired actions of the herbal constituents. Phytosomes can be prepared by various methods similar to the preparation of liposomes for synthetic drugs. They have huge scope of delivery of phytomedicines in coming future. The present book chapter elucidates the spectrophotometric evaluation, methods of preparation, physicochemical properties, characterization, applications, structural features of phytosomes along with advantages as well as disadvantages as herbal drug carriers. It also highlights some reported literature on phytosomes, including their future prospects as carries of herbal drugs.

13.1 INTRODUCTION

Conventional oral medications like tablets, capsules, and liquid preparations including liquid orals, suspension, and emulsion are widely acceptable dosage forms to patients due to their ease of administration and manufacturability. However, many a time, these dosage forms suffer from their inherent biopharmaceutical features like low gastrointestinal absorption, chemical instability in variable pH environment of gastrointestinal tract, low therapeutic index, short half-life, poor aqueous solubility, and others. The concept of designing novel drug delivery system (NDDS) has emerged to overcome or address these problems. NDDS results in a new life of an existing drug molecule, i.e., older drug molecule in newer clothes, and thereby increasing market value, and competitiveness (Bhagwat and Vaidhya, 2013). Among various advantages, some important ones are mentioned below (Malaterre et al., 2009):

- Simplified drug administration protocols;
- Smaller dose size compared to conventional dosage regimen for producing desire effects;
- Increased efficacy and therapeutic index (Saraf, 2010);
- Improved bioavailability;
- Ability of drug targeting by coupling with site specific ligands.

In spite of many potential benefits, synthetic drugs are infamous due to their associated potential adverse effects which have drawn huge attention worldwide. As an alternative strategy, medical practitioners are shifting towards the use of plant based medicinal products (phytomedicines) or herbal drugs because they are considered free or with minimum toxicity or side effects. At present, herbal drugs have overtaken a significant amount of market share. The worldwide market of herbal medicine is going to establish a huge demand in coming years, and according to experts, it will reach a market value of USD 1,29,689 million until 2023 with a compound annual growth rate (CAGR) of 5.88%. This highlights the importance of herbal drugs and its contribution of global healthcare system in near future.

In line with NDDS of synthetic drugs, many innovative formulation approaches have been researched for herbal drugs to overcome or engineer their inherent poor biopharmaceutical properties, phytosome is one of them. Phytosomes contain water-soluble bioactive phytoconstituents of herbs bounded and surrounded by phospholipids. They are little cell like structures. The word phytosomes is composed of a combination of two words, 'phyto' and 'somes,' where 'phyto' means plants and 'somes' means cell-like (Pk and Wahile, 2006). Indena developed a patented method to incorporate standardized plant material extract into lipid vesicles to increase its absorption and named them as phytosomes (Sharma and Roy, 2010).

13.2 STRUCTURAL FEATURES OF PHYTOSOMES

Representative structure of phytosomes is given in Figure 13.1. It is composed of phospholipids such as phosphatidyl (choline, inositol, serine, ethanolamine), among them phosphatidylcholine is used widely due to its certain therapeutic values. Phospholipids serve as vesicles forming component. Various solvents such as acetone, methanol, ethanol, n-hexane, methylene chloride is used for the preparation of phytosomes. Figure 13.2 highlights some of the excipients commonly used for preparation of phytosomes. Phytosomes are usually available in nano form within a range of 50 nm to a few 100 μm enclosing the herbal drugs within lipid cores. The degradation of active constituent of herbal extract or drug by bacteria and digestive secretion is avoided due to coating, also referred to as envelope, around it. The first phytosomal preparation was flavonognan Silybin (silymarin) (Bhattacharya and Ghosh, 2009) obtained from milk thistle fruit that has antioxidant, liver detoxification and anti-inflammatory properties (Moscarella et al., 1993). Hydrophilic compounds such as glycosides, flavonoids are basically molecules of interest for the preparation of phytosomes.

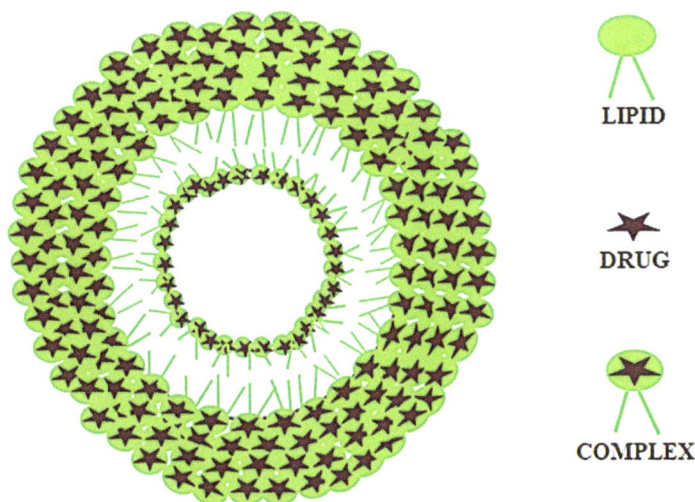

LIPID

DRUG

COMPLEX

FIGURE 13.1 Representative structure of drug loaded phytosomes.

13.3   ADVANTAGES OF PHYTOSOMES AS HERBAL DRUG CARRIERS

Phytosomes are structurally similar to liposomes or modified liposomes like transferosomes and ethosomes (Mahmood et al., 2014; Mahmood et al., 2018). The following advantages have been documented for phytosomes (Sharma and Roy, 2010; Manthena and Srinivas, 2010):

- Phospholipids used in preparations of phytosomes provide synergistic effect with hepatoprotective agents, act as carrier or vehicle and provide many health benefits.
- Phytosomes enhance the absorption of active constituents resulting requirement of minimum dose to produce the desired therapeutic actions (Raju et al., 2011).
- Phystosomes result in formation of chemical bonds between phospholipids and herbal extracts, thereby showing better stability.
- Phytosomes, because of their lipidic nature, become easily soluble in bile salts which help in liver targeting of many herbal constituents.
- Phytosomes possess lipid layer around phytoconstituents which are responsible for phytosomes to permeate through skin and increase their effectiveness.
- Method of preparation of phytosomes is simple, easy, and convenient.
- During formulation, the drug moiety conjugates with lipids and forms vesicles which provide increased entrapment efficiency at a predetermined rate.
- Phytosomes show better bioavailability by increasing the absorption of polar herbal extracts through topical and oral routes.
- Phytosomes contain phosphatidylcholine which provides nourishment to the skin when applied topically (Bombardelli, 1991).
- Phytosomes result easy systemic transfer of herbal constituents from hydrophilic environment of body to lipophilic environment of cell resulting in systemic targeting (Sharma and Correspondence Morali, 2005).

13.4   DISADVANTAGES OF PHYTOSOMES

The basic disadvantage of phytosomes is that the phytoconstituents are rapidly eliminated from the body and results in reduction of the desired drug content which illustrates their unstable nature (Chivte et al., 2017).

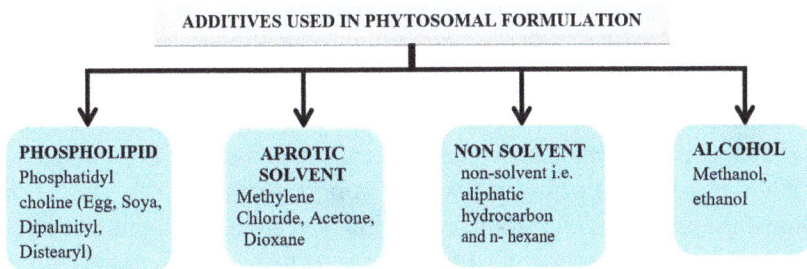

FIGURE 13.2 Commonly used excipients for preparation of phytosomes.

13.5 PREPARATION OF PHYTOSOMES

Some of the methods commonly used for the preparation of phytosomes are discussed in subsections.

13.5.1 ROTARY EVAPORATION METHOD

This method involves the use of rotary round bottom flask (RBF) in which desired quantity of lipid (example: soya lecithin) and phyto drug are mixed in definite volume of organic solvent (example: tetrahydrofuran, dichloromethane, chloroform, ethanol, and their suitable mixture) by stirring at temperature more than 40°C for 3 hrs (Awasthi et al., 2011). After evaporation, a thin film of sample is formed around the inner surface of RBF. The dried precipitate is taken out, transferred to another collection bottles (if light-sensitive, use amber color glass bottle), stored at desired storage condition for future analysis (Yu et al., 2016). As part of optimization of the formulation composition, quality by design (QBD) approach may be adopted and accordingly various critical parameters like critical quality attributes (CQA), critical material attributes (CMA) and critical process parameters (CPP) need to be identified (Table 13.1).

TABLE 13.1 Critical Formulation and Process Parameters for Phytosome Preparation

Critical Material Attributes (CMA)	Critical Process Parameters (CPP)	Critical Quality Attributes (CQA)
• Lipid content	• Speed of stirrer	• Particle size
• Phyto drug content	• Temperature	• Particle shape
• Organic solvent content	• Time of operation	• Entrapment efficiency
		• Drug content

13.5.2   ANTI-SOLVENT PRECIPITATION METHOD

First, an RBF is loaded with a weighed amount of soya lecithin and drug. The content is refluxed for 2 hrs at a temperature more than 60°C with 20 ml of dichloromethane. After concentrating, the content is precipitated with the addition of 20 ml of hexane with continuous stirring. The sample thus obtained is subjected to filtration, collection, and storage in vacuum desiccators for overnight. The obtained dried mass is further crushed, passed through 00 mesh sieve and collected in amber colored glass bottles for future storage at room temperature (Hüsch et al., 2013).

13.5.3   SOLVENT EVAPORATION METHOD

Natural or synthetic phospholipid and phytoconstituents are suspended in an appropriate solvent. The sample is refluxed for 2 hrs at 50–60°C. The obtained mass is filtered, dried, and collected in amber colored glass bottles for future storage at room temperature (Mazumder et al., 2016).

13.6   PHYSICOCHEMICAL PROPERTIES OF PHYTOSOMES

13.6.1   PHYSICOCHEMICAL PROPERTIES

- When phytosomes are treated with water, it results in the formation of micelle like shape which is similar to that of liposomes. Structural properties are revealed by the use of photon correlation spectroscopy (PCS) (Kumar et al., 2017).
- Phytosomes are freely soluble in aprotic solvents, sparingly soluble in fats and insoluble in water. It is generally unstable in alcohol.
- From spectroscopic techniques, it can be determined that the unchanged signals are obtained due to fatty chain both in free phospholipid and in complex, which specifies that the active principle is surrounded by long aliphatic chains, forming lipophilic envelope.
- When an appropriate quantity of phospholipid is reacted with the botanical extract as substrate, it leads to the formation of complex called phytosomes. By analysis, it can be specified that the formation of hydrogen bond within the polar functionalities of the substrate and polar head (i.e., ammonium, and phosphate group) results in interaction between phospholipid and substrate (Manach et al., 2004).

13.7   CHARACTERIZATION OF PHYTOSOMES

13.7.1   MICROSCOPIC STUDIES

Surface morphology and size are important parameters with respect to formulation of phytosomes and they need to be evaluated by suitable microscopic studies. Scanning electron microscope (SEM) is routinely used for this evaluation. However, advanced version of this instrument which is transmission electron microscope (TEM) gives rather accurate results with additional information. In SEM, phytosomal vesicles are coated with a very thin layer of gold and visualized at an appropriate magnification. The spherical shape of the phytosomes can be confirmed through the spherical bulging generally obtained on the surface. TEM studies determine the internal environment in which the drug is entrapped and their distributions within the lipid core is visualized (Semalty et al., 2010; Gupta and Dixit, 2011).

13.7.2   PARTICLE SIZE AND SURFACE CHARGE

The effective zeta potential and particle size of phytosomes can be checked by dynamic light scattering technique based on the electrophoresis and electrical conductivity which uses PCS and computerized inspection system (Dayan and Touitou, 2000). Zeta potential can be defined as the difference of charge across interface of liquid and solid surfaces. The diluted phytosome sample could be placed in clear disposable zeta cells and results can be recorded. The significance of zeta potential is that its value correlates to the short and long-term stability of the formulation (Gabetta et al., 1989).

13.7.3   ENTRAPMENT EFFICIENCY

The percentage of drug encapsulated is the amount of drug entrapped/encapsulated in a liquid vesicle. Ultracentrifugation technique or disruption of lipid vesicles by organic solvents is used to determine the total amount of drug entrapped within the phytosomal formulation (El-Maghraby et al., 2000). The phytoconstituent trapped within the vesicles is separated out and estimated by suitable analytical techniques.

13.7.4   MEASUREMENT OF SURFACE TENSION

Measure of surface tension of any colloidal preparation is important in view of its physical stability. Amount of surface tension should be optimum to avoid the incident of particle aggregation or coalescence. Du Nouy ring tensiometer is used to determine the surface tension of the drug in aqueous solution.

13.7.5   STABILITY STUDIES

These studies are performed to maintain physical, chemical, therapeutic, microbiological, and toxicological specifications of a particular formulation kept in a specific container closure system throughout its shelf-life. By determining the structure and particle size of vesicles kept over time, the stability can be checked. It is done to develop stable dosage form and to ensure the safety, efficacy, and quality of active drug substances and dosage forms.

13.7.6   DRUG CONTENT

Various spectroscopic techniques such as UV and HPLC can be used to analyze the drug content in phytosomal formulation if the reference standard of marker compound present in the herbal material is available. Weighed accurately the desire amount of phytosomal complex and dissolved in solvent. The absorbance of the sample is determined after suitable dilution using the spectroscopic method and the drug content is calculated (Zhang et al., 2013).

13.8   SPECTROPHOTOMETRIC EVALUATIONS

13.8.1 ^{1}H-NMR

The NMR spectrum is used for estimation of complex formed within the active phytoconstituents and phosphatidylcholine molecule. During complex formation, a noticeable alteration in ^{1}H-NMR signal is observed. In the case of phytoconstituents, signals due to proton are widened. An up-field shift corresponds to N-$(CH_3)_3$ of choline, whereas phospholipids show broadening of signals (Gabetta et al., 1989; Malandrino and Pifferi, 1990).

13.8.2 ^{13}C-NMR

In this technique, all the phytoconstituents carbons are invisible when phytoconstituents and phosphatidylcholine complex are recorded in room temperature. The original sharp line shape represents resonance of the fatty acid chains of phosphatidylcholine, but the signals of choline portion and glycerol are widened, and some are shifted.

13.8.3 FT-IR

FTIR can be preferred to confirm the stability of phytosomal complex. Individual phytoconstituents, excipients, and their physical mixtures are studied, and the spectrums of the same are compared against that of the phytosome preparations.

13.9 APPLICATION OF PHYTOSOMES

13.9.1 FOR TREATMENT OF CANCER

The chemical components like coumarins, flavones, flavonoids, isoflavones, lignins, anthocyanins, catechins, and isocatechin have been reported to be effective against cancer. Antioxidant properties of these phytoconstituents are responsible for such activities (Raina et al., 2014). Shalini et al. (2015) investigated the antiproliferative activity of methanolic extract of *Terminalia arjuna* bark and its phytosome preparation. Human breast cancer cell line MCF-7 was used, and the researchers carried out to MTT assay and compared antiproliferative activities of quercetin, active constituent of *Terminalia arjuna* bark and the developed phytosome preparation. The IC50 values of the extract and its phytosome were 25 µg/ml and 15 µg/ml respectively, which suggests that phytosomal preparation exerts more antiproliferative effect as compared to free drug (Shalini et al., 2015).

13.9.2 ANTI-HEPATOTOXIC OR PROTECT LIVER DAMAGE

The leaf extract of *Ginkgo biloba* is known to have cardioprotective, anti-diabetic, anti-asthmatic, anti-oxidant, hepatoprotective, and potent CNS activities (Panda and Naik, 2008). The group experiment *Ginko biloba*-based phytosomal preparation on rifampicin treated rats for its hepatotoxicity and reported its probable mechanism.

13.9.3 ANTIOXIDANT

Moscarella et al. (1993) studied the antioxidant and free radical scavenging activity of Silipide which is phytosome of *Silybum marianum* plant against liver oxidative damage induced by paracetamol and CCl_4 (high dosages) in rats. Toxic effects of drug (paracetamol) and chemical (CCl_4) cause lipid peroxidation by generated reactive oxygen species (ROS). Authors suggested that the silipide is responsible to avert oxidative damage of hepatocytes by inhibiting this lipid peroxidation.

13.9.4 WOUND HEALING ACTIVITY

Devi and Divakar (2012) investigated the comparative effects of ethanolic extracts of *Wrightia arborea* leaves and its phytosomes. The phytosomes exhibited about 90.40% healing while the ethanolic extract alone could heal only 65.63% of the wound.

13.9.5 BIOAVAILABILITY ENHANCEMENT

Evodiamine, a quinoline alkaloid, (*Evodia rutaecarpa*) possess a number of pharmacological activities, such as anti-obesity, anti-tumor, anti-nociceptive, anti-inflammatory, and thermoregulatory effects. Evodiamine shows anti-tumor property by inducing apoptosis, inhibiting proliferation and reducing metastasis and invasion. The AUC (1772.35 µg h^{-1} L^{-1}) and $t^{1/2}$ (1.33 hours) of evodiamine increased to 3787.24 µg h^{-1} L^{-1} and 2.07 hours, respectively because of phytosomal preparation (Tan et al., 2012).

13.9.6 TRANSDERMAL APPLICATION

Das and Kalita (2104) investigated Rutin (*Ruta graveolens*) for the treatment of capillary fragility, hypertension, ultraviolet radiation-induced cutaneous oxidative stress, hepatic, and blood cholesterol, cataract, cardiovascular disease and possess antioxidant, anti-inflammatory, antithrombotic, antineoplastic, and antiplatelet activity. It was observed that the rutin phytosomes were penetrated easily through the stratum corneum than its free form. Skin uptake of Rutin phytosomes was $33 \pm 1.33\%$ whereas that of Rutin was $13 \pm 0.87\%$ (Das and Kalita, 2014).

13.10 HIGHLIGHT OF SOME REPORTED LITERATURES ON PHYTOSOMES

Hashemzehi et al. (2018) formulated phytosomes by interacting CST (purity 98%) and soy phosphatidylcholine (SPC) phospholipid, at different molar ratios CST: SPC (1:3, 1:2, and 1:1), by Solvent evaporation technique. For characterization of phytosomes, *in-vitro* and *in-vivo* studies were carried out and it was confirmed that CST-PHY complex enhanced the herbal drug absorption. Antitumor activity of novel formulation of Curcumin along with 5-fluorouracil in breast cancer was studied (Hashemzehi et al., 2018).

Freag et al. (2017) prepared the self-assembled phytosomal nano-carriers of celastrol (CST) for enhancing its bioavailability and solubility. CST, isolated from the root extract of *Celastrus reglii* studied as an anticancer surrogate against different types of cancer cell lines including, melanoma, human prostate cancer, pancreatic cancer cells, lung cancer, and breast MCF-7 cells. CST has limited applications due to low aqueous solubility and bioavailability (Freag et al., 2018).

Dhase et al. (2015) prepared the phytosome from the root extract of *Clerodendron paniculatum* L. To determine the active constituents, phytochemical studies were carried out. These phytosome acts against cancer cells such as MCF-7. The solvent evaporation method was used to formulate Luteolin-loaded phytosomes. Luteolin, a flavonoid present in the phytosomes, basically inhibits Nrf2 and sensitizes cancer cells against the chemotherapeutic agents. The flower of *Butea monosperma is known to* be used traditionally for the treatment of diabetes and hepatoprotective activity. However, *B. monosperma* has low bioavailability because of its limited gastrointestinal absorption. Gahandule et al. (2016) formulated phytosomal preparation with aqueous extract of *B. monosperma* and soya lecithin. The developed preparation had all the required physic-chemical attributes. Free radical scavenging activity was studied by DPPH model and the group reported synergistic activity of soya lecithin and *B. monosperma* with respect to hepatoprotective activity.

Pereira and Mallya (2015) developed a phospholipid complex containing amla extract for transdermal application. Authors reported improved delivery of phytoconstituents of amla extract which are mainly polyphenols into the skin. The characterization studies showed that the complex was formed successfully using the constituents of amla extract along with phospholipids and the entrapment efficiency was found to be 94.03 ± 0.10%. Further, the developed cream resulted in improved antioxidant property as compared to its conventional counterpart. Similarly, the *ex-vivo* diffusion studies of cream produced higher skin retention then the marketed cream.

Sumathi and Senthamarai (2015) developed one phytosomal preparation with *Nymphaea nouchal* and *Trichosanthes dioica* (Td). Formulation was prepared by solvent evaporation technique by reacting phosphatidylethanol-amine (PE) in tetrahydrofuran in dioxane: methanol (7:3) solvent system. Various formulations were prepared with molar ratios of 1:10, 1:8, 1:6, 1:4, 1:2 and 1:1 for *Nymphaea nouchal* (Nn) and Td, respectively. Various characterizations such as particle size, IR spectroscopy, DSC, drug content, diffusion, and stability studies were performed. The mean particle size was found to be 268 nm for the selected best formulation with *Nymphaea nouchal* and Td ratio of 1:8. The formulation had an entrapment efficiency of 89%, and it was found to be stable for a significant period of time when tested with specific storage conditions. As compared to standard (Levamisole) and crude drug mixture, the developed phytosomal preparation exhibited significant increase in diffusion rate. The developed formulation had favorable *in vitro* release characteristics which might be is promising for decreasing the effect of exogenous factors and increasing drug delivery.

Allam et al. (2015) formulated curcumin phytosomes by solvent evapora-tion method to increase curcumin content in soft gels. The physicochemical characteristics of phytosomes such as drug content and zeta potential were determined. Various oils (castor oil, oleic acid and Miglyol 812), bioactive surfactants (KLS P 124, Cremophor EL) were used to develop the formula-tion. PEG 400 was used in the formulation as a hydrophilic vehicle. The formulation was characterized by *in vitro* dissolution and stability studies. TEM Microscopic evaluation proved the existence of and a spherical, self-closed structure of the phytosomal formulation. The developed formulation achieved a decrease and controlled release of curcumin from the complex (Allam et al., 2015).

Arora and Kaur (2013) formulated and characterized phytosomal *Phyl-lanthus amarus* complex tablets for sustained delivery of drug. By using silica gel column chromatography, phyllanthin (active lignin) was isolated from the aerial parts. In comparison to other reported procedures, it provides high yield, i.e., 1.23% and the purity was checked by HPTLC technique.

Various characterizations such as melting point determination, FT-IR, UV-spectroscopy, HPTLC, and NMR studies were carried of Phyllanthin. Surface morphology of the developed tablet was evaluated by scanning electron microscopy (SEM). An HPTLC study was carried out and R_f factor was found to be 0.25. Drug release kinetics was evaluated by USP-type I dissolution apparatus. Vacuum drying of phytosome preparation of Phyllanthus had maximum drug content for 1:1 ratio of drug and excipient. The optimized formulation had resulted in extended drug release, 88.1% ± 4.1% drug got released in a span of 12 hrs (Arora and Kaur, 2013).

Demir et al. (2012) prepared photosomes by encapsulating the extracts of *C. officinalis* and gold nanoparticles using traditional film hydration method. Gold nanoparticles act as anticancer upon living cells and used for wound healing. *Calendula officinalis* L. has anti-tumoral, pharmacological, anti-inflammatory, antioxidant, and wound healing activities and in 200 cosmetic products in extracted form. The resulting phytosomes were evaluated by atomic force microscopy (AFM), particle size measurement by DLS and surface charge, respectively. The phytosome had high encapsulation efficiency and major constituent of *C. officinalis* extract (Demir et al., 2014).

Sangeeta et al. (2012) developed phytosomes using *Prosopis cineraria* extract in combination with phospholipids by rotary evaporator method to improve its lipophilic properties and to reduce the problem of absorption and bioavailability. The physicochemical properties of the phytosomes such as solubility, % yield, infrared spectrophotometry, drug content, apparent partition coefficient and *in vitro* dissolution studies were determined. The results of IR spectra showed no new characteristic absorption peaks, indicating that no new covalent bonds were formed but some interaction between drug (*Prosopis cineraria* methanolic extract) and phospholipid (soya lecithin) in the complex (phytosomes) were observed (Manral et al., 2019).

Bombardelli et al. (2005) prepared phytosomes using silymarin and reported higher specific activity as well as showed longer-lasting action in comparison to the single constituent, with respect to inhibition of myeloperoxidase activity, % reduction of edema, suppression of free radical scavenging and antioxidant activity.

Maiti et al. (2005) formulated quercetin phytosome and later indicated the enhanced bioavailability. *In vivo* studies carried on injured rat liver showed better therapeutic efficacy than the uncomplexed molecule (Maiti et al., 2005). Further, the developed andrographolide herbosome, studied on rats, has been found to show hepatoprotective activity. Additionally, researchers have reported an increased activity of phytosomal formulation as compared to uncomplexed andrographolide (Maiti et al., 2010).

Jiang et al. (2001) formulated phytosomes using herbaepimedii flavonoids (EPF) through solvent evaporation technique and performed the dissolution studies using different ratios of EPF-PVP precipitate. The researchers reported the higher dissolution of the precipitate as compared to that of its physical mixture and tablets of herbaepimedii extract (Jiang et al., 2001).

13.11   FUTURE PROSPECT OF PHYTOSOMES AS CARRIES OF HERBAL DRUGS

Phytosomes are considered advanced or drug delivery system that overcomes shortcomings of conventional drug delivery system containing herbal medicine. This novel formulation aims to achieve maximum absorption and permeation of phytoconstituents into systemic circulation which is otherwise challenging for conventional formulations. Phytosomes have evidenced enhanced pharmacokinetic and pharmacodynamics attributes which have broader implications and huge scopes in cosmeticology. The method of preparation of phytosomes is simple, non-convenient, and reproducible which include use of phospholipids that have their own beneficial effect on the body. It is considered an advanced version of dosage form than its conventional counterpart with improved attributes for delivery of active phytoconstituents. Phytosomes based several formulations have already marked their footsteps in the commercial arena and many more are on the way. It is expected that in near future, photosomes as novel carriers will have huge impact for effective delivery of phytomedicines.

KEYWORDS

- applications
- characterization
- evaluation
- herbal drug carrier
- physicochemical properties
- phytosomes
- preparation
- structural features

REFERENCES

Allam, A. N., Komeil, I. A., & Abdallah, O. Y., (2015). Curcumin phytosomal soft gel formulation: Development, optimization and physicochemical characterization. *Acta Pharm., 65*(3), 285–297.

Arora, S., & Kaur, P., (2013). Preparation and characterization of phytosomal-phospholipid complex of *P. amarus* and its tablet formulation. *JPTRM, 1*(1), 1–18.

Awasthi, R., Kulkarni, G. T., & Pawar, V. K., (2011). Phytosomes: An approach to increase the bioavailability of plant extracts. *Int. J. Pharm. Pharm. Sci., 3*(2), 1–3.

Bhagwat, R. R., & Vaidhya, I. S., (2013). Novel drug delivery systems: An overview. *Int. J. pharm. Sci. Res., 4*(3), 970.

Bhattacharya, S., & Ghosh, A., (2009). Phytosomes: The emerging technology for enhancement of bioavailability of botanicals and nutraceuticals. *The Int. J. Aest. Antiaging Med., 2*(1), 141–153.

Bombardelli, E., (1991). Phytosome: New cosmetic delivery system. *Boll. Chim. Farm., 130*(11), 431–438.

Bombardelli, E., Della, L. R., Sosa, S., Spelta, M., & Tubaro, A., (1991). Aging skin: Protective effect of silymarin-phytosome. *Fitoterapia., 62*(2), 115–122.

Chivte, P. S., Pardhi, V. S., Joshi, V. A., & Rani, A., (2017). A review on therapeutic applications of phytosomes. *J. Drug Deliv. Ther., 7*(5), 17–21.

Das, M. K., & Kalita, B., (2014). Design and evaluation of phyto-phospholipid complexes (phytosomes) of rutin for transdermal application. *J. Appl. Pharm. Sci., 4*(10), 51–57.

Dayan, N., & Touitou, E., (2000). Carriers for skin delivery of trihexyphenidyl HCl: Ethosomes vs. liposomes. *Biomaterials, 21*(18), 1879–1885.

Demir, B., Barlas, F. B., Guler, E., Gumus, P. Z., Can, M., Yavuz, M., & Timur, S., (2014). Gold nanoparticle loaded phytosomal systems: Synthesis, characterization and *in vitro* investigations. *RSC Adv., 4*(65), 34687–34695.

Devi, S. L., & Divakar, M. C., (2012). Wound healing activity studies of *Wrightia arborea* phytosome in rats. *Hygeia J. D. Med., 4*, 87–94.

El Maghraby, G. M. M., Williams, A. C., & Barry, B. W., (2000). Oestradiol skin delivery from ultra deformable liposomes: Refinement of surfactant concentration. *Int. J. Pharm., 196*(1), 63–74.

Freag, M. S., Saleh, W. M., & Abdallah, O. Y., (2018). Self-assembled phospholipid-based phytosomal nanocarriers as promising platforms for improving oral bioavailability of the anticancer celastrol. *Int. J. Pharm., 535*(1, 2), 18–26.

Gabetta, B., Zini, G. F., & Pifferi, G., (1989). Spectroscopic studies on IdB 1016, a new flavanolignan complex. *Planta Med., 55*(07), 615.

Gahandule, M. B., Jadhav, S. J., Gadhave, M. V., & Gaikwad, D. D., (2016). Formulation and development of hepato-protective butea monosperma-phytosome. *Int. J. Res. Pharm. Pharm. Sci., 1*, 21–27.

Gupta, N. K., & Dixit, V. K., (2011). Development and evaluation of vesicular system for curcumin delivery. *Arch. Dermatol. Res., 303*(2), 89–101.

Hashemzehi, M., Avan, A., Hasanzadeh, M., Shahid, S. S., Yousefi, Z., Kadkhodayan, S., & Hassanian, S. M., (2018). Effects of the novel formulated forms of curcumin on tumor growth inhibition in breast cancer. *Iran. J. Obstet. Gynecol. Infertil., 21*(2), 75–84.

Hüsch, J., Bohnet, J., Fricker, G., Skarke, C., Artaria, C., Appendino, G., & Abdel-Tawab, M., (2013). Enhanced absorption of *Boswellic* acids by a lecithin delivery form (Phytosome®) of Boswellia extract. *Fitoterapia., 84*, 89–98.

Jiang, Y. N., Yu, Z. P., Yang, Z. M., & Chen, J. M., (2001). Studies on preparation of herba epimedii total flavonoids phytosomes and their pharmaceutics. *Zhongguo Zhong Yao Za Zhi., 26*(2), 105–108.

Kumar, A., Kumar, B., Singh, S. K., Kaur, B., & Singh, S., (2017). A review on phytosomes: Novel approach for herbal phytochemicals. *Asian J. Pharm. Clin. Res., 10*(10), 41.

Mahmood, S., Mandal, U. K., & Chatterjee, B., (2018). Transdermal delivery of raloxifene HCl via ethosomal system: Formulation, advanced characterizations and pharmacokinetic evaluation. *Int. J. Pharm., 542*(1, 2), 36–46.

Mahmood, S., Taher, M., & Mandal, U. K., (2014). Experimental design and optimization of raloxifene hydrochloride loaded nanotransfersomes for transdermal application. *Int. J. Nanomed., 9*, 4331.

Maiti, K., Mukherjee, K., Gantait, A., Nazeer, A. H., Saha, B. P., & Kumar, M. P., (2005). Enhanced therapeutic benefit of quercetin phospholipid complex in carbon tetrachloride-induced acute liver injury in rats: A comparative study. *Iran. J. Pharm. Ther., 4*(2), 80–84.

Maiti, K., Mukherjee, K., Murugan, V., Saha, B. P., & Mukherjee, P. K., (2010). Enhancing bioavailability and hepatoprotective activity of andrographolide from *Andrographis paniculata*, a well known medicinal food, through its herbosome. *J. Sci. Food Agric., 90*(1), 43–51.

Malandrino, S., & Pifferi, G., (1990). IdB-1016Silybin phosphatidylcholine Complex. *Drugs Future., 15*, 226–227.

Malaterre, V., Ogorka, J., Loggia, N., & Gurny, R., (2009). Oral osmotically driven systems: 30 years of development and clinical use.*Eur. J. Pharm. Biopharm., 73*(3), 311–323.

Manach, C., Scalbert, A., Morand, C., Rémésy, C., & Jiménez, L., (2004). Polyphenols: Food sources and bioavailability. *Am. J. Clin. Nutr., 79*(5), 727–747.

Manral, K., Singh, A. K., & Sah, V., (2019). Development and characterization of morin loaded phytosomes for its anti-oxidant activity. *J. Drug Deliv. Ther., 9*(4), 30–36.

Manthena, S., Srinivas, P., & Sadanandam, (2010). Phytosome in Herbal drug delivery. *J. Nat. Pharm., 1*(1), 16.

Mazumder, A., Dwivedi, A., Du Preez, J. L., & Du Plessis, J., (2016). In vitro wound healing and cytotoxic effects of sinigrin-phytosome complex. *Int. J. Pharm., 498*(1, 2), 283–293.

Moscarella, S., Giusti, A., Marra, F., Marena, C., Lampertico, M., Relli, P., & Buzzelli, G., (1993). Therapeutic and anti-lipoperoxidant effects of silybin-phosphatidylcholine complex in chronic liver disease: Preliminary results. *Curr. Ther. Res., 53*(1), 98–102.

Naik, S. R., & Panda, V. S., (2008). Hepatoprotective effect of ginkgoselect phytosome® in rifampicin induced liver injury in rats: Evidence of antioxidant activity. *Fitoterapia., 79*(6), 439–445.

Panda, V. S., & Naik, S. R., (2008). Cardioprotective activity of Ginkgo biloba phytosomes in isoproterenol-induced myocardial necrosis in rats: A biochemical and histoarchitectural evaluation. *Exp. Toxicol. Pathol., 60*(4, 5), 397–404.

Pereira, A., & Mallya, R., (2015). Formulation and evaluation of a photoprotectant cream containing *Phyllanthus emblica* extract-phospholipid complex. *J. Pharmacogn. Phytochem., 4*(2).

Pk, M., & Wahile, A., (2006). Integrated approach towards drug development from Ayurveda and other Indian systems of medicine. *J. Ethnopharmacol., 103*, 25–35.

Raina, H., Soni, G., Jauhari, N., Sharma, N., & Bharadvaja, N., (2014). Phytochemical importance of medicinal plants as potential sources of anticancer agents. *Turk. J. Bot., 38*(6), 1027–1035.

Raju, T. P., Reddy, M. S., & Reddy, V. P., (2011). Phytosomes: A novel phyto-phospholipid carrier for herbal drug delivery. *Int. Res. J. Pharm., 2*(6), 28–33.

Saraf, S., (2010). Applications of novel drug delivery system for herbal formulations. *Fitoterapia, 81*(7), 680–689.

Semalty, A., Semalty, M., Rawat, M. S. M., & Franceschi, F., (2010). Supramolecular phospholipids-polyphenolics interactions: The PHYTOSOME® strategy to improve the bioavailability of phytochemicals. *Fitoterapia., 81*(5), 306–314.

Shalini, S., Kumar, R. R., & Birendra, S., (2015). Antiproliferative effect of phytosome complex of methanolic extract of terminalia arjuna bark on human breast cancer cell lines (MCF-7). *Int. J. Drug. Dev. Res., 7*(1), 173–182.

Sharma, M. D., Morali, D. S., (2005). Phytosome: A review. *Planta Indica.* Cite seer.

Sharma, S., & Roy, R. K., (2010). Phytosomes: An emerging technology. *Int. J. Pharm. Res. Dev., 2*(5), 1–7.

Sumathi, A., & Senthamarai, R., (2015). Design and development of phytosomes containing methanolic extracts of *Nymphaea nouchali* and *Trichosanthes dioica. World J. Pharm. Res.*

Tan, Q., Liu, S., Chen, X., Wu, M., Wang, H., Yin, H., & Zhang, J., (2012). Design and evaluation of a novel evodiamine-phospholipid complex for improved oral bioavailability. *AAPS PharmSciTech., 13*(2), 534–547.

Yu, F., Li, Y., Chen, Q., He, Y., Wang, H., Yang, L., & Xue, M., (2016). Monodisperse microparticles loaded with the self-assembled berberine-phospholipid complex-based phytosomes for improving oral bioavailability and enhancing hypoglycemic efficiency. *Eur. J. Pharm. Biopharm., 103*, 136–148.

Zhang, J., Tang, Q., Xu, X., & Li, N., (2013). Development and evaluation of a novel phytosome-loaded chitosan microsphere system for curcumin delivery. *Int. J. Pharm., 448*(1), 168–174.

CHAPTER 14

SYNTHETIC SEEDS *VIS-A-VIS* CRYOPRESERVATION: AN EFFICIENT TECHNIQUE FOR LONG-TERM PRESERVATION OF ENDANGERED MEDICINAL PLANTS

MD. NASIM ALI[1] and SYANDAN SINHA RAY[2]

[1]*Department of Agricultural Biotechnology, Faculty of Agriculture, Bidhan Chandra KrishiViswavidyalaya, Mahanpur, Nadia, West Bengal, India, E-mail: nasimali2007@gmail.com*

[2]*IRDM Faculty Center, Ramakrishna Mission Vivekananda Educational and Research Institute, Ramakrishna Mission Ashrama, Narendrapur, Kolkata – 700103, West Bengal, India*

ABSTRACT

Medicinal plants are the primary source of pharmaceutical products. These plants have become a soft target of pharmaceutical industries due to their economic and medicinal value. Ignorance and mismanagement lead to the destruction of natural sources of these medicinal plant. Therefore, conservation is mostly needed to keep these valuable plant resources alive. Conservation may be done following *ex-situ* and *in-situ* methods. *In vitro* conservation method is much more advantageous and cost-effective since it requires less space. Contamination-free long-term preservation is possible through cryopreservation. Nevertheless, the major problem is the toxicity of cryoprotectant on the plant sample, which may be overcome by using synthetic seed. As the plant samples are protected by artificial beads, it could be easy for inter-laboratories exchange of germplasm avoiding mechanical injury. The presence of artificial endosperm in synthetic seed provides proper nutrition to the growing plant material. This chapter focuses on different factors affecting synthetic seed production as well as its importance in germplasm conservation with special reference to endangered medicinal plants.

14.1 INTRODUCTION

According to WHO (World Health Organization), plants contain/synthesize any curative compounds essentially required to manufacture the useful drugs are called medicinal plants (Banu and Nagarajan, 2014). These plants are the major resource for therapeutic drugs. Presently, the demand for medicinal plants is increasing due to the overdoing of herbal drugs and /or medicinal products over the globe (Cole et al., 2007; Chen et al., 2016). Pharmaceutical industries thereby are intensifying both the quantity and quality of these plants. India holds rank second after China to export medical plants of about 32,600 tons to all over the world (Dhar et al., 2000).

The modern agriculture reinstates landraces with high yielding varieties in the agricultural system (Altieri and Merrick, 1987). Besides, deforestation, industrialization, and urbanization, results in the reduction of plant species related to key sources of economically and agronomically important traits/genes. Due to such activities, the annual loss of forest land is about 15 million hectares (Rao, 2004). As a result, several plant species including medicinal plants are now likely to be extinct in the future. The red list of IUCN (International Union for Conservation of Nature) is a global diversity indicator that highlights the endangered species. During 1996–2004, more than 8,000 plant species were included in the red list of IUCN (http://lib. riskreductionafrica.org/bitstream/handle/123456789/423/a%20global%20 species%20assessment.%202004.pdf?sequence=1).

According to Botanical Survey of India (BSI), 53 species out of 8,000 medicinal plants are under threatened categories in India (http://pib.nic.in/ newsite/PrintRelease.aspx?relid=137143). Improper management and ignorance lead to a reduction in the natural resources of these endangered plant species and create imbalance between demand and supply.

14.1.1 IMPORTANCE OF GERMPLASM CONSERVATION

Plant germplasm is a set of existing cells from which new plants can be generated. Loss of germplasm results loss of genetic resources from nature. Hence the basic challenge of germplasm conservation is to keep the germplasm in its native form (Miller, 1993). The agricultural productivity of a single plant variety may be under risk when it solely covers a huge area. To overcome this problem, agronomists, and plant biologists have attempted to store germplasms so that plant breeders will use these germplasm for improvement of plants in the future (Plucknett et al., 1983). The concept of "germplasm conservation" does not only to keep balance in agro-biodiversity in nature (Benito et al., 2004) but also to keep them alive for future purposes.

14.1.2   CONSERVATION METHODS

Effective conservation of germplasm depends upon several factors such as physiological status of germplasm, storage methods, and techniques (Villalobos and Engelmann, 1995). In a broad sense, the germplasm is conserved either through *in situ* or *ex-situ* conservation methods.

14.1.2.1   IN SITU CONSERVATION

The conservation of germplasm under its natural habitat (Paunescu, 2009) by creating reserved forests, biosphere reserves, eco-parks, etc. (Siddiqui and Shukla, 2015) are termed as *in situ* conservation. *In situ* conservation allows the conservation of ecosystems and natural habitats. It also maintains and recovers the viable populations of species in their natural surroundings (https://www.cbd.int/convention/articles/default.shtml?a=cbd-02) which is more applicable for the conservation of landraces (Engelmann and Engels, 2002). *In situ* conservation may be done in following ways depending upon the mode of practices and situations, i.e., either: (i) preserve the landraces in a farmhouse under natural environment through traditional ways of culti-vation; or (ii) on-farm conservation of the germplasm using support from sponsoring agency (Brush, 1999). So, traditional endogenous knowledge on local germplasm may play a significant role to conserve the germplasm under their natural habitat. Since the objective of conservation is to keep the present genetic structure intact and, thus, *in situ* conservation is usually the preferred form of conservation than other conservation methods (McIlwrick et al., 2000). But the major constrains of the *in-situ* conservation method is the loss of wild areas (Engelmann, 1991). A combined approach of G.B. Pant Institute of Himalayan Environment and Development, Department of Forest and several agencies have been reported for *in situ* conservation of endangered medicinally important plants such as *Aconitum heterophyllum*,

Podophyllum hexandrum, *Picrorhiza kurroa* in Sikkim Himalaya (Rai et al., 2000). Conservation of endangered medicinal plant *Coptis teeta* through *in situ* conservation was suggested by Pandit and Babu (1998) because of its specific microsite requirement.

14.1.2.2   EX SITU CONSERVATIONS

In this method the germplasm is conserved out of its natural habitat (Paunescu, 2009). *Ex-situ* conservation permits the conservation of crops and their wild types (Engelmann and Engels, 2002). It is the only way to conserve the germplasm where *in situ* conservation does not possible. Plants species having a low population or restricted to small geographic locations or facing its alarming stage (due to human activity and abiotic factors), or quite diverse from its taxonomical common plant species are most appropriate for *ex situ* conservation (Cochrane et al., 2007). Problems during storage and poor emphasis on minor crops having multipurpose importance for the improvement of germplasm are common drawbacks of *ex situ* conservation (Altieri and Merrick, 1987).

In *ex situ* conservation, plant germplasm is conserved through several methods such as *seed storage, botanical garden, field genebank, pollen storage, DNA storage*, and *in vitro storage* method (Engelmann and Engels, 2002). All these conservations and its types with special reference to endangered medicinal plants are discussed in subsections.

14.1.2.2.1   Seed Bank

One of the most convenient ways of long-term *ex situ* conservation is storing the seed under low moisture and temperature (Paunescu, 2009). In a seed bank, the storage of seeds is carried under the cold and dry conditions to sustain the viability of seeds (Schoen and Brown, 2001). This method is the easiest and inexpensive conservation method (Phartyal et al., 2002). Seeds as "storing material" are gainful for their small size which can be easily distributed and transported from place to place. But it is restricted to 'Orthodox seed' as 'recalcitrant seeds' are unable to survive under low temperature and desiccation (Engelmann and Engel, 2002). This conservation technique provides quick access to plant samples for research work, also permits researchers to get information which could be helpful to conserve the remaining germplasm of plant sample and finally plants conserved in seed banks are free from territory demolition, diseases, and predators (Schoen and Brown, 2001). The duration of seed bank-based conservation depends on temperature and moisture content of seed (Roberts, 1972; Rao and Jackson, 1996). Seed based storage of endemic medicinal plants, i.e., *Hypericum sinaicum* and *Plantago sinaica* for long-duration were reported by Moustafa et al. (2015).

14.1.2.2.2 Botanical Garden

Plant seeds that are not feasibly stored under seed bank may be conserved through the botanical garden (Dulloo et al., 1998) which plays an important role in the conservation of plants (Li et al., 2002). In addition to conservation, another advantage of the botanical garden is its influential capacity to increase public awareness regarding the conservation, utility, and importance of plant species (Hurka, 1994). The fundamental principle depends in growing the plants under the greenhouse or out of door or conservatories. They are used to grow and display plants primarily for scientific and educational purposes (Kasso and Balakrishnan, 2013). However, this conservation method permits the conservation of a small number of plant samples (Brütting et al., 2013). For conservation of small population major constrains are genetic drift and inbreeding depression (Francisco-Ortega et al., 2000). The combined approach of the Tropical Botanic Garden and Research Institute, Trivandrum has developed a gene pool of 650 medicinal plant species (Heywood, 1991). Earth Ethnobotanic Garden of Costa Rica was developed to conserve and analyze the potential use of medicinal plants (Waylen, 2006).

14.1.2.2.3 Pollen Bank

Pollen bank stores pollen at 4°C to −20°C for short term (Hanna and Towill, 1995) or at −149°C in liquid nitrogen (cryopreservation) for long term storage (Bajaj, 1987). The report on the cryopreservation of pollen of the germplasm is very less. Cryopreservation of pollen for one week of endangered medicinal plants, i.e., *Celastrus paniculatus*, *Oroxylum indicum* were reported by Rajasekharan et al. (2013). Though the small size of pollen makes itself suitable for storage purposes (Borokini, 2013) but this conservation permits conservation of half of the whole genome of germplasm (Wang et al., 1993). Their short viability in comparison to seed, make pollen conservation method limited for large scale plant germplasm conservation (Hoekstra, 1995).

14.1.2.2.4   Field Gene Bank

Field gene bank permits conservation of "recalcitrant" plant species (Noor et al., 2011). Hence, clones are multiplied and preserved in the organized form (i.e., trees, roots, tubers, corms, etc.). This type of conservation allows visual evaluation of plants that are grown in the field. Hence the continuation of germplasm under field gene banks method is labor-intensive and costly (Kartha, 1985; Jarret and Florkowski, 1990). Plants are difficult to maintain, and due to their presence in an open environment, they are susceptible to disease, which may be considered as a major threat for the germplasm being conserved (Withers, 1991).

14.1.2.2.5   DNA Bank

DNA is the coding language of life that can be stored. Here, the total genomic DNA of germplasm is used as storage materials. Due to the advent of molecular biology techniques, DNA storage is considered as complementary to *ex-situ* conservation (Kasso and Balakrishnan, 2013). In terms of applicability, this method overcomes all the above-mentioned restrictions stated earlier for other conservation methods. Dried DNA samples in small vials can also be stored for an indefinite period without any damage. Since DNA has less weight, requires less space to store, it permits the easiest way of transferring germplasm from place to another (Vijayan et al., 2011). To conserve a good quality sample after isolation, it is always mandatory to quantify the sample DNA prior to conservation. However, this technique is expensive.

14.1.2.2.6   In Vitro Conservation

Plant tissue culture is *in vitro* cultivation of cell, tissue or organ in a defined media under aseptic condition (Thorpe, 2007). A large number of pathogen-free plants can be regenerated from a single source through the *in vitro* propagation method (Cruz-Cruz et al., 2013). Besides clonal propagation, *in vitro* propagation permits the conservation of germplasm for a reasonable duration. This approach of conservation has gained importance because of its wider application, cost-effectiveness, and least requirement of space (Matsumoto, 2001). *In vitro* conservation of germplasm can be done either for short-mid term or long-term storage (Villalobos et al., 1991). The basic principle for short-mid-term storage under *in vitro* condition is to slow down the growth rate of the plant (Kaviani, 2011).

On the contrary, cryopreservation is the most widely used method for long-term storage of germplasm under *ex-situ* condition at ultra-low temperature (–150 to –196°C) using liquid nitrogen (Chudhury and Malik, 2004). This is the only method to ensure the safe and cost-efficient long-term conservation of various types of plants (Engelmann, 2011). This method has been widely used for long time conservation because the metabolic activity of cells, cell divisions are ceased at an ultra-low temperature as well as there is no scope of any genetic modification which may happen during when they are maintained by serial subculturing (Cruz-Cruz et al., 2013). Optimum responses of plant propagules after cryopreservation are depending on the status of the plant, cryopreservation techniques and re-growth conditions (Uchendu and Reed, 2008). A convenient way of cryopreservation leads to the formation of ice and increases the solute concentration within the cell which causes cell damage. To counter this problem, cryoprotectants are used to reduce the amount of ice that crystallizes at any given temperature and thereby limit the solute concentration factor (Fahy et al., 1984).

14.2   CRYOPRESERVATION

Cryopreservation may be done through either conventional method (freeze induced dehydration: slow cooling to –40°C followed by immersion in liquid nitrogen) or vitrification (elimination of freezable water by dehydration followed by ultra-rapid freezing to prevent ice crystals) (Rao, 2004). Cryo-preservation technique is broadly subdivided into the following subsections.

14.2.1   SLOW FREEZING

Slow freezing is known as equilibrium freezing due to the exchange of fluids between the extra- and intracellular spaces and results in safe freezing without serious osmotic and deformation effects to cells (Mazur, 1990). The slow freezing method at the initial stage replaced the intercellular water content with cryoprotectants to reduce cell damage and adjust the cooling rate in accordance with the permeability of the cell membrane (Jang et al., 2017). This technique is considered as a safe procedure, because of the use of relatively low concentration of cryoprotectants, which makes the procedure less toxic and reduces the scope of osmotic damage (Valojerdi et al., 2009). Basic problems of preservation under refrigerator are its high cost, samples have limited shelf life and they are susceptible to contamination (Karlsson and Toner, 1996).

14.2.2   VITRIFICATION

In this method, the concentrated aqueous solution converted into a glassy state instead of ice crystal within the tissue at a sufficiently low tempera-ture (Engelmann, 1991). Use of vitrification for cryopreservation was first invented by Luyet in 1937 (Kalita et al., 2012). The objective of the vitrification-based method is preventing ice crystallization within the cell using cryoprotectants. These cryoprotectants are termed as "vitrification solution" in the presence of which, cells can be cooled down to below the glass transition temperature without appreciable ice formation (Fahy et al., 1987). Basic factors for effective vitrification in cells are: concentrations of cryoprotectants, dehydration of cells and rapid freezing rate (El-Danasouri and Selman, 2005). During the vitrification method, the glassy state is achieved through increasing cellular liquid content viscosity followed by the fast cooling of the system (Pinto et al., 2016). Cell dehydration prior to rapid cooling is done by exposing the sample to concentrated cryoprotective media or airflow to avoid intracellular ice formation (Dixit et al., 2004). So, there is less chance of ice-related injury within the cell in comparison to the slow freezing method and there is no need for any programed freezer (Tavukcuoglu et al., 2012). The most widely used vitri-fication solutions are PVS2 (consists of glycerol, ethylene glycol, dimethyl sulfoxide, sucrose), PVS3 (consists of glycerol and sucrose, basal culture medium) (Sakai and Engelmann, 2007). Vitrification method is further modified into encapsulation vitrification-involves use of encapsulating media to encapsulate the plant sample. Osmoprotectants are already added in encapsulating media for the treatment of osmoprotective chemicals such as sugars (Tanaka et al., 2004). Another modified version of vitrifica-tion is droplet vitrification. In droplet vitrification, plant samples treated with vitrification solutions are put as drop-in aluminum foil followed by immersion in liquid nitrogen. Due to the presence of fewer amounts of cryoprotectants, it permits rapid cooling/warming during the process of cryopreservation (Sakai and Engelmann, 2007). Direct exposure of plant samples to a high concentration of vitrification solutions may damage the sample due to the toxic effect of vitrification solutions (Matsumoto et al., 2001). Reports based on vitrification-based conservation are very less in compared to encapsulated vitrification (Discuss later). Vitrification based conservation of shoot tip using PVS2 was reported for endangered medicinal plant *Picrorrhiza kurroa Royle ex Benth* (Sharma and Sharma, 2003); *Centaurea ultreiae* (Compositae) (Mallón et al., 2008). Another study based on vitrification-based conservation reported for *in vitro* shoot tips of *Dioscorea deltoidea* WALL (Mandal and Dixit-Sharma, 2007).

14.2.3   DEHYDRATION

In dehydration method, explants (plant part used to initiate the *in vitro* culture) are dehydrated using a high concentration of osmoticum followed by dehydration under sterile air. In general, dehydration of samples pretreated with a high concentration of osmoticum (sucrose in most of the cases) is done using laminar airflow. Sucrose is commonly used to induce dehydration and freezing tolerance in the cell, is also commonly used as a cryoprotectant (Dumet et al., 1993). Among the sugars, sucrose was found effective to enhance resistance against dehydration during the storage of banana under glucose and fructose under liquid nitrogen (Helliot et al., 2002). Preculturing the sample with a high concentration of sucrose was found effective for cryopreservation of shoot tips of several plant species (Matsumoto et al., 1994; Pennycooke and Towill, 2000). This method is also modified into encapsulation dehydration. In this method before immersion to liquid nitrogen, the encapsulated explants are precultured in media having a high sugar level to improve the resistance capacity against dehydration and freezing under liquid nitrogen (Shatnawi and Johnson, 2004).

14.3   SYNTHETIC SEED

Synthetic seed technology is considered as an alternative option for *in situ* conservation (Baskaran et al., 2015). Alginate-encapsulation of plant organs has been used to produce synthetic seeds, has gained interest as a tool for storage of germplasm as well as conservation, and direct distribution of planting materials for propagation (Germana et al., 2011). Synthetic seed-based conservation has several disadvantages such as it is relatively difficult to get a viable seed after long term storage, while lack of oxygen inside the matrix, production of phenolics/secondary plant metabolites may interfere with the growth of plant propagule (Pehwal et al., 2013). Despite these problems, this technology is considered as one of the promising parts of plant tissue culture because of advantages such as its cost-effectiveness and transportable capacity (Zych et al., 2005). Since these synthetic seeds are alternative to natural seeds but non-zygotic in nature, so they are "converted" instead of "germinated" under proper conditions (Adriani et al., 2000). Because of this advantage, the synthetic seed has gained the attention of the researchers in the early 1980s.

14.3.1 SYNTHETIC SEED: HISTORICAL BACKGROUND

The concept of "synthetic seed" or "artificial seed" was first proposed by Murashige in 1977 (Reddy et al., 2012). According to Murashige (1978), the artificial seed is defined as "an encapsulated single somatic embryo" (https://www.biotecharticles.com/Agriculture-Article/What-are-Synthetic-Seeds-Their-Need-Uses-and-Types-3315.html). At earlier stage, purpose of this technique was to use the somatic embryo as "seed material" for storage and transport of plant materials without any difficulty. This definition was again modified by Bapat et al. (1987) as the encapsulation of "*in vitro*-derived propagules" instead of somatic embryos. The addition of the term "*in vitro*-derived propagules" has become a major breakthrough for this technique as it removes the restriction on "type of explants to be used for the production of synthetic seed." The most updated definition was given by Aitken-Christie et al. (1995) as "artificially encapsulated somatic embryos, shoots or other tissues which can be used for sowing under *in vitro* or *ex vitro* condi-tions." In the modern era of tissue culture, *in vitro* derived shoot tips have gained an attractive option for synthetic seed production because of high mitotic activity in the apical meristem (Ballester et al., 1997). To date, the protocol for synthetic seed production is standardized for several medicinal plant species by scientists/researchers using different types of explants (in most cases, explants types are restricted to shoot tips, nodes, or somatic embryos; Table 14.1).

TABLE 14.1 Types of Explants in Synthetic Seed Production for Endangered Medicinal Plants

Type of Explants	Plants
Cotyledon: *Arnebia euchroma* (Manjkhola et al., 2005)	
Microshoot: *Picrorhiza kurrooa* (Mishra et al., 2011); *Rauvolfia serpentina* (Faisal et al., 2012); *Rauvolfia tetraphylla* (Alatar and Faisal, 2012).	
Shoot tip: *Cineraria maritime* (Srivastava et al., 2009)	
Somatic embryo	*Tylophora indica* (Burm.f.) Merrill (Devendra et al., 2011); *Swertia chirayita* (Kumar and Chandra, 2014); *Rhinacanthus nasutus* (L.) Kurz. (Cheruvathur et al., 2013); *Clitoria ternatea* Linn (Kumar and Thomas, 2012); *Mondia whitei* (Baskaran et al., 2015)
Node	*Bacopa monnieri* (L.) (Ramesh et al., 2009);
	Tylophora indica (Burm. f.) Merrill (Faisal and Anis. 2007);
	Cineraria maritima (Srivastava et al., 2009)

14.3.2 TYPES OF SYNTHETIC SEEDS

Synthetic seed may be either hydrated or desiccated in nature. The first hydrated synthetic seed was developed by Redenbaugh et al. (1984) for alfalfa and celery while desiccated synthetic seed was developed by Kitto and Janick (1985) for carrot (Ara et al., 2000). The hydrated artificial seeds are made up of encapsulating plant materials in hydrogel coats while the desiccated seeds are either naked or encapsulated in polyoxyethylene glycol followed by its desiccation (Kikowska and Thiem, 2011). Desiccation may be done either slowly over a period of one or two weeks sequentially decreasing relative humidity or rapidly by unsealing the petri dishes and leaving them on the bench overnight to dry under airflow. These types of synthetic seeds are prepared for desiccation tolerance while encapsulated seeds are produced for desiccation susceptible plants (Ara et al., 2000).

14.3.3 BASIC COMPONENTS OF SYNTHETIC SEED

Structurally, synthetic seeds are capsules with a gel envelope containing plant materials (Vdovitchenoko and Kuzovkina, 2011). In synthetic seed, the plant materials are protected by a protective coat, i.e., "bead." The addition of the coating agent over the plant sample provides stability and protects the plant material from external damage during handling (Ravi and Anand, 2012). Alginate is reported as the most effective and suitable coating agent among several other gelling agents (agar, polyco 2133, carboxymethyl cellulose, carrageenan, gelrite (Kelko. Co.), guargum, sodium pectate, etc.), for preparation of synthetic seed (Saiprasad, 2001). Biochemically this chemical is polymers of β-D-mannuronic and α-L-gluronic acids, extracted from brown algae (Helmiyati and Aprilliza, 2017). Alginate is anionic in nature and widely used for gelling purposes because of several advantages such as biocompatibility, less toxicity, less expensive and mild gelation by the addition of divalent cations such as Ca^{2+} (Lee and Mooney, 2012). Formation of bead is depending upon the ionic exchange between the Na^+ of sodium alginate with Ca^{2+} of calcium chloride solution (sodium alginate droplets containing the somatic embryos/any *in vitro* derived plant propagule form round and firm bead in presence of calcium chloride).

14.3.3.1   ROLE OF CALCIUM CHLORIDE AND SODIUM ALGINATE IN SYNTHETIC SEED FORMATION

Effects of sodium alginate and calcium chloride on synthetic seed production have been studied elaborately to date. Major influential parameters for generating effective beads are considered to be the concentration and polymerization time of both of these chemicals. In general, most of the cases, 3% sodium alginate coupled with 100 mM of calcium chloride are found to be most effective and promising for the production of synthetic seed for several plant species, i.e., *Rauvolfia tetraphylla* L. (Faisal et al., 2006); *Tylophora indica (Burm. f.) Merrill* (Faisal and Anis, 2007); *Cassia angustifolia* VAHL (Bukhari et al., 2014). Concentrations of both of these chemicals are also subjected to change for getting optimum response as suggested by findings of Andlib et al. (2011) for *Stevia rebaudiana* Bertoni; Haque et al. (2015) for *Bacopa chamaedryoides*.

14.3.3.1.1   Effects of Concentration

Fragile seed coat was obtained through a low concentration of sodium alginate during synthetic seed production of *Cassia angustifolia* VAHL (Bukhari et al., 2014). This may be due to loss of solidifying capacity of alginate (at low concentration) because of autoclaving prior to use (Larkin et al.,1988; Faisal and Anis, 2007). Beads prepared using high concentrations (4–5%) of sodium alginate were found hard in nature and delayed the germination/ shoot emergence (Singh et al., 2009). A similar study was conducted for medicinal plant *Catharanthus roseus* (L.) G. Don by Maqsood et al. (2012). They found a combination of 2.5% sodium alginate and 100 mM calcium chloride was most effective among the selected concentrations of calcium chloride and sodium alginate for generating suitable isodiametric beads. 75 mM calcium chloride and 2.5% sodium alginate were suitable to form uniform isodiametric beads for *Rauvolfia serpentina* (L.) Benth. ex Kurz (Gantait et al., 2017).

14.3.3.1.2 *Effect of Polymerization Time*

Duration of polymerization of both of these chemicals (sodium alginate and calcium chloride) during synthetic seed production is also considered as the decisive factor to get the good and proper shape of synthetic seed as suggested by several authors. Shape, as well as germination rate, is also affected by the polymerization duration. This time period may also vary from plant to plant. In most of the cases, time duration ranges from 15–45 minutes depending upon the concentration of both sodium alginate and calcium chloride as well as the status of plant propagule. Long time exposure of beads of sodium alginate under calcium chloride made the beads hard and toxic. Exposure of 2.5% sodium alginate coated embryo in 100 mM calcium chloride for 15 minutes formed firm, uniform, and round beads with respect to more or less than 15 minutes of polymerization for *Catharanthus roseus* (L.) G. Don (Maqsood et al., 2012). Though Lata et al. (2009) found effective beads after 30 minutes of polymerization time for 50 mM calcium chloride and 5% sodium alginate for *Cannabis sativa* L. So, both the concentration as well as the polymerization time of both of above-mentioned chemicals influence the formation of synthetic seed. Using both of these chemicals, synthetic seeds are generated for several plant species, for example, Cassava (Danso and Ford-Lloyd, 2003); *Paulownia elongates* (Ipekci and Gozukirmizi, 2003); *Withania somnifera* (Singh et al., 2006); *Olea europaea* L. cv. Moraiolo (Micheli et al., 2007); *Tylophora indica (Burm. f.) Merrill* (Faisal and Anis, 2007); *Clitoria ternatea* (Kumar and Thomas, 2012); *Cassia angustifolia* VAHL (Bukhari et al., 2014); *Centella asiatica* (L.) (Prasad et al., 2014).

In addition to coating agents, artificial endosperm (made up of nutrients, plant growth regulators, carbon source, etc.), is provided to plant materials to support its sprouting and rooting or its conversion to whole plants (Helal, 2011). In addition to growth regulators, vitamins to the medium were found effective for the high rate of germination of synthetic seed (Kumar et al.,

2005). Among the carbon sources, sucrose is most widely used though it depends on explants type. Huda et al. (2007) found sucrose as an effective carbon source during encapsulation of nodal explants while sucrose: sorbitol (1:1) was effective for encapsulation of somatic embryo of eggplant. The addition of root induction treatment to explants prior to encapsulation was found effective for earliest germination, i.e., formation of root from encapsulating explants as suggested by Chand and Singh (2004) for *Dalbergia Sissoo* Roxb.

14.4   ENCAPSULATION BASED CONSERVATION

Zygotic embryos are desiccated during its maturation phase and remain viable during its dormant stage. Since somatic embryo (regenerated through plant tissue culture) has a similar morphology to zygotic embryo (except cotyledon), if they are modified to follow such mechanism (inactive for some time), then they may act as the true seed in terms of storage for certain duration (Senaratna, 1990). Based on this principle, the desiccated synthetic seed of carrot was prepared by Kitto and Janick (1985) using the gelling agent "polyex" wafer (Janick et al., 1989).

Encapsulation of explants using alginate for cryopreservation has several advantages such as it reduces the chance of mechanical injury and oxidative stress as well as comparatively easier in handling in comparison to non-encapsulated ones (Niino and Sakai, 1992; Suzuki et al., 2005). The synthetic seed has accepted a suitable material for the storage of germplasm because of its small size. Besides, a synthetic seed-based approach for germplasm conservation is inexpensive and easily transportable in nature (Zych et al., 2005). These facts strongly suggested that the encapsulated explants are most preferred material forcryopreservation.

14.4.1   EXPLANT TYPES FOR GERMPLASM CONSERVATION THROUGH SYNTHETIC-BASED APPROACH

Response of encapsulated materials during cryopreservation is explant specific. Different types of explants have been reported for that purpose. For storage of germplasm, "shoot tips" is a viable choice as Castillo et al. (2010) found shoot tips were genetically more stable than somatic embryos for cryopreservation using the molecular markers. Because of its availability all over the year as well as easy to cultivate and cryoprotective treatment can be applied to *in vitro* grown tip, shoot tip of the plant is a desirable choice for cryopreservation (Benelli et al., 2016). Cryopreservation of meristem is considered as the best choice for long term storage because of stable phenotypic and genotypic uniqueness of stored germplasm (https://www.nap.edu/read/2116/chapter/11).

14.4.2   ENCAPSULATION BASED CRYOPRESERVATION TECHNIQUES

Storage of encapsulated plant materials in most of the cases done through either of encapsulation vitrification or encapsulation dehydration method.

14.4.2.1   ENCAPSULATION VITRIFICATION

The basic principle of vitrification is based on converting the cellular water level to an amorphous state to avoid the ice crystallization within the cell (Halmagyi et al., 2010). But basic problems of vitrification method are chemical toxicity, i.e., long exposure of plant materials under vitrification solution may be adversely affected due to toxicity of chemicals (Lambardi et al., 2000). So, in practical view dehydration method is less toxic compared to the vitrification method of cryopreservation. In spite of this problem, encapsulation vitrification-based conservation is reported for several plant species, i.e., *Eruca sativa* Mill., *Astragalus membranaceus* and *Gentiana macrophylla* Pall using hairy roots (Xue et al., 2008); *Dioscorea bulbifera* L using embryogenic callus (Ming-Hua and Sen-Rong, 2010).

14.4.2.2   ENCAPSULATION DEHYDRATION

Cryopreservation through encapsulation-dehydration based method was first reported by Fabre and Dereuddre (1990) for *Solanum phureja* (See Gonzalez-Arnao and Engelmann (2006). The encapsulation-dehydration technique is easy to handle and simplifies the dehydration process (Niino and Sakai, 1992). It is based on the encapsulation of plant material followed by the treatment of a high concentration of sucrose and desiccation of the sample under sterile air and finally immersed in liquid nitrogen (Reed et al., 2005). This method has high survivability than the conventional method of cryopreservation (Villalobos and Engelmann, 1995). That may be due to the presence of a bead over the sample that protects the sample from liquid nitrogen (Martinez and Revilla, 1999). The basic advantages of this technique are the use of nontoxic cryoprotectants and explants are protected from damage during dehydration (Verleysen et al., 2005). From all of these aspects, anyone can prefer encapsulation dehydration to get toxic-free plant germplasm conservation because of the simplicity of this technique. Encapsulation-dehydration based approach using different explants reported by several authors such as *Siberian ginseng* using somatic embryo (Choi and Jeong, 2002); axillary shoot meristems for *Indigofera tinctoria* (L.) (Nair and Reghunath, 2009); shoot tip for *Rabdosia rubescens* (Ai et al., 2012).

14.5   CONCLUSION

Endangered medicinal plants, the valuable gift from nature is present in its alarming stage. So, conservation of these plant germplasm is most essential to keep it live on earth. Though *in situ* conservation is advantageous over other conservation methods but the basic problem is lack of land. Among *ex situ* conservation, *in vitro* conservation permits conservation of large-scale germplasm within short space. The synthetic seed-based approach of germplasm conservation is most widely popular due to the simplicity of this technique as well as transportable nature. The addition of artificial endosperm provides the food while the seed coat protects the plant material from external damage. The problem of hard seed coat may be overcome using the treatment of potassium nitrate to increase the germination rate. From this point of view, coupled application of both of these techniques (synthetic seed and cryopreservation) makes the conservation technique easy and economically viable since plant propagules can be stored at minimum space. So, these techniques have a bright future and can play a significant role in germplasm conservation of endangered medicinal plants.

KEYWORDS

- **conservations**
- **cryopreservation**
- **ex-situ**
- **in situ**
- **medicinal plants**
- **synthetic seed**

REFERENCES

Adriani, M., Piccioni, E., & Standard, A., (2000). Effect of different treatments on the conversion of 'Hayward' kiwifruit synthetic seeds to whole plants following encapsulation of *in vitro*-derived buds. *New Zeal. J. Crop. Hort., 28*, 59–67.

Ai, P. F., Lu, L. P., & Song, J. J., (2012). Cryopreservation of *in vitro*-grown shoot-tips of *Rabdosia rubescens* by encapsulation-dehydration and evaluation of their genetic stability. *Plant Cell Tissue Organ Cult., 108*(3), 381–387.

Aitken-Christie, J., Kozai, T., & Takayama, S., (1995). *Automation in plant tissue culture— general introduction and overview*. In: Aitken-Christie, J., Kozai, T., & Smith M. A. L., (eds.), *Automation and Environmental Control in Plant Tissue Culture* (pp. 1–18). Springer, Netherlands.

Alatar, A. A., & Faisal, M., (2012). Encapsulation of *Rauvolfia tetraphylla* micro shorts as artificial seeds and evaluation of genetic fidelity using RAPD and ISSR markers. *J. Med. Plant Res., 6*(7), 1367–1374.

Altieri, M. A., & Merrick, L., (1987). *In situ* conservation of crop genetic resources through maintenance of traditional farming systems. *Eco. Bot., 41*(1), 86–96.

Andlib, A., Verma, R. N., & Batra, A., (2011). Synthetic seeds an alternative source for quick regeneration of a zero-calorie herb-*Stevia rebaudiana* bertoni. *J. Pharm. Res., 4*(7), 2007–2009.

Ara, H., Jaiswal, U., & Jaiswal, V. S., (2000). Synthetic seed: Prospects and limitations. *Curr. Sci., 78*(12), 1438–1444.

Bajaj, Y. P. S., (1987). Cryopreservation of pollen and pollen embryos, and the establishment of pollen banks. In: Giles, K. L., & Prakash, J., (eds.), *Pollen Cytology and Development-International Review of Cytology* (Vol. 107, p 397–420). Academic Press, INC: Orlando, Florida.

Ballester, A., Janeiro, L. V., & Vieitez, A. M., (1997). Cold storage of shoot cultures and alginate encapsulation of shoot tips of *Camellia japonica* L. and *Camellia reticulata* Lindley. *Sci. Hort., 71*(1, 2), 67–78.

Banu, H. R., & Nagarajan, N., (2014). Phytochemical investigation of *Wedelia chinensis* (Osbeck.) Merrill. *International Journal of Pharmaceutical and Chemical Sciences, 3*(1), 40–46.

Bapat, V. A., Mhatre, M., & Rao, P. S., (1987). Propagation of *Morus indica* L.(mulberry) by encapsulated shoot buds. *Plant Cell Rep., 6*(5), 393–395.

Baskaran, P., Kumari, A., & Van, S. J., (2015). Embryogenesis and synthetic seed production in *Mondia whitei. Plant Cell Tissue Organ Cult., 121*(1), 205–214.

Benelli, C., (2016). Encapsulation of shoot tips and nodal segments for *in vitro* storage of "Kober 5BB" grapevine rootstock. *Horticulturae., 2*(3), 10. https://www.mdpi.com/2311-7524/2/3/10/htm (accessed on 01 November 2021).

Benito, M. G., Clavero-Ramírez, I., & López-Aranda, J. M., (2004). The use of cryopreservation for germplasm conservation of vegetatively propagated crops. *Span. J. Agric. Res., 2*(3), 341–351.

Borokini, T. I., (2013). The state of *ex-situ* conservation in Nigeria. *Int. J. Conserv. Sci., 4*(2), 197–212.

Brush, S. B., (1999). *The issues of in situ conservation of crop genetic resources*. In: *Genes in the Field. On-Farm Conservation of Crop Diversity* (pp. 3–26). Brush S.B., Ed.; IPGRI, IDRC, Lewis Publishers, Boca Raton.

Brütting, C., Hensen, I., & Wesche, K., (2013). *Ex-situ* cultivation affects genetic structure and diversity in arable plants. *Plant Biol., 15*(3), 505–513.

Bukhari, N., Siddique, I., Perveen, K., Siddiqui, I., & Alwahibi, M., (2014). Synthetic seed production and physio-biochemical studies in *Cassia angustifolia* vahl. —a medicinal plant. *Acta Biol. Hung., 65*(3), 355–367.

Castillo, N. R. F., Bassil, N. V., Wada, S., & Reed, B. M., (2010). Genetic stability of cryopreserved shoot tips of Rubus germplasm. *In vitro Cell Dev. Biol. Plant., 46*(3), 246–256.

Chand, S., & Singh, A. K., (2004). Plant regeneration from encapsulated nodal segments of *Dalbergia sissoo* roxb., a timber-yielding leguminous tree species. *J. Plant Physiol., 161*(2), 237–243.

Chaudhury, R., & Malik, S. K., (2004). Genetic conservation of plantation crops and spices using cryopreservation. *Indian J. Biotechnol., 3*, 348–358.

Chen, S. L., Yu, H., Luo, H. M., Wu, Q., Li, C. F., & Steinmetz, A., (2016). Conservation and sustainable use of medicinal plants: Problems, progress, and prospects. *Chinese Medicine, 11*, 37. https://cmjournal.biomedcentral.com/articles/10.1186/s13020-016-0108-7 (accessed on 01 November 2021).

Cheruvathur, M. K., Kumar, G. K., & Thomas, T. D., (2013). Somatic embryogenesis and synthetic seed production in *Rhinacanthus nasutus* (L.) Kurz. *Plant Cell Tissue Organ Cult., 113*(1), 63–71.

Choi, Y., & Jeong, J., (2002). Dormancy induction of somatic embryos of *Siberian ginseng* by high sucrose concentrations enhances the conservation of hydrated artificial seeds and dehydration resistance. *Plant Cell Rep., 20*(12), 1112–1116.

Cochrane, J. A., Crawford, A. D., & Monks, L. T., (2007). The significance of *ex-situ* seed conservation to reintroduction of threatened plants. *Aust. J. Bot., 55*(3), 356–361.

Cole, I. B., Saxena, P. K., & Murch, S. J., (2007). Medicinal biotechnology in the genus *Scutellaria. In vitro Cell Dev. Biol. Plant., 43*(4), 318–327.

Cruz-Cruz, C. A., González-Arnao, M. T., & Engelmann, F., (2013). Biotechnology and conservation of plant biodiversity. *Resources, 2*(2), 73–95.

Danso, K. E., & Ford-Lloyd, B. V., (2003). Encapsulation of nodal cuttings and shoot tips for storage and exchange of cassava germplasm. *Plant Cell Rep., 21*(8), 718–725.

Devendra, B. N., Srinivas, N., & Naik, G. R., (2011). Direct somatic embryogenesis and synthetic seed production from *Tylophora indica* (Burm. f.) Merrill an endangered, medicinally important plant. *Int. J. Bot., 7*(3), 216–222.

Dhar, U., Rawal, R. S., & Upreti, J., (2000). Setting priorities for conservation of medicinal plants—a case study in the Indian Himalaya. *Biol. Conserv., 95*(1), 57–65.

Dixit, S., Ahuja, S., Narula, A., & Srivastava, P. S., (2004). Cryopreservation: A potential tool for long-term conservation of medicinal plants. In: Srivasta, S., Narula, A., & Srivasta, S., (eds.), *Plant Biotechnology and Molecular Markers* (pp. 278–288). Springer, Dordrecht.

Dulloo, M. E., Guarino, L., Engelmann, F., Maxted, N., Newbury, J. H., Attere, F., & Ford-Lloyd, B. V., (1998). Complementary conservation strategies for the genus *Coffea*: A case study of *Mascarene Coffea* species. *Genet. Resour. Crop Ev., 45*(6), 565–579.

Dumet, D., Engelmann, F., Chabrillange, N., & Duval, Y., (1993). Cryopreservation of oil palm (*Elaeis guineensis* Jacq.) somatic embryos involving a desiccation step. *Plant Cell Rep., 12*(6), 352–355.

El-Danasouri, I., & Selman, H., (2005). DEBATE-Vitrification versus conventional cryopreservation technique. *Middle East Fertil. Soc. J., 10*(3), 205–206.

Engelmann, F., & Engels, J. M. M., (2002). Technologies and strategies for ex situ conservation. In: Engels, J. M. M., Ramanatha, R. V., Brown, A. H. D., & Jackson, M. T., (eds.), *Managing Plant Genetic Diversity* (pp. 89–103). IPGRI, UK.

Engelmann, F., (1991). *In vitro* conservation of tropical plant germplasm—a review. *Euphytica, 57*(3), 227–243.

Engelmann, F., (2011). Use of biotechnologies for the conservation of plant biodiversity. *In vitro Cell Dev. Biol. Plant., 47*(1), 5–16.

Fahy, G. M., Levy, D. I., & Ali, S. E., (1987). Some emerging principles underlying the physical properties, biological actions, and utility of vitrification solutions. *Cryobiology, 24*(3), 196–213.

Fahy, G. M., MacFarlane, D. R., Angell, C. A., & Meryman, H. T., (1984). Vitrification as an approach to cryopreservation. *Cryobiology, 21*(4), 407–426.

Faisal, M., & Anis, M., (2007). Regeneration of plants from alginate-encapsulated shoots of *Tylophora indica* (Burm. f.) Merrill, an endangered medicinal plant. *J. Hortic. Sci. Biotech., 82*(3), 351–354.

Faisal, M., Ahmad, N., & Anis, M., (2006). *In vitro* plant regeneration from alginate-encapsulated microcuttings of *Rauvolfia tetraphylla* L. *Am Eur J Agric Environ Sci, 1*, 1–6.

Faisal, M., Alatar, A. A., Ahmad, N., Anis, M., & Hegazy, A. K., (*2012*). Assessment of genetic fidelity in *Rauvolfia serpentina* plantlets grown from synthetic (encapsulated) seeds following *in vitro* storage at 4 C. *Molecules, 17*(5), 5050–5061.

Francisco-Ortega, J., Santos-Guerra, A., Kim, S. C., & Crawford, D. J., (2000). Plant genetic diversity in the Canary Islands: A conservation perspective. *Am. J. Bot., 87*(7), 909–919.

Gantait, S., Kundu, S., Yeasmin, L., & Ali, M. N., (2017). Impact of differential levels of sodium alginate, calcium chloride and basal media on germination frequency of genetically true artificial seeds of *Rauvolfia serpentina* (L.) benth. ex kurz. *J. Appl. Res. Med. Aroma. Plants., 4*, 75–81.

Germana, M. A., Micheli, M., Chiancone, B., Macaluso, L., & Standardi, A., (2011). Organogenesis and encapsulation of *in vitro*-derived propagules of Carrizo citrange [*Citrus sinensis* (L.) Osb.× *Poncirius trifoliata* (L.) Raf]. *Plant Cell Tissue Organ Cult., 106*(2), 299–307.

Gonzalez-Arnao, M. T., & Engelmann, F., (2006). Cryopreservation of plant germplasm using the encapsulation-dehydration technique: Review and case study on sugarcane. *Cryo Letters, 27*(3), 155–168.

Halmagyi, A., Deliu, C., & Isac, V., (2010). Cryopreservation of malus cultivars: Comparison of two droplet protocols. *Sci. Hort., 124*(3), 387–392.

Hanna, W. W., & Towill, L. E., (1995). Long-term pollen storage. In: Janick, J., (ed.), *Plant Breed Reviews* (Vol. 13, pp. 179–207). John Wiley & Sons. Inc. Canada.

Haque, S. M., Kundu, S., Das, A., & Ghosh, B., (2015). *In vitro* mass propagation and synthetic seed production combined with phytochemical and antioxidant analysis of *Bacopa chamaedryoides*: An ethno-medicinally important plant. *Asian J. Pharm. Clin. Res., 8*(2), 377–383.

Helal, N. A. S., (2011). The green revolution via synthetic (artificial) seeds: A review. *Res. J. Agric. Biol. Sci., 7*(6), 464–477.

Helliot, B., Panis, B., Poumay, Y., Swennen, R., Lepoivre, P., & Frison, E., (2002). Cryopreservation for the elimination of cucumber mosaic and banana streak viruses from banana (*Musa spp.*). *Plant Cell Rep., 20*(12), 1117–1122.

Helmiyati, & Aprilliza, M., (2017). Characterization and properties of sodium alginate from brown algae used as an ecofriendly superabsorbent. In: *IOP Conference Series: Materials Science and Engineering* (Vol. 188, No. 1, p. 012019). https://iopscience.iop.org/article/10.1088/1757-899X/188/1/012019 (accessed on 01 November 2021).

Heywood, V., (1991). Botanic gardens and the conservations of medicinal plants. In: Akerele, O., Heywood, V., & Synge, H., (eds.), *Conservation of Medicinal Plants* (pp. 213–228). Cambridge. Cambridge University Press.

Hoekstra, F. A., (1995). Collecting pollen for genetic resources conservation. In: Guarino, L., Ramanantharao, V., & Reid, R., (eds.), *Collecting plant Genetic Diversity—Technical Guidelines* (pp. 527–550). CABI, Wallingford.

http://lib.riskreductionafrica.org/bitstream/handle/123456789/423/a%20global%20species%20assessment.%202004.pdf?sequence=1 (accessed on 01 November 2021).

http://pib.nic.in/newsite/PrintRelease.aspx?relid=137143 (accessed on 01 November 2021).

https://www.biotecharticles.com/Agriculture-Article/What-are-Synthetic-Seeds-Their-Need-Uses-and-Types-3315.html (accessed on 01 November 2021).

https://www.cbd.int/convention/articles/default.shtml?a=cbd-02 (accessed on 01 November 2021).

https://www.nap.edu/read/2116/chapter/11 (accessed on 01 November 2021).

Huda, A. K. M. N., Rahman, M., & Bari, M. A., (2007). Effect of carbon source in alginate bead on synthetic seed germination in eggplant (*Solanum melongena* L.). *J. Plant Sci., 2,* 538–544.

Hurka, H., (1994). Conservation genetics and the role of botanical gardens. In: Loeschcke, V., Jain, S. K., & Tomiuk, J., (eds.), *Conservation Genetics* (pp. 371–380). Birkhäuser, Basel, Denmark, AG.

Ipekci, Z., & Gozukirmizi, N., (2003). Direct somatic embryogenesis and synthetic seed production from *Paulownia elongata. Plant Cell Rep., 22*(1), 16–24.

Jang, T. H., Park, S. C., Yang, J. H., Kim, J. Y., Seok, J. H., Park, U. S., Choi, C. W., et al., (2017). Cryopreservation and its clinical applications. *Integr. Med. Res., 6*(1), 12–18.

Janick, J., Kitto, S. L., & Kim, Y. H., (1989). Production of synthetic seed by desiccation and encapsulation. *In vitro cell Dev. Biol., 25*(12), 1167–1172.

Jarret, R. L., & Florkowski, W. J., (1990). *In vitro* active vs. field gene bank maintenance of sweet potato germplasm: Major costs and considerations. *Hort. Science, 25*(2), 141–146.

Kalita, V., Choudhury, H., Kumaria, S., & Tandon, P., (2012). Vitrification-based Cryopreservation of Shoot-tips of *Pinus kesiya* royle ex. gord. *Cryo Letters, 33*(1), 58–68.

Karlsson, J. O., & Toner, M., (1996). Long-term storage of tissues by cryopreservation: Critical issues. *Biomaterials, 17*(3), 243–256.

Kartha, K.K. (1985). Meristem culture and germplasm preservation. In: K.K. Kartha (ed.). Cryopreservation of plant cells and organs (pp.115–134.). CRC Press, Boca Raton, Florida

Kasso, M., & Balakrishnan, M., (*2013*). Ex-situ conservation of biodiversity with particular emphasis to Ethiopia. *ISRN Biodiversity*. https://www.hindawi.com/journals/isrn/2013/985037/ (accessed on 01 November 2021).

Kaviani, B., (2011). Conservation of plant genetic resources by cryopreservation. *Aust. J. Crop Sci., 5*(6), 778–800.

Kikowska, M., & Thiem, B., (2011). Alginate-encapsulated shoot tips and nodal segments in micropropagation of medicinal plants. A review. *Herba Pol., 57*(4), 45–57.

Kumar, G. K., & Thomas, T. D., (2012). High frequency somatic embryogenesis and synthetic seed production in *Clitoria ternatea* Linn. *Plant Cell Tissue Organ Cult., 110*(1), 141–151.

Kumar, M. A., Vakeswaran, V., & Krishnasamy, V., (2005). Enhancement of synthetic seed conversion to seedlings in hybrid rice. *Plant Cell Tissue Organ Cult., 81*(1), 97–100.

Kumar, V., & Chandra, S., (2014). High frequency somatic embryogenesis and synthetic seed production of the endangered species *Swertia chirayita. Biologia, 69*(2), 186–192.

Lambardi, M., Fabbri, A., & Caccavale, A., (2000). Cryopreservation of white poplar (*Populus alba* L.) by vitrification of *in vitro*-grown shoot tips. *Plant Cell Rep., 19*(3), 213–218.

Lange, D.,(1997). Trade figures for botanical drugs world-wide. *Medicinal Plant Conservation Newsletter.* 3: 16–17.

Larkin, P. J., Davies, P. A., & Tanner, G. J., (1988). Nurse culture of low numbers of Medicago and Nicotiana protoplasts using calcium alginate beads. *Plant Science, 58*(2): 203–210.

Lata, H., Chandra, S., Khan, I. A., & ElSohly, M. A., (2009). Propagation through alginate encapsulation of axillary buds of *Cannabis sativa* L.—an important medicinal plant. *Physiol. Mol. Bio. Plants, 15*(1), 79–86.

Lee, K. Y., & Mooney, D. J., (2012). Alginate: Properties and biomedical applications. *Prog Polym Sci., 37*(1), 106–126.

Li, Q., Xu, Z., & He, T., (2002). *Ex-situ* genetic conservation of endangered *Vatica guangxiensis* (Dipterocarpaceae) in China. *Biol. Conserv, 106*(2), 151–156.

Mallón, R., Bunn, E., Turner, S. R., & González, M. L., (2008). Cryopreservation of *Centaurea ultreiae* (Compositae) a critically endangered species from Galicia (Spain). *Cryo Letters, 29*(5), 363–370.

Mandal, B. B., & Dixit-Sharma, S., (2007). Cryopreservation of *in vitro* shoot tips of *Dioscorea deltoidea* Wall., an endangered medicinal plant: Effect of cryogenic procedure and storage duration. *Cryo Letters, 28*(6), 461–470.

Manjkhola, S., Dhar, U., & Joshi, M., (2005). Organogenesis, embryogenesis, and synthetic seed production in *Arnebia euchroma*—a critically endangered medicinal plant of the Himalaya. *In Vitro Cell Dev. Biol. Plant, 41*(3), 244–248.

Maqsood, M., Mujib, A., & Siddiqui, Z. H., (2012). Synthetic seed development and conversion to plantlet in *Catharanthus roseus* (L.) G. don. *Biotechnol., 11*(1), 37–43.

Martinez, D., Tamés, R. S., & Revilla, M. A., (1999). Cryopreservation of *in vitro*-grown shoot-tips of hop (*Humulus lupulus* L.) using encapsulation/dehydration. *Plant Cell Rep., 19*(1), 59–63.

Matsumoto, T., (2001). Cryopreservation of in vitro-cultured meristems of wasabi. In: Engelmann, F., & Takagi, H., (eds.), *Cryopreservation of Tropical Plant Germplasm* (pp. 212–216). JIRCAS, Japan.

Matsumoto, T., Sakai, A., & Yamada, K., (1994). Cryopreservation of *in vitro*-grown apical meristems of wasabi (*Wasabia japonica*) by vitrification and subsequent high plant regeneration. *Plant Cell Rep., 13*(8), 442–446.

Mazur, P., (1990). Equilibrium, quasi-equilibrium, and nonequilibrium freezing of mammalian embryos. *Cell Biophys., 17*(1), 53–92.

McIlwrick, K., Wetzel, S., Beardmore, T., & Forbes, K., (2000). *Ex-situ* conservation of American chestnut (*Castanea dentata* (Marsh.) Borkh.) and butternut (*Juglans cinerea* L.), a review. *Forest. Chron., 76*(5), 765–774.

Micheli, M., Hafiz, I. A., & Standardi, A., (2007). Encapsulation of *in vitro*-derived explants of olive (*Olea europaea* L. cv. Moraiolo): II. Effects of storage on capsule and derived shoots performance. *Sci. Hort., 113*(3), 286–292.

Millar, C. I., (1993). Conservation of germplasm in forest trees. In: Ahuja, M. R., Libby, W. J., (eds.), *Clonal Forestry II. Conservation and Application* (pp. 42–65). Berlin: Springer.

Ming-Hua, Y., & Sen-Rong, H., (2010). A simple cryopreservation protocol of *Dioscorea bulbifera* L. embryogenic Calli by encapsulation-vitrification. *Plant Cell, Tissue and Organ Cult., 101*(3), 349–358.

Mishra, J., Singh, M., Palni, L. M. S., & Nandi, S. K., (2011). Assessment of genetic fidelity of encapsulated microshoots of *Picrorhiza kurrooa*. *Plant Cell Tissue Organ Cult., 104*(2), 181–186.

Moustafa, A. R. A., Zaghloul, M. S., & Al-Sharkawy, D. H., (2015). Seed bank approach for conservation of two threatened endemic medicinal plant species; *Hypericum sinaicum* Hocsht. & Steud ex Boiss. and *Plantago sinaica* (Barneoud) Decne. *American-Eurasian J. Agric. & Environ. Sci., 15*(12), 2512–2520.

Murashige T (1977). Plant cell and organ culture as horticultural practice. *Acta Hortic.* 78:17–30.

Nair, D. S., & Reghunath, B. R., (2009). Cryoconservation and regeneration of axillary shoot meristems of *Indigofera tinctoria* (L.) by encapsulation-dehydration technique. *In Vitro Cell Dev. Biol. Plant, 45*(5), 565–573.

Niino, T., & Sakai, A., (1992). Cryopreservation of alginate-coated *in vitro*-grown shoot tips of apple, pear and mulberry. *Plant Sci., 87*(2), 199–206.

Noor, N. M., Kean, C. W., Vun, Y. L., & Mohamed-Hussein, Z. A., (2011). *In vitro* conservation of Malaysian biodiversity—achievements, challenges and future directions. *In Vitro Cell Dev. Biol. Plant, 47*(1), 26–36.

Pandit, M. K., & Babu, C. R., (1998). Biology and conservation of *Coptis teeta* wall. –an endemic and endangered medicinal herb of Eastern Himalaya. *Environ. Conserv., 25*(3), 262–272.

Paunescu, A., (2009). Biotechnology for endangered plant conservation: A critical overview. *Rom. Biotechnol. Lett., 14*(1), 4095–4103.

Pehwal, A., Vij, S. P., Pathak, P., & Attri, L. K., (2013). Augmented shelf-life and regeneration competence of activated charcoal (AC) supplemented synthetic seeds in *Cymbidium pendulum* (Roxb.) Sw. *Curr. Bot., 3*(5), 30–34.

Pennycooke, J. C., & Towill, L. E., (2000). Cryopreservation of shoot tips from *in vitro* plants of sweet potato [*Ipomoea batatas* (L.) Lam.] by vitrification. *Plant Cell Rep., 19*(7), 733–737.

Phartyal, S. S., Thapliyal, R. C., Koedam, N., & Godefroid, S., (2002). *Ex-situ* conservation of rare and valuable forest tree species through seed-gene bank. *Curr. Sci., 83*(11), 1351–1357.

Pinto, M. D. S., Paiva, R., Silva, D. P. C. D., Santos, P. A. A., Freitas, R. T. D., & Silva, L. C., (2016). Cryopreservation of coffee zygotic embryos: Dehydration and osmotic rehydration. *Ciênc. Agrotec., 40*(4), 380–389.

Plucknett, D. L., Smith, N. J. H., Williams, J. T., & Anishetty N. M., (1983). Crop germplasm conservation and developing countries. *Sci., 220*(4593), 163–169.

Prasad, A., Singh, M., Yadav, N. P., Mathur, A. K., Mathur, A., (2014). Molecular, chemical and biological stability of plants derived from artificial seeds of *Centella asiatica* (L.) Urban—An industrially important medicinal herb. *Ind. Crop Prod., 60*, 205–211.

Rai, L. K., Prasad, P., & Sharma, E., (2000). Conservation threats to some important medicinal plants of the Sikkim Himalaya. *Biol. Conserv., 93*(1), 27–33.

Rajasekharan, P. E., Ravish, B. S., Kumar, T. V., & Ganeshan, S., (2013). Pollen cryobanking for tropical plant species. In: Normah, M. N., Chin, H. F., Reed, B. M., (eds.), *Conservation of Tropical Plant Species* (pp. 65–75). Springer, New York.

Ramseh, M., Marx, R., Mathan, G., & Pandian, S. K., (2009). Effect of Bavistin on *in vitro* plant conversion from encapsulated uninodal microcuttings of micropropagated *Bacopa monnieri* (L.)–An ayurvedic herb. *J. Environ. Biol., 30*(3), 441–444.

Rao, N. K., (2004). Plant genetic resources: Advancing conservation and use through biotechnology. *Afr. J. Biotechnol., 3*(2), 136–145.

Rao, N. K., Jackson, M. T., (1996). Seed longevity of rice cultivars and strategies for their conservation in genebanks. *Ann. Bot., 77*(3), 251–260.

Ravi, D., & Anand, P., (2012). Production and applications of artificial seeds: A review. *Int. Res. J. Biol. Sci., 1*(5), 74–78.

Reddy, M. C., Murthy, K. S. R., & Pullaiah, T., (2012). Synthetic seeds: A review in agriculture and forestry. *Afr. J. Biotechnol., 11*(78), 14254–14275.

Reed, B. M., Schumacher, L., Dumet, D., & Benson, E. E., (2005). Evaluation of a modified encapsulation-dehydration procedure incorporating sucrose pretreatments for the cryopreservation of ribes germplasm. *In Vitro Cell Dev. Biol. Plant, 41*(4), 431–436.

Roberts, E., (1972). Storage environment and the control of viability. In: Roberts, E. H., (ed.), *Viability of Seeds* (pp. 14–58). Springer, Dordrecht.

Roberts, E. H., (1973). Predicting the viability of seeds. *Seed Science and Technology,* 1: 499–514.

Saiprasad, G. V. S., (2001). Artificial seeds and their applications. *Resonance, 6*(5), 39–47.

Sakai, A., & Engelmann, F., (2007). Vitrification, encapsulation-vitrification and droplet-vitrification: A review. *CryoLetters, 28*(3), 151–172.

Schoen, D. J., & Brown, A. H., (2001). The Conservation of Wild Plant Species in Seed Banks: Attention to both taxonomic coverage and population biology will improve the role of seed banks as conservation tools. *Bioscience, 51*(11), 960–966.

Senaratna, T., McKersie, B. D., & Bowley, S. R., (1990). Artificial seeds of alfalfa (*Medicago sativa* L.). Induction of desiccation tolerance in somatic embryos. *In Vitro Cell Dev. Biol., 26*(1), 85–90.

Sharma, N., & Sharma, B., (2003). Cryopreservation of shoot tips of *Picrorhiza kurroa* royle ex Benth., an indigenous endangered medicinal plant, through vitrification. *CryoLetters, 24*(3), 181–190.

Shatnawi, M. A., & Johnson, K. A., (2004). Cryopreservation by encapsulation-dehydration of 'Christmas bush' (*Ceratopetalum gummiferum*) shoot tips. *In Vitro Cell Dev. Biol. Plant, 40*(2), 239–244.

Siddiqui, A., & Shukla, S., (2015). Conservation of plant genetic resources and their utilization in global perspective. *LS–An International Journal of Life Sciences., 4*(1), 46–61.

Singh, A. K., Varshney, R., Sharma, M., Agarwal, S. S., & Bansal, K. C., (2006). Regeneration of plants from alginate-encapsulated shoot tips of Withania somnifera (L.) Dunal, a medicinally important plant species. *Journal of plant physiology, 163*(2): 220–223.

Singh, S. K., Rai, M. K., Asthana, P., Pandey, S., Jaiswal, V. S., & Jaiswal, U., (2009). Plant regeneration from alginate-encapsulated shoot tips of *Spilanthes acmella* (L.) Murr., a medicinally important and herbal pesticidal plant species. *Acta Physiol. Plant., 31*(3), 649–653.

Srivastava, V., Khan, S. A., & Banerjee, S., (2009). An evaluation of genetic fidelity of encapsulated microshoots of the medicinal plant: *Cineraria maritima* following six months of storage. *Plant Cell Tissue Organ Cult., 99*(2), 193–198.

Suzuki, M., Akihama, T., & Ishikawa, M., (2005). Cryopreservation of encapsulated gentian axillary buds following 2 step-preculture with sucrose and desiccation. *Plant Cell Tissue Organ Cult., 83*(1), 115–121.

Tanaka, D., Niino, T., Isuzugawa, K., Hikage, T., & Uemura, M., (2004). Cryopreservation of shoot apices of *in-vitro* grown gentian plants: Comparison of vitrification and encapsulation-vitrification protocols. *CryoLetters, 25*(3), 167–176.

Tavukcuoglu, S., Al-Azawi, T., Khaki, A. A., & Al-Hasani, S., (2012). Is vitrification standard method of cryopreservation. *Middle East Fertil. Soc. J., 17*(3), 152–156.

Thorpe, T. A., (2007). History of plant tissue culture. *Mol. Biotechnol., 37*(2), 169–180.

Uchendu, E. E., & Reed, B. M., (2008). A comparative study of three cryopreservation protocols for effective storage of *in vitro*-grown mint (*Mentha spp.*). *CryoLetters., 29*(3), 181–188.

Valojerdi, M. R., Eftekhari-Yazdi, P., Karimian, L., Hassani, F., & Movaghar, B., (2009). Vitrification versus slow freezing gives excellent survival, post warming embryo morphology and pregnancy outcomes for human cleaved embryos. *Journal of Assisted Reproduction and Genetics, 26*(6):347–354.

Vdovitchenko, M. Y., & Kuzovkina, I. N., (2011). Artificial seed preparation as the efficient method for storage and production of healthy cultured roots of medicinal plants. *Russ. J. Plant Physl., 58*(3), 461–468.

Verleysen, H., Van Bockstaele, E., & Debergh, P., (2005). An encapsulation-dehydration protocol for cryopreservation of the azalea cultivar 'Nordlicht' (*Rhododendron simsii* Planch.). *Sci. Hort., 106*(3), 402–414.

Vijayan, K., Saratchandra, B., & Da Silva, J. A. T., (2011). Germplasm conservation in mulberry (*Morus spp.*). *Sci Hort., 128*(4), 371–379.

Villalobos, V. M., & Engelmann, F., (1995). *Ex-situ* conservation of plant germplasm using biotechnology. *World J Microbiol. Biotechnol., 11*(4), 375–382.

Villalobos, V. M., Ferreira, P., & Mora, A., (1991). The use of biotechnology in the conservation of tropical germplasm. *Biotechnology Advances, 9*(2), 197–215.

Wang, B. S., Charest, P. J., & Downie, B., (1993). *Ex Situ Storage of Seeds, Pollen and in Vitro Cultures of Perennial Woody Plant Species* (No. 113). Food & Agriculture Org. Rome, Italy. http://www.fao.org/3/T0824e/T0824e00.pdf (accessed on 01 November 2021).

Waylen, K., (2006). Botanic gardens: Using biodiversity to improve human wellbeing. *Medicinal Plant Conservation, 12*, 4–8.

Withers, L. A., (1991). *In-vitro* conservation. *Biol. J. Linnean Soc., 43*(1), 31–42.

Xue, S. H., Luo, X. J., Wu, Z. H., Zhang, H. L., & Wang, X. Y., (2008). Cold storage and cryopreservation of hairy root cultures of medicinal plant *Eruca sativa* mill., *Astragalus membranaceus* and *Gentiana macrophylla* pall. *Plant Cell Tissue Organ Cult., 92*(3), 251–260.

Zych, M., Furmanowa, M., Krajewska-Patan, A., Łowicka, A., Dreger, M., & Mendlewska, S., (2005). Micropropagation of *Rhodiola kirilowii* plants using encapsulated axillary buds and callus. *Acta Bio. Cracov. Bot., 47*(2), 83–87.

CHAPTER 15

USE OF MICROCOMPUTED TOMOGRAPHY AND IMAGE PROCESSING TOOLS IN MEDICINAL AND AROMATIC PLANTS

YOGINI S. JAISWAL,[1] YANLING XUE,[2] TIQIAO XIAO,[2] and LEONARD L. WILLIAMS[1]

[1]*Center for Excellence in Post-Harvest Technologies, North Carolina Agricultural and Technical State University, The North Carolina Research Campus, 500 Laureate Way, Kannapolis, NC – 28081, USA, E-mails: yoginijaiswal@gmail.com; ysjaiswa@ncat.edu (Y. S. Jaiswal); llw@ncat.edu (L. L. Williams)*

[2]*Shanghai Synchrotron Radiation Facility (SSRF), Shanghai Advanced Research Institute, Chinese Academy of Sciences, Pudong, Shanghai – 201203, P.R. China*

ABSTRACT

X-ray micro-computed tomography (X-Ray μCT) has become a versatile and valuable tool for non-invasive analysis of materials including plant tissues. This technique has been recently used to study Spatio-temporal, morphological, and functional characteristics of tissues of plants. The high-resolution synchrotron X-ray μCT enables scientists to study the quantitative aspects of plant anatomy and relate them to the metabolic functions. Laboratory-based miniature μCT devices are designed for benchtop scale; however, the resolution and signals are lower compared to a synchrotron X-Ray μCT system.

The capabilities of this non-invasive technique complement the information obtained from other imaging and metabolomics techniques such as magnetic resonance imaging (MRI), scanning electron microscopy (SEM), mass spectrometry imaging (MSI), Liquid chromatography-mass spectrometry (LC-MS), and gas chromatography-mass spectrometry (GC-MS). These techniques in combination have served as powerful tools for quantitative and qualitative investigations of plant structure and function. While the ability of non-invasive 3D imaging makes this technique indispensable, there is a lot of progress to be made in the image processing methods and software, for exploiting the benefits of this technique. Currently only a few commercially available software which are cost-prohibitive provide extensive data analysis capabilities. In this chapter, the theoretical and functional parameters of the X-Ray μCT system and its applications in plant phenomics are discussed, to make readers aware of this invaluable technique and its capabilities.

15.1   INTRODUCTION TO 3D IMAGING

In the past couple of decades, plant "genotyping" has made great strides in the study of interlinks between the environmental factors, growth conditions, stress, and disease tolerance of plants with their genetic makeup. With the advent of high throughput genotyping techniques, generation of data and analysis has become an inexpensive process (Pellerin et al., 2004; McMullen et al., 2009). Agricultural and plant sciences now demand the need for selection of plant species based not only on the genetic information, but also on phenotypic characters. Before the development of genetic techniques, farmers carried out the selection of species based on phenotypic characteristics (McMullen et al., 2009). Plant phenotyping initially involved scoring and observation of target characteristics by experts for a specific number of growth cycles. Phenotyping has now grown into a field that involves the merger of expertise from several disciplines such as computer science, botany, biology, physics, and engineering (Fiorani and Schurr, 2013). Robotics and imaging technologies now form the important pillars of phenotyping studies. There is a need for application of phenotyping methods to be extended from model species such as *Arabidopsis* to other plants of commercial and medicinal importance (Deikman, Petracek, and Heard, 2012; Yang et al., 2013; 2016).

For the study of plants by application of phenotyping techniques, several factors need to be critically considered, and protocols for data acquisition need to be optimized. The factors that need to be considered include the effect of environmental factors, stress conditions, and gene expression, on the phenotypic characteristic to be studied (Walter, Studer, and Kölliker, 2012).

For data acquisition, the imaging equipment hardware settings need optimization for obtaining the desired resolution. Post image analysis challenges include the selection of a software appropriate for datasets generated and sorting of the raw data for use in the selected software. Phenotyping studies with the application of imaging tools can be carried out in the laboratory or on the field, to study dynamic processes or growth characteristics for pre- and post-harvest periods. Earlier, most studies using imaging technologies involved quantitative analysis in real-time. However, with the expansion of applications of imaging techniques, studies including qualitative aspects are also carried out (White et al., 2012; Berger, Parent, and Tester, 2010).

Imaging techniques usually involve measurements of interactions between target plant tissues and light photons. Plant tissues have varying absorbance wavelengths which can be measured using visible, fluorescence, spectroscopic, infrared or other imaging techniques. Other imaging techniques include magnetic resonance imaging (MRI), computed tomography (CT) and positron emission tomography (PET) (Li, Zhang, and Huang, 2014; Zuo et al., 2010; Li et al., 2018).

15.2 INTRODUCTION TO SYNCHROTRON RADIATION (SR) TECHNIQUES

Synchrotron radiation instruments are designed to accelerate electrons in a very high-speed trajectory and utilize the produced energy to generate beams. The generated light beams have energy levels from infrared to X-rays. These are very high energy beams which cannot be generated in a conventional setup (Vijayan et al., 2015). Synchrotron instrumentation setups are very cost-intensive due to the large area required for the installation and the cost of the machinery. Synchrotron setups may vary in their ability of energy generation, based on whether they are optimized for generation of soft or hard X-rays. There are only few synchrotron instruments available in research laboratories, globally. Typically, in a synchrotron instrument, an electron gun is used to produce electrons that are collected and passed through a linear accelerator. The electrons are accelerated by the linear accelerator up to certain energy. The electrons are accelerated further and passed through a booster ring followed by passing through a storage ring. During their passage from the storage ring, electron beams pass through varying types of magnetic devices and release radiant energy. There is a loss of energy created by the electrons during collision and movement along the storage ring walls.

The lost energy is constantly restored by providing new injections. The magnetic devices that are used for generation of synchrotron radiation are either flattened, undulators, or bending type magnets. Electromagnetic radiation is generated when the passage of electrons between the dipoles of these magnets takes place. By use of devices such as slits, the electromagnetic radiation can be used for extracting ultraviolet, hard X-ray, infrared, and soft X-rays. Before the beams are used for focusing on target samples placed in a microscope or some other instrument, they are collimated. Magnetic dipole devices are used to produce discrete spectral bands. The size of a synchrotron instrument depends on the number of magnetic devices and the arrangement of different components. Electromagnetic radiations are carried by 'beamlines' to the 'end station' where the radiations are focused on the sample material. Data can be collected in 2D or 3D for specific regions of interest-based on the positioning of the detector (Miller and Dumas, 2006; Graceffa et al., 2013). A diagrammatic representation of a typical synchrotron facility is shown in Figure 15.1 (illustration with Shanghai synchrotron radiation facility (SSRF), as an example).

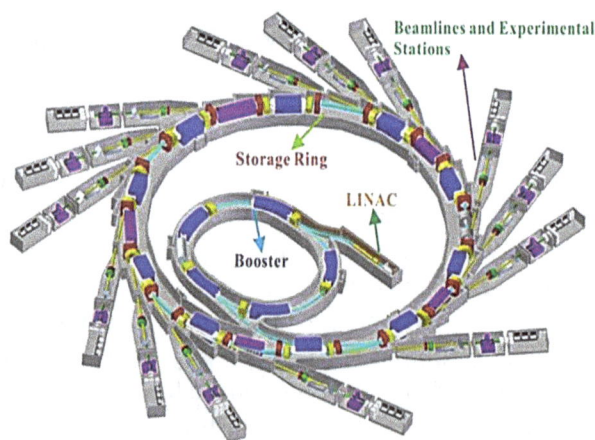

FIGURE 15.1   Diagrammatic representation of a typical synchrotron facility.

Application of SR provides merits of combining nanosecond pulses, high intensity brightness, wide spectral range for selection, and polarization which is difficult to obtain in conventional instruments (Miller and Dumas, 2006; Duncan and Williams, 1983). SR, when focused on a target tissue of plant specimen, should be able to interact with constituents within the tissues, without causing any physicochemical changes to them. The alignment of components in the instrument is optimized to capture the emergent radiation without causing significant loss or distortion (Shapiro et al., 2014). In the mid-infrared region, a resolution ranging from 1–10 μm can be obtained, and with soft-X-rays, a resolution of up to 5 nm can be obtained for SR devices.

There are several types of Synchrotron techniques available for imaging which include: (1) synchrotron radiation-Fourier transforms infrared (SR-FTIR) spectroscopy; (2) X-ray absorption spectroscopy (XAS); (3) X-ray micro fluorescence (μ-XRF) and X-ray computed tomography and phase-contrast imaging. With use of Synchrotron Radiation-Fourier Transform Infrared (SR-FTIR) Spectroscopy, research can identify and quantitate plant constituents within tissues and cells (Goff et al., 2013). The transmission or fluorescence of samples can be recorded by XAS. In an extended fine structure absorption spectrum, the generated spectrum can be used for quantification of absorption by atoms of various species and distances. Thus, this technique finds its application in studying uptake and distribution of nutrients in plants (Kopittke et al., 2012, 2014; Sarret et al., 2013). μ-XRF is used to study the uptake of metals within different plant tissues. X-ray computed tomography and Phase Contrast Imaging techniques scan samples and generate images of virtual slices of the samples with millisecond intervals (Moore et al., 2010). Integration of these SR techniques with other analysis techniques helps in the exploration of biological systems.

15.2.1 BASIC PRINCIPLES OF MICRO-COMPUTED TOMOGRAPHY

Technologies used for morphological analysis of biological samples have considerably advanced in the last decade. Non-invasiveness of the methods gives them added advantage to the already existing techniques. CT is one of these imaging techniques, which offers its non-invasive feature with versatility in the kind of biological samples that can be analyzed.

Tomography involves imaging of samples, where the images are created from the projections of the samples. The projections are made at a specified angle, and these projections are integrals of images created in a direction at the selected angle (Kak, Slaney, and Wang, 2002). In other words, the illumination of objects at a specific angle causes the generation of transmission energies. These transmission energies are recorded as diffracted projections, which are used for image construction. The recorded two-dimensional (2D) X-ray images are reconstructed to 3D images by use of various commercially available software (Goerne and Rajiah, 2018; Hampel, 2015).

15.2.2   *INSTRUMENTATION AND SAMPLE ANALYSIS PROCEDURE FOR MICRO-COMPUTED TOMOGRAPHY*

Micro-computed tomography can be realized either with synchrotron radiation or on X-ray tube. The beamline of X-ray imaging and biomedical applications (BL13W1) at SSRF is one of the typical instruments used for micro-computed tomography based on synchrotron radiation (Xie et al., 2015). The light source is a hybrid-type wiggler of eight periods in periodic length of 14 cm. The maximum K-value is 24.8 at minimum gap (17 mm) of the wiggler magnet. Energy range of the synchrotron radiation is 8–72.5 keV, corresponding to the gaps from 17 mm to 35 mm. A white beam slit is placed at 20 m away from the source point. The maximum aperture is 30 mm × 4 mm. The maximal beam size is 45 mm (H) × 5 mm (V) @32m@20 keV.

In a typical CT laboratory instrument, electron beams are generated by a vacuum tube with a voltage of up to 240 kV. These electron beams are focused on a metal target like tungsten. The metal target reacts with electrons, and this interaction causes the generation of X-rays. These X-rays are then focused on a sample, and the generated projections are recorded as 2D images by the detector (Miller and Dumas, 2006 Kak, Slaney, and Wang, 2002; Hampel, 2015).

The basic parts of an industrial CT instrument setup include: (1) target sample manipulator (2) X-ray detector and (3) ionizing radiation. The sample manipulator adjusts the position of the target sample and places it in the path of the light beam in an angle. The diffracted radiation after passing through the sample is converted into 2D images, by the detector. Several hundreds to thousands of such 2D images are produced during the scanning process and are used to reconstruct 3D images. In the generated 2D images, the summation of all the volumetric pixels represents the x-ray density of the sample (Miller and Dumas, 2006; Kopittke et al., 2012, 2014).

15.2.2.1   *PROCEDURE FOR SAMPLE ANALYSIS*

Sample analysis by micro-CT analysis involves five steps which include: (i) mounting or positioning of the sample; (ii) optimization or setup of parameters for scanning; (iii) scanning; (iv) reconstruction of 3D images from generated 2D projections; (v) 3D visualization of data.

> ➤ **Sample Preparation:** The samples to be mounted for analysis do not require any pre-treatment prior to analysis. However, positioning

(mounting) of the sample is a critical step for scanning, as the sample is placed on a rotating chamber. To avoid sample movement during scanning, the samples are affixed to the rotating chamber by use of a low-density material such as cardboard or glass. It is advisable to have the sample staged in an angle and not parallel to the direction of the x-ray beam. This caution is necessary as the x-rays do not penetrate the surfaces which are parallel to them and this can lead to variations in the generated images. The movement of the sample during scanning can cause the obtained images to be blurred. Long scanning times can also lead to drying or shrinking of samples. Thus, it is essential to optimize scanning time based on the physiochemical nature of the sample or pre-treat the sample adequately to avoid sample damage during scanning. Some researchers prefer wrapping of samples with paper or cloth pre-soaked in water, isopropanol or ethyl alcohol to avoid dehydration of the sample. Fragile samples can be processed by placing them in glass tubes or containers, taking care that the edges of the container do not touch the sample. If the lids or edges touch the sample, they may affect their integrity and lead to defects in the 2D images. For delicate tissue samples that are scanned in liquid filled containers, it is advisable to use staining to enhance the contrast of the sample with respect to the surrounding liquid.

➢ Optimization of Scanner Settings:
  • Resolution of Sample Images: Selection of proper resolution is an important step in micro-CT analysis as it considerably affects the quality and processing of data sets post-analysis. To avoid artifacts in resolution due to sample size, it is suggested that a resolution of factor 1000 smaller than the diameter of the sample be used.

    Analysts suggest that the cone-beam geometry is such that its construction is not conducive for high resolution away from the center of the sample, and its intensity is reduced along the edges. With the increase in pixel size up to 2000 pixels, magnification can be improved. However, it can lead to an increase in the size of processed images and longer processing times.

  • Effect of X-Ray Spots and Voxel Sizes: Voxel size is described as the width of one pixel in 3D. The voxel size depends on the target sample size, magnification, and the distance between the detector and the x-ray source (x-ray spot) (Schoeman et al., 2016). Voxel size is often misunderstood for spatial resolution of the scanning system. The actual resolution is dependent on the X-ray spot size. X-ray spot size is critical for optimum spatial resolution. Commercially available scanners have a precalculated voxel size and it is recommended to use the given value for selection of X-ray spot size. If the x-ray spot size is significantly higher than the voxel size value, it leads to poor resolution images. For in-house built scanners, standards, and reference standards are available to maintain spatial resolution. Resolution can differ significantly from scan to scan on the same instrument, and between scans of the same sample on two different instruments. The resolution of CT scan images is dependent on a multitude of factors including the X-ray spots, scan parameters, and voxel size. To ascertain the scan quality, one can identify a small region of interest with known area and check its visibility in the obtained 3D images (Du Plessis et al., 2017).

- **Parameters Used for Scanning:** The density of the material determines the x-ray voltage or energy to be used during scanning. For example, of X-ray tube, samples like metals and heavy rocks require high voltages ranging from 160–240 kV. Small and low-density samples require low x-ray tube voltages for scanning. To identify optimum settings for scanning, the sample should be mounted and rotated to obtain a 2D projection image with the darkest wide region. The x-ray penetration ratio should then be calculated based on the darkest region (area of minimum penetration) and gray value counts. Penetration values ranging between 10–90% are reported to provide good resolution images. The x-ray energies may face a decrease in intensity or distortion in their path due to high density of the whole sample or high density of specific regions of the sample. This effect is called "beam hardening." Beam hardening can lead to brightening effect along the periphery of the whole high-density samples (termed as 'cupping') or striated distortions in specific dense parts of the sample. Filtration is a technique that can reduce beam hardening effects. This can be done by placing filters between the sample and the x-ray source (beam filtration) and/ or between the sample and the x-ray detector (detector filtration). Beam filtration reduces polychromaticity and reduces distortions in images caused due to dense spots in samples. Detector filtration reduces the scattering of x-rays caused due re-emission of x-rays from dense samples. A beam filter is also used to prevent saturation of detector with scattered x-rays. Scan time can vary from detector to detector and sample to sample. Scan times can vary from several milliseconds per image to several seconds per image. Low scanning times can result in grainy, low-quality images. To optimize scanning time, the dynamic full scan range is used. Some scanners are equipped with a continuous scanning system where an average of images taken at various positions is used to reduce noise and obtain good quality images. The difference between the sample size and magnification determines the number of pixels and projection steps. For a good post-analysis reconstruction, high numbers of images are helpful.

Before scanning is initiated, it is important to normalize the background and adjust any fluctuations in the x-ray intensities. Normalization need not be repeated for the sample. It is required only when the acquisition parameters are changed. Beam centering is also done before scans are performed to confirm the focus spot is the narrow with the highest obtainable emission. After the scanning settings are entered and the sample is positioned, the scanner performs the scanning in a fully automated manner. It is important to periodically monitor the process to ensure the sample is positioned in place, and there are no changes in x-ray intensity changes. Care during the process can avoid loss of machine time and post processing data analysis issues. High quality images can also be obtained with low scanning times if averaging is avoided and numbers of images are adequately reduced. The nature of the sample and goals of the analysis determine if low scan times or long scan times are essential for the study.

15.3   APPLICATIONS OF SYNCHROTRON RADIATION TECHNIQUES IN IMAGING

The applications of SR imaging techniques have been extended from food products to biomedicine, archaeology, pharmaceuticals, biomedicine, and plants. The section below provides a brief description of these applications:

1. **Biomedicine Therapy and Diagnosis:** SR imaging techniques have been used in medicine for dynamic and *in-vivo* imaging of animal soft tissues and bone structures. They have been used for detection of tumors, neurological, and skeletal issues in clinical

therapies (Yang et al., 2013, 2016; Tang et al., 2011; Yang, 2013). Challenging investigations such as the study of osseous defects and cerebral artery occlusions have been carried out by the application of SR techniques. Figure 15.2 shows further study of the morphology of lateral surface area (LSAs). Evaluation of these reconstructed images revealed three types of LSAs in adult mouse. Performance of surgical implants, scaffolds, and medicinal sponges within bodies of experimental rabbits was studied by application of SR imaging. These exploratory studies have opened avenues for the application of SR techniques in biomedical therapies (Yang et al., 2013, 2016; Cao et al., 2014; Dai et al., 2011).

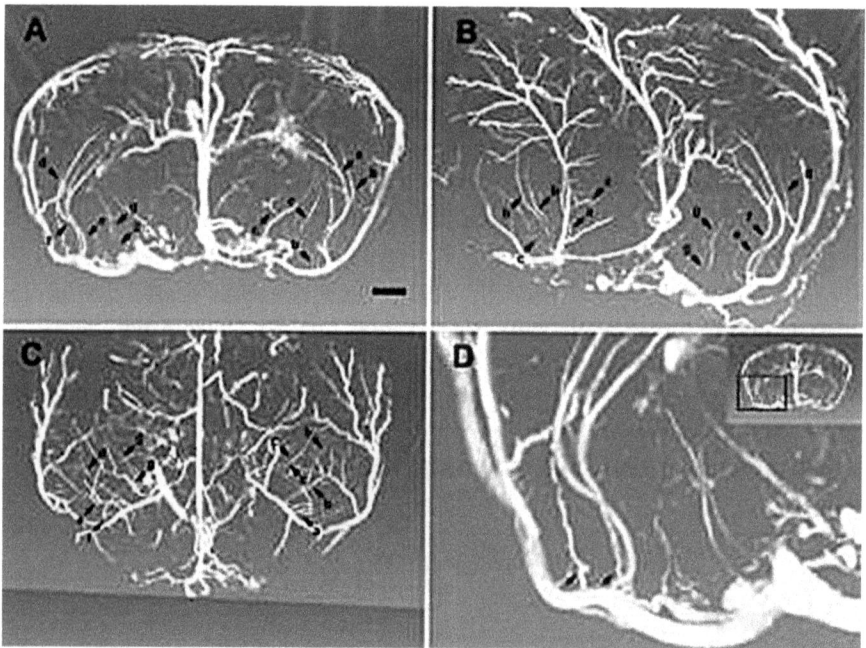

FIGURE 15.2 Image reconstruction of angiography of vasculature of forebrain. (A) Coronal view of the brain LSAs derived from the MCA stem trunk are indicated by arrows b and e. (B) A sagittal view of the brain shows LSAs derived from the secondary branch of MCA, which are indicated by arrows a, d, and f. (C) A superior view of the brain shows LSAs derived from the circle of Willis, which are indicated by arrows c and g. (D) Enlargement of image A. Arrows indicate the spiral pattern of LSAs [LSA: lenticulostriate artery; MCA: middle cerebral artery]. Scale bar = 1 mm.
Source: Reprinted with permission from Yuan et al., 2013.

2. **Investigation of Archeological and Paleontological Samples:** SR imaging techniques find their use in imaging archeological and paleontological samples due to their non-invasive nature. Valuable samples are benefited from such techniques, as no sample preparation or physiochemical changes are required prior to analysis. SR imaging techniques have been recently reported to be used in the study of parasitoid biology, taxonomic identification of specimens found in fossils, study of vasculature development in extinct species and study of evolutionary aspects in animal species.

3. **Pharmaceutical Industry:** The structure of pharmaceutical formulations affects their bioavailability and function. In the design of controlled and sustained released formulations, biphasic preparations or coated nano-formulations, the distribution, size, and efficiency of particles plays a critical role. Several drugs have been analyzed by imaging techniques to estimate they are *in-vivo* bioavailability, stability, and function (Li, Zhang, and Huang, 2014; Zuo et al., 2010; Li et al., 2018; Douglas et al., 2018; Limsitthichaikoon et al., 2018; Priprem et al., 2018). Wu et al. studied the material distributions and functional structures in probiotic microcapsules and the quantitative analysis and characterization of internal microstructures has been done (Wu and Becker, 2012; Wu et al., 2018).

4. **Material Sciences:** SR imaging techniques are used in the study of morphological and functional characteristics of many synthetic and natural materials. These techniques have been reported to study the internal structure of composites (ceramic, cement or natural materials). Alloys, metals, and soft foams have been studied by application of imaging techniques for calculation of their porosity, microstructure, and structural changes due to physical stress. Scanning electron microscopy (SEM) in combination with ultramicrotomy has been used in the study of polymer matrices (Green et al., 2017; Takao et al., 2015). Synchrotron radiation imaging technique can also be used to observe the dendrite growth of a solidifying alloy under a direct current electric field. Wang et al. studied the evolution of dendrite morphology of a binary alloy under an applied electric current *in situ,* as indicated in Figure 15.3 (Wang et al., 2010, 2013).

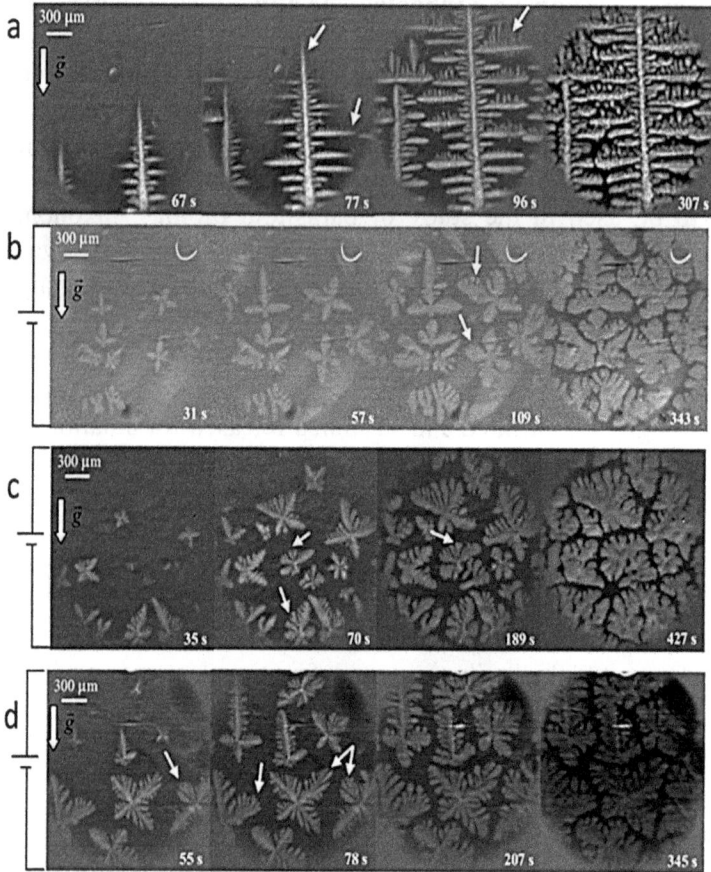

FIGURE 15.3 *In situ* observations on the dendritic growth of a solidifying Sn-Bi alloy under dc field. (a) Without DC. *Columnar dendritic* grains; thin primary, secondary, and tertiary dendrite arms with sharp tips (denoted by arrows). (b) DC density: 7 A/cm². Equiaxed cellular grains; thick primary arms, degenerate secondary arms with round tips (denoted by arrows); no tertiary dendrite branching. (c) DC density: 19 A/cm². Equiaxed dendritic grains; some primary dendrite tips split for branching (denoted by arrows); no tertiary dendrite branching. (d) DC density: 32 A/cm². Equiaxed dendritic grains; some primary dendrite tips split for branching (denoted by arrows); no tertiary dendrite branching.

Source: Reprinted with permisison from Yang et al., 2010. © 2010 American Physical Society.

15.4 APPLICATIONS OF SYNCHROTRON RADIATION TECHNIQUES IN IMAGING OF PLANTS

Due to the non-invasive nature of SR techniques, they have been used widely to study the structure and function characteristics of plants. Macro and microstructures of plant parts and living whole plants have been investigated by 3D spatiotemporal analysis. SR techniques are more advantageous in plant analysis compared to other available techniques due to their polarization, brightness, and pulse properties (Miller and Dumas, 2006). SR techniques provide spatial resolutions close to 5 nm and in soft X-ray machines and from 1–10 mm in mid-infrared region, in contrast to other techniques which can provide spatial resolution only up to 20 mm (Pellerin et al., 2004; Shapiro et al., 2014). During selection of SR techniques for analysis, it is important to select the energy levels that can interact with constituents in plants without significantly affecting their physicochemical nature. After penetration of the incident radiation, it is important that the emergent radiation does not undergo significant distortions. X-rays are used to study cellular, sub-cellular aspects and metabolic pathways of plant tissues as they penetrate the tissues without causing considerable damage. The medicinal plants of traditional Chinese medicine (TCM), have been studied by using quantitative X-ray microtomography (Li, Zhang, and Huang, 2014; Wei et al., 2005).

For plant tissue samples prepared with specific treatment protocols, the metabolic and developmental changes can be studied by application of X-rays and infrared radiations (Brodersen, Knipfer, and McElrone, 2018; Brodersen et al., 2013; Holbrook et al., 2001; Lee and Kim, 2008). Integration of SR techniques with microscopy or other analysis methods helps analysts to extensively explore biological questions (Wu and Becker, 2012; Wu et al., 2018; Lombi and Susini, 2009; Willmott, 2011). Analysis of trace elements in plant at low concentration was challenging prior to the introduction of SR X-rays. Conventional X-ray analysis faces challenges in the analysis of trace elements due to the overlap of absorption bands of different elements. Higher sensitivity and resolution of SR-X rays over-come this disadvantage and can be effectively used for trace metal analysis (Scheenen et al., 2007; Voegelin, Weber, and Kretzschmar, 2007; Shen, 2014). The accumulation of trace metals in plants can be detected either by the surface analysis [X-ray fluorescence (XRF)] or passing X-rays through the sample (XAS). The inter-atomic distances and species of atoms in plant tissues can be detected with an EXAFS (extended X-ray absorption fine structure) spectrum. Due to these attributes, the above-mentioned techniques are applied in the study of plant biology, morphological characteristics and metabolic pathways (Kopittke et al., 2012, 2014; Sarret et al., 2013; Harada et al., 2010; Maher et al., 2013).

A list of some representative applications of SR techniques in various disciplines of science are listed in Table 15.1.

TABLE 15.1 Examples of Applications of SR Techniques in Study of Materials

Discipline of Study	Technique	Application
Archaeology and paleontology	Synchrotron FTIR micro-spectroscopy	Study of collagen Jurassic sauropodomorph dinosaur (Karunakaran et al., 2015).
	Phase-contrast X-ray synchrotron microtomography	Study of gross morphology and histology of conifer tissues dated to be hundreds of million years old (Withana-Gamage et al., 2013).
	X-ray computed micro-tomography	Study of DNA in sub-fossilized bones (Yu et al., 2003).
	Phase-contrast X-ray synchrotron microtomography	Study of braincase morphology of primitive gnathostome (Heraud et al., 2005).
	X-ray computed micro-tomography	Study of amphibious ecomorphology of maniraptorans (Akhter et al., 2014).
	X-ray computed micro-tomography	Study of host-parasitoid interactions in fossilized flies (Naftel et al., 2001).
	X-ray computed micro-tomography	3D anatomical analysis of mineralized arthropods (Feldkamp, Davis, and Kress, 1984).
	X-ray microtomography	Investigation of ostrich eggshell beads (Yang et al., 2016).
Biomedicine	X-ray computed micro-tomography	Study of renal circulation and vascular geometry in experimental rabbits and rats (Ngo et al., 2017).
	X-ray computed micro-tomography	Investigation of cortical porosity and osteocyte lacunar density in iliac crest in men and women (Bach-Gansmo et al., 2016).
	Small-angle X-ray analysis	Study of crystal structures of enzymes supporting Cyclic N6-threonylcarbamoyladenosine ('cyclic t6A,' ct(6)A) in *E. coli* (López-Estepa et al., 2015).
	X-ray computed micro-tomography	Study of structural changes in labeled asthmatic lung tissues in mice (Dullin et al., 2015).

TABLE 15.1 *(Continued)*

Discipline of Study	Technique	Application
Pharmaceuticals	X-ray computed micro-tomography	Study of efficacy of self-gelling injectable composites (Douglas et al., 2018).
	Nano-computed tomography (nano-CT)	Study of effect of hydrogelators containing alkaline phosphatase in bacteria (Zheng et al., 2016).
	X-ray computed micro-tomography	Study of drug dissolution and structure in polymer-coated granules (Noguchi et al., 2013).
	X-ray computed micro-tomography	Study of osteocyte-lacunae and micro parasite characteristics on restricting estrogen supplements (Tommasiniet al., 2012).
	X-ray computed micro-tomography	Study of delivery efficacy of drug nanocarriers (Nilsson et al., 2013).
	X-ray computed micro-tomography	Post-mortem detection of gold-loaded micro-capsules in rats (Astolfoet al., 2014).
	X-ray computed micro-tomography	Study of efficacy of gastro-floating granules against *H. pylori* infections (Green et al., 2017).
	Nano-computed tomography (nano-CT)	Study of burst release efficacy of porous microspheres (Huang et al., 2015).
	X-ray computed micro-tomography	Studying *in-vivo* and *ex-vivo* vasculature using phase-contrast (Blery et al., 2016).
	X-ray computed micro-tomography	Study of ventilation mechanism in birds and flies (Martín-Vega, et al., 2017).
Material sciences	X-ray computed micro-tomography	Study of pores in carbonate rock (Qin et al., 2017).
	X-ray absorption fine structure (XAFS) spectroscopy and X-ray computed micro-tomography	Study of distribution of catalysts in polymer electrolyte fuel cells (Matsui et al., 2018).
	X-ray computed micro-tomography	Study of internal structures of probiotic microcapsules (Wu et al., 2018).
	X-ray diffraction computed tomography	Study of porosity and mineralogical changes in cement paste (Claret et al., 2018).

TABLE 15.1 *(Continued)*

Discipline of Study	Technique	Application
	X-ray microscopy tomography	Assessment of morphological features of lithium-ion battery electrodes (Li et al., 2018).
	X-ray computed micro-tomography	Study of mineralization patterns of sheep tooth (Wang et al., 2010).
	Operando 3D computed-tomography imaging	Study of degradation of catalysts in fuel cells (Gilbert et al., 2015).
	X-ray computed tomography	Micro damage analysis in reinforced composites (Hu et al., 2016).
	X-ray computed tomography	Mineralogical and chemical profiling of wellbore cement (Mason et al., 2014).
	X-ray computed tomography	Microstructure analysis of titanium and silicone composites (McDonald et al., 2003).
	X-ray dynamic imaging	Observation of the evolution of dendrite morphology of alloy *in situ* (Wei et al., 2005).
Plant sciences	X-ray computed tomography	Study of root hair structure in barley (Koebernick et al., 2018).
	4D X-ray computed tomography	Study of soil deformation around plant growth area (Keyes et al., 2016, 2017).
	X-ray computed tomography	Determination of oil content in soybeans (Zonget al., 2017).
	X-ray microtomography	Detection of embolism in conducting vessels (Nolf et al., 2017).
	X-ray microtomography and X-ray micro fluorescence	Study of distribution of metals in *Phragmites australis* (Feng et al., 2016).
	X-ray synchrotron microtomography	Study of leaf histology and male cones of *Glenrosa carentonensis* (Moreau et al., 2015).
	X-ray absorption near-edge structure, X-ray synchrotron microtomography and synchrotron X-ray fluorescence	Study of distribution of metals in roots of *Spartina alterniflora* (Feng et al., 2015).

TABLE 15.1   *(Continued)*

Discipline of Study	Technique	Application
	X-ray computed tomography	Study of changes in transport of nutrients under stress conditions (Choat et al., 2015).
	X-ray microtomography	Effect of infections on wood quality of pines (Sedighi et al., 2014).
	High resolution x-ray computed tomography	3D imaging of plant vasculature (McElrone et al., 2013).
	X-ray microtomography	Non-destructive investigation to Chinese medicinal materials (Holbrook et al., 2001).
	Quantitative X-ray microtomography	Identification of ginseng root (Brodersen et al., 2013).

15.5   LIMITATIONS OF SYNCHROTRON RADIATION TECHNIQUES IN ANALYSIS OF PLANTS

There are several factors that may pose limitations to the use of SR techniques in analysis of plants. Due to the penetrating characteristic of X-rays, prolonged exposure to tissues may cause changes in elemental distribution and concentrations. Soft X-ray may cause disassociation of structures of constituents present within the tissues. The sample size, the water content, scanning duration and speed are other factors that may affect the amount of damage that may be caused by the X-rays. Cooling of samples with liquid helium is suggested to reduce the damage caused by X-rays (Zhao et al., 2014). *In-vivo* studies on intact samples should be designed carefully considering the penetrating effect of rays using SR techniques (Scheckel et al., 2004, 2007). Long exposure to X-rays can cause damage to the protein structure due to heating and for imaging experiments; this issue should be considered critically (Lombi and Susini, 2009). Effects caused due to heating can be avoided by maintaining moisture levels of the sample via water filled glass vials or by sealing. Researchers have also designed humidity-controlled chambers to overcome this limitation (Kopittke et al., 2012, 2014; Wang et al., 2010, 2013). The differences in chemistry of constituents, and thus their differences in sensitivities to X-rays should be considered in the optimization of the parameters for a SR technique. Constituents such as cellulose may have an increase in the intensities of keto and enol group peaks due to radiation damage. The damage to a specific region of tissue can be estimated by the difference in peak intensities prior to scanning and after scanning. A background region can also be selected as the blank area for comparison (Karunakaran et al., 2015). As discussed earlier, it is also important to choose the most suitable beam width and sample spot to ensure uniformity in beam intensity. A single point array may provide better 3D projections in samples where beam intensity across the section is not uniform. For absorbance-based studies, the desired thickness of samples is from several 100 nanometers to 5–10 mm for X-ray and mid-IR radiations, respectively. For thicker samples use of XRF imaging is suggested. Post scanning methods involves the removal of background noise caused by the sample holder and chamber (Withana-Gamage et al., 2013; Yu et al., 2003).

Mid-IR analysis is suitable for fresh samples. However, samples with high water content can cause masking of absorbance peaks (Heraud et al., 2005). Samples with high water content can be frozen or dehydrated to avoid masking of the absorbance peaks. Samples that have a fragile physical nature should be cryo-sectioned to avoid unwanted effects caused due to dehydration and fixation with chemicals. Ice crystals may get formed inside the tissues, if samples are flash-frozen at −80°C and stored for a long duration. Another method used for sample preparation is, embedding of samples in paraffin wax or resin. Utmost care must be taken while removing off paraffin prior to scanning, as residual paraffin can cause masking of signals from the sample when SR-FTIR is used (Akhter et al., 2014; Naftel et al., 2001). Cells are designed for placing samples, where water content is a cause of concern during scanning. In these chambers, specially designed windows allow replacement of water with deuterium. These chambers are useful for experiments performed in the mid-IR region (Goff et al., 2013).

15.6   IMAGE PROCESSING TOOLS FOR SYNCHROTRON RADIATION TECHNIQUES

After scanning of samples, the 2D images are reconstructed into 3D images. Reconstruction involves the creation of 3D datasets from the 2D projections. Reconstruction is also referred to as *visualization*. During the reconstruction process, every voxel is mapped, and from different angles, the projections of the same voxel are created. The mapping is carried out by using an algorithm that is inbuilt in the commercially available software. The algorithm used in such software is called the Feldkamp filtered back-projection algorithm. Several software is commercially available, and these include: General

Electric, Datos, Avizo®, Amira, Solid works, Blender, Octopus Reconstruction, etc. Some software in addition to the inbuilt algorithm, provide modules which can be applied in various kinds of image analysis goals. The volumetric data are significantly different from a computer aided design (CAD) software and require high power computers for processing and storage.

Image analysis software is based on complex steps where the user processes the images using various operations such as segmentation, thresholding, selection of region of interest by manual or automated software options, extraction of processed images, etc. Segmentation involves optimization of various threshold values, color coding of target tissue regions and calculations of geometries in 2D or 3D images (Li, Zhang, and Huang, 2014; Zuo et al., 2010; Li et al., 2018). Thresholding is one of the most commonly used operations in image processing. It involves setting up a threshold value for one gray region, and all the values greater than the selected gray value are used by the software for further analysis. With the use of different modules, one can create axial slices of an object and observe selected regions of these sections in different colors for differentiation. Filters such as Gaussian filter can be used to smooth the image and reduce background noise. In segmentation, one can select a region of interest and create a binary (black and white) image of the region by assigning voxel values of 1 and 0. Steps performed in analysis depend on the objective of the study and the features available in the software. The image analysis software can be used for quantitative and qualitative analysis of datasets (Feldkamp, Davis, and Kress, 1984). Pre-made modules for specific image analysis goals are provided by some software. Design of modules for customized projects goals is a time-consuming process as it involves the creation of flowcharts using various operations available. Overall, the advent of commercially available software with in-built modules, has given a great advantage to SR techniques and their application in various fields of science.

KEYWORDS

- **3D imaging**
- **biomedicines**
- **image processing**
- **metabolomics**
- **X-ray micro-computed tomography (X-ray μCT)**

REFERENCES

Akhter, M. F., Omelon, C. R., Gordon, R. A., Moser, D., & Macfie, S. M., (2014). Localization and chemical speciation of cadmium in the roots of barley and lettuce. *Environmental and Experimental Botany, 100*, 10–19.

Astolfo, A., Qie, F., Kibleur, A., Hao, X., Menk, R.H., Arfelli, F., Rigon, L., Hinton, T.M., Wickramaratna, M., Tan, T., et al. (2014). A simple way to track single gold-loaded alginate microcapsules using x-ray CT in small animal longitudinal studies.*Nanomedicine Nanotechnology, Biol. Med. 10*(8), 1821–1828.

Bach-Gansmo, F. L., Brüel, A., Jensen, M. V., Ebbesen, E. N., Birkedal, H., & Thomsen, J. S. (2016). Osteocyte lacunar properties and cortical microstructure in human iliac crest as a function of age and sex. *Bone, 91*, 11–19.

Berger, B., Parent, B., & Tester, M., (2010). *High-Throughput Shoot Imaging to Study Drought Responses. J Exp Bot. 61*, 3519–3528.

Blery, P., Pilet, P., Vanden-Bossche, A., Thery, A., Guicheux, J., Amouriq, Y., Espitalier, F., Mathieu, N., & Weiss, P. (2016). Vascular imaging with contrast agent in hard and soft tissues using microcomputed-tomography. *J. Microsc., 262*(1), 40–49.

Brodersen, C. R., Knipfer, T., & McElrone, A. J., (2018). In vivo visualization of the final stages of xylem vessel refilling in grapevine (*Vitis vinifera*) stems. *New Phytol, 217*, 117–126.

Brodersen, C. R., McElrone, A. J., Choat, B., Lee, E. F., Shackel, K. A., & Matthews, M. A., (2013). In vivo visualizations of drought-induced embolism spread in *Vitis vinifera*. *Plant Physiol., 161*, 1820–1829.

Cao, L., Wang, J., Hou, J., Xing, W., & Liu, C., (2014). Vascularization and bone regeneration in a critical-sized defect using 2-N,6-O-sulfated chitosan nanoparticles incorporating BMP-2. *Biomaterials, 35*, 684–698.

Choat, B., Brodersen, C. R., & Mcelrone, A. J. (2015). Synchrotron X-ray microtomography of xylem embolism in Sequoia sempervirens saplings during cycles of drought and recovery. *New Phytol., 205*(3), 1095–1105.

Claret, F., Grangeon, S., Loschetter, A., Tournassat, C., De Nolf, W., Harker, N., Boulahya, F., Gaboreau, S., Linard, Y., Bourbon, X., et al. (2018). Deciphering mineralogical changes and carbonation development during hydration and ageing of a consolidated ternary blended cement paste. *IUCrJ, 5*(Pt 2), 150–157.

Dai, C., Guo, H., Lu, J., Shi, J., Wei, J., & Liu, C., (2011). Osteogenic evaluation of calcium/magnesium-doped mesoporous silica scaffold with incorporation of rhBMP-2 by synchrotron radiation-based muCT. *Biomaterials, 32*, 8506–8517.

Deikman, J., Petracek, M., & Heard, J. E., (2012). Drought tolerance through biotechnology: improving translation from the laboratory to farmers' fields. *Current Opinion in Biotechnology, 23*, 243–250.

Douglas, T. E. L., Schietse, J., Zima, A., Gorodzha, S., Parakhonskiy, B. V., KhaleNkow, D., Shkarin, R., et al., (2018). Novel self-gelling injectable hydrogel/alpha-tricalcium phosphate composites for bone regeneration: Physiochemical and microcomputer tomographical characterization. *J. Biomed. Mater. Res. A, 106*, 822–828.

Du Plessis, A., Broeckhoven, C., Guelpa, A., & Le Roux, S. G., (2017). Laboratory x-ray micro-computed tomography: a user guideline for biological samples. *Gigascience*. Jun 1; *6*(6), 1–11. doi: 10.1093/gigascience/gix027. PMID: 28419369; PMCID: PMC5449646.

Dullin, C., Dal Monego, S., Larsson, E., Mohammadi, S., Krenkel, M., Garrovo, C., Biffi, S., Lorenzon, A., Markus, A., Napp, J., et al. (2015). Functionalized synchrotron in-line phase-contrast computed tomography: A novel approach for simultaneous quantification of structural alterations and localization of barium-labelled alveolar macrophages within mouse lung samples. *J. Synchrotron Radiat.*, *22*(Pt 1), 143–155.

Duncan, W. D., & Williams, G. P., (1983). Infrared synchrotron radiation from electron storage rings. *Appl. Opt., 22*, 2914.

Feldkamp, L. A., Davis, L. C., & Kress, J. W., (1984). Practical cone-beam algorithm. *Journal of the Optical Society of America A*, 1.

Feng, H., Qian, Y., Gallagher, F. J., Zhang, W., Yu, L., Liu, C., Jones, K. W., & Tappero, R. (2016). Synchrotron micro-scale measurement of metal distributions in Phragmites australis and Typha latifolia root tissue from an urban brownfield site. *J. Environ. Sci. (China)*, *22*, 18933–18944.

Feng, H., Zhang, W., Liu, W., Yu, L., Qian, Y., Wang, J., Wang, J. J., Eng, C., Liu, C. J., Jones, K. W., et al. (2015). Synchrotron micro-scale study of trace metal transport and distribution in Spartina alterniflora root system in Yangtze River intertidal zone. *Environ. Sci. Pollut. Res.*, *22, 23*, 18933–18944.

Gilbert, J. A., Kropf, A. J., Kariuki, N. N., DeCrane, S., Wang, X., Rasouli, S., Yu, K., Ferreira, P. J., Morgan, D., Myers, D. J. (2015). In-Operando Anomalous Small-Angle X-ray Scattering Investigation of Pt_3 Co Catalyst Degradation in Aqueous and Fuel Cell Environments. *J. Electrochem. Soc., c. 167,* 100558.

Goerne, H., & Rajiah, P., (2018). Computed tomography. In: *Right Heart Pathology* (pp. 601–612).

Goff, K. L., Headley, J. V., Lawrence, J. R., & Wilson, K. E., (2013). Assessment of the effects of oil sands naphthenic acids on the growth and morphology of *Chlamydomonas reinhardtii* using microscopic and Spectro microscopic techniques. *Sci. Total Environ., 442*, 116–122.

Graceffa, R., Nobrega, R. P., Barrea, R. A., Kathuria, S. V., Chakravarthy, S., Bilsel, O., & Irving, T. C., (2013). Sub-millisecond time-resolved SAXS using a continuous-flow mixer and x-ray microbeam. *J. Synchrotron Radiat., 20*, 820–825.

Green, D. R., Green, G. M., Colman, A. S., Bidlack, F. B., Tafforeau, P., & Smith, T. M., (2017). Synchrotron imaging and Markov chain Monte Carlo reveal tooth mineralization patterns. *PLoS One, 12*, e0186391.

Hampel, U., (2015). X-ray computed tomography. In: *Industrial Tomography* (pp. 175–196).

Harada, E., Hokura, A., Takada, S., Baba, K., Terada, Y., Nakai, I., & Yazaki, K., (2010). Characterization of cadmium accumulation in willow as a woody metal accumulator using synchrotron radiation-based X-ray microanalyses. *Plant Cell Physiol., 51*, 848–853.

Heraud, P., Wood, B. R., Tobin, M. J., Beardall, J., & McNaughton, D., (2005). Mapping of nutrient-induced biochemical changes in living algal cells using synchrotron infrared microspectroscopy. *FEMS Microbiol. Lett., 249*, 219–225.

Holbrook, N. M., Ahrens, E. T., Burns, M. J., & Zwieniecki, M. A., (2001). In vivo observation of cavitation and embolism repair using magnetic resonance imaging. *Plant Physiol., 126*, 27–31.

Hu, X., Fang, J., Xu, F., Dong, B., Xiao, Y., & Wang, L. (2016). Real internal microstructure based key mechanism analysis on the micro-damage process of short fibre-reinforced composites. *Sci. Rep., 6*, 34761.

Huang, X., Li, N., Wang, D., Luo, Y., Wu, Z., Guo, Z., Jin, Q., Liu, Z., Huang, Y., Zhang, Y., et al. (2015). Quantitative three-dimensional analysis of poly (lactic-co-glycolic acid) microsphere using hard X-ray nano-tomography revealed correlation between structural parameters and drug burst release. *J. Pharm. Biomed. Anal.*, *10*(112), 43–49.

Kak, A. C., Slaney, M., & Wang, G., (2002). Principles of Computerized Tomographic Imaging. *Medical Physics, 29*, 99–107.

Karunakaran, C., Christensen, C. R., Gaillard, C., Lahlali, R., Blair, L. M., Perumal, V., Miller, S. S., & Hitchcock, A. P., (2015). Introduction of soft X-ray Spectromicroscopy as an advanced technique for plant biopolymers research. *PLoS One, 10*, e0122959.

Keyes, S. D., Cooper, L., Duncan, S., Koebernick, N., McKay Fletcher, D. M., Scotson, C. P., Van Veelen, A., Sinclair, I., & Roose, T. (2017). Measurement of micro-scale soil deformation around roots using four-dimensional synchrotron tomography and image correlation. *J. R. Soc. Interface, 14*(136), 20170560.

Keyes, S. D., Gillard, F., Soper, N., Mavrogordato, M. N., Sinclair, I., Roose, T. (2016). Mapping soil deformation around plant roots using in vivo 4D X-ray Computed Tomography and Digital Volume Correlation. *J. Biomech., 49*(9), 1802–1811.

Koebernick, N., Daly, K. R., Keyes, S. D., Bengough, A. G., Brown, L. K., Cooper, L. J., George, T. S., Hallett, P. D., Naveed, M., Raffan, A., et al. (2018). Imaging microstructure of the barley rhizosphere: particle packing and root hair influences. *New Phytol., 221*(4), 1878–1889.

Kopittke, P. M., De Jonge, M. D., Menzies, N. W., Wang, P., Donner, E., McKenna, B. A., Paterson, D., et al., (2012). Examination of the distribution of arsenic in hydrated and fresh cowpea roots using two- and three-dimensional techniques. *Plant Physiol., 159*, 1149–1158.

Kopittke, P. M., De Jonge, M. D., Wang, P., McKenna, B. A., Lombi, E., Paterson, D. J., Howard, D. L., et al., (2014). Laterally resolved speciation of arsenic in roots of wheat and rice using fluorescence-XANES imaging. *New Phytol., 201*, 1251–1262.

Lee, S. J., & Kim, Y., (2008). In vivo visualization of the water-refilling process in xylem vessels using X-ray micro-imaging. *Ann. Bot., 101*, 595–602.

Li, L., Zhang, Q., & Huang, D., (2014). A review of imaging techniques for plant phenotyping. *Sensors (Basel)*. Nov; *14*(11), 20078–20111.

Li, T., Kang, H., Zhou, X., Lim, C., Yan, B., De Andrade, V., De Carlo, F., & Zhu, L., (2018). Three-dimensional reconstruction and analysis of all-solid li-ion battery electrode using synchrotron transmission x-ray microscopy tomography. *ACS Appl Mater Interfaces, 10*, 16927–16931.

Li, T., Kang, H., Zhou, X., Lim, C., Yan, B., De Andrade, V., De Carlo, F., & Zhu, L. (2018). Three-Dimensional Reconstruction and Analysis of All-Solid Li-Ion Battery Electrode Using Synchrotron Transmission X-ray Microscopy Tomography. *ACS Appl. Mater. Interfaces*.

Limsitthichaikoon, S., Khampaenjiraroch, B., Damrongrungruang, T., Limphirat, W., Thapphasaraphong, S., & Priprem, A., (2018). Topical oral wound healing potential of anthocyanin complex: Animal and clinical studies. *Ther. Deliv., 9*, 359–374.

Lombi, E., & Susini, J., (2009). Synchrotron-based techniques for plant and soil science: opportunities, challenges and future perspectives. *Plant and Soil, 320*, 1–35

López-Estepa, M., Ardá, A., Savko, M., Round, A., Shepard, W. E., Bruix, M., Coll, M., Fernández, F. J., Jiménez-Barbero, J., Vega, M. C. (2015). The crystal structure and small-angle X-ray analysis of CsdL/TcdA reveal a new tRNA binding motif in the MoeB/E1 superfamily. *PLoS One, 10*(7), e0134070.

Maher, W., Foster, S., Krikowa, F., Donner, E., & Lombi, E., (2013). Measurement of inorganic arsenic species in rice after nitric acid extraction by HPLC-ICPMS: Verification using XANES. *Environ. Sci. Technol., 47*, 5821–5827.

Martín-Vega, D., Simonsen, T. J., & Hall, M. J. R. (2017). Looking into the puparium: Micro-CT visualization of the internal morphological changes during metamorphosis of the blowfly, Calliphora vicina, with the first quantitative analysis of organ development in cyclorrhaphous dipterans. *J. Morphol., 278*(5), 629–651.

Mason, H. E., Walsh, S. D. C., Dufrane, W. L., & Carroll, S. A. (2014). Determination of diffusion profiles in altered wellbore cement using X-ray computed tomography methods. *Environ. Sci. Technol., 48*(12), 7094–7100.

Matsui, H., Maejima, N., Ishiguro, N., Tan, Y., Uruga, T., Sekizawa, O., Sakata, T., & Tada, M. (2018). Operando XAFS Imaging of Distribution of Pt Cathode Catalysts in PEFC MEA. *Chem. Rec., 19*(7), 1380–1392.

McDonald, S. A., Preuss, M., Maire, E., Buffiere, J. Y., Mummery, P. M., & Withers, P. J. (2003). X-ray tomographic imaging of Ti/SiC composites. *J. Microsc., 209*(Pt 2), 102–112.

McElrone, A. J., Choat, B., Parkinson, D. Y., MacDowell, A. A., & Brodersen, C. R. (2013). Using High Resolution Computed Tomography to Visualize the Three Dimensional Structure and Function of Plant Vasculature. *J. Vis. Exp., 5* (74), 50162.

McMullen, M. D., Kresovich, S., Villeda, H. S., Bradbury, P., Li, H., Sun, Q., Flint-Garcia, S., et al., (2009). Genetic properties of the maize nested association mapping population. *Science, 325*, 737–740.

Miller, L. M., & Dumas, P., (2006). Chemical imaging of biological tissue with synchrotron infrared light. *Biochimica et Biophysica Acta (BBA) – Biomembranes, 1758*, 7, 846–857

Moore, K. L., Schroder, M., Lombi, E., Zhao, F. J., McGrath, S. P., Hawkesford, M. J., Shewry, P. R., & Grovenor, C. R., (2010). NanoSIMS analysis of arsenic and selenium in cereal grain. *New Phytol., 185*, 434–445.

Moreau, J.D., Néraudeau, D., Tafforeau, P., & Dépré, É. (2015). Study of the histology of leafy axes and male cones of Glenrosa carentonensis sp. nov. (cenomanian flints of charente-maritime, France) using synchrotron microtomography linked with palaeoecology. *PLoS One, 10*(8), e0134515.

Naftel, S. J., Martin, R. R., Sham, T. K., Macfie, S. M., & Jones, K. W., (2001). Micro-synchrotron X-ray fluorescence of cadmium-challenged corn roots. *Journal of Electron Spectroscopy and Related Phenomena, 119*, 235–239.

Ngo, J. P., Le, B., Khan, Z., Kett, M. M., Gardiner, B. S., Smith, D. W., Melhem, M. M., Maksimenko, A., Pearson, J. T., Evans, R. G. (2017). Micro-computed tomographic analysis of the radial geometry of intrarenal artery-vein pairs in rats and rabbits: Comparison with light microscopy. *Clin. Exp. Pharmacol. Physiol., 44*(12), 1241–1253.

Nilsson, C., Barrios-Lopez, B., Kallinen, A., Laurinmäki, P., Butcher, S. J., Raki, M., Weisell, J., Bergström, K., Larsen, S.W., & Østergaard, J., et al. (2013). SPECT/CT imaging of radiolabeled cubosomes and hexosomes forpotential theranostic applications. *Biomaterials, 34*(33), 8491–8503.

Noguchi, S., Kajihara, R., Iwao, Y., Fujinami, Y., Suzuki, Y., Terada, Y., Uesugi, K., Miura, K., & Itai, S. Investigation of internal structure of fine granules by microtomography using synchrotron X-ray radiation. *Int. J. Pharm.*2013, 445(1–2), 93–98.

Nolf, M., Lopez, R., Peters, J. M. R. R., Flavel, R. J., Koloadin, L. S., Young, I. M., & Choat, B. (2017). Visualization of xylem embolism by X-ray microtomography: a direct test against hydraulic measurements. *New Phytol., 214*(2), 890–898.

Pellerin, C., Snively, C. M., Chase, D. B., & Rabolt, J. F., (2004). Performance and application of a new planar array infrared spectrograph operating in the mid-infrared (2000–975 cm(-1)) fingerprint region. *Appl. Spectrosc, 58*, 639–646.

Priprem, A., Damrongrungruang, T., Limsitthichaikoon, S., Khampaenjiraroch, B., Nukulkit, C., Thapphasaraphong, S., & Limphirat, W., (2018). Topical niosome gel containing an anthocyanin complex: a potential oral wound healing in rats. *AAPS PharmSciTech, 19*, 1681–1692.

Qin, T., Javanbakht, G., Goual, L., Piri, M., & Towler, B. (2017). Microemulsion-enhanced displacement of oil in porous media containing carbonate cements. *Colloids Surfaces A Physicochem. Eng. Asp., 10*, 530.

Sarret, G., Smits, E. A. H. P., Michel, H. C., Isaure, M. P., Zhao, F. J., & Tappero, R., (2013). Use of synchrotron-based techniques to elucidate metal uptake and metabolism in plants. *Advances in Agronomy.*

Scheckel, K. G., Hamon, R., Jassogne, L., Rivers, M., & Lombi, E., (2007). Synchrotron X-ray absorption-edge computed microtomography imaging of thallium compartmentalization in Iberis intermedia. *Plant and Soil, 290*, 51–60.

Scheckel, K. G., Lombi, E., Rock, S. A., & McLaughlin, M. J., (2004). In vivo synchrotron study of thallium speciation and compartmentation in Iberis intermedia. *Environ. Sci. Technol., 38*, 5095–5100.

Scheenen, T. W., Vergeldt, F. J., Heemskerk, A. M., & Van, A. H., (2007). Intact plant magnetic resonance imaging to study dynamics in long-distance sap flow and flow-conducting surface area. *Plant Physiol, 144*, 1157–1165.

Schoeman, L., Williams, P., Du Plessis, A., & Manley, M., (2016). X-ray micro-computed tomography (µCT) for non-destructive characterization of food microstructure. *Trends in Food Science & Technology, 47*, 10–24.

Sedighi Gilani, M., Boone, M. N., Mader, K., & Schwarze, F. W. M. R. (2014). Synchrotron X-ray micro-tomography imaging and analysis of wood degraded by Physisporinus vitreus and Xylaria longipes. *J. Struct. Biol., 187*, 149–157.

Shapiro, D. A., Yu, Y. S., Tyliszczak, T., Cabana, J., Celestre, R., Chao, W., Kaznatcheev, K., et al., (2014). Chemical composition mapping with nanometre resolution by soft X-ray microscopy. *Nature Photonics, 8*, 765–769.

Shen, Y., (2014). Distribution and speciation of lead in model plant *Arabidopsis thaliana* by synchrotron radiation X-ray fluorescence and absorption near edge structure spectrometry. *X-Ray Spectrometry, 43*, 146–151.

Takao, S., Sekizawa, O., Samjeske, G., Nagamatsu, S., Kaneko, T., Yamamoto, T., Higashi, K., et al., (2015). Same-view nano-XAFS/STEM-EDS imagings of Pt chemical species in Pt/C cathode catalyst layers of a polymer electrolyte fuel cell. *J. Phys. Chem. Lett., 6*, 2121–2126.

Tang, R., Xi, Y., Chai, W. M., Wang, Y., Guan, Y., Yang, G. Y., Xie, H., & Chen, K. M., (2011). Microbubble-based synchrotron radiation phase-contrast imaging: Basic study and angiography applications. *Phys. Med. Biol., 56*, 3503–3512.

Tommasini, S. M., Trinward, A., Acerbo, A. S., de Carlo, F., Miller, L. M., & Judex, S. (2012). Changes in intracortical microporosities induced by pharmaceutical treatment of osteoporosis as detected by high resolution micro-CT. *Bone, 50*(3), 596–604.

Vijayan, P., Willick, I. R., Lahlali, R., Karunakaran, C., & Tanino, K. K., (2015). Synchrotron radiation sheds fresh light on plant research: the use of powerful techniques to probe structure and composition of plants. *Plant and Cell Physiology, 56*(17), 1252–1263.

Voegelin, A., Weber, F. A., & Kretzschmar, R., (2007). Distribution and speciation of arsenic around roots in a contaminated riparian floodplain soil: Micro-XRF element mapping and EXAFS spectroscopy. *Geochimica et Cosmochimica Acta, 71*, 5804–5820.

Walter, A., Studer, B., & Kölliker, R., (2012). Advanced phenotyping offers opportunities for improved breeding of forage and turf species. *Ann Bot. 110*(6), 1271–1279.

Wang, P., Menzies, N. W., Lombi, E., McKenna, B. A., De Jonge, M. D., Paterson, D. J., Howard, D. L., et al., (2013). In situ speciation and distribution of toxic selenium in hydrated roots of cowpea. *Plant Physiol., 163*, 407–418.

Wang, P., Menzies, N. W., Lombi, E., McKenna, B. A., De Jonge, M. D., Donner, E., Blamey, F. P., et al., (2013). Quantitative determination of metal and metalloid spatial distribution in hydrated and fresh roots of cowpea using synchrotron-based X-ray fluorescence microscopy. *Sci. Total Environ., 463, 464*, 131–139.

Wang, T., Xu, J., Xiao, T., Xie, H., Li, J., Li, T., & Cao, Z., (2010). Evolution of dendrite morphology of a binary alloy under an applied electric current: An in-situ observation. *Phys. Rev. E Stat. Nonlin. Soft Matter Phys., 81*, 042601.

Wei, X., Xiao, T. Q., Liu, L. X., Du, G. H., Chen, M., Luo, Y. Y., & Xu, H. J., (2005). Application of x-ray phase-contrast imaging to microscopic identification of Chinese medicines. *Phys. Med. Biol, 50*, 4277–4286.

White, J. W., Andrade-Sanchez, P., Gore, M. A., Bronson, K. F., Coffelt, T. A., Conley, M. M., Feldmann, K. A., et al., (2012). Field-based phenomics for plant genetics research. *Field Crops Research, 133*, 101–112.

Willmott, P., (2011). *An Introduction to Synchrotron Radiation. 1*, 15–37.

Withana-Gamage, T. S., Hegedus, D. D., Qiu, X., Yu, P., May, T., Lydiate, D., & Wanasundara, J. P., (2013). Characterization of Arabidopsis thaliana lines with altered seed storage protein profiles using synchrotron-powered FT-IR Spectromicroscopy. *J. Agric. Food Chem., 61*, 901–912.

Wu, B., & Becker, J. S., (2012). Imaging techniques for elements and element species in plant science. In: *Proceedings of the Metallomics*; *4*, 403–416.

Wu, L., Qin, W., He, Y., Zhu, W., Ren, X., York, P., Xiao, T., Yin, X., & Zhang, J., (2018). Material distributions and functional structures in probiotic microcapsules. *Eur J. Pharm. Sci., 122*, 1–8.

Xie, H., Deng, B., Du, G., Fu, Y., & Chen, R., (2015). Latest advances of X-ray imaging and biomedical applications beamline at SSRF. *Nuclear.*

Yang, F., Wang, J., Hou, J., Guo, H., & Liu, C., (2013). Bone regeneration using cell-mediated responsive degradable PEG-based scaffolds incorporating with rhBMP-2. *Biomaterials, 34*, 1514–1528.

Yang, W., Duan, L., Chen, G., Xiong, L., & Liu, Q., (2013). *Plant Phenomics and High-Throughput Phenotyping: Accelerating Rice Functional Genomics Using Multidisciplinary Technologies.*

Yang, Y., Wang, C., Gao, X., Gu, Z., Wang, N., Xiao, T., & Wang, C., (2016). Micro-CT investigation of ostrich eggshell beads collected from locality 12, the shuidonggou site, China. *Archaeological and Anthropological Sciences, 10*, 305–313.

Yu, P., McKinnon, J. J., Christensen, C. R., Christensen, D. A., Marinkovic, N. S., & Miller, L. M., (2003). Chemical imaging of microstructures of plant tissues within cellular dimension using synchrotron infrared microspectroscopy. *J. Agric. Food Chem., 51*, 6062–6067.

Yuan F, Wang Y, Guan Y, Ren Y, Lu H, Xiao T, Xie H, Vosler PS, Chen J, Yang GY. Real-time imaging of mouse lenticulostriate artery following brain ischemia. Front Biosci (Elite Ed). 2013 Jan 1;5:517-24. doi: 10.2741/e633. PMID: 23277007.

Zhao, F. J., Moore, K. L., Lombi, E., & Zhu, Y. G., (2014). Imaging element distribution and speciation in plant cells. *Trends Plant Sci. 19*(3), 183–192.

Zheng, Z., Tang, A., Guan, Y., Chen, L., Wang, F., Chen, P., Wang, W., Luo, Y., Tian, Y., & Liang, G. (2016). Nanocomputed tomography imaging of bacterial Alkaline phosphatase activity with an iodinated hydrogelator. *Anal. Chem., 88*(24), 11982–11985.

Zong, Y., Yao, S., Crawford, G.W., Fang, H., Lang, J., Fan, J., Sun, Z., Liu, Y., Zhang, J., Duan, X., et al. (2017). Selection for Oil Content During Soybean Domestication Revealed by X-Ray Tomography of Ancient Beans. *Sci. Rep., 7,* 43595.

Zuo, Y., Yang, F., Wolke, J. G., Li, Y., & Jansen, J. A., (2010). Incorporation of biodegradable electrospun fibers into calcium phosphate cement for bone regeneration. *Acta Biomater, 6,* 1238–1247.

CHAPTER 16

POSTHARVEST CARE OF MEDICINAL AND AROMATIC PLANTS: A RESERVOIR OF MANY HEALTH BENEFITING CONSTITUENTS

ANKAN DAS[1] and A. B. SHARANGI[2]

[1]Deptartment of Horticulture, Institute of Agricultural Science, University of Calcutta, 51/2 Hazra Road, Kolkata – 700019, West Bengal, India

[2]Department of Plantation, Spices, Medicinal, and Aromatic Crops, Faculty of Horticulture, Bidhan Chandra Krishi Viswavidyalaya, Mohanpur, Nadia – 741252, West Bengal, India, E-mail: absharangi@gmail.com

ABSTRACT

Group of plants with specific active constituents having the ability to heal or to provide aroma and fragrance-rich residues are categorized under medicinal and aromatic plants (MAPs). Numerous species of these groups of plants develop in the wild or are cultivated in our country. Globally many developed and developing countries now are shifting their interest towards these MAPs as because the products obtained from them possesses extreme utilities with huge market demand. Pharmaceutical and cosmetic industries develop many commodities which contains extract obtained from them. So efficient cultivation as well as management, especially, with respect to the post-harvest aspect becomes very important. Scientific protocols are needed to be followed in order to get proper and judicious extraction of the desired component from the plants. Proper handling and modern ways of preservation are required, so that these plants can be processed and withheld for a long time. So, keeping in mind the extreme significance of these plants and the requirement of proper post-harvest infrastructure, the present chapter is provided giving an insight about the MAPs and the technologies which can be used for efficient recovery and long-term preservation.

16.1   INTRODUCTION

If we talk about medicinal and aromatic plants (MAPs) we can say that these are those categories of horticultural crops which are mainly used for their inbuilt curative and odoriferous characteristic especially in the pharmaceutical and cosmetic industries in the developed as well as third world countries (Overwalle, 2006; Guleria et al., 2014). Medicinal plants according to World Health Organization (WHO) can be said as a crop or herb in which single or multiple plant parts possesses essential ingredients which are used for remedial cause (Malik, 2007). The internal chemical component synthesized by the medicinal plants also gives them a natural upper hand for protecting them from the attack of different animals of herbivore category. One such example is the production of salicylic acid which acts as a hormone and enriches the plant defense mechanism (USDA, 2017; Hayat and Ahmad, 2007). As per the Secretariat of the Convention on Biological Diversity, in the year 2002, the earnings from the vending of medicinal as well as herbal products across the planet have been calculated to be 600 U.S. million dollars (WHO, 2003; Hishe et al., 2016).

In today's world, considering the strong pharmaceutical ability of the inert components of plant-based chemicals of medicinal plants, they are widely preferred and used in the medicine industry as they possess the capacity to be developed into different medicines helping in treating different ailments (Raju, 2019). It has been found that in the current day 80% of inhabitants in third world countries depend in a maximum amount for their medical care on drugs isolated from plants. Today one-third of the entire medicine sold and marketed all over the sphere contains components which are extracted from plants (Hishe et al., 2016).

Medicinal plant contains different important group of chemicals like alkaloids which are unsweetened components available in different plant parts and stem is one of them (Jaume et al., 2006; Drugs.com, 2017; Briks, 2006). These medicinal plants are compensating the requirements of the conventional drugs providing a helping hand to the local and foreign markets and also improving socio-economic as well as ethnic and biological aspects of different groups of people (Hishe et al., 2016). Polyphenols is another group of chemicals associated with medicinal plants. The polyphenols may be further categorized into phytoestrogens which are beneficial against gynecological problems like infertility and menopause (Dietland, 2006) and terpenes and terpenoids are the other groups which are aroma-rich and utilized in aromatherapy (Elumalai et al., 2012; Tchen, 1965; Singsaas, 2000). Aromatic crops on the other hand are those groups of plants which mainly yield us with different essential oils (EOs). These oils though are scented but are extremely volatile which are generally present in specific cells or channels in variable areas of crop like radicle, trunk, blossom, and fruit (Malik, 2007). Growing of aromatic plants for the farmers may sometimes become very challenging due to environmental variability's and many other biotic and abiotic factors (Craker, 2007). Oils inside aromatic plants is as a result of some metabolic processes and chemical reactions which talks place at the cellular or internal levels of the plant involved and are released out in the environment in the form of some fragrance rich by-product, The development of the oil in these plants is in a very less or minute quantity and we can say that the total aggregate of final extracted oil would only encompass a very little snippet of the whole plant biomass as such (Malik, 2007).

The plants irrespective of their primitive origin, still attain a stature of a fundamental pillar for native health care as well as modern day treatment. According to a report of WHO (2003) medicinal plants yet in the present century are used by a maximum share of population of the underdeveloped countries (Hishe et al., 2016). For aromatic plants the volatile oils present in them are not available as such, but exist in the form of some aroma less component which are called as glycosides. Now when these plants are subjected to various processes during oil extraction like maceration, an enzymatic reaction does takes place in the respective plant cells and the glycosides thus present experiences a synthetic alteration which results in the formation of the required oil (Malik, 2007).

16.2   INDIAN SCENARIO

A large number of MAPs is found to be grown in developed in India, which is having variable climatic and geographical regimes (Kumar and Jnanesha, 2016). It has been found that around 17,000 different upper plants are present in our country and out of which 7,500 plants are believed to have therapeutic characteristics (Shiva, 1996). Various conditions prevalent in our country like its position with respect to latitude and longitude, the existence of herbs of earlier age and innumerable living and non-living conditions are favorable for the development of different categories of plants (Kumar and Jnanesha, 2016). According to Rao et al. (2004) near about a quarter percentage of medicines present in the market today are procured from herbs, and some drugs, if not completely or directly using herbal extracts may contain artificial derivatives which are developed from antecedent components which are again extracted from plants itself. The Himalayan region of our country is highly rich in different medicinal and aromatic plant species and also is a home for countless wild species which has not been explored yet.

Our country is an arena for an uncountable number of plants of different genus and MAPs holds a major share in it (Kumar and Jnanesha, 2016). Till date, from the sacred Himalayan region of India, around 8,000 angiosperm species, 600 pteridophytes plant species and 44 gymnosperm plant species have been found (Singh and Hajra, 1996) and from this total bulk of plants 1,748 plants are medicinal or therapeutic type (Samant et al., 1998; Guleria et al., 2014). Many traditional medicinal systems have been used and followed in our country and 'Ayurveda' is the prominent name of one such example. 'Ayurveda' in our country has itself documented more than 2,000 different types of plants having medicinal use. A very ancient and popular document of our country called 'Charak Samhita' is purely established on utilization of medicinal and herbal plants for treatment. In this document, there are 340 curative medicines derived from plants and their uses have been mentioned (Prajapati et al., 2003).

16.3   POST-HARVEST AND VALUE ADDITION

Now, as mentioned above that our country hosts a huge number of medicinal and aromatic plant diversities. But in order for their effective utilization, higher longevity and better consumer acceptance, efficient post-harvest management system is very vital (Yahia, 2019). The age-old systems which are used for post-harvest management as well as extraction of absolute from the plant and value addition requires many modifications and abatements in order to derive complete utility from such an important group of plants. Changes especially in the sectors of processing in products and value addition are very much demanded (Raju, 2019). The inevitable process of respiration which continues even after harvest results in breaking down of complex substances into simpler products along with liberation of energy continues which ultimately cause loss and leaching of various important components from the plants like its functional ingredients, pigments, volatiles, loss in moisture and more importantly becomes feast of various micro-organisms which cause rapid deterioration of the produce.

The plants in which the leaves and stem are of economic importance uttermost care has to be taken as in this region's the bio-chemical processes are very high which becomes further elevated during and after harvesting. There proper post-harvest handling is very much essential for the sustenance of this treasured output of the country (Yahia, 2019). Thus, systematic handling and management after harvest from trained and skilled personnel becomes very important for increasing the post-harvest shelf life and utility of the produce for a considerable period of time.

Improvement in this segment of post-harvest handling can be attained by taking care of the targeted plant at the field level only than proper quality checking in order to receive the genuine material can be incorporated and finally processing steps are needed to be upgraded to develop a satisfying commodity (Tcheknavorian and Wijesekera, 1982; Raju, 2019). In order for required mercantile squeezing and increase the necessary demand of the herbal products in the market, proper, and systematic value addition of the MAPs becomes very useful (Kumar et al., 2014). All the necessary postulates and prepositions which otherwise applied for other horticultural produce are also incorporated for MAPs. But only difference is that the care after harvest for these curative and odoriferous crops becomes furthermore demanding as they because of their huge variation, different utilization and very less amount of principle component needed, which if not given proper and trained attention can get spoiled (Yahia, 2019).

Today many verified crop components are not meeting the prerequisite standards of quality and the desired nutraceutical ingredients are also very less as per the benchmark of pharmacopeial grades or demand of various manufacturing companies. This results in providing a financial crisis to the framers (Kumar et al., 2014). Thus, innovations with respect to post-harvest handling are very much needed to be implemented for these categories of plants. Following of protocols for post-harvest management would help in increase of the practicality of the produce and the consumer would also become more and more aware of using maximum herbal derivatives (Yahia, 2019).

Value addition thus as mentioned above becomes a very critical part of pot harvest life which help in increasing the shelf life also enhances the profit to the growers. Value addition for MAPs can be achieved broadly by two approaches. One of them is value addition by direct means and value addition in indirect way is another form (Kumar et al., 2014).

16.4   VARIOUS STEPS OF POST-HARVEST MANAGEMENT

16.4.1   HARVESTING TIME AND MATURITY

For MAPs, if harvesting is done prior to their optimum stage, then it would result in insufficient or improper development of the essential therapeutic components required to be present in it. And if harvesting is delayed then again there would be chance of loss of the volatiles or deterioration of the active ingredient due to biotic nada biotic factors (Raju, 2019). Similarity harvesting time is also very important. In general, it is recommended that harvesting should be carried out during the cooler hours of the day which would result in lesser accumulation of field heat, causing minimum spoilage and would ultimately lead to a better post-harvest life (Yahia, 2019).

16.4.2   GRADING, SIZING, AND SORTING

These are very simple and effective ways by which value addition can be obtained and products can be sold at higher market prices. The yield is generally sorted out for the presence of any disease, damages from physical injuries like abrasion and bruising or damages caused by the attack of insects or pests (Yahia, 2019). Grading can be followed thereafter, but as in the case of MAPs, there is so much variation, therefore the grading is required to be done according to the target market requirements. But whatever grading procedures are followed, care should be taken that these medicinal plants should hold their characteristic freshness and there should not be any loss in their flavor and aroma (Raju, 2019; Kumar et al., 2014).

16.4.3   WASHING

Cleaning procedure if is not properly followed, can render the freshly harvested herbs susceptible to rapid attack of microorganism. Sometimes due to wounds or injury caused during harvesting or handling the plant gets more effected. From these cut or injured areas, the entry of pathogens takes place which therefore cause decay of the plants due to this secondary infection.

Hence it is best recommended that proper washing of the yield should be done in chlorinated water which will help in cleaning as well as primary disinfection (Yahia, 2019). This is a very easy but an extremely vital step in post-harvest handling of fresh produce. Proper cleaning helps in the removal of outside particles, inert matters and dusts (Raju, 2019; Kumar et al., 2014).

16.4.4   DRYING AND DEHYDRATION

Majority of the plant portion of medicinal and aromatic crops contains moisture which becomes one of the sound reasons of post-harvest decay. More the moisture or water content means more rate of respiration, transpiration, and more affinity of microorganism towards the produce. Thus, removal of moisture with the help of natural and artificial ways becomes one of the most important techniques successfully utilized in preservation of commodities for a considerable period of time.

16.4.5   MEDICINAL AND AROMATIC PLANTS (MAPS)

MAPs which are hence dried or dehydrated have a better and longer post-harvest life. According to Esper and Mühlbauer (1998), this process of drying and dehydration can also be said as a post-harvest method where the water content which is available for biological activity is minimized which helps in checking the development of pathogens. Drying and dehydration not only helps in reducing the decay but also as the bulk volume of the biomass is lowered, it further helps in facilitating the transit from one place to another and the cost involved in this also gets minimized (Dikbasan, 2007). During when the drying process is being carried out a precaution should be followed that the biomass should not be subjected to the drying condition for a very long time as because it would result in decay or deterioration of the produce due to limitless living and nonliving factors present in the open environment, which would ultimately cause in lowering the financial output of the commodity (Kostaropoulos and Saravacos, 1995; El-Beltagy et al., 2007; Akbulut and Durmus, 2009).

The moisture content of the fresh produce is lowered to the safe acceptable limit it results in a reduction in the activity of the microorganism as well as the material and biological changes taking place at the internal tissues which helps in refining the steadiness of the herbs (Hatamipour et al., 2007; Das and Sharangi, 2018). To get a better status of the final output, it is thus required that the orthodox systems used for moisture removal must be changed to modern or innovative ways of dehydration. Vacuum, osmotic, and freeze-drying can be brought into use. For example, by the application of freeze-drying method very high rated dehydrated products can be expected (Muthukumaran et al., 2008). However high capital required for undertaking these types of drying innovations into implementation, often restricts their utilizations (Shishehgarha et al., 2002).

16.4.6 CURING

It is a terminology that is used when a plant is exposed to drying conditions for partial removal of moisture to enhance the post-harvest life. Traditional curing methods are those where the produce is kept under shade in field condition only for the moisture removal. However, present day curing for MAPs can be done closed cabins where hot air is forcefully drawn in and the humidity and temperature are precisely controlled (Yahia, 2019).

16.4.7 PACKAGING

It forms the next very crucial step in the post-harvest handling process where the produces raw or processed is packed by some standard packaging substance. Packaging of MAPs is required to be done in a material which is well suited to the produce. The material for packaging should be as such that it would help to reduce the transpiration loss and lower down the process of aging (Yahia, 2019). Packaging of the medicinal and aromatic herbs helps them in many ways. First of all, through the help of efficient packaging the chances of microbial infestation, decay, and spoilage are reduced (Wills et al., 1989; Irtwenge, 2006). The temperature becomes a very vital factor for packed produce during storage as inside the packaging material a microenvironment is created. Therefore, it is thus required that either the material inside which packaging is carried should be having certain levels of lacerations and if not, then the material should be semi or partially permeable to moisture and certain gasses (Yahia, 2019).

Thus, packaging material selection should be done strictly according to the requirements of the produce to be packed inside it. Packaging material taken should be able to handle the necessary wear and tear during transportation and should also be able to lower the biochemical activity taking inside the produce to a minimum (Wills et al., 1989; Irtwenge, 2006). Also, during the time of packaging the herbs should be properly managed as otherwise abrasion or bruising injury-causing physical damage to the inner tissues would reduce their post-harvest life. For packaging of fresh MAPs hard plastic vessels can be used. Modern packaging materials viz. "Pillow packs" where bags become relatively filled with air, helping in providing a cushioning support can be used (Yahia, 2019).

16.4.8   STORAGE

It becomes another very vital step of post-harvest handling as the therapeutic plants are needed to be kept in a very product specific condition otherwise chances of deterioration and loss becomes very high (Kumar et al., 2014). The condition of the storage environment is very important. Undesirable ambiance would only result in losses. Contamination by the infestation of molds would result in the accumulation of aflatoxins which is very much undesirable. For most of the MAPs storage in low temperature conditions is recommended which helps in maintaining various quality related parameters and stops the loss of active ingredients or accumulation of unwanted photochemical (Kumar et al., 2014). Then coming after temperature, relative humidity becomes an important parameter. Generally, it has been seen that for the majority of the fresh commodity the relative humidity percentage should be very high at a range above 85% (Kader, 2013). Also, the maintenance of relative humidity during storage is very crucial. Humidity below the acceptable limit would cause accelerated water loss and placidness similarly humidity percentage above the optimum would increase the microbial attack and infestation. In case of those categories of MAPs which are photo-sensitive, care should be taken that entry of light should be completely blocked and packaging and storage should be done strictly in light absent environment (Kumar et al., 2014).

16.5   VALUE ADDITION

16.5.1   VALUE ADDITION IN DIRECT MANNER

Value addition by straight or direct ways can be undertaken by different post-harvest steps which ultimately would help in maintain or withhold the quality for a longer period of time and also allow the growers or producers to sell the commodity in domestic as well as foreign markets with higher profitable returns. Following are the ways by which value addition through direct means can be reached (Kumar et al., 2014).

16.5.2   VALUE ADDITION IN INDIRECT MANNER

It is another broader way in which the value addition for MAPs. As per Kumar et al. (2014), indirect value addition can be undertaken as follows. First of all, purity testing is done to see that the material is genuine or not, then the foreign particle if any are discarded, thereafter the amount of moisture content is recorded and finally amount of active ingredient present in the sample is judged.

16.5.3   VALUE ADDITION BY PROCESSING

This step is mainly followed in the industries or companies where the MAPs are subjected to various scientific and innovative extraction procedures (TNAU, 2020a; TNAU, 2020b) for collecting their desired valuable chemical constituents along with further necessary refinement for selling market at reasonable prices (Raju, 2019). Some of the latest procedures for extraction and processing of MAPs are as follows.

16.6   DIFFERENT EXTRACTION PROCESSES

16.6.1   MACERATION

This is technology which is mainly followed for those groups of MAPs which contains temperature-sensitive active constituents. Hence here the lot of plants either as such or in grinded form is mixed with some organic solvent and kept for 72 hrs. Then the organic solvent containing the chemical ingredient is collected. Thereafter the solvent is cleared by proper filtration or decantation can also be used (Handa, 2008; Pandey and Tripathi, 2014). Different solvents can be used for the process. As per the works of (Al-Mansoub et al., 2014) when methanol was used as a solvent at the ratio of 1:10 w/v for *Garnicia atriviridis*, the extract showed better antioxidant properties whereas the aqueous extract of 1:10 w/v ratio exhibited anti-hyperlipidemic properties on a higher side (Azwanida, 2015).

16.6.2   SOXHLET EXTRACTION

This method is mainly used for those groups of plants which possesses a very little solubility of their active ingredients in the menstruum. Equipment called as the 'Soxhlet apparatus' is used here (Handa, 2008). It is mainly laboratory equipment (Harwood, Laurence, and Moody, 1989) which was invented by Franz von Soxhlet in the year 1879 (Soxhlet et al., 1879). The plant portions are subjected to heat. The desired constituent from the plants gets dissolved in the hot rising steam, which is then condensed by the help of a condenser and thereafter the condensed liquid is extracted out (Handa, 2008). It was seen that by the help of Soxhlet extraction many phyto-chemicals were received from leaf powder extracts of *Azadirachta indica* in methanol ~1:5 w/v (Hossain et al., 2013). This process of Soxhlet extraction is continued until and unless full extraction is achieved (Rassem et al., 2016). In the study conducted by Anuradha et al. (2010), it was observed that the technique of Soxhlet extraction yielded 2.2% w/w lypodial components from the powdered flowers of *Clitorea ternate* with utilization of petroleum ether at a temperature of 60°C–80°C (Azwanida, 2015).

16.6.3   INFUSION

This is nothing but a solution or mixture containing the active chemical constituent of medicinal plants. It is generally prepared by putting the plant parts in hot or cold water for a standard period of time (Raju, 2019; Handa, 2008; Pandey and Tripathi, 2014). It was seen that when *Centella asiatica* was boiled at a temperature of 90°C, it resulted in the better obtainment of antioxidant and content of phenols, however the pH of the extracts was affected as a resulted prolonged time used in extraction (Yung et al., 2010; Azwanida, 2015).

16.6.4   SUPER CRITICAL FLUID EXTRACTION

Here one active constituent is isolated from another by using special solvents called as supercritical fluids (Rassem et al., 2016). As the name itself indicated a supercritical fluid-like carbon dioxide is employed in the extraction of desired constituents from the plants (Taylor, 1996; Kiran et al., 1998; Naik et al., 2014). Supercritical-CO_2 (SC-CO_2) is very much used for this process as it is an excellent medium for solubilizing nonpolar analytes and also as carbon dioxide has lower levels of toxicity and easy availability (Azwanida, 2015). This method results in fast recovery of the active constituents in a very short time. But the technology is very capital intensive and can be successfully used for those substances only which are having very high molecular weight (Taylor, 1996; Kiran et al., 1998; Naik et al., 2014. Patil et al., 2013) reported that use of Supercritical-CO_2 on *Wadelia calendulacea* with parameters like temperature of 25°C, 90 minutes time for extraction and 10% modifier concentration resulted in optimum yield of 25 MPa.

16.6.5   PERCOLATION

A container called a percolator having a thin cone like appearance with opening from both the distal sides is used here. The lower opening of the percolator is kept closed during this period and the plant produce inside is kept to be macerated for a period of 24 hours. Then the lower end of the percolator is opened which allows the solvent containing the extracts of the plant to ooze out slowly. The mixture is then strained (Cowman, 1999; Handa, 2008; Pandey and Tripathi, 2014).

16.6.6   SONICATION

Here the desired plant parts are treated with ultrasound waves in between 20 kHz to 2,000 kHz which helps in elevating the penetrability of their cell walls, facilitating the process of extraction strained (Cowman, 1999; Handa, 2008; Pandey and Tripathi, 2014). Final output having very demandable values can be obtained from this technique (Bhaskaracharya et al., 2009; Rassem et al., 2016). However, the high cost as well as chances of formation of unwanted chemical components inside the plants due to sound waves, limits the use of the technology strained (Cowman, 1999; Handa, 2008; Pandey and Tripathi, 2014). In this process, oil constituents from leaves, seeds or flowers can be extracted (Sereshti et al., 2012; Rassem et al., 2016). With respect to the process of sonication it was observed that when ultrasound waves of 45 kHz along with 50.33% v/v ethanol and temperature of 65°C for a period of 15 minutes was used for extraction from *Cratoxylum formosum*, resulted in yielding phenolics with better efficacy (Yingngam et al., 2014; Azwanida, 2015).

16.6.7   AQUEOUS ALCOHOLIC EXTRACTION BY FERMENTATION

In this process the unpurified medicament especially in grounded form is mixed with a solvent and kept undisturbed for a considerable period. During this tenure fermentation does take place in the mixture and alcohol is generated which results in the better drawing out of the wanted chemical constituents (Handa, 2008).

16.6.8   DECOCTION

Here the biomass is subjected to boiling water for a time duration of 15 minutes which results in the solubilization of water dissolvable components which are not affected by heat. Thereafter the mixture is cooled and filtered and diluted with cold water to get the required quantity of the final produce (Raju, 2019; Pandey and Tripathi, 2014).

16.7   EXTRACTS FROM AROMATIC PLANTS

Aromatic plants can be used to derive different categories of extracts. Handa in his work in 2008, mentioned the following different types. Concrete viscous and gloomy containing different important chemical components, absolutes concrete mixed with alcohol, resinoids containing resinous contents and essential oil contains some oxygenated compounds which forms the principal agent for fragrance.

16.7.1   ESSENTIAL OIL EXTRACTION

The aromatic groups of plants are mainly used for getting essential or volatile oils from them. Various machines and equipment can be used for getting out these oils. Various small-scale setups can be made in rural and urban areas for extraction of EOs which would benefit the growers as well as the producers in many ways (Raju, 2019). Some of the technologies used for essential oil extraction are mentioned hereunder.

16.7.1.1   DISTILLATION

This is a process where the plant materials are heated and the steam coming out carrying the desired constituents is passed through condensation, and then the condensed volume is filtered or decanted to get the final extract (Handa, 2008). Distillation can be done according to the following subsections.

16.7.1.1.1 Hydro Distillation

It is a very ancient and easiest method of performing the distillation process (Meyer-Warnod et al., 1984). This particular process is mainly adopted for extraction of EOs from grounded materials of plant parts (Öztekin and Martinov, 2007; Munir, 2010). In this process, the plant materials are submerged in water which is then heated to get out the steam along with the necessary components. Different plant substances like powder of cinnamon bark or spices can be incorporated to hydrodistillation for essential oil extraction. Extraction from rose or orange can be done by the help of this technique (Öztekin and Martinov, 2007; Munir, 2010).

16.7.1.1.2 Water and Steam Distillation

Plant materials are kept separated from water by the help of a punctured platform. The water underneath is then boiled, resulting in the development of the steam which rises upward, passing through the crop parts. The steam then containing the essentialities is condensed and the oil is separated (Handa, 2008). As per the works of Oyen and Dung (1999), the technique can be successfully incorporated for extraction from different plant materials like thyme (*Thymus vulgaris*), peppermint (*Mentha piperita*) and lavender (*Lavandula* sp.).

16.7.1.1.3 Direct Steam Distillation

It is mainly followed for those plants which are very much sensitive to higher temperatures. This process is still is very much used in many industries (Fahlbusch et al., 2003; Rassem et al., 2016). Direct steam distillation is hence is a process which can be utilized for plant materials fresh in nature but having high point of boiling though. Seed, wood, and root from different plants come under this category (Öztekin and Martinov, 2007; Munir, 2010). Here only stem is used for extraction which is generated by the help of some machines outside the distillation unit. The stem then created is forced inside the distillation unit over the plant parts. The stem later is condensed and subjected to decantation for extraction of the essential oil (Handa, 2008). This process can also be used for extraction from fresh plant materials of spearmint (*Mentha spicata*), peppermint (*Mentha piperita)* and chamomile (*Matricaria chamomilla)* (Öztekin and Martinov, 2007; Munir, 2010).

16.7.1.1.4   Cold Pressing Method

Here the outward tissues of the plant which contains the oil are subjected to scrubbing. Thereafter the entire biomass is pressed to get the complete extraction of the oil. Then the oils which come up are isolated from the plant portion by the help of the centrifugation process (Rassem et al., 2016).

16.7.1.1.5   Cohobation

This procedure is carried out as an additional technique during water distillation or water and steam distillation. Here when the essential oil is separated from the condensed water by decantation, the leftover water is again pushed back into the distillation unit to be boiled again for generation of steam (Handa, 2008). It is a practice which is very ordinarily used in case of extraction from flowers of rose, as the water obtained from distillation, i.e., the distillate which is a very vital product of this process of distillation and also very much important for 'attars' development (Oyen and Dung, 1999).

16.7.1.1.6   Solvent Extraction

Here extraction is done by the help of some solvent in which the active constituent of the plant may get dissolved. It helps in producing a good quantity of oil and the cost of extraction is also less (Chrissie et al., 1996). But disadvantage like more solvent and time requirement for extraction and restricts its use (Dawidowicz et al., 2008).

16.7.1.1.7   Hydrolytic Maceration Distillation

In this technique maceration of the plants selected are done in warm water for getting out their EOs. The target chemical component in this group of plants is joined by the help of glycosidic bonds, so hot water helps in the better release (Handa, 2008). It has been seen that for *Gaultheria procumbens* which is also commonly called wintergreen, the warm water used herein the technique of Hydrolytic Maceration Distillation shows its activity over gaulther in a precursor and helps in the liberation of primeverose and free methyl salicylate (TNAU Agritech Portal).

16.7.1.1.8   Microwave-Assisted Hydrodistillation (MAHD)

It is a modern and innovative process where a microwave oven is used for isolation. It can be used as an alternative to hydrodistillation (Rassem et al., 2016). The effectiveness of the process depends on the dielectric constant of the sample as well as water (Brachet et al., 2002). In case of *Dioscorea hispida* Microwave-Assisted Extraction using 100 Watts of energy for a period of 20 minutes by utilizing ethanol 85% at a sample-solvent ratio of 1:12.5 provided the highest yield (Kumoro and Hartati, 2015).

16.7.1.1.9   Liquid CO_2 Extraction

In this method, liquid carbon dioxide of temperature $22 \pm 2°C$ of 62 ± 2 bar pressure is used for the extraction. The plant materials are placed in the top of the equipment Soxhlet kind instrument with a narrow tube connecting to the bottom where the liquid gas is placed. The liquid is CO_2 is forced to the top which comes in contact of the plant parts and the residue thus formed again moves down in the chamber of liquid CO_2 and is collected over there. Later the residues are collected and strained (Rout et al., 2007; Naik et al., 2014).

16.7.1.1.10   Enfleurage

The process of enfleurage helps in preservation of odor obtained from exquisite flowers for a considerable period of time (Gildemeister and Hoff-mann, 1956–1966; Oyen and Dung, 1999). Here cold fat possessing huge absorption capability is principally employed for getting the fragrance. The fresh lots of flowers like tuberose, jasmine, etc., are harvested and spread over a layer of fat. During harvesting, care should be taken that the flowers are picked at their optimum requisite standards. Then flowers are kept for a certain duration of time in contact with the fat until the aroma from them gets absorbed in the fat. After and when the fat becomes saturated with aroma, it is removed out and mixed with alcohol to get the necessary desired components (Handa, 2008). Different flowers which can be undertaken for the process of enfleurage are jasmine (*Jasminum grandiflorurn*), heliotrope (*Heliotropium peruvianum*), cassie flower *Acacia farnesiana* sour or bitter orange blossom (*Citrus aurantium* violet (*Viola odorata*) and tuberose (*Polianthes tuberosa*) (Gildemeister and Hoffmann, 1956–1966; Oyen and Dung, 1999).

16.8 CONCLUSION

The geographical diversity and wide climatic variation of our country makes it a harbor of innumerable MAPs. Many of these plants are still not identified yet. It is well understood that these group of plants contains chemical constituents which are extremely beneficial for the human body helping it in curing and fighting against an array of diseases and ailments. Furthermore, with the increase of awareness of the present-day consumers and accelerated interest towards these naturally derived medicaments, the importance of MAPs increases in an exponential manner. So today what we need is to take care of the precious natural reserves which our country possesses. Proper cultivation, harvesting after fulfillment of requisite standards and efficient post-harvest handling through modern and innovative means is the need of present-day century. This would result in an increase of the market demand of these plants as well as the products derived from them. Their loss after harvest would be minimized and the stakeholders at all levels would be benefitted.

KEYWORDS

- constituents
- extraction
- medicinal and aromatic plants
- utility
- value-addition

REFERENCES

Akbulut, A., & Durmus, A., (2009). Thin layer solar drying and mathematical modeling of mulberry. *International Journal of Energy Research, 33*, 687–695.

Al-Mansoub, M. A., Asmawi, M. Z., & Murugaiyah, V., (2014). Effect of extraction solvents and plant parts used on the antihyperlipidemic and antioxidant effects of *Garcinia atroviridis*, a comparative study. *Journal of the Science of Food and Agriculture, 94*, 1552–1558.

Anjum, M., (2010). *Design, Development and Modeling of a Solar Distillation System for the Processing of Medicinal and Aromatic Plants*. Dissertation Witzenhausen.

Anuradha, M., Pragyandip, P. D., Richa, K., & Murthy, P. N., (2010). Evaluation of neuropharmacological effects of ethanolic Extract of *Clitoria ternatea* flowers. *Pharmacologyonline, 1*, 284–292.

Azwanida, N. N., (2015). A review on the extraction methods used in medicinal plants, principle, strength and limitation. *Medicinal and Aromatic Plants., 4*, 196. doi 10.4172/2167-0412.1000196.

Bhaskaracharya, R. K., Kentish, S., & Ashokkumar, M., (2009). Selected applications of ultrasonics in food processing. *Food Engineering Reviews., 1*, 31–49.

Birks, J., (2006). Cholinesterase inhibitors for Alzheimer's disease. *The Cochrane Database of Systematic Reviews, 1*. CD005593. doi,10.1002/14651858.

Brachet, A., Christen, P., & Veuthey, J. L., (2002). Focused microwave-assisted extraction of cocaine and benzoylecgonine from coca leaves. *Phytochemical Analysis, 13*, 162–169.

Chrissie, W., (1996). *The Encyclopedia of Aromatherapy* (pp. 16–21). Vermont, Healing Arts Press.

Cowan, M. M., (1999). Plant products as antimicrobial agents. *Clinical Microbiology Reviews, 12*, 564–582.

Craker, L. E., (2007). Medicinal and Aromatic Plants—Future Opportunities. In: Janick, J., &. Whipkey, A., (eds.), *Issues in the New Crops and New Uses*. ASHS Press, Alexandria, VA. https://hort.purdue.edu/newcrop/ncnu07/pdfs/craker248-257.pdf (accessed on 1 November 2021).

Das, A., & Sharangi, A. B., (2018). Post-harvest technology and value addition of spices. In: Sharangi, A. B., (ed.), *Indian Spices, The Legacy, Production & Processing of India's Treasured Export* (249–276). Springer International Publication, Springer Nature.

Dawidowicz, A. L., Rado, E., Wianowska, D., Mardarowicz, M., & Gawdzik, J., (2008). Application of PLE for the determination of essential oil components from *Thymus vulgaris* L. *Talanta, 76*, 878–884.

Dietland, M. S., (2006). Chemical Ecology of Vertebrates (p. 287). Cambridge University Press. ISBN 978-0-521-36377-8.

Dikbasan, T., (2007). *Determination of the Effective Parameters for Drying of Apples*. Master of Science in Energy Engineering, Izmir Institute of Technology, Izmir.

Drugs.com. (2017). *Galantamine*. https://www.drugs.com/monograph/galantamine.html (accessed on 1 November 2021).

El-Beltagy, A., Gamea, G. R., & Amer, E. A. H., (2007). Solar drying characteristics of strawberry. *Journal of Food Engineering, 78*, 456–464.

Elumalai, A., & Chinna, E. M., (2012). Herbalism- A Review. *International Journal of Phytotherapy, 2*(2), 96–105.

Esper, A., & Mühlbauer, W., (1998). Solar drying-an effective means of food preservation. *Renew Energy, 15*, 95–100.

Fahlbusch, K. G., Franz-Josef, H., Johannes, P., Wilhelm, P., Dietmar, S., Kurt, B., Dorothea, G., & Horst, S., (2003). *Flavors and Fragrances.* Ullmann's Encyclopedia of Industrial Chemistry. doi,10.1002/14356007.a11_141.

Gildemeister, E., & Hoffmann, F., (1956–1966). *Die ätherischen Öle [The Essential Oils]* (4th edn., Vol. 8). Akademie Verlag, Berlin, Germany.

Guleria, C., Vaidya, M. K., Sharma, R., & Dogra, D., (2014). Economics of Production and Marketing of important medicinal and aromatic plants in mid-hills of Himachal Pradesh. *Economic Affairs, 59*(3), 363–378.

Handa, S. S., (2008). An overview of extraction techniques for medicinal and aromatic plants. In: *Book- Extraction Technologies for Medicinal and Aromatic Plants* (pp. 21–54).

Harwood, L. M., & Moody, C. J., (1989). *Experimental organic chemistry, Principles and Practice* (pp. 122–125). Illustrated ed. Wiley-Blackwell. ISBN 0-632-02017-2.

Hatamipour, M. S., Kazemi, H. H., Nooralivand, A., & Nozarpoor, A., (2007). Drying Characteristics of six varieties of sweet potatoes in different dryers. *Food and Bioproduct Processing, 85*(3), 171–177.

Hayat, S., & Ahmad, A., (2007). *Salicylic Acid - a Plant Hormone.* Springer Science and Business Media. ISBN 978-1-4020-5183-8.

Hishe, M., Asfaw, Z., & Giday, M., (2016). Review on value chain analysis of medicinal plants and the associated challenges. *Journal of Medicinal Plants Studies, 4*(3), 45–55.

Hossain, M. A., Al-Toubi, W. A. S., Weli, A. M., Al-Riyami, Q. A., & Al-Sabahi, J. N., (2013). Identification and characterization of chemical compounds in different crude extracts from leaves of Omani neem. *Journal of Taibah University for Science, 7*, 181–188.

Irtwange, S. V., (2006). Application of modified atmosphere packaging and related technology in postharvest handling of fresh fruits and vegetables. *Agricultural Engineering International, 4*, 1–12.

Jaume, B., Rodolfo, L., Viladomat, V. F., & Cordell, G. A., (2006). *Chemical and biological aspects of "Narcissus" alkaloids. The Alkaloids, Chemistry and Biology, 63*, 87–179. doi,10.1016/S1099-4831.

Kader, A. A., (2013). Postharvest technology of horticultural crops - an overview from farm to fork. *Ethiop. Journal of Applied Science and Technology, 1*, 1–8.

Kiran, E., Debenedetti, P. G., & Peters, C. J., (1998). *Supercritical Fluids--Fundamentals and Applications.* Academic Publications, Boston, Kluwer.

Kostaropoulos, A. E., & Saravacos, G. D., (1995). Microwave pre-treatment for sun-dried raisins. *Journal of Food Science, 60*, 344–347.

Kumar, A., & Jnanesha, A. C., (2016). Medicinal and Aromatic Plants Biodiversity in India and Their Future Prospects--A Review. *Unani Medicine., 9*, 10–17. https://www.researchgate.net/publication/314724944 (accessed on 1 November 2021).

Kumar, V., Ajeesh, R., Revale, A. A., & Nayak, M. R., (2014). Medicinal plants: Cultivation to value addition, problems and issues--research and reviews. *Journal of Agriculture and Allied Sciences, 3*, 63–71.

Kumoro, C., & Hartati, I., (2015). Microwave assisted extraction of dioscorin from gadung Dioscorea hispida dennst tuber Flour. *Procedia Chemistry, 14*, 47–55.

Malik, R. P. S., (2007). *Cultivation of Medicinal and Aromatic Crops as a Means of Diversification of Agriculture in Uttaranchal* (pp. 1–105). Research Study No. 5.

Meyer-Warnod, B., (1984). Natural essential oils, extraction processes and application to some major oils. *Perfume. Flavorist, 9*, 93–104.

Muthukumaran, A., Ratti, C., & Raghavan, V. G. S., (2008). Foam-mat freeze-drying of egg white—mathematical modeling. Part II. Freeze drying and modelling. *Drying Technology, 26*, 513–518.

Naik, S. N., Jadeja, G. C., Pradhan, R. C., & Rout, P. K., (2014). Extraction of natural products using supercritical fluids and pressurized liquids. *Pharmaceutical and Biological Evaluations, 1*, 9–24.

Overwalle, G. V., (2006). Intellectual property protection for medicinal and aromatic plants. In: Bogers, R. J., Craker, L. E., &. Lange, D., (eds.), *Medicinal and Aromatic Plants* (pp. 121–128). Chapter 9. Netherlands.

Oyen, L. P. A., & Dung, N. X., (1999). Plant Resources of South-East Asia No. 19. Essential-oils plants. Backhuys Publishers. Leiden. P.O Box 321, 2300 AH Leiden, the Netherlands.

Öztekin, S., & Martinov, M., (2007). *Medicinal and Aromatic Crops, Harvesting, Drying and Processing.* Haworth Food & Agricultural Products Press TM, An Imprint of the Haworth Press, Inc., 10 Alice Street, Binghamton, New York 13904-1580 USA.

Pandey, A., & Tripathi, S., (2014). Concept of standardization, extraction and pre phytochemical screening strategies for herbal drug. *Journal of Pharmacognosy and Phytochemistry, 2*(5), 115–119.

Patil, Sachin, B. S., Wakte, P. S., & Shinde, D. B., (2013). Optimization of supercritical fluid extraction and HPLC identification of wedelolactone from *Wedelia calendulacea* by orthogonal array design. *Journal of Advanced Research, 5*, 629–635.

Prajapati, N. D., Purohit, S. S., Sharma, A. K., & Kumar, T., (2003). *A Handbook of Medicinal Plants.* Jodhpur, Agrobios.

Raju, S., (2019). *Value Addition in Medicinal and Aromatic Plants MAPs: An Overview.* https//www.researchgate.net/publication/266081140 (accessed on 1 November 2021).

Rao, M. R., Palada, M. C., & Becker, B. N., (2004). Medicinal and aromatic plants in agroforestry systems. *Advances in Agroforestry*, 107–122.

Rassem, H. H. A., Nour, A. H., & Yunus, R. M., (2016). Techniques for extraction of essential oils from plants: A review. *Australian Journal of Basic and Applied Sciences, 10*(16), 117–127.

Rout, P. K., Naik, S. N., Rao, Y. R., Jadeja, G., & Maheshwari, R. C., (2007). Extraction and composition of volatiles from *Zanthoxylum rhesta*, comparison of subcritical CO_2 and traditional processes. *Journal of Supercritical Fluids, 42*, 334–341.

Samant, S. S., Dhar, U., & Palni, L. M. S., (1998). *Medicinal Plants of Indian Himalayan, Diversity Distribution Potential Values.* Almora, G.B. Pant Institute of Himalayan Environment and Development.

Sereshti, H., Rohanifar, A., Bakhtiari, S., & Samadi, S., (2012). Bifunctional ultrasound-assisted extraction and determination of *Elettaria cardamomum* Maton essential oil. *Journal of Chromatography A, 1238*, 46–53. doi,http,//dx.doi.org/10.1016/j. chroma.2012.03.061.

Shishehgarha, F., Makhlouf, J., & Ratti, C., (2002). Freeze-drying characteristics of strawberries. *Drying Technology, 20*, 131–145.

Shiva, M. P., (1996). *Inventory of Forestry Resources for Sustainable Management and Biodiversity Conservation.* Indus Publishing Company, New Delhi, India.

Singh, D. K., & Hajra, P. K., (1996). Floristic diversity. In: *Biodiversity Status in the Himalaya* (pp. 23–38). British Council, New Delhi, India.

Singsaas, E. L., (2000). Terpenes and the thermotolerance of photosynthesis. *New Phytologist, 146*, 1–4. doi10.1046/j.1469-8137.2000.00626.x.

Soxhlet, F., (1879). The weight analysis of milk fat. *Dingler's Polytechnic. Journal in German, 232*, 461–465.

Taylor, L. T., (1996). *Supercritical Fluid Extraction.* New York, John Wiley & Sons Inc.

Tcheknavorian, A. A., & Wijesekera, R. O. B., (1982). *Industrial Utilization of Medicinal and Aromatic Plants.* UNIDO IO.505.

Tchen, T. T., (1965). The biosynthesis of steroids, terpenes and acetogenins. *American Scientist, 53*(4), 499A–500A. JSTOR 27836252.

TNAUa. (2012). TNAU Agritech Portal. http://agritech.tnau.ac.in/horticulture/extraction_methods_natural_essential_oil.pdf (accessed on 1 November 2021).

TNAUb. (2012). TNAU Agritech Portal. http://agritech.tnau.ac.in/horticulture/extraction_techniques%20_medicinal_plants.pdf (accessed on 1 November 2021).

United States Department of Agriculture, (2017). *Active Plant Ingredients Used for Medicinal Purposes.* https://www.fs.fed.us/wildflowers/ethnobotany/medicinal/ingredients.shtml (accessed on 1 November 2021).

Wills, R. B. H., McGlasson, W. B., Graham, D., Lee, T. H., & Hall, E. G., (1989). Postharvest-An introduction to the physiology and handling of fruit and vegetables (3rd edn., p. 45). New York, U.S.A., Van Nostrand Reinhold.

World Health Organization, ((2003),). WHO guidelines on good agricultural and collection practices *GACP for Medicinal Plants*, 1. Geneva.

Yahia, E. M., (2019). *Postharvest Handling of Aromatic and Medicinal Plants.* https://www.researchgate.net/publication/277954793 (accessed on 1 November 2021).

Yingngam, B., Monschein, M., & Brantner, A., (2014). Ultrasound-assisted extraction of phenolic compounds from *Cratoxylum formosum* ssp. *formosum* leaves using central composite design and evaluation of its protective ability against H_2O_2-induced cell death. *Asian Pacific Journal of Tropical Medicine, 7*, S497–S505.

Yung, O. H., Maskat, M. Y., & Wan, M. W. A., (2010). Effect of extraction on polyphenol content, antioxidant activity and pH in pegaga *Centella asiatica. Sains. Malaysiana, 39*, 747–752.

CHAPTER 17

PROSOPIS CINERARIA (KHEJRI): ETHANOPHARMACOLOGY AND PHYTOCHEMISTRY

TARUN KUMAR UPADHYAY,[1] MANAS MATHUR,[2]
RAKESH KUMAR PRAJAPAT,[2] SUNIL KUMAR NAGAR,[2]
KULVEER SINGH,[2] FAHAD KHAN,[3] PRATIBHA PANDEY,[3]
and MOHAMMAD MUSTUFA KHAN[4]

[1]*Parul Institute of Applied Sciences and Animal Cell Culture and Immunobiochemistry Lab, Parul University, Vadodara, Gujarat – 391760, India, E-mails: tarun_bioinfo@yahoo.co.in; tarunkumar.upadhyay18551@paruluniversity.ac.in*

[2]*School of Agriculture, Suresh Gyan Vihar University, Jaipur, Rajasthan – 302017, India*

[3]*Department of Biotechnology, Noida Institute of Engineering Technology, 19, Knowledge Park-II, Institutional Area, Greater Noida, Uttar Pradesh – 201306, India*

[4]*Department of Basic Medical Sciences, Integral Institute of Allied Health Sciences & Research (IIAHS&R) and Department of Biochemistry, Integral Institute of Medical Sciences & Research (IIMS&R), Integral University, Lucknow, Uttar Pradesh – 226026, India*

ABSTRACT

It is traditionally used as an ayurvedic medicine because of its therapeutic potentials with pharmacological properties like free radical scavenging, pain-relieving, antipyretic, anticancer, antidiabetic, anti-hypercholesterolemia, and nootropic activities. Various plant parts are traditionally recommended in healing of several disorders. Flowers are recommended to combat dermatophytes infections, as coolant and along with that it assists in phagocytosis thus removing impurities from blood. *Prosopis cineraria* is recommended as a protectant in pregnancy by inhibiting lapse in pregnancy. Dehydrated pods of the plants are known as sangri, and it is the main sustenance of some Rajasthani dishes and also has a broader range of ethnopharmacological relevance to combat pain, high cholesterol level, and diabetes, anemia, kidney, and liver disorders. The leaves are recommended in mouth ulcer and eye trouble; along with that it is having antibacterial, antihyperglycemic, antihyperlipidemic, and antioxidant activity. Key search engines like Science Direct, Scopus, JSTOR, PubMed, and Google Scholar were cited to search for traditional literatures related to the ethnopharmacology, biological activity, toxicology, and phytochemistry of *Prosopis cineraria*. In this book chapter, we aim to report an inclusive update on the ethnopharmacology, phytochemistry, and therapeutic potentialities of *Prosopis cineraria* and their phytochemical constituents.

17.1   INTRODUCTION

In the current scenario, there have been many reasons to divert from synthetic to herbal medicines that have proved themselves as a gift of life. Natural products have proven their worth in a lot of researches in the last few decades and are consequently, much valued globally as a basis of healing source for the cure of many metabolic disorders (Sharma et al., 2008). Expedition for healthy as well as prolonged life led human beings to find a library of therapeutic agents in their immediate natural habitat. This warehouse of the healing powers of medicines has accumulated over many years as a result of human intrusive nature. Nowadays, we have many valuable techniques for confirming the health care benefits of plants. The worth of medicinal plants and their value in remedying the fitness need is gaining a lot of attraction globally. Therefore, renewed research on plants that possess bioactive compounds is gaining a lot of attention at an astounding rate.

The significance of this plant has gained keen interest due to the socioeconomic upliftment in the parched habitat of our country mainly Thar Desert in the Rajasthan. The tree can tolerate an extreme range of heat conditions till 48°C and height reaches up to medium sized plant. The plant is known by its common name *Ghaf, Kandi, Jand, Khejri, Shemi, Shami, Khejado, and Jambi*. It is identified by regional name as "Kalpatru," which means "the king of desert" due to its food, feed, and medicinal value. The plant is worshipped by a number of communities, and it is practiced globally, but it is mainly confined in regions of western and southern Asia including India, Saudi Arabia, Iran, Pakistan, and Afghanistan. The crude extracts of this plant show intuition result in increasing the physical and mental conditions of humans and recommended in curing of many metabolic disorders like protein and mineral deficiency. This tree is comprehensively recommended as rapid growing plant which has potentiality to bear abiotic stress like and practiced as fuel and fodder by some communities and it has been found as bellicose unwanted plant in certain region of world. The stem bark is an excellent source of fuel, firewood, and charcoal which are playing a vital role in improving the economic conditions of financially weak farmers residing in the urban part of the country. Different stem branches of the tree are recommended as poles and fence posts in the building of homes and lodgings. Sawn wood is used for making furniture and flooring. Honey produced on this plant has prominent superiority with extensive and adequate flowering. However, it has been found that gum extracted from the bark bears prominent similarity with gum Arabic. Leaves harvested by the farmers are consumed as compost in their cultivable land and it also possesses some fungicidal and insecticidal activity. Bark is used as a source of tannin, dye, and fibers therefore recommended in preparation of medicines mostly for eye, skin, and used to combat infections in stomach. *P. cineraria* help in fixation of atmospheric nitrogen, so it is valuable for soil as it improves its physical features and fertility (Pareek et al., 2015).

17.2 BOTANICAL DESCRIPTION

It is a tree that reaches a height up to 7 m with straight bowl reaching up to 2 m and a circular pinnacle which is consumed for fodder. There are some reports which reveal that it shows some variations in pod size, wide seed collection and growth rate on the basis of different species. Physiologically it is an evergreen tree and flowering and fruiting starts at an early age. Young juvenile leaves develop when the mature leaves degrade in the summer. The tiny yellow flowers grow during March to May. The pods are matured and consumed in the month of June to August (Orwa, 2009; Pasiecznik et al., 2004).

Natural products present in this plant have a number of chemical constituents that have nutritional value as well as certain action in the prevention and treatment of multiple diseases.

17.3   GEOGRAPHICAL LOCATION

It is inhabitant to arid portions of the Asian subcontinent, including India, Oman, Pakistan, Iran, Saudi Arabia, Afghanistan, the United Arab Emirates, and Yemen. Initially, this plant was expanded geographically to the southern part of Asia, covering Indonesia. In India, it founds in the various parts of Rajasthan, Gujarat, Haryana, Uttar Pradesh, and Tamil Nadu (Dharani et al., 2011).

17.4   NUTRITIONAL ANALYSIS

In this report, potential benefits have been described in Sangri pods. Moisture content and dry matter analysis is very vital because it directly affects the nutritional content. The moisture content was quite low (8.55%) which may be beneficial in view of the sample's shelf life. The pods of this plant were found to be rich in carbohydrates (51.01%). The plant contains adequate amount of protein (28.42%) making it as a good source of protein, along with that it also possesses prominent quantity of fibers. Various literatures provide the evidences for the indigestibility of dietary fiber with a large number of beneficial effects. Pods have very low amount of fat (2.30) which make them an ideal diet for overweight people (Rani et al., 2013).

17.5   TRADITIONAL USES OF *P. CINERARIA*

It has been reported by Kirtikar et al. (1935) that all parts of the plant are traditionally used by indigenous people for curing various ailments. Aqueous extracts of leaves and bark are conventionally recommended for ailment of cure mouth and throat infections including bronchitis and ulcers; internal diseases infected with parasites and urinary diseases and dermatitis (Pasiecznik, 1999). The Indian Council of Forestry Research and Education (ICFRE) revealed in 1993 medicinal uses of native *Prosopis* species in Asia. Flowers were found to be anti-abortifacient and stem bark was found to be in controlling the effect of tumors, bronchitis, asthma, leucoderma, rheumatism, leprosy, and dysentery. It has been recommended that eye infections are cured by application of Leaf smoke and extracts are conventionally recommended for use against snakebite and scorpion sting (Pimental, 1960). Hairs are removed by use of ashes of bark by applying on skin which is rubbed over it. Unsullied leaves juice assorted with lemon juice and it is used for dyspepsia, crushed pods is recommended for pain relief, toothache, earache and healing of fractured bones (Garg and Mittal, 2013). They are also reported for their potent pharmacological applications like antihelminthic, antiviral, antitumor, and antimicrobial activities. Paste of leaves of *P. cineraria* is used in combating the effect of ulcers in the mouth of animals and rashes which appears in the form of boils and blisters. The smoke of the leaves is considered to be a good remedy for ailments of the eye (Bhansali et al., 2012). The bark is recommended for scorpion stings.

P. cineraria flower is pulverized mixed with sugar and used during pregnancy as a safeguard against miscarriage (Khatri et al., 2010). The pod is considered as stringent in Punjab. The smoke of the leaves is good for eye problems. The plant is recommended for the treatment of snakebite (Dharani et al., 2011).

17.6 PHARMACOLOGICAL EFFECTS OF *P. CINERARIA*

17.6.1 ANTIBACTERIAL ACTIVITY

It was reported that the presence of phytochemicals like flavonoids and tannins are responsible for antibacterial activity. The polar extracts like water and methanol prepared from stem bark show moderate antibacterial activity at a dose level of 250 µg/ml. Against bacterial strains of *K. pneumoniae, E. coli, P. aeruginosa, S. typhi* it was found to be resistant at same concentration against aqueous and chloroform extracts (Sharma et al., 2012). Different medicinal uses of the *P. cinenaria* parts are listed in Table 17.1.

TABLE 17.1 Various Reports on Medicinal Uses of Different Parts of *Prosoposis cinenaria*

SL. No.	Activity	Plant Part	Dose	References
1.	Antibacterial activity	Stem bark	250 µg/ml	Sharma et al. (2012)
2.	Antihyperglycemic activity	Stem bark	300 mg/kg	Sharma et al. (2013); Soni et al. (2018)
3.	Analgesic activity	Root	200 mg/Kg b.wt*. and 300 mg/kg	Joseph et al. (2011)
4.	Anticonvulsant activity	Stem bark	200 and 400 mg/kg	Velmurugan et al. (2012)

TABLE 17.1 *(Continued)*

SL. No.	Activity	Plant Part	Dose	References
5.	Antihyperlipidemic effect	Bark	500 mg/Kg body weight per day	Preeti et al. (2015)
6.	Antifungal activity	Seed	Antifungal protein with a molecular mass of 38.6 kDa	Solanki et al. (2018)
7.	Antidepressant effect	Leaves	200 mg/kg	George et al. (2012)
8.	Antihelminitic activity	Stem bark	160 mg/ml	Velmurugan et al. (2011)
9.	Apoptotic activity	Leaves	20 mg/20 µl., 65.27 µg/ml and 37.02 µg/ml	Sumathi et al. (2013); Jinu et al. (2017)
10.	Antioxidant and anti-inflammatory activity	Ethyl acetate, chloroform, and butanol fractions of PC hydroethanolic extract of whole plants	NA	Yadav et al. (2018)
11.	Respiratory and gastrointestinal activity	stem bark	Phenylephrine at (11 µM)	Sumitra et al. (2013)

17.6.2 ANTI-HYPERGLYCEMIC ACTIVITY

Sharma et al. (2013) reported antihyperglycemic and antioxidant activities of 50% Hydro-alcoholic extract of stem bark in alloxan-induced
(AI) mice. They have reported that fasting blood glucose (FBG) level
reduced by 27.3%, in comparison of 49.3% as reduced by Glibenclamide
also called glyburide is taken as standard drug and glycogen level was
enhanced in liver at dose level of 300 mg/kg. When compared to non-
treated group.

The antidiabetic activity of chloroform fraction of stem bark of *P.
cineraria* was reported by Soni et al. (2018) against streptozotocin-induced
diabetes. The doses of plant at 50 and 100 mg/kg b.wt were induced in rats
for 21 days which are already treated with STZ at a dose level of 55 mg/
kg b.wt. It was observed that after induction of plant dose there was reduction in blood glucose level, glycosylated hemoglobin and also reestablished

liver glycogen content, serum insulin level and body weight, exponentially in a dose-dependent manner. Plant extract is useful for reduction in serum lipid profile markers and also exhibit a high level of HDL-C after treatment, which showed the protective effects in diabetes-associated complications. Further, it was observed that plant dose at IC_{50} value of 40.29 µg/ml reduced significantly inhibition of α-amylase enzyme. It was concluded that this plant is recommended as anodyne harmonizing medicine in the control of diabetes and its related disorders.

17.6.3   ANALGESIC ACTIVITY

Joseph et al. (2011) reported the analgesic activity of aqueous extract of leaves and ethanolic extract of root at a dose of (200 mg/Kg b.wt.) and 300 mg/kg respectively in Swiss albino mice. They reported that extract had better activity as compared to control. The plant possessed potent antipyretic efficiency at similar treatment in Brewer's yeast induced hyperpyrexia animal model.

17.6.4   ANTI-HYPERLIPIDEMIC EFFECT

Preeti et al. (2015) reported Hypo-lipidemic and anti-atherosclerotic effects of bark extract of *P. cineraria* is evaluated in hyperlipidemic rabbits. The administration of 70% ethanolic extract of bark significantly reduced serum total cholesterol, LDL-C, triglyceride, VLDL-C, and also ischemic indices (Total cholesterol/LDL-C and LDL-C/HDL-C).

17.6.5   ANTICONVULSANT ACTIVITY

Velmurugan et al. (2012) showed Anticonvulsant activity of the methanolic extract of *P. cineraria* stem barks against induced maximal electroshock (MES) and pentylenetetrazole (PTZ) convulsions in mice. They reported that extract curbed hind limb tonic extensions (HLTE) induced by MES and also exhibited protector effect in PTZ Induced Seizures in a dose dependent manner. The activity was potent at doses of 200 mg/kg and 400 mg/kg along with Phenytoin (25 mg/kg).

17.6.6 ANTIMICROBIAL ACTIVITY

Evaluation of plant-based materials against the bacteria and fungus play a vital part for innovation of targeted drugs as therapeutics for benefits of manhood suffering from different complications. Solanki et al. (2018) reported antifungal activity of a novel seed protein of *P. cineraria*. They reported that purified protein had potent activity against *Lasiodiplodia theobromae* and *Aspergillus fumigatus*. Studies reported by Girase et al. (2016) that ethyl ether and alcoholic leaves extracts were screened for antimicrobial activity by using 3 microorganisms such as *Staphylococcus aureus* (Gram-positive), *Escherichia coli* (Gram-negative) and *Candida albicans* (Fungal pathogen).

17.6.7 ANTIDEPRESSANT EFFECT

Chaudhary et al. (2018) reported the antidepressant effect of *P. cineraria* against depression by (to overcome depression) of aqueous extract of leaves of *P. cineraria in* skeletal muscle relaxant activity. It was observed that dose level of 200 mg/kg tremendously reduced the time interval of immobility time when carried by forced swim assay.

17.6.8 ANTIHELMINITIC ACTIVITY

Velmurugan et al. (2011) reported anti-parasitic activity of different isolates of stem bark of *P. cineraria*. They reported that the methanolic extract at a dose of 160 mg/ml induced paralysis in 25 min and death in 62 min against *Phretima Posthuma* when compared with standard drug piperazine citrate (10 mg/ml) which showed significant reduction at 23 min and 61 min, respectively.

17.6.9 APOPTOTIC ACTIVITY

To check the cell death stimulation of *P. cineraria,* extract studies conducted by Sumathi et al. (2013) showed methanolic extract of leaves was tested in breast cancer cell line MCF-7 and non-cancerous cell line such as HBL 100. They found that plant extract caused a steep increase in apoptotic cell ratio in cancer cell line and not in HBL 100 which is healthy cell line.

Jinu et al. (2017) reported antimicrobial and cytotoxic activities of nanoparticles prepared from *P. cineraria* leaf extract. They reported that these nanoparticles had 50% inhibition with inhibitory concentrations (IC_{50}) of 65.27 μg/ml and 37.02 μg/ml respectively against a commonly used breast cancer cell line MCF-7.

17.6.10   ANTIOXIDANT AND ANTI-INFLAMMATORY ACTIVITY

Yadav et al. (2018) reported that due to adequate amount of phenolic rich ointment which is used in wound healing the plant possess potent antioxidant and anti-inflammatory potentials. They reported that butanol extracts possessed noteworthy *in vitro* antioxidant and anti-inflammatory efficacy.

17.6.11   RESPIRATORY AND GASTROINTESTINAL ACTIVITY

Methanolic extract isolated from stem bark of *P. cineraria* was tested for bronchodilator, spasmolytic, and vasodilator actions and it can be used for treatment of such problems. Studies reported by Sumitra et al. (2013) and it was observed that bronchodilator and vasodilator activities which were possibly mediated through blockade of Ca^{2+} channels.

17.6.12   IN VIVO CYTOTOXIC EVALUATION OF P. CINERARIA

Previous studies reported that when 50% hydrochloric extract of leaves and stem were orally administered to Wistar rats at a time interval of 28 days, it was observed that LD50 of the extract was higher than 2,000 mg/kg dose level. At the end of the 28th day, there were no variations in parameters like body weight, behavior, hematological parameters including biochemical analysis. There was not any noticeable malfunctioning when examined histopathologically. There was no case of any mortality when rats were administrated with dose level of 1,000 mg/kg. It was overall concluded that the plant dose was deficient in subacute for toxicity studies. Female rats were treated with 50% hydroalcoholic extract of leaves and stem bark at a dose of 200, 500, 1,000 mg/Kg b.wt. It was observed that in various hematological parameters like erythrocyte, leukocytes, platelets, Hb, PCV, clotting, and ESR, there were no variations in extract-treated animals when compared to control. The death rate was almost nil in one day after induction of dose. Further in breathing, sensory nervous system, cutaneous effects and in behavior responses no optimum variations were observed (Robertson et al., 2013).

17.7   PHYTOCHEMISTRY OF *P. CINERARIA*

Leaves of *P. cineraria* have various classes of phytochemicals like sitosterol, campesterol, cholesterol, and actacosanol, stigmasterol, methyldocosanoate, hentriacontane, Tricosan-1-ol, Diisopropyl-10, 11-dihydroxyicosane-1,20-dioate, and 7,24-Tirucalladien-3-one along with a piperidine alkaloid spicigerine. Amino acids purified from leaves are Threonine, Aspartic acid, Glycine, Serine, Histidine, Glutamic acid, Arginine, Alanine, Proline, Tyrosine, Cystine, Isoleucine, Valine, Methionine, Leucine, Phenylalanine, and Lysine (Gupta et al., 2014), phenolic acid derivatives (Malik and Kalidhar, 2007; Khan et al., 2006). Flowers of *P. cineraria* hold patuletin glycoside, spicigerine, patulitrin, sitosterol, flavone derivatives Prosogerin A and Prosogerin B.

The leaves possess high content of unsaturated fatty acids, with linoleic acid and oleic acid (Malik and Kalidhar, 2007). Fresh, ripe pods contain calcium and phosphorus (Murthy, 1975). They are rich in carbohydrates along with a good source of protein (Robertson et al., 2014). The dry pods are a rich source of manganese, copper, and zinc, yielded fatty oils (Murthy, 1975). Dried pods of this plant also contain maslinic acid 3-glucoside, 3-benzyl-2-hydroxy-urs-12-en-28-oic acid, linoleic acid, prosphylline, 5,5'-oxybis-1,3-benzendiol, 3,4,5, trihydroxycinnamic acid 2-hydroxy ethyl ester, and 5,3,'4'-trihydroxyflavanone 7-glycoside (Liu et al., 2012). When hot aqueous extract of pods is fractionated using methanol and trichloromethane, different phytochemicals like such as 3-benzyl-2-hydroxy-urs-12-en-28-oic acid and maslinic acid-3-glucoside (triterpenoids); linoleic acid (fatty acid); 5,3',4'-trihydroxyflavanone 7-glycoside (polyphenols); 5,5'-oxybis-1,2-benzanediol; 3,4,5-trihydroxycinnamic acid 2-hydroxyethyl ester; and prosophylline (piperidine alkaloid) are obtained (Karim et al., 2012). Broad classes of phytochemicals like tannins (gallic acid), steroids (stigmasterol, sitosterol, campestral), alkaloids (spicigerine, prosophylline), Flavone derivatives (Prosogerin A, B, C, D, and E), etc., have been isolated from the pods (Gehlot et al., 2008). Dried unripe pods of confirmed the presence of tannins, alkaloids, flavonoids, and glycosides (Sharma et al., 2012).

The bark contains glucose, rhamnose, sucrose, and starch which have been proved by various researchers (Gupta et al., 2014; Sumitra et al., 2013). The chloroform extract contains Methyl 5-tridecyloctadec-4-enoate, nonacosan-8-one, lupeol, β-sitosterol and stigmasterol (Duke, 1994).

Seeds contain 6,7-dimethoxy-2-(3,4,5-trimethoxyphenyl)-4H-chromen-4-one, 7-hydroxy-6-methoxy-2-(3,4,5-trimethoxyphenyl)chromen-4-one,3, 5,3,4-tetrahydroxy-6-methoxyflavone-7-O-β-Dglucopyranoside, -(3,4-Dihydroxyphenyl)-5,7-dihydroxy-4-chromenone,3,4,5-Trihy-droxybenzoic acid, 2-(3,4-dihydroxyphenyl)-5,7-dihydroxy-3-[(2S,3R,4S, 5S,6R)-3,4,5-trihydroxy-6-[[(2R,3R,4R,5R,6S)-3,4,5-trihydroxy-6-methyloxan-2-yl]oxymethyl]oxan-2-yl]oxychromen-4-one, and 6-Methoxyquercetin 519-96-0 Quercetagetin 6-methyl ether, all are having potential to act as anticancerous agents (Garg and Mittal, 2013). The seeds contain protein, carbohydrates (Murthy, 1995). Seed protein is constituted of 2-Aminobutanedioic acid, 2-Aminopentanedioic acid, 2-Amino-3-(1H-imidazol-4-yl)propanoic acid, 2,6-Diaminohexanoic acid, 2-amino-4-(methylthio)butanoic acid, 2-Amino-3-phenylpropanoic acid, 2-Aminoethanoic acid-2-Amino-3-hydroxypropanoic acid, 2-Aminopropa-noic acid, 2-Amino-5-guanidinopentanoic acid, 2-amino-3-methylpentanoic acid, 2-Amino-4-methylpentanoic acid, 2-Amino-3-(4-hydroxyphenyl) propanoic acid, Pyrrolidine-2-carboxylic acid, 2-Amino-3-methylbutanoic acid, and minute quantities of 2-amino-3-(1H-indol-3-yl) propanoic acid (Rani et al., 2013) also contains fixed oils, fatty acid like palmitic acid, stearic acid, oleic acid and linoleic acid, sterols like campstool, stigmasterol, β-sitosterol, stimasta-5, 24(28)-dien-3 β-ol, stimasta-1,3,5-triene, stimasta-4,6-dien-3-one (Robertson et al., 2011). The seed bears a huge amount of unsaturated fatty acids, in which majority are linoleic and oleic acids (Gangal et al., 2009; Rastogi and Mehrotra, 1995).

There are some research reports which confirmed the presence of fatty acids, glycosides, alkaloids, and phytosterols, glucosides, and flavones from different plants like flowers and seeds (Gangal et al., 2009). Physio-chemical assays confirmed the presence of hydrocarbons and phenolic acid (Khan et al., 2006; Malik and Kalidhar, 2007). The leaves also showed the presence of a large fraction of unsaturated fatty acids like cis, cis-9, 12-Octadecadienoic acid and cis-9-octadecenoic acid. The presence of phytochemicals like flavonoids, tannins, alkaloids, and glycosides were confirmed in dehydrated immature pods of *P. cineraria* (Sharma et al., 2012; Purohit et al., 1979).

17.8   SOCIOECONOMIC IMPORTANCE OF THE *P. CINERARIA*

P. cineraria is one of the most prominent flora for the population residing in desert areas of our country. This plant gives fodder, fuelwood, small timber, medicines, and also improves the soil structure. Farmers have spatial attention toward this tree and provide protection. It is highly compatible with agricultural crops outstanding to a deep root system, nitrogen-fixing ability, and high efficiency of recharging the soil with organic matter. Based on the experimental data, we exhibited that *P. cineraria* should be preferred as a species for the development of degraded landscapes in arid areas. Recently due to heavy pressure on this species, its natural regeneration has been checked to a great extent, and therefore planting of seedlings of Khejri by the farmers has become essential to conserve this important native tree.

17.9   FUTURE PROSPECTS

The keen attention has been devoted to maximize the consumption of natural products in the exponentially increasing communities globally, the urge for drugs and dietary supplements isolated from plants have gained interest in the current scenario. The enhanced consumption and rapidly developing market of natural products and extensive use of herbal medicines is expanding at a rapid rate globally in coming decades with appropriate scientific proof of their eminence, effectiveness, and safety as per reports of certain scientific communities. The available data on *P. cineraria* can provide evidential support for the clinical development as adjuvant therapy. Overall, we recommend that this plant fulfills the criteria for its selection based on its therapeutic potential and toxicity profile, and also availability of the plant. It is observed from various studies that this plant has numerous pharmaceutical and medicinal properties. Therefore, it is recommended as an active medicinal cradle to combat a number of metabolic disorders. It can be assumed that the biomedical importance of *P. cineraria* could be coordinated, towards a probable amalgamation into the healthcare schemes.

17.10   CONCLUSIONS

P. cineraria are extremely tailored to severe natural environment and physiologically develop in a broad geographic territory. It can be concluded that *P. cineraria* is a promising medicinal plant having a broad spectrum of therapeutic applications which are recommended conventionally *viz*, anti-diabetic, hepatotoxicity, antimicrobial, anti-hypertensive, antioxidant, reduction in lipid, anti-inflammatory, and anticancer. Besides this, *P. cineraria* have tremendous nourishing features. The present review is aimed to summarize the latest knowledge on the conventional practices, therapeutic applications, and phytochemical investigations of *P. cineraria*. Several scanty reports are available on innovative potentials therefore this plant is attracted a lot of attention of scientific community for research in future perspectives, keeping in mind its multipurpose ethnopharmacological applications, there is an ample scope for future research on *P. cineraria*, Alongside innovation in orthodox chemistry and pharmacology in innovating potent drugs, the medicinal flora might provide a useful source of new medicines and may be used in place of existing drugs.

KEYWORDS

- ayurvedic medicines
- ethnopharmacology
- Kalpatru
- Khejri plant
- pharmacological effects

REFERENCES

AGRIS-FAO, (1999). *Prosopis-Pest or Providence, Weed or Wonder Tree?* By Pasiecznik, N., http://agris.fao.org/agris-search/search.do?recordID=GB2012100242 (accessed on 01 November 2021).

Aparna, P., Deepika, S., & Pareek, L. K., (2012). In-vitro micropropagation through cotyledonary nodal segments in *Prosopis cineraria* L. *Research Journal of Pharmaceutical, Biological and Chemical Sciences, 3*(3), 309–313.

Ashok, P., & Heera, R., (2012). Hypolipidemic and anti-atherosclerotic effects of *Prosopis cineraria* bark extract in experimentally induced hyperlipidemic rabbits. *Asian Journal of Pharmaceutical and Clinical Research, 5*(3), 106–109.

Bahuguna, U., & Shukla, R. N., (2010). A study on investigation of the chemical constituents and milled wood lignin analysis of *Lantana camara* and *Prosopis chilensis. International Journal of Applied Biology and Pharmaceutical Technology, 1*(3), 830–839.

Bhansali, R. R., (2012). Development of flower galls in *Prosopis cineraria* trees of Rajasthan. *The Journal of Plant Protection Sciences, 4*(1), 52–56.

Chaudhary, K. K., Kumar, G., Varshney, A., Meghvansi, M. K., Ali, S. F., Karthik, K., & Kaul, R. K., (2018). Ethnopharmacological and phytopharmaceutical evaluation of Prosopis cineraria: An overview and future prospects. *Current Drug Metabolism, 19*(3), 192–214.

Dharani, B., Sumathi, S., Sivaprabha, J., & Padma, P. R., (2011). In vitro antioxidant potential of *Prosopis cineraria* leaves. *J. Nat. Prod. Plant Resour., 1*, 26–32.

Duke, J., & Bogenschutz, M. J., (1994). *Dr. Duke's Phytochemical and Ethnobotanical Databases* (pp. 1–8). USDA, Agricultural Research Service.

Gangal, S., Sharma, S., & Rauf, A., (2009). Fatty acid composition of *Prosopis cineraria* seeds. *Chemistry of Natural Compounds, 45*(5), 705.

Garg, A., & Mittal, S. K., (2013). Review on *Prosopis cineraria*: A potential herb of Thar desert. *Drug Invention Today, 5*(1), 60–65.

Gehlot, P., Bohra, N. K., & Purohit, D. K., (2008). Endophytic mycoflora of inner bark of *Prosopis cineraria*-a keystone tree species of Indian desert. *Am. Eur. J. Bot., 1*(1), 01–04.

George, M., Joseph, L., & Sharma, A., (2012). Antidepressant and skeletal muscle relaxant effects of the aqueous extract of the *Prosopis cineraria. Brazilian J. Pharmaceutical Sci., 48*(3), 577–582.

Girase, M. V., Jadhav, M. L., & Jain, A. S., (2016). Prosopis *Spicigera*: A nature's gift. *International Journal of Pharmaceutical Chemistry and Analysis, 3*(1), 49–52.

Gupta, A., Sharma, G., Pandey, S., Verma, B., Pal, V., & Agrawal, S. S., (2014). *Prosopis cineraria* and its various therapeutic effects with special reference to diabetes: A novel approach. *Int. J. Pharm. Sci. Rev. Res., 27*(2), 328–333.

Jinu, U., Gomathi, M., Saiqa, I., Geetha, N., Benelli, G., & Venkatachalam, P., (2017). Green engineered biomolecule-capped silver and copper nanohybrids using *Prosopis cineraria* leaf extract: Enhanced antibacterial activity against microbial pathogens of public health relevance and cytotoxicity on human breast cancer cells (MCF-7). *Microbial Pathogenesis., 105*, 86–95.

Joseph, L., George, M., Sharma, A., & Gopal, N., (2011). Antipyretic and analgesic effects of the aqueous extracts of *Prosopis cineraria. Global J. Pharmacol., 5*(2), 73–77.

Karim, A. A., & Azlan, A., (2012). Fruit pod extracts as a source of nutraceuticals and pharmaceuticals. *Molecules, 17*(10), 11931–11946.

Khan, S. T., Riaz, N., Afza, N., Nelofar, A., Malik, A., Ahmed, E., & Hussain, S., (2006). Studies on the chemical constituents of Prosopis cineraria. *Journal of the Chemical Society of Pakistan, 28*(6), 619–622.

Khatri, A., Rathore, A., & Patil, U. K., (2010). *Prosopis cineraria* (L.) Druce: A boon plant of desert—an overview. *International Journal of Biomedical and Advance Research, 1*(5), 141–149.

Kirtikar, K. R., & Basu, B. D., (1918). *Indian Medicinal Plants Vol-3*. Bishen Singh Mahendra Pal Singh and Periodical Experts.

Liu, Y., Singh, D., & Nair, M. G., (2012). Pods of khejri (Prosopis cineraria) consumed as a vegetable showed functional food properties. *Journal of Functional Foods, 4*(1), 116–121.

Malik, A., & Kalidhar, S. B., (2007). Phytochemical examination of *Prosopis cineraria* L. (Druce) leaves. *Indian Journal of Pharmaceutical Sciences, 69*(4), 576.

Pasiecznik, N. M., Harris, P. J., & Smith, S. J., (2004). *Identifying Tropical Prosopis Species: A Field Guide* (p. 29). Coventry: HDRA Publishing.

Pimental, M. D. L., (1960). *P. juliflora* (SW) (DC). In: *1 "Simposio Brasilerios obre Algarobera,"* (Vol. 1, p. 330e5).

Purohit, S. D., Ramawat, K. G., & Arya, H. C., (1979). Phenolics, peroxidase and phenolase as related to gall formation in some arid zone plants. *Current Science, 714*–716.

Rani, B., Singh, U., Sharma, R., Gupta, A. A., Dhawan, N. G., Sharma, A. K., & Maheshwari, R. K., (2013). *Prosopis cineraria* (L) Druce: A desert tree to brace livelihood in Rajasthan. *Asian Journal of Pharmaceutical Research and Health Car., 5*(2), 58–64.

Rastogi, R. P., & Mehrotra, B. N., (1993). *Compendium of Indian Medicinal Plants* (Vol. 2, p. 864). 1970–1979 Central Drug Research Institute, Lucknow and Publications & Information Directorate, New Delhi, India. ISBN 13:9788185042084.

Robertson, S., Narayanan, N., & Raj, K. B., (2011). Antitumor activity of *Prosopis cineraria* (L.) Druce against Ehrlich ascites carcinoma-induced mice. *Natural Product Research, 25*(8), 857–862.

Robertson, S., Narayanan, N., Deattu, N., & Nargis, N. R., (2010). Comparative anatomical features of *Prosopis cineraria* (L.) Druce and *Prosopis juliflora* (Sw.) DC (Mimosaceae). *International Journal of Green Pharmacy, 4*(4).

Sharma, B., Balomajumder, C., & Roy, P., (2008). Hypoglycemic and hypolipidemic effects of flavonoid rich extract from *Eugenia jambolana* seeds on streptozotocin induced diabetic rats. *Food and Chemical Toxicology, 46*(7), 2376–2383.

Sharma, D., & Singla, Y. P., (2013). Evaluation of antihyperglycemic and antihyperlipidemic activity of *Prosopis cineraria* (Linn.) in Wistar rats. *Journal of Scientific and Innovative Research, 2*(4), 751–758.

Sharma, R., Jodhawat, N., Purohit, S., & Kaur, S., (2012). Antibacterial activity and phytochemical screening of dried pods of *Prosopis cineraria*. *Int. J. Pharm. Sci. Rev. Res., 14*(1), 15–17.

Solanki, D. S., Kumar, S., Parihar, K., Tak, A., Gehlot, P., Pathak, R., & Singh, S. K., (2018). Characterization of a novel seed protein of *Prosopis cineraria* showing antifungal activity. *International Journal of Biological Macromolecules, 116*, 16–22.

Soni, L. K., Dobhal, M. P., Arya, D., Bhagour, K., Parasher, P., & Gupta, R. S., (2018). In vitro and in vivo antidiabetic activity of isolated fraction of *Prosopis cineraria* against streptozotocin-induced experimental diabetes: A mechanistic study. *Biomedicine Pharmacotherapy, 108*, 1015–1021.

Sumathi, S., Dharani, B., Sivaprabha, J., Raj, K. S., & Padma, P. R., (2013). Cell death induced by methanolic extract of *Prosopis cineraria* leaves in MCF-7 breast cancer cell line. *Int J Pharmacol. Sci. Invent., 2*, 21–26.

Sumitra, S., Vijay, N., & Sharma, S. K., (2013). Isolation of novel phytoconstituents from the bark of *Salvadora oleoides* decne. *International Journal of Herbal Medicine, 1*(2), 9–13.

Velmurugan, V., Arunachalam, G., & Ravichandran, V., (2010). Antibacterial activity of stem bark of *Prosopis cineraria* (Linn.) Druce. *Archives of Applied Science Research, 2*(4), 147–150.

Velmurugan, V., Arunachalam, G., & Ravichandran, V., (2012). Anticonvulsant activity of methanolic extract of *Prosopis cineraria* (Linn) Druce stem barks. *Int. J. Pharm. Tech. Res., 4*(1), 89–92.

Yadav, E., Singh, D., Yadav, P., & Verma, A., (2018). Antioxidant and anti-inflammatory properties of *Prosopis cineraria* based phenolic rich ointment in wound healing. *Biomedicine Pharmacotherapy, 108*, 1572–1583.

CHAPTER 18

MITIGATION OF OBESITY: A PHYTOTHERAPEUTIC APPROACH

A. B. SHARANGI AND SUDDHASUCHI DAS

Department of Plantation, Spices, Medicinal, and Aromatic Crops, Faculty of Horticulture, Bidhan Chandra Krishi Viswavidyalaya (Agricultural University), Mohanpur – 741252, West Bengal, India, E-mail: absharangi@gmail.com (A. B. Sharangi)

ABSTRACT

Obesity is a recognized global epidemic all throughout the globe with its dangerous dent in almost every nook and corner. It is an increasingly common phenomenon all over the world and the whole scientific community, governments, and organizations worldwide are impulsively extra attentive to address this issue. This apparently peaceful malady not only affects human life in a negative way slowly, but imposes unwarranted implications in the overall health system. Obesity is often associated with diabetes, dyslipidemia, osteoarthritis, musculoskeletal disturbances, and even some types of cancer, such as endometrial, colon, and breast cancer. Apart from many life-style related requirements of behavioral changes as well as quite a few chemical and synthetic options, the phytotherapeutic horizons of mitigating obesity are opening up rapidly and consistently. Comprehensive research practices are continued around the world over time with the studies on phytotherapeutic usage profile, action mechanism, possible limitations, etc. A new hope has already been ushered through the wide ranges of medicinal plants opening new windows for further research validation and confirmation. Additional synergy on chemical, biological, and clinical aspects are essential on the effectiveness of such plants, including those used as spices and condiments in our daily diet, in developing and treating obesity in humans. Such anti-obesity findings would suggest food and drug manufacturers to develop newer products, and to governments to control food products as a step forward to improve and enhance public health. The findings of this review may be useful in streamlining obesity research through plants and providing a roadmap for future studies to pave the way for more desirable and greener phytotherapeutic options.

18.1   INTRODUCTION

Any undesirable imbalance between energy intake and expenditure results in obesity. When dietary energy intake exceeds energy spending, surplus energy is converted to triglyceride which is stored in adipose tissue, thereby increasing body fat and causing weight gain. Obesity is assessed by means of body mass index (BMI) which is obtained by dividing the body weight (kg) with the square of height (m). A value of and over 30 kg/m² indicates obesity. Nearly 1.9 billion adults (18 years or more) around the world are overweight and about 600 million of them are clinically obese. That is why obesity is recognized as one of the major health related threats throughout the globe (WHO, 2020). This malady, initially a concern for higher-income countries, is now on the rise in low- and middle-income countries also, especially in urban areas. The characteristic symptom of obesity is an increase in adipose cell size as quantified by the amount of fat accumulation at the cytoplasm of adipocytes (Devlin et al., 2000). Enzymes namely fatty acid synthase, lipoprotein lipase and adipocyte fatty acid-binding protein controls this metabolic change in the adipocytes (Rosen et al., 2000).

Altered lipid metabolic processes together with lipogenesis and lipolysis facilitate the development of obesity (Pagliassotti et al., 1997). Synthetic moieties and surgical procedures are the universal therapy of obesity, but have detrimental side effects and likelihood of severe recurrence (Karri et al., 2019). Lipogenesis stores free fatty acids in the form of triglyceride (Mandrup and Lane, 1997); whereas in lipolysis, the stored triglyceride is metabolized to free fatty acids and glycerol (Ducharme and Bichel, 2008). Obesity is accompanied by an abnormally high concentration of lipids in blood, i.e., hyperlipidemia (Akiyama et al., 1996). The adipose tissue secretes several biologically active adipokines and thereby regulates metabolism and homeostasis (Yudkin et al., 1999). Three key transcription factors like peroxisome proliferator-activated receptor (PPAR), CCAAT/enhancer-binding protein (C/EBP) and sterol regulatory element-binding protein (SREBP) regulate the expression of these lipid-metabolizing enzymes during adipose tissue development (Freytag and Utter, 1983). 5' AMP-activated protein kinase

(AMPK) plays a major role in lipid and glucose metabolism by inactivating acetyl-CoA carboxylase (ACC) and Through up-regulating the expression of carnitine palmitoyl transferase-1 (CPT-1), PPAR, and uncoupling protein, stimulation of fatty acid oxidation is done (Kim et al., 2007).

This review summarizes the present understanding on obesity, the underlying causes of the expansion of obesity, its epidemiology, pathophysiology, anti-obesity preparations, anti-obesity mechanisms of natural dietary or herbal products, plant-based bioactive chemical components, progress of anti-obesity foods and the challenges ahead towards futuristic research on phytotherapeutic options in handling obesity.

18.2   CAUSES OF OBESITY

18.2.1   HEREDITY

Obesity is a composite, heritable feature influenced by the interaction of genetics and the environment (Thaker, 2017). Heredity influences the fat tissue distribution. Generally, if parent is overweight, it is enough probable that the heavy newborns grow into heavy adolescents. Weight regulation in the human body depends upon diverse genetically deciding factors such as hormones. Any irregularity in these factors could be ended with considerable weight gain. This is said to be an inherited character for the majority of (approximately 60%) obese people. So, the idea that genetic influence can contribute to weight gain cannot be ignored.

18.2.2   ENDOCRINOLOGY

Several endocrine alterations due to changes in the hypothalamic-pituitary hormone axes are reported (Sidhu et al., 2017). Some of them are considered as causative factors for obesity development, whereas others are secondary effects of obesity (usually restored after weight loss). In rare cases, hormonal imbalance or glandular problems are responsible for some people to be genetically predisposed to obesity. Different syndromes like hypothyroidism, Cushing's syndrome, hypogonadism in men and polycystic ovarian syndrome in women are observed in obesity. Hypothalamic lesions like tumors, infections or severe traumas that are known to lead to obesity are ascribed to be developed genetically.

18.2.3   MEDICATION

Bodyweight can be greater than before through certain drugs such as cortico-steroids, diabetes medication (e.g., insulin; sulfonylureas viz., Glimepiride, Gipizide, Glyburide, etc.; thiazolidinedione viz., Pioglitazone; others viz., Nateglinide, Repaglinide), steroidal contraceptives and anticonvulsants such as valproate used in epileptic treatment. Mood stabilizers like antipsychotics, older antidepressants (e.g., Amitriptyline, Imipramine, Nortriptyline, Trazo-done, Monoamine oxidase inhibitors-MAOIs, etc.), lithium, benzodiaz-epines, heartburn drugs, hormone therapy/contraceptives, anti-seizure drugs, anticonvulsants/anti-migraine/neuropathic pain (Gabapentin, Pregabalin, Valproic acid, Carbamazepine, Divalproex, etc., are also identified to have the same weight increasing properties (Verhaegen and Van Gaal, 2019).

18.2.4   PSYCHOLOGICAL CAUSES

The relationship between one's emotional fluctuations and obesity is now extensively accredited. Feelings of sadness, anxiety or stress led to negative emotions as well as low self-esteem. To cope up with depressive symptoms, quite a few patients eat a lot which results in substantial weight gain. This habit subsequently becomes a repetitive process over time and sooner or later results in obesity (Değirmenci et al., 2015).

18.2.5   DIETARY FACTORS

Today's world is more affluent than it ever was. In spite of having a stan-dard prescribed food for a sustainable healthy lifestyle, majority of people have diverse dietary options. Nowadays, people are less energetic than their predecessors, keeping the calorific content of their daily di*et al*most intact, even increased. The diet style has drastically changed over time around the world. A significant transformation to a high-carbohydrate, high-fat diet from a high protein, high-fat diet is evident. The over-consumption of empty-calorie foods like aerated drinks, alcohol, candies, etc., has also risen sharply. All of these empty-calorie foods, coupled with an inactive lifestyle, make the perfect combination for vulnerability to diabetes and obesity. It is further linked to augmented incidence of hypertension, type 2 diabetes mellitus, arthritis, coronary heart disease, sleep apnea, and certain forms of cancer (Ogden et al., 2006).

18.3   EPIDEMIOLOGY OF OBESITY

In Western countries and later on worldwide, obesity gradually emerged as a significant health issue, whose prevalence has sharply increased in the last few decades. It has been defined as a pandemic and one of the momentous health nuisances ever. Obesity represents a health challenge since it considerably increases the menace like type 2 diabetes, fatty liver, hypertension, stroke, dementia, osteoarthritis, obstructive sleep apnoea, several cancers and contributes to a declining life quality and life expectancy. On the other side, it is also associated with unemployment, social disadvantages and reduced socio-economic productivity (Blüher, 2019). Overweight is greater than 25% in the case of children, while in adults, it is more than 50% (Barquera et al., 2013a). In the past 30 years, Mexico witnessed the incidence of obesity most rapidly, where female is mostly affected (approximate 1.5% points) and the preschool children have shown the least morbidity (0.3% points) (Barquera et al., 2013b). This pervasiveness is attributed to the severe changes of dietary food in Western countries. An increased consumption of non-nutritional carbohydrates, especially sugar-sweetened beverages often lead to obesity preceded by cardiovascular diseases (CVD) and diabetes.

18.4   PATHOPHYSIOLOGY OF OBESITY

When energy expenditure and calorific intake are imbalanced, obesity is an obvious consequence. Human adipose tissue is generally of two types-brown and white. Brown adipocytes (which are found only in mammals) mainly regulates thermogenesis and expresses high concentration of uncoupling protein 1 (UCP-1) (Dulloo et al., 2010). The UCP-1 dissipates the proton gradient across the inner mitochondrial membrane and generates heat at the expense of ATP. White adipose tissue, on the other hand, plays a decisive role in whole-body energy homeostasis. In general, adipocytes are the major energy storage sites of the body in the form of fat storage, and having critical endocrine functions. The adipose tissue structure includes fibroblasts, macrophages, pre, and mature adipocytes. In humans, brown adipose tissue surrounds the heart. High caloric diet promotes hypertrophy and hyperplasia of adipocytes. Hypoxia results as an occurrence of hypertrophy when the size of adipocytes increases and the diffusion of oxygen is affected (Poulain-Godefroy et al., 2008). As a result, adipocytes express the factor hypoxia-inducible (HIF-1a) and the unfolded protein response in the endoplasmic reticulum. The genes involved with the expression of pro-inflammatory cytokines, viz., leptin, vascular endothelial growth factor (VEGF) is regulated by HIF-1a (Goossens, 2008). As a consequence of obesity, the primary attribute of hypertrophic adipocytes is reduced sensibility to insulin, due to the reported affectation of membrane receptors. This results in inflammation through diapedesis of monocytes to visceral stroma (Deng and Scherer, 2010). The non-esterified fatty acids, glycerol, hormones, and other factors released by these cells partly contribute to the sensitivity of lower insulin in hypertrophic adipocytes. Even type 2 diabetes may occur as a consequence of alterations association in pancreatic islet β-cells and insulin resistance in insulin-dependent tissues (Kahn et al., 2006).

18.5   ANTI-OBESITY PREPARATIONS: GENERAL MECHANISM OF ACTION

Several mechanisms are responsible for inducing weight loss through natural anti-obesity preparations. The antiobesity functions can be classified into five major categories, as given in Table 18.1. Depending on the inhibition of pancreatic lipase activity (Birari and Bhutani, 2007), the intake of some medicinal plants prevents the absorption of lipids in the intestine. By increasing the basic metabolic rate certain bioactive components can advance energy expenditure through thermogenesis (Hansen et al., 2010). This function will help to burn excess body fat and additional calories. Adipogenesis and the formation of fat cells in adipose tissues are inhibited through prevention of adipocyte differentiation due to the consumption of medicinal plants (Uto-Kondo et al., 2009). Furthermore, some medicinal plant products can augment lipolysis through inducing β-oxidation or noradrenaline secretion in fat cells based on enhancing lipid metabolism (lipolysis) (Okuda et al., 2001). Other anti-obesity ingredients can provoke satiety and diminish appetite (Geoffroy et al., 2011), which will facilitate to defend appetite. Ultimately, these anti-obesity medicinal plants will help to reduce food and energy intake (Haaz et al., 2006). Through a number of mechanisms, natural anti-obesity preparations can induce weight loss.

TABLE 18.1 Different Functions of Anti-Obesity Medicinal Plants in Humans

SL. No.	Anti-Obesity Function	Anti-Obesity Preparations
1.	Inhibiting pancreatic lipase activity	Chitosan (Bondiolotti et al., 2007, Jun et al., 2010), green tea (Koo and Noh, 2007), mate tea (Martins et al., 2009), oolong tea (Hsu et al., 2006) jasmine tea (Okuda et al., 2001), levan (Kang et al., 2006)
2.	Enhancing thermogenesis	Seaweed (Maeda et al., 2007, Maeda et al., 2005, Maeda et al., 2008), bitter orange (Dallas et al., 2008, Haaz et al., 2006, Roberts et al., 2007), soybean (Ishihara et al., 2003)
3.	Preventing adipocyte differentiation	Turmeric (Ahn et al., 2010), capsicum (Hsu et al., 2007), palm oil (Van Rooyenet al., 2008), banana leaf (Bai et al., 2008, Klein et al., 2007), flaxseed (Udani et al., 2004), black soybean (Kim et al., 2007), garlic (Ambati et al., 2009), brown algae (Maeda et al., 2006)
4.	Enhancing lipid metabolism	Cinnamon (Smyth et al., 2006), herb teas (Okuda et al., 2001)
5.	Decreasing appetite	Hoodia gordonii (Walsh et al., 1984), pomegranate leaf (Lei et al., 2007), ginseng (Kim et al., 2005), pine nut (Pasman et al., 2008)

Certain bioactive components can boost the metabolic rate (Hansen et al., 2010) through increased thermogenesis and thereby helps burn calories and surplus body fat. Adipocyte differentiation prevention through medicinal plants may hinder adipogenesis and development of fat cells, (Van Heerden, 2008). Several medicinal plants can boost lipolysis through inducing β-oxidation or nor-adrenaline secretion in fat cells (Okuda et al., 2001). Other anti-obesity ingredients can decrease the desire for food and encourage satiety (Geoffroy et al., 2011), allowing for appetite control. These conflicting functions of anti-obesity medicinal plants will ultimately reduce food and energy intake (Haaz et al., 2006). The values of BMI and the associated complications determine the new definition of obesity (Table 18.2).

TABLE 18.2   The New Definition of Obesity from the AACE*

Diagnosis	Body Mass Index (BMI)	Clinical Component (Complications)
Overweight	≥25–29.9	No complications
Obesity stage 0	≥30	No complications
Obesity stage 1	≥25	One or more mild-to-moderate complications
Obesity stage 2	≥25	One or more severe complications

*AACE (2020; https://www.aace.com/disease-state-resources/nutrition-and-obesity).

18.6   ANTI-OBESITY MECHANISMS OF NATURAL DIETARY OR HERBAL PRODUCTS

18.6.1   INCREASE IN ENERGY EXPENDITURE

More adiposity, as a consequence of excessive food intake coupled with absence of energy expenditure, leads to an imbalance in energy homeostasis (Aydin, 2014). Therefore, an efficient weight management demands the building of a negative energy balance by means of increasing energy expenditures. It can be possible by three ways viz., obligatory energy expenditure, physical activity and adaptive thermogenesis. Most anti-obesity products characteristically control body weight through raising mandatory energy expenditure. In the human body, brown adipose tissue is mainly responsible for transferring energy from food into heat. It plays a pivotal role in thermogenic effect through UCP-1 (also known as *thermogenin*). Thus, increasing energy expenditure to upregulate UCP-1 gene expression could be a prospective approach for achieving an anti-obesity effect (Kajimura and Saito, 2014).

18.6.2   APPETITE SUPPRESSANT EFFECT

A complex interaction of neurological and hormonal signals regulates the biological mechanisms of appetite and satiety. Many research confirmed that some particular food ingredients could provide satiety beneficial for weight control (Chambers et al., 2015). The mechanism which enhances the noradrenaline level and succeeding commencement of sympathetic nervous system activity, leads to an augmentation in satiety and energy expenditure, elevation in fat oxidation, and suppression of appetite (Belza et al., 2007). Serotonin, histamine, dopamine, and their associated receptor activities are neural signal peptides found to be associated with satiety regulation and could be potential target areas to the development of supplement products (Morton et al., 2014).

18.6.3 LIPASE INHIBITORY EFFECT

The best way to manage obesity is to impede fat absorption down the gastro-intestinal tract directly by developing inhibitors for digestion of nutrient and assimilation. Enzymatic break down of any dietary fat by the action of pancreatic lipase is very much essential to be absorbed in human intestine This is the vital indicator for the anti-obesity potential of natural products (Marrelli et al., 2013). Pancreatic lipase hydrolyzes triglyceride to mono-glyceride and fatty acids for absorption of dietary triglyceride. A derivative of the naturally-occurring lipase inhibitor, tetrahydrolipstatin (orlistat), is isolated from *Streptomyces toxytricini* (Zhu et al., 2014). To block the absorption of dietary fat, a synthetic drug is designed to take action through a covalent bond to the active site serine of pancreatic lipase (Mulzer et al., 2006; Tsujita et al., 2006).

18.6.4 REGULATORY EFFECT ON ADIPOCYTE DIFFERENTIATION

Adipocytes release fatty acid, which are used as fuel by organs in times of limited glucose. These fatty acids are the outcomes from triacylglycerol breakdown, which contain more energy per unit mass compared to carbo-hydrates. Lipid homeostasis and energy balance is centrally regulated by adipocytes. According to changing energy demands they release free fatty acids from stored triglycerides. The hyperplasia and hypertrophy of adipocytes both are involved with adipocyte tissue growth, which led to the development of natural products which helps in anti-obesity therapy that exclusively target adipogenesis inhibition. Some research has also proposed that through blockade of several transcription factors like C/EBP_ (CCAAT/ enhancer-binding protein beta) and PPAR (peroxisome proliferator-activated receptor-gamma) adipocyte differentiation could be inhibited (Kang et al., 2013).

18.6.5   REGULATORY EFFECT ON LIPID METABOLISM

Triglyceride hydrolysis is stirred by increasing rate of lipolysis leading to reduced fat storage and ultimately reduced obesity. For example, lipolysis in white adipocytes and thermogenesis in brown fat are triggered by the adrenergic receptor (Bordicchia et al., 2014). Activation of adenosine monophosphate-activated protein kinase (AMPK) resulting in enhanced glucose transport and fatty acid oxidation in skeletal muscle is another instance (Kola et al., 2008, O'Neill et al., 2013). Transcription factors simulated lipolysis system can turn out to be a significant aspect towards development of an anti-obesity product. Adipogenesis are found to be activated through the up-regulation of the AMPK pathway by flavonoids, specifically flavonols (e.g., quercetin). Moreover, quercetin activates the apoptotic pathway is fully grown adipocytes (Table 18.3) (Ahn et al., 2008).

TABLE 18.3   Functional Compounds in Natural Antiobesity Products

Groups	Active Ingredients	Structures	References
Phenolic acids	O-Coumaric acid		Hsu et al. (2009)
Lignans	Podophyllotoxin		Kim et al. (2016)
Isoflavonoids	Genistein		Behloul et al. (2013); Cha et al. (2014); Yao et al. (2010)
Flavones	Apigenin		Ono et al. (2011)
Flavans-3-ol	Catechin		Rains et al. (2011)

TABLE 18.3 *(Continued)*

Groups	Active Ingredients	Structures	References
Anthocyanins	Malvidin		Hossain et al. (2016)
Phytosterols	Diosgenin		Mohamed et al. (2014)
Alkaloids	Caffeine		Mohamed et al. (2014)

18.7 ACTIVE COMPONENTS FROM PLANT SOURCES

Fruits, vegetables, cereal, legumes, and spices contain an assortment of bioactive components in various quantities. The role of these active components and mechanism of action in obesity management are extensively studied by various researchers. In this way, these plant sources provide a fitting and practicable approach for the management of obesity (Table 18.4).

TABLE 18.4 Active Components Present in Various Plants and Their Possible Mechanisms

Plants and Parts Used	Active Components	Mechanism of Action	References
Achyranthes aspera L. (Chaff flower) seeds	Total phenols; flavonoids; saponins	Delays intestinal absorption of fat in the diet by inhibition of pancreatic amylase and activity of the enzyme lipase	Rani et al. (2012); Mythili Avadhani (2013)
Acorus calamus L. (Sweet flag) rhizome, root, and leaf	Rhizomes: β-asarone; Aerial parts: choline, acorin glycosides; Fresh leaves: oxalic acid.	Ethyl acetate extract suppresses α-glucosidase activity.	Karmase et al. (2013)

TABLE 18.4   *(Continued)*

Plants and Parts Used	Active Components	Mechanism of Action	References
Aegle marmelos (L.) Corrêa. (Golden apple/bael) leaf	Cumarins	Reduces triglyceride and cholesterol levels of lipid metabolism modulation	Karmase et al. (2013)
Allium sativum (Garlic) cloves	S-allyl-l-cysteine; Sulphoxide; S-allyl cysteine	• Decreases relative masses of liver and fat tissues, serum triacylglyceride levels, hepatic oxidative stress; • Increases fecal lipid contents in high fat diet rats; • Upregulates adenosine monophosphate-activated protein kinase, Sirtuin1, adipose triacylglyceride lipase, hormone-sensitive lipase, Acyl-CoA oxidase, palmitoyl transferase 1; • Downregulates cluster of differentiation.	Chen et al. (2014a)
Alpinia galanga L. (Thai ginger/Galangal) rhizome	Galangin	Decreases serum lipids, liver weight, lipid peroxidation and accumulation of hepatic TGs.	Kumar and Alagawadi (2013)
Boerhaavia diffusa L. (Punarnava/Red spiderling) root	β-sitosterol	Reduces cholesterol by lowering the level of LDL-cholesterol	Khalid and Siddiqui (2012)
Capsicum annuum L. (Pepper) fruit	Capsinoids, Capsicoside-G	Activation of adenosine monophosphate-activated protein adipogenesis is suppressed Through uncoupling protein 1-dependent mechanism reduces the diet-induced obesity	Okamatsu-Ogura et al. (2015); Sung and Lee (2016)
Carica papaya L. (Papaya) leaf	Saponins	Suppresses appetite stimulus signals in the hypothalamus	Hamao et al. (2011)

TABLE 18.4 *(Continued)*

Plants and Parts Used	Active Components	Mechanism of Action	References
Carica papaya L. (Papaya) fruit	Alkaloids, saponins, tannins, anthraquinones, flavonoids (anthocyanidins)	Reduces levels of triglycerides, LDL-C E VLDL-C	Moro and Basile (2000); Adeneye and Olagunju (2009)
Carum carvi L. (Caraway) seed	α-pinene, β-ocimene, p-cymine, α-terpineol, carvone	Reduces weight, body mass index, body fat percentage, and waist-to-hip ratio.	Kazemipoor et al. (2013)
Coffea arabica (Coffee) beans/ seeds	Polyphenols, caffeine	• Suppresses postprandial hyperglycemia, and hyperlipidemia; • Inhibits fatty acid absorption; • Reduces leptin levels; • Inhibited lipogenesis by down-regulating sterol regulatory element-binding protein, acetyl-CoA carboxylase-1 and -2, stearoyl-CoA desaturase-1 and pyruvate dehydrogenase kinase-4 in the liver.	Murase et al. (2012); Xu et al. (2015)
Coleus forskohlii (Coleus) root	Forskolin (7 β-acetoxy-8,13-epoxy-1α,6β,9α-trihydroxylabd-14-en-11-one)	Inhibits dyslipidemia.	Shivaprasad (2014)
Corchorus olitorius L. (Jute/ Jew's Mallow) leaves	Oleic-, palmitic-, linoleic acid, β-sitosterol	• Down-regulates liver tissue gene expression of gp91phox (NOX2) involved in oxidative stress; • Up-regulates genes related to the activation of β-oxidation like PPARα and CPT1A.	Wang et al. (2011)
Crocus sativus (Saffron) stamen	Crocin	Significantly reduced plasma levels of triacylglycerol and total cholesterol	Mashmoul et al. (2014)

TABLE 18.4 *(Continued)*

Plants and Parts Used	Active Components	Mechanism of Action	References
Cucurbita moschata D. (Pumpkin) fruit, stalk	Terpenes	Reduces triglyceride and cholesterol levels of lipid metabolism modulation	Choi et al. (2007)
Curcuma longa (Turmeric) rhizome	Curcumin	Regulation of inflammatory reactions and oxidative stress-induced overweight	Jarzab and Kukula-Koch (2018)
Eugenia caryophyllus (Clove) flower bud	Eugenol, acetyl eugenol, caryophyllene, and humulene, fatty acid synthase	• Inhibits the S-phase DNA replication of HepG2 cells; • Adipocyte differentiation of OP9 cells.	Ding et al. (2017)
Fragaria ananassa (Strawberry), *Rubus idaeus* (Raspberry) fruits	Tiliroside	• Enhances the liver and skeletal muscle fatty acid oxidation; • Suppresses the obesity-induced hepatic and muscular triglyceride accumulation, inflammation	Goto et al. (2012)
Ginkgo biloba (Maidenhair tree) leaves	Terpene trilactones, including ginkgolides and bilobalide	Hypolipidemic activity by inhibiting pancreatic lipase	Bustanji et al. (2011)
Glycine max L. (Black soybeans) seed	Anthocyanin	• Significantly reduces the expression of lipogenesis genes (acetyl-CoA carboxylase) and fat accumulation; • Enhances the levels of lipolysis proteins (lipoprotein lipase, hormone-sensitive lipase, and adenosine monophosphate-activated protein kinase) in mesenteric fat.	Kim et al. (2015)

TABLE 18.4 *(Continued)*

Plants and Parts Used	Active Components	Mechanism of Action	References
Gymnema sylvestre (Australian Cow plant/Gurmaar) leaves	Deacyl gymenemic acid	• Controls diabetes-induced obesity; • Decreases body weight gain; • Lowers food and energy efficiency ratio; • Lowers the serum levels of total cholesterol, triglycerides, LDL, VLDL.	Kim et al. (2016); Kanetkar et al. (2007)
Hordeum vulgare (Barley) seed	Coumaric acid, ferulic acid	Inhibits adipocyte differentiation, prevents body weight gain, and dysregulates lipid profiles	Seo et al. (2015b)
Morinda citrifolia L. (Noni) fruit	Anthraquinones, iridoid glucosides, citrifolinin B epimer a and b, cytidine	• Increases glucose tolerance; • Reduces plasma triglycerides level.	Saminathan (2013)
Moringa oleifera (Drumstick tree/ Moringa) leaves	Leaves: glycine, leucine, valine, threonine, alanine, aspartic acid, glutamic acid, phenylalanine, arginine, tryptophan, isoleucine, histidine, lysine, cysteine, and methionine.	• Reduces total lipid content from body; • Reduces body weight.	Asolkar et al. (1992)
Morus sp. (Mulberry) leaf	Polyphenol, quercetin, caffeic acid, hydroxyflavin, hesperetin	Suppresses the expression of sterol regulatory element-binding proteins-1c, PPARc proteins, target genes adipocyte-specific fatty acid-binding protein and fatty acid synthase	Chang et al. (2016)
Murraya koenigii (L.) Spreng (curry leaf) leaves	Leaves: essential oil, tannins, koenigin, koenigicine, koenidine, koenimbine, cyclomahanimbine, koemine, koenigine, mahanine, mahanimbidine and scopolin.	Decreases weight gain, triglyceride, and cholesterol levels.	Ahn et al. (2013)

TABLE 18.4 *(Continued)*

Plants and Parts Used	Active Components	Mechanism of Action	References
Nephelium lappaceum L. (Rambutan) fruit	β-damascenone, vanillin, cinnamic acid, δ-decalactone, m-cresol	Reduces the expression of Igf-1 and Igf-1R	Zhao et al. (2011)
Olea europaea L. (Olive) leaves	Oleanolic acid, maslinic acid, erythrodiol, and uvaol	• Reverses HFD-induced upregulation of WNT10b- and galanin-mediated signaling molecules and key adipogenic genes; • Induces downregulation of thermogenic genes involved in uncoupled respiration and mitochondrial biogenesis.	Poudyal et al. (2010)
Oryza sativa germinated brown rice, germinated black rice, seed	Catechin, myrecitin, cinnamic acid, p-coumaric acid	• Decreases body weight gain and lipid accumulation in the liver and epididymal adipose tissue; • Decreases CCAAT enhancer-binding protein (C/EBP)-α, SREBP(SREBP)-1c, and peroxisome proliferator-activated receptors (PPAR)-γ, and related genes (aP2, FAS).	Ho et al., 2012
Panax ginseng (Asian Ginseng) root	Saponins I	• Suppresses body weight; • Controls plasma triglycerols by regulating pancreatic lipase.	Ono et al. (2006)
Phaseolus vulgaris (Common beans) fruit	(-)-epigallocatechin Phytohemagglutnin	Alpha-amylase inhibition	Obiro et al. (2008)
Premna integrifolia Linn. (Brihad Agnimantha/ (Headache tree) roots	β-sitosterol, linalool, premnine, iridoids glycoside	Decrease in the levels of serum glucose, triglyceride, total cholesterol, LDL, and VLDL	Mali et al. (2013)

TABLE 18.4 *(Continued)*

Plants and Parts Used	Active Components	Mechanism of Action	References
Punica granatum (Pomegranate) PEELS	Camphor, benzaldehyde, phenolic compounds, flavonoids, gallic acid, catechins	• Reduces lipase activity	Hadrich et al. (2014)
Rosmarinus officinalis (Rosemary) leaves	Carnosic acid and carnosol	• Reduces body weight gain; • Serum triglycerides, cholesterol, and insulin Inhibiting pancreatic lipase.	Vaquero et al. (2012)
Salix matsudana (Chinese willow) leaves	Apigenin-7-O-D-glucoside	• Reduces plasma triglycerol levels and hepatic total cholesterol content; • Enhances nor-epinephrine induced lipolysis in cells.	Han et al. (2003)
Tamarindus indica L. (Tamarind) fruit pulp, seed coat.	Fruit pulp: tartaric, citric, malic, and acetic acids. Leaves: glycosides Bark: tannins	Decreases total cholesterol, LDL-C, and triglyceride and elevates the level of HDL.	Shidfar et al. (2015)
Theobroma cacao (Cocoa) fruit	Polyphenols	Lowers lipid in the liver, genes in lipid catabolism, primarily in fatty acid oxidation, was upregulated, whereas genes in lipid synthesis pathways were down-regulated, helps to manage obesity-induced steatosis markers.	Ali et al. (2015)
Vaccinium myrtillus (Bilberry) fruit, leaf	Anthocyanidins	• Reduces the adipocyte differentiation by promoting the gene expressions of insulin pathway; • Reduces PPAR, sterol regulatory element-binding protein 1c and tyrosine residues of insulin receptor substrate 1 phosphorylation.	Suzuki et al. (2011)

TABLE 18.4   *(Continued)*

Plants and Parts Used	Active Components	Mechanism of Action	References
Vitis vinifera L. (Grape) seed flours, peel, roots, fruit	Tannins, flavonoids, procyanidins	• Up-regulates hepatic genes related to cholesterol (CYP51) and bile acid (CYP7A1) synthesis and LDL cholesterol uptake; • Down-regulates lipid metabolism-associated genes (Mlxp1, Stat5a, Hsl, Plin1, and Vdr); • Regulates the lipid metabolism.	Jeong et al. (2011)
Wasabia japonica (Miq.) Matsum (Wasabi/Japanese Horseradish) leaves	Not clear	• Lowers body weight gain; • Reduces liver weight, epididymal WAT; • Enhances the levels of adiponectin and PPARα; • Suppresses SREBP-1c; • In WAT-expression of leptin PPARγ and C/EBPα were suppressed.	Yamasaki et al. (2013)
Zingiber officinale (Ginger) rhizome	Gingerol, Paradol, Shojail	Enhances lipid profile	Mahmoud and Elnour (2013)

Adapted from: Sun et al. (2016); de Freitas and de Almeida (2017); Karri et al. (2019); Patra et al. (2015); Mahmudur and Mahfuzur (2017).

Natural ingredients and medicinal plant preparations available in the market can improve satiety, trigger metabolism, and accelerate weight loss (Larson et al., 2009). But, regardless of a mounting global market for satiety, fat burning, dietary supplements and other weight managing therapies, patient consciousness of these products is entirely inadequate. In the following paragraph few more natural medicinal plants and their anti-obesity potential are discussed in detail, which could aid obesity patients in selecting a particular or range of botanical products to develop a healthy body (Kazemipoor et al., 2012).

18.7.1   ALOE VERA

Aloe vera belongs to the family Liliaceae. The major chemical composition of *A. vera* includes phytosterols, anthraquinones, chromones, enzymes, tannins, amino acids, proteins, vitamins, pectins, hemicelluloses, glucomannan, acemannan, and mannose derivatives (Misawa et al., 2012a). *A. vera* gel powder in Sprague-Dawley rats with diet-induced obesity decreased body weight (Misawa et al., 2012a). Misawa et al. (2012b) reported that feeding of *A. vera to* Zucker diabetic fatty rats which produces lophenol and cycloartenol (two types of phytosterol), significantly reduced visceral fat weights. Stimulation of energy expenditure is one of the proposed anti-obesity mechanisms of *A. vera* (Misawa et al., 2012a), other mechanism being the regulation of expression levels of hepatic genes encoding to lipogenic enzymes (ACC, FAS), and transcriptor factor SREBP-1, which, by the administration of aloe sterols, is found to be decreased drastically; and to the increased of hepatic β-oxidation enzymes ACO, CPT1, PPARα (Misawa et al., 2012b).

18.7.2   ARACHIS HYPOGAEA

Peanut is a legume or "bean" belonging to the Fabaceae family and free from transfats. Germinated peanut contains lots of resveratrol in addition to polyphenols, isoflavones, and essential amino acids. Peanut sprout extract has anti-obesity potential by reducing the PPARγ expressions which in turn regulates expression of adiponectin (Kang et al., 2014). So, it reduces body weight gain, liver triglyceride content and liver size in addition to increased fecal lipid excretion, suggesting an inhibitory mechanism on lipid absorption (Ranjbar et al., 2012).

18.7.3   BAUHINIA PURPUREA

Bauhinia purpurea is a flowering plant belonging to the family Fabaceae and native to South China as well as Southeast Asia. A high fat diet in rats was resulted in increasing triglycerides, total cholesterol and low-density lipoprotein LDL along with a decline in serum level of high-density lipoprotein (HDL). Oral administration of methanolic extract of *Bauhinia purpurea* (200 mg/kg w/w) to obese rats was, however, found to decrease total cholesterol triglycerides, LDL, but to increase HDL (Ramgopal et al., 2010).

18.7.4   CAMELLIA SINENSIS

The dried leaves of black tea (*Camellia sinensis*) contain polyphenols such as theaflavins and the red-brown thearubigins that are oxidation products of flavan-3-ols during fermentation. These are quite dissimilar from those found in green tea, theanine, catechins, and caffeine (Scharbert, 2005). A Keemun black tea extract via oral administration was successfully found to reduce food intake, body weight and plasma triglyceride levels in diet-induced obese rats (Du et al., 2005). Fatty acid synthase inhibited through the black tea extract. This effect was mostly reduced with boiling water (Plantenga et al., 2006). In addition to the leaf of *C. sinensis* having an anti-obesity effect, the fruit peel is also is recognized as an agricultural waste (Chaudhary et al., 2014). The chemical compounds with the acknowledged anti-obesity potential are principally catechin type polyphenols.

18.7.5   CITRUS AURANTIUM

This plant is belongs to the Rutaceae family. Antiobesity effect of *C. aurantium* contains synephrine, a stimulant with comparable characteristics as caffeine and ephedrine. It is observed to have similar effects by increasing metabolism and energy expenditure and suppressing appetite (Haaz et al., 2006). *C. aurantium* aided in weight loss and increase thermogenesis to some extent. On the contrary, the loss of fat mass in the test group was appreciably superior compared to the placebo and control groups (Suryawanshi et al., 2011).

18.7.6   CITRUS PARADISI

Grapefruit (*Citrus paradisi*) is a subtropical citrus tree of Rutaceae. It is one of the extensively cultivated fruits in the United States, predominantly in Florida, California, and the other semitropical Southern states. Grapefruits are traditionally used for losing weight. Active compounds reported for *C. paradise* includes flavonoids and furanocoumarins (De Castro et al., 2006; Gattuso et al., 2007). Treatment with *C. paradisi* infusion on obese rats fed with a high-saturated-fat-diet resulted in adipocyte size and volume reduction. It regulates the lipid metabolism, inducing relative expression of carnitine palmitoyl-transferase 1a (CPT1a) in obese rats compared with the control (Gamboa-Gómez et al., 2014).

18.7.7 DOLICHOS BIFLORUS AND PIPER BETLE

Dolichos biflorus, belonging to family Leguminosae, is a twining herb of Old-World tropics and cultivated in India for food and fodder. *Piper betle* belongs to the Piperaceae family, which includes pepper and kava also. It is observed that the combined extract of the above two mentioned plants is used to prepare the herbal formulation LI10903F which shows considerable adipogenesis having the capacity to reduce lipid accumulation in 3T3-L1 adipocytes and demonstrate lipolysis (Sengupta et al., 2012).

18.7.8 HIBISCUS SABDARIFFA

H. sabdariffa has great potential to reduce obesity. The main phytochemicals reported in *H. sabdariffa* are phenolic and flavonoids compounds, whereas; the chemical composition includes delphinidin-3-sambubioside, cyanidin-3-sambubioside, kaempferol-3-glucoside, protocatechuic acid, and chlorogenic acid (Peng et al., 2011). Gamboa-Gómez et al. (2014) reported that infusions (1% w/w) of *H. sabadariffa* for 16 weeks in diet-induced obese rats reduced body (10%) and adipose tissue weights (29%) compared with the obese controls.

18.7.9 GARCINIA CAMBOGIA

The *Garcinia cambogia* is a fruit that belongs to the family Guttiferae. It is commonly known as brindle berry, brindall berry, garcinia, malabar tamarind, gambooge, gorikapuli, uppagi, garcinia kola, mangosteen oil tree and distributed all throughout South East Asia including India. The fruit rinds contain hydroxycitric acid (HCA) which helps in weight loss by reducing fat production and suppressing appetite. Garcinia is also rich in citrine (an extract with 50–60% HCA) which inhibits an enzyme that helps the body manufacture fat for storage in adipose tissue. HCA produce energy, inhibits lipogenesis, reduces the production of cholesterol and fatty acids, enhances the production of glycogen in the liver, and reduces appetite (Sethi et al., 2011). *Garcinia cambogia* derived hydroxycitric acid extract effects the liberation and availability of 5-HT, which is responsible for controlling appetite (Ohia et al., 2002).

18.7.10   HOODIA GORDONII

This plant belongs to Apocynaceae family (VanHeerden et al., 2002) and distributed in Northern Cape, Kimberley, Western Cape, the Southmost parts of the Free State as well as in Southwestern Namibia. It is consumed for its purported anti-obesity effect. Reduction in food intake, increased water consumption, reduced mean body mass gain, and body mass loss was evident in rats by a purified extract of *Hoodia gordonii*, as per one US patent (Vermaak et al., 2011). P57 has a likely mechanism of action in the central nervous system and is involved in the control of hunger, appetite, and temperature (MacLean and Luo, 2004).

18.7.11   HYPERICUM PERFORATUM

St John's wort (*Hypericum perforatum* L.) is an herbaceous perennial plant, native to Europe and Asia, and afterwards introduced into America. Compounds with biological activity for *H. perforatum* includes hyperforin, hypericin, flavonoids (kaempferol, quercetin, luteolin, isoquercitrin, quercitrin, rutin, among others), and condensed tannins (proanthocyanidins) are also present (Nahrstedt and Butterweck, 1997). Several studies report that *H. perforatum* has anti-obesity activity. Hernández-Saavedra et al. (2013) established that body weight gain was prevented (8%) in obese rats fed with fructose and high saturated fat diet by *H. perforatum* infusion treatment for 12 weeks.

18.7.12   MURRAYA KOENIGII

Murraya koenigii is a tropical to sub-tropical tree of Rutaceae and native to India and Sri Lanka. A study confirmed the capability of *Murraya koenigii* leaves to demonstrate a potent improvement of glucose intolerance. A potent anti-hyperglycemic activity was found with repeated oral administration of *Murraya koenigii* leaves in high fat diet obese rats. Whereas, high fatty diet group increased both the total cholesterol and triglycerides levels as compared to control (Tembhurne et al., 2012).

18.7.13   NELUMBO NUCIFERA

Nelumbo nucifera is an aquatic plant, resembling the water lily with large flowers. It is usually known as Indian lotus, sacred lotus, bean of India, and belongs to the Nelumbonaceae family. To treat obesity in China, *Nelumbo nucifera* leaf extract is used. Anti-obesity effect of *Nelumbo nucifera* essentially involves inhibition of alpha-amylase and lipase activity and regulated lipid metabolism. It also accelerates the lipid metabolism by expression of UCP3 mRNA in C2C12 myotubes (Ono et al., 2006). *Nelumbo nucifera* leaf extract was found to prevent the increase in body weight, parametrial adipose tissues weight and liver triacylglycerol level (Kumar et al., 2011).

18.7.14 *PERSEA AMERICANA*

Avocado (*Persea americana*) belongs to Lauraceae and is native from Central and South America. Its cultivation has spread throughout Africa, Asia, Europe, and United States. Major chemical constituents include alkanols ("aliphatic acetogenins"), terpenoid glycosides, various furan ring-containing derivatives, flavonoids, and a coumarin. The highly functionalized alkanols of avocado have exhibited quite diverse biological properties thus far (Yasir et al., 2010). Anti-obesity effects have been reported for both the leaf and fruit. Treatment with aqueous and methanolic extracts of *P. americana* leaves (10 mg/Kg) for 8 weeks in hypercholesterolemic albino rats caused a 25% reduction in the body weight gain (Brai et al., 2007).

18.7.15 *ZIZIPHUS MAURITIANA/ZIZIPHUS JUJUBE*

These shrubs belong to the Rhamnaceae family and mostly habited in warm temperate zone from Western Africa to India. For treating hyperlipidemic and hyperglycemic conditions, seeds, and leaves of these plants are used as folkloric medicine (Jarald, 2009). High fat diet HFD induced obese rats normally showed an increase in body weights, body fat and insulin resistance. But after 90 days schedule of *Ziziphus mauritiana* bark powder administration, they showed a significant reduction in body weight gain. The anti-obesity activities have been attributed to increase fecal fat excretion via the inhibition of lipase activity (Deshpande et al., 2013).

18.8 DEVELOPMENT OF ANTI-OBESITY FOODS

Development of functional foods for weight control involves the knowledge of the bodyweight control system. By incorporating active compounds into the food systems, limiting the bioavailability of nutrients, stimulating energy expenditure (thermogenesis) and modifying the composition of the gut microbiota, we can precisely control the body weight (Trigueros et al., 2013). Fortified foods with active compounds may be an approachable innovative strategy due to their sensitivity to a range of chemical and physical factors. Different technologies viz., encapsulation, change in food formulation (reformulation), and adaptation of the processing conditions ensure release of active ingredients like polyphenols, flavonoids, and quercetin in foods (McClements, 2015).

18.9   CHALLENGES AHEAD

Now a days, there is an overabundance of so-called anti-obesity products all throughout the market outlets, grocery stores, shopping malls, etc. (Jacobs and Gundling, 2009). They are not only costly, but also exhibited quite a few side effects, such as gastrointestinal and kidney problems. Moreover, these products do not have satisfactorily impact on weight loss or are not tolerated by the body, especially in patients with cardiovascular disorders. Hence, their long-term consumption is not at all suggested (Jacobs and Gundling, 2009; Rucker et al., 2007). For example, among the varieties of anti-obesity drugs (Orlistat, Fluoxetine, Sertraline, Topiramate, Sibutramine, etc.), only Orlistat and Sibutramine can be used long-term among the varieties of anti-obesity drugs. Therefore, the idea of using of natural/ plant-based remedies for weight loss is coming up rapidly to cope up with this burgeoning challenge. Scientists believe that botanical sources seem more reliable, safer, and also cheaper than current conventional methods, such as synthetic drugs (Chang, 2000) or surgical procedures (Clegg et al., 2003) having negative effects and limited duration in effectiveness (Mahan and Raymond, 2016).

18.10   CONCLUSION

Obesity is the sum total of many contributing factors, which include dietary, lifestyle, genetic, and environmental factors. Appropriate lifestyle and behavior interventions may be fundamental in alleviating this complex, chronic disorder mediated mainly by weight loss, but maintaining such a healthy lifestyle is extremely challenging. Multiple natural products could confer a synergistic activity through increasing the anti-obesity action on multiple targets as well as offering advantages over chemical treatments in terms of serious side effects. Phytotherapeutical approaches effect in anti-obesity and also offer other health benefits like anti-diabetic and anti-hyperlipidemic activities, simultaneously. However, the development of evidence-based public policies is necessary for the formulations. It will contribute a beneficial and sustainable approach for novel anti-obesity products and open up new research insights towards validation and confirmation of all the positive results time-tested through natural medicinal plants. Translational research should promote the exchange of knowledge between producers, researchers, developers, and industrialists to result in the much-needed synergy and harmony.

KEYWORDS

- **anti-obesity herbal food**
- **antiobesity**
- **control**
- **diseases**
- **heredity**
- **lifestyle**
- **medicinal plants**
- **obesity**
- **pathophysiology**

REFERENCES

AACE: American Association of Clinical Endocrinologists. (2020). https://www.aace.com/disease-and-conditions/nutrition-and-obesity (accessed on 01 November 2021).

Adeneye, A. A., & Olagunju, J. A., (2009). Preliminary hypoglycemic and hypolipidemic activities of the aqueous seed extract of *Carica papaya* Linn. in Wistar rats. *Biol. Med., 1*, 1–10.

Ahn, J. H., Kim, E. S., Lee, C., et al., (2013). Chemical constituents from *Nelumbo nucifera* leaves and their anti-obesity effects. *Bioorg. Med. Chem. Lett., 23*, 3604–3608.

Ahn, J., Lee, H., & Kim, S., (2010). Curcumin-induced suppression of adipogenic differentiation is accompanied by activation of Wnt/β-catenin signaling. *Am. J. Physiol. Cell Physiol., 298*(6), C1510- C1516.

Ahn, J., Lee, H., Kim, S., Park, J., & Ha, T., (2008). The anti-obesity effect of quercetin is mediated by the AMPK and MAPK signaling pathways. *Biochem. Biophys. Res. Commun., 373*, 545–549.

Akiyama, T., Tachibana, I., Shirohara, H., Watanabe, N., & Otsuki, M., (1996). High-fat hypercaloric diet induces obesity, glucose intolerance and hyperlipidemia in normal adult male Wistar rat. *Diabetes Res. Clin. Pract., 31*, 27–35.

Ali, F., Ismail, A., Esa, N. M., Pei, C. P., & Kersten, S., (2015). Hepatic genome-wide expression of lipid metabolism in diet-induced obesity rats treated with cocoa polyphenols. *J. Funct. Foods, 17*, 969–978.

Ambati, S., Yang, J. Y., & Rayalam, S., (2009). Ajoene exerts potent effects in 3T3-L1 adipocytes by inhibiting adipogenesis and inducing apoptosis. *Phytotherapy Res., 23*(4), 513–518.

Asolkar, L. V., Kakkar, K. K., & Chakre, O. J., (1992). *Second Supplement to Glossary of Indian Medicinal Plants with Active Principles*. Part-1 (A-K), CSIR, Publications & Information Directorate, New Delhi, India. ISBN: 9788172360481.

Aydin, S., (2014). Three new players in energy regulation: Preptin, adropin and irisin. *Peptides, 56*, 94–110.

Bai, N., He, K., & Roller, M., (2008). Active compounds from *Lagerstroemia speciosa*, insulin-like glucose uptake stimulatory/inhibitory and adipocyte differentiation-inhibitory activities in 3T3-L1 cells. *J. Agr. Food. Chem., 56*(24), 11668–11674.

Barbalho, S. M., Soares De, S. M. D. S., Dos, S. B. P. C., Guiguer, E. L., Farinazzi-Machado, F. M. V., Araújo, A. C., Meneguim, C. O., et al., (2012). *Annona montana* fruit and leaves improve the glycemic and lipid profiles of Wistar rats. *J Med Food., 15*, 917–922.

Barquera, S., Campos, I., & Rivera, J., (2013b). Mexico attempts to tackle obesity: The process, results, pushbacks and future challenges. *Obes Rev., 14*(Suppl 2), 69–78.

Barquera, S., Campos-Nonato, I., Hernandez-Barrera, L., Pedroza, A., Rivera-Dommarco, J. A., (2013a). Prevalencia de obesidad en adultosmexicanos, ENSANUT. 2012. *Salud Pública de Mexico, 55*, S151–S160.

Behloul, N., & Wu, G., (2013). Genistein: A promising therapeutic agent for obesity and diabetes treatment. *Eur. J. Pharmacol., 698*, 31–38.

Birari, R. B., & Bhutani, K. K., (2007). Pancreatic lipase inhibitors from natural sources: Unexplored potential. *Drug Discovery Today., 12*(19, 20), 879–889.

Blüher, M., (2019). Obesity: Global epidemiology and pathogenesis. *Nature Rev. Endocrinology, 15*, 288–298.

Bondiolotti, G., Bareggi, S. R., & Frega, N. G., (2007). Activity of two different polyglucosamines, L1120 and FF450, on body weight in male rats. *Eur. J. Pharmacol., 567*(1, 2), 155–158.

Bordicchia, M., Pocognoli, A., D'Anzeo, M., Siquini, W., Minardi, D., Muzzonigro, G., Dessì-Fulgheri, P., & Sarzani, R., (2014). Nebivolol induces, via _3 adrenergic receptor, lipolysis, uncoupling protein 1, and reduction of lipid droplet size in human adipocytes. *J. Hypertens., 32*, 389–396.

Brai, B. I. C., Odetola, A. A., & Agomo, P. U., (2007). Effects of *Persea americana* leaf extracts on body weight and liver lipids in rats fed hyperlipidaemic diet. *Afr. J Biotech., 6*, 1007–1011.

Bustanji, Y., Al-Masri, I. M., Mohammad, M., Hudaib, M., Tawaha, K., Tarazi, H., & AlKhatib, H. S., (2011). Pancreatic lipase inhibition activity of trilactone terpenes of *Ginkgo biloba*. *J. Enzyme Inhib. Med. Chem., 26*, 453–459.

Cha, Y. S., Park, Y., Lee, M., Chae, S. W., Park, K., Kim, Y., & Lee, H. S., (2014). Doenjang, a Korean fermented soy food, exerts anti-obesity and antioxidative activities in overweight subjects with the PPAR-γ2 C1431T polymorphism: 12-week, double-blind randomized clinical trial. *J. Med. Food, 17*, 119–127.

Chambers, L., McCrickerd, K., & Yeomans, M. R., (2015). Optimizing foods for satiety. *Trends Food Sci. Technol., 41*, 149–160.

Chang, J., (2000). Medicinal herbs: Drugs or dietary supplements? *Biochemical Pharmacology., 59*(3), 211–219.

Chang, Y. C., Yang, M. Y., Chen, S. C., & Wang, C. J., (2016). Mulberry leaf polyphenol extract improves obesity by inducing adipocyte apoptosis and inhibiting preadipocyte differentiation and hepatic lipogenesis. *J. Funct. Foods., 21*, 249–262.

Chaudhary, N., Bhardwaj, J., Seo, H. J., Kim, M. Y., Shin, T. S., & Kim, J. D., (2014). Camellia sinensis fruit peel extract inhibits angiogenesis and ameliorates obesity induced by high-fat diet in rats. *J. Funct. Foods., 7*, 479–486.

Chen, Q., Wu, X., Liu, L., & Shen, J., (2014b). Polyphenol-rich extracts from oil tea camellia prevent weight gain in obese mice fed a high-fat diet and slowed the accumulation of triacylglycerols in 3T3-L1 adipocytes. *J. Funct. Foods, 9*, 148–155.

Chen, Y. C., Kao, T. H., Tseng, C. Y., Chang, W. T., & Hsu, C. L., (2014a). Methanolic extract of black garlic ameliorates diet-induced obesity via regulating adipogenesis, adipokine biosynthesis, and lipolysis. *J. Funct. Foods, 9*, 98–108.

Choi, H., Eo, H., Park, K., Jin, M., Park, E. J., Kim, S. H., Park, J. E., & Kim, S., (2007). A water-soluble extract from Cucurbita moschata shows anti-obesity effects by controlling lipid metabolism in a high fat diet-induced obesity mouse model. *Biochem. Biophys. Res. Commun., 359*, 419–425.

Clegg, A., Colquitt, J., Sidhu, M., Royle, P., & Walker, A., (2003). Clinical and cost-effectiveness of surgery for morbid obesity: A systematic review and economic evaluation. *International Journal of Obesity, 27*(10), 1167–1177.

Dallas, C., Gerbi, A., Tenca, G., et al., (2008). Lipolytic effect of a polyphenolic citrus dry extract of red-orange, grapefruit, orange (SINETROL) in human body fat adipocytes. Mechanism of action by inhibition of cAMP phosphodiesterase (PDE). *Phytomedicine., 15*(10), 783–792.

De Castro, W. V., Mertens-Talcott, S., Rubner, A., Butterweck, V., & Derendorf, H., (2006). Variation of flavonoids and furanocoumarins in grapefruit juices: A potential source of variability in grapefruit juice-drug interaction studies. *J Agric Food Chem., 54*, 249–255.

De Freitas, Jr. L. M., & de Almeida, Jr. E. B., (2017). Medicinal plants for the treatment of obesity: Ethnopharmacological approach and chemical and biological studies. *Am. J. Transl. Res., 9*(5), 2050–2064. www.ajtr.org /ISSN: 1943-8141/AJTR0051320.

Değirmenci, T., Kalkanoğlu, N., Sözeri-Varma, G., Özdel, O., & Fenkci, S., (2015). Psychological symptoms in obesity and related factors. *Noro Psikiyatr Ars., 52*(1), 42–46.

Deng, Y., & Scherer, P. E., (2010). Adipokines as novel biomarkers and regulators of the metabolic syndrome. *Ann. NY Acad. Sci., 1212*, E1–E19.

Deshpande, M. S., Shengule, S., Apte, K. G., Wani, M., Piprode, V., & Parab, P. B., (2013). Anti-obesity activity of *Ziziphus mauritiana*: A potent pancreatic lipase inhibitor. *Asian J. Pharm. Clin. Res., 6*, 168–173.

Devlin, M. J., Yanovski, S. Z., & Wilson, G. T., (2000). Obesity: What mental health professionals need to know. *Am. J. Psychiatry, 157*, 854–866.

Ding, Y., Gu, Z., Wang, Y., Wang, S., Chen, H., Zhang, H., Chen, W., & Chen, Y. Q., (2017). Clove extract functions as a natural fatty acid synthesis inhibitor and prevents obesity in a mouse model. *Food Funct., 8*, 2847–2856.

Du, Y. T., Wang, X., Wu, X. D., & Tian, W. X., (2005). Keemun black tea extract contains potent fatty acid synthase inhibitors and reduces food intake and body weight of rats via oral administration. *J. Enzyme Inhib. Med. Chem., 20*(4), 349–356.

Ducharme, N. A., & Bickel, P. E., (2008). Lipid droplets in lipogenesis and lipolysis. *Endocrinology, 149*, 942–949.

Dulloo, A. G., Jacquet, J., Solinas, G., Montani, J. P., & Schutz, Y., (2010). Body composition phenotypes in pathways to obesity and the metabolic syndrome. *Int. J. Obes., 34*, S4–S17.

Gamboa-Gómez, C., Salgado, L. M., González-Gallardo, A., Ramos-Gómez, M., Loarca-Piña, G., & Reynoso-Camacho, R., (2014). Consumption of *Ocimum sanctum* L. and *Citrus paradisi* infusions modulates lipid metabolism and insulin resistance in obese rats. *Food Funct., 5*, 927–935.

Gattuso, G., Barreca, D., Gargiulli, C., Leuzzi, U., & Caristi, C., (2007). Flavonoid composition of citrus juices. *Molecules, 12*, 1641–1673.

Geoffroy, P., Ressault, B., & Marchioni, E., (2011). Synthesis of hoodigogenin A, aglycone of natural appetite suppressant glycosteroids extracted from *Hoodia gordonii. Steroids, 76*(7), 702–708.

Goossens, G. H., (2008). The role of adipose tissue dysfunction in the pathogenesis of obesity-related insulin resistance. *Physiol. Behav., 94*, 206–218.

Goto, T., Teraminami, A., Lee, J. Y., Ohyama, K., Funakoshi, K., Kim, Y. I., Hirai, S., Uemura, T., Yu, R., Takahashi, N., & Kawada, T., (2012). Tiliroside, a glycosidic flavonoid, ameliorates obesity-induced metabolic disorders via activation of adiponectin-signaling followed by enhancement of fatty acid oxidation in liver and skeletal muscle in obese-diabetic mice. *J. Nutr. Biochem., 23*(7), 768–776.

Haaz, S., Fontaine, K., Cutter, G., Limdi, N., Perumean-Chaney, S., & Allison, D., (2006). Citrus aurantium and synephrine alkaloids in the treatment of overweight and obesity: An update. *Obesity Reviews, 7*(1), 79–88.

Hadrich, F., Cher, S., Gargouri, Y. T., & Adel, S., (2014). Antioxidant and lipase inhibitory activities and essential oil composition of pomegranate peel extracts. *J. Oleo Sci., 63*, 515–525.

Hamao, M., Matsuda, H., Nakamura, S., Nakashima, S., Semura, S., Maekubo, S., Wakasugi, S., Yoshikawa, M., (2011). Anti-obesity effects of the methanolic extract and Chaka saponins from the flower buds of *Camellia sinensis* in mice. *Bioorganic Med. Chem., 19*, 6033–6041.

Han, L., Sumiyoshi, M., Zheng, Y., Okuda, H., & Kimura, Y., (2003). Anti-obesity action of *Salix matsudana* leaves (Part 2). Isolation of anti-obesity effectors from polyphenol fractions of *Salix matsudana. Phytother. Res., 17*, 1195–1198.

Hansen, J. C., Gilman, A. P., & Odland, J. Ø., (2010). Is thermogenesis a significant causal factor in preventing the "globesity" epidemic? *Medical Hypotheses, 75*(2), 250–256.

Hernández-Saavedra, D., Hernández-Montiel, H. L., Gamboa-Gómez, C. I., Salgado, L. M., & Reynoso-Camacho, R., (2013). The effect of Mexican herbal infusions on dietinduced insulin resistance. *Nutrafoods, 12*, 55–63.

Ho, J. N., Son, M. E., Lim, W. C., Lim, S. T., & Cho, H. Y., (2012). Anti-obesity effects of germinated brown rice extract through down-regulation of lipogenic genes in high fat diet-induced obese mice. *Biosci. Biotechnol. Biochem., 76*, 1068–1074.

Hossain, M. K., Dayem, A. A., Han, J., Yin, Y., Kim, K., Saha, S. K., Yang, G. M., Choi, H. Y., & Cho, S. G., (2016). Molecular mechanisms of the anti-obesity and anti-diabetic properties of flavonoids. *Int. J. Mol. Sci., 17*, 569.

Hsu, C. L., & Yen, G. C., (2007). Effects of capsaicin on induction of apoptosis and inhibition of adipogenesis in 3T3- L1 cells. *Journal of Agricultural and Food Chemistry, 55*(5), 1730–1736.

Hsu, C. L., Wu, C. H., Huang, S. L., & Yen, G. C., (2009). Phenolic compounds rutin and *o*-coumaric acid ameliorate obesity induced by high-fat diet in rats. *J. Agric. Food Chem., 57*, 425–431.

Hsu, T., Kusumoto, A., & Abe, K., (2006). Polyphenol-enriched oolong tea increases faecal lipid excretion. *Eur J Clin Nutr., 60*(11), 1330–1336.

Ishihara, K., Oyaizu, S., & Fukuchi, Y., (2003). A soybean peptide isolate diet promotes postprandial carbohydrate oxidation and energy expenditure in type II diabetic mice. *Eur. J. Nutr., 133*(3), 752–757.

Jacobs, B., & Gundling, K., (2009). *ACP Evidence-Based Guide to Complementary and Alternative Medicine* (pp. 289–325). Amer College of Physicians Press.

Jarald, E. E., Joshi, S. B., & Jain, D. C., (2009). Anti-diabetic activity of extracts and fractions of *Ziziphus mauritiana. Pharm Biol., 47*(4), 328–334.

Jarzab, A., & Kukula-Koch, W., (2018). Recent advances in obesity: The role of turmeric tuber and its metabolites in the prophylaxis and therapeutical strategies. *Curr. Med. Chem., 25*(37), 4837–4853.

Jeong, Y. S., (2011). Anti-obesity effect of grape skin extract in 3T3-L1 adipocytes. *Food Sci and Biotechnology, 20*, 635–642.

Jun, S., Jung, E., Kang, D., et al., (2010). Vitamin C increases the fecal fat excretion by chitosan in guinea-pigs, thereby reducing body weight gain. *Phytotherapy Research, 24*(8), 1234–1241.

Kahn, S. E., Hull, R. L., & Utzschneider, K. M., (2006). Mechanisms linking obesity to insulin resistance and type 2 diabetes. *Nature, 444*(7121), 840–846.

Kajimura, S., & Saito, M., (2014). A new era in brown adipose tissue biology: Molecular control of brown fat development and energy homeostasis. *Annu. Rev. Physiol., 76*, 225–249.

Kanetkar, P., Singhal, R., & Kamat, M., (2007). Recent advances in Indian herbal drug research. In: Thomas, P., & Asir, D., (eds.), *Gymnema sylvestre: A Memoir: J. Clin. Biochem. Nutr.* (Vol. 41, pp. 77–81).

Kang, H. J., Seo, H. A., Go, Y., Oh, C. J., Jeoung, N. H., Park, K. G., & Lee, I. K., (2013). Dimethyl fumarate suppresses adipogenic differentiation in 3T3-L1 preadipocytes through inhibition of STAT3 activity. *PLoS One, 8*, e 61411.

Kang, N. E., Ha, A. W., Woo, H. W., & Kim, W. K., (2014). Peanut sprouts extract (*Arachis hypogaea* L.) has anti-obesity effects by controlling the protein expressions of PPARγ and adiponectin of adipose tissue in rats fed a high-fat diet. *Nutrition Res. Prac., 8*(2), 158–164.

Kang, S. A., Hong, K., Jang, K. H., et al., (2006). Altered mRNA expression of hepatic lipogenic enzyme and PPARα in rats fed dietary levan from *Zymomonas mobilis. The Journal of Nutritional Biochemistry., 17*(6), 419–426.

Karmase, A., Birari, R., & Bhutani, K. K., (2013). Evaluation of anti-obesity effect of *Aegle marmelos* leaves. *Phytomedicine, 20*, 805–812.

Karri, S., Sharma, S., Hatware, K., & Patil, K., (2019). Natural anti-obesity agents and their therapeutic role in management of obesity: A future trend perspective. *Biomedicine and Pharmacotherapy, 110*, 224–238.

Kazemipoor, M., Radzi, C. W. J. W. M., Cordell, G. A., & Yaze, I., (2012). Potential of traditional medicinal plants for treating obesity: A review. *International Conference on Nutrition and Food Sciences IPCBEE., 39*, 1–6. IACSIT Press, Singapore.

Kazemipoor, M., Radzi, C. W., Hajifaraji, M., Haerian, B. S., Mosaddegh, M. H., et al., (2013). Anti-obesity effect of caraway extract on overweight and obese women: A randomized, triple-blind, placebo-controlled clinical trial. *Evid. Based Complement Alternat Med., 2013,* 928582.

Khalid, M., & Siddiqui, H. H., (2012). Evaluation of weight reduction and anti-cholesterol activity of punarnava root extract against high fat diets induced obesity in experimental rodent. *Asian Pacific Journal of Tropical Biomedicine, 2,* S1323–S1328.

Kim, E. J., Jung, S., Son, K. H., Kim, S. R., & Ha, T. Y., (2007). Antidiabetes and anti-obesity effect of cryptotanshinone via activation of AMP- activated protein kinase. *Mol. Pharmacol., 72,* 62–72.

Kim, H. J., Hong, S. H., Chang, S. H., Kim, S., Lee, A. Y., Jang, Y., Davaadamdin, O., et al., (2016). Effects of feeding a diet containing *Gymnema sylvestre* extract: Attenuating progression of obesity in C57BL/6J mice. *Asian Pac. J. Trop. Med., 9,* 437–444.

Kim, J. H., Hahm, D. H., & Yang, D. C., (2005). Effect of crude saponin of Korean red ginseng on high fat diet-induced Obesity in the rat. *J. Pharmacol Sci., 97*(1), 124–131.

Kim, M., Lee, Y. J., Jee, S. C., Choi, I., & Sung, J. S., (2016). Anti-adipogenic effects of sesamol on human mesenchymal stem cells. *Biochem. Biophys. Res. Commun., 469,* 49–54.

Kim, S. Y., Wi, H. R., Choi, S., Ha, T. J., Lee, B. W., & Lee, M., (2015). Inhibitory effect of anthocyanin-rich black soybean testa (Glycine max (L.) Merr.) on the inflammation-induced adipogenesis in a DIO mouse model. *J. Funct. Foods., 14,* 623–633.

Klein, G., Kim, J., Himmeldirk, K. et al., (2007). Anti-diabetes and anti-obesity activity of Lagerstroemia speciosa. *Evidence-Based Complimentary and Alternative Medicine, 4*(4), 401–408.

Kola, B., Grossman, A., & Korbonits, M., (2008). The role of AMP-activated protein kinase in obesity. *Front. Horm. Res., 36,* 198–211.

Koo, S. I., & Noh, S. K., (2007). Green tea as inhibitor of the intestinal absorption of lipids: Potential mechanism for its lipid-lowering effect., *J. Nutr. Biochem., 18*(3), 179–183.

Kumar, S., & Alagawadi, K. R., (2013). Anti-obesity effects of galangin, a pancreatic lipase inhibitor in cafeteria diet-fed female rats. *Pharm Biol., 51,* 607–613.

Kumar, Y. S., (2011). Herbs used in the management of obesity. *International Journal of Institutional Pharmacy and Life Sciences, 1*(1), 7–17.

Lei, F., Zhang, X. N., & Wang, W., (2007). Evidence of anti-obesity effects of the pomegranate leaf extract in high-fat diet induced obese mice. *Int. J. Obes. (Lond)., 31*(6), 1023–1029.

MacLean, D. B., & Luo, L. G., (2004). Increased ATP content/production in the hypothalamus may be a signal for energy-sensing of satiety: Studies of the anorectic mechanism of a plant steroidal glycoside. *Brain Res., 1020,* 1–11.

Maeda, H., Hosokawa, M., & Sashima, T., (2005). Fucoxanthin from edible seaweed, Undariapinnatifida, shows antiobesity effect through UCP1 expression in white adipose tissues. *Biochemical and Biophysical Research Communications, 332*(2), 392–397.

Maeda, H., Hosokawa, M., & Sashima, T., (2006). Fucoxanthin and its metabolite, fucoxanthinol, suppress adipocyte differentiation in 3T3-L1 cells. *Int. J. Mol. Med., 18*(1), 147–152.

Maeda, H., Hosokawa, M., & Sashima, T., (2007). Dietary combination of fucoxanthin and fish oil attenuates the weight gain of white adipose tissue and decreases blood glucose in obese/diabetic KK-AY mice. *J. Agr. Food. Chem., 55*(19), 7701–7706.

Maeda, H., Tsukui, T., & Sashimaet, T., (2008). Seaweed carotenoid, fucoxanthin, as a multifunctional nutrient. *Asia Pac. J Clin. Nutr., 17*(S1), 196–199.

Mahan, L. K., & Raymond, J. L., (2016). *Krause's Food and Nutrition Care Process* (14th edn., p. 1152), Saunders/Elsevier. ISBN 9780323340755.

Mahmoud, R. H., & Elnour, W. A., (2013). Comparative evaluation of the efficacy of ginger and orlistat on obesity management, pancreatic lipase and liver peroxisomal catalase enzyme in male albino rats. *Eur. Rev. Med. Pharmacol. Sci., 17*, 75–83.

Mahmudur, R. A. H. M., & Mahfuzur, R. M., (2017). Medicinal plants having anti-obesity potentiality available in Bangladesh: A review. *Biol. Med. Case Rep., 1*(2), 4–11.

Mali, P. Y., Bigoniya, P., Panchal, S. S., & Muchhandi, I. S., (2013). Anti-obesity activity of chloroform-methanol extract of *Premna integrifolia* in mice fed with cafeteria diet. *J Pharm Bioallied Sci., 5*, 229–236.

Mandrup, S., & Lane, M. D., (1997). Regulating adipogenesis. *J. Bio.l Chem., 272*, 5367–5370.

Marrelli, M., Loizzo, M. R., Nicoletti, M., Menichini, F., & Conforti, F., (2013). Inhibition of key enzymes linked to obesity by preparations from Mediterranean dietary plants: Effects on amylase and pancreatic lipase activities. *Plant Foods Hum. Nutr., 68*, 340–346.

Martins, F., Noso, T. M., & Porto, V. B., (2009). Mate tea inhibits in vitro pancreatic lipase activity and has hypolipidemic effect on high-fat diet-induced obese mice. *Obesity, 18*(1), 42–47.

Mashmoul, M., Azlan, A., Yusof, B. N. M., Khazaai, H., Mohtarrudin, N., & Boroushaki, M. T., (2014). Effects of saffron extract and crocin on anthropometrical, nutritional and lipid profile parameters of rats fed a high fat diet. *J. Funct. Foods, 8*, 180–187.

McClements, D. J., Li, F., & Xiao, H., (2015). The nutraceutical bioavailability classification scheme: Classifying nutraceuticals according to factors limiting their oral bioavailability. *Annual Review of Food Science and Technology, 6*, 299–327.

Misawa, E., Tanaka, M., Nabeshima, K., Nomaguchi, K., Yamada, M., Toida, T., et al., (2012a). Administration of dried Aloe vera gel powder reduced body fat mass in diet induced obesity (DIO) rats. *J. Nutr. Sci. Vitaminol., 58*, 195–201.

Misawa, E., Tanaka, M., Nomaguchi, K., Nabeshima, K., Yamada, M., Toida, T., et al., (2012b). Oral ingestion of Aloe vera phytosterols alters hepatic gene expression profiles and ameliorates obesity-associated metabolic disorders in Zucker diabetic fatty rats. *J. Agric. Food Chem., 60*, 2799–2806.

Mohamed, G. A., Ibrahim, S. R., Elkhayat, E. S., & El Dine, R. S., (2014). Natural anti-obesity agents. *Bull. Fac. Pharm. Cairo Univ., 52*, 269–284.

Moro, C. O., & Basile, G., (2000). Obesity and medicinal plants. *Fitoterapia., 71*(1), S73–82.

Morton, G. J., Meek, T. H., & Schwartz, M. W., (2014). Neurobiology of food intake in health and disease. *Nat. Rev. Neurosci., 15*, 367–378.

Mulzer, M., Tiegs, B. J., Wang, Y., Coates, G. W., & O'Doherty, G. A., (2014). Total synthesis of tetrahydrolipstatin and stereoisomers via a highly regio- and diastereo-selective carbonylation of epoxyhomoallylic alcohols. *J. Am. Chem. Soc., 136*, 10814–10820.

Murase, T., Yokoi, Y., Misawa, K., Ominami, H., Suzuki, Y., Shibuya, Y., & Hase, T., (2012). Coffee polyphenols modulate whole-body substrate oxidation and suppress postprandial hyperglycaemia, hyper-insulinaemia and hyperlipidaemia. *Br. J. Nutr., 107*(12), 1757–1765.

Mythili, A. M. N., (2013). The sweetness and bitterness of sweet flag (*Acorus calamus* L.) – A review. *Res J Pharm Biol Chem Sci., 4*, 598–610.

Nahrstedt, A., & Butterweck, V., (1997). Biologically active and other chemical constituents of the herb of *Hypericum perforaturn* L. *Pharmacopsychiatry, 30*, 129–134.

O'Neill, H. M., Holloway, G. P., & Steinberg, G. R., (2013). AMPK regulation of fatty acid metabolism and mitochondrial biogenesis: Implications for obesity. *Mol. Cell. Endocrinol., 366*, 135–151.

Obiro, W. C., Zhang, T., & Jiang, B., (2008). The nutraceutical role of the Phaseolus vulgaris α- amylase inhibitor. *Br. J. Nutr., 100*, 1–12.

Ogden, C. L., Carroll, M. D., Curtin, L. R., McDowell, M. A., Tabak, C. J., & Flegal, K. M., (2006). Prevalence of overweight and obesity in the United States. *J. Amer. Med. Assoc., 295*(13), 1549–1555.

Ohia, S. E., Opere, C. A., LeDay, A. M., Bagchi, M., Bagchi, D., & Stohs, S. J., (2002). Safety and mechanism of appetite suppression by a novel hydroxycitric acid extract (HCASX). *Mol. Cell. Biochem., 238*, 89–103.

Okamatsu-Ogura, Y., Tsubota, A., Ohyama, K., Nogusa, Y., Saito, M., & Kimura, K., (2015). Capsinoids suppress diet-induced obesity through uncoupling protein 1- dependent mechanism in mice. *J. Funct. Foods, 19*, 1–9.

Okuda, H., Han, L., Kimura, Y., Saito, M., & Murata, T., (2001). Anti-obesity action of herb tea(Part 1). Effects or various herb teas on Noradrenaline-induced lipolysis in rat fat cells and pancreatic lipase activity. *Japanese Journal of Constitutional Medicine., 63*(1/2), 60–65.

Ono, M., & Fujimori, K., (2011). Antiadipogenic effect of dietary apigenin through activation of AMPK in 3T3-L1cells. *J. Agric. Food Chem., 59*, 13346–13352.

Ono, Y., Hattori, E., Fukaya, Y., Imai, S., & Ohizumi, Y., (2006). Anti-obesity effect of *Nelumbo nucifera* leaves extract in mice and rats, *J. Ethnopharmacol., 106*, 238–244.

Pagliassotti, M. J., Gayles, E. C., & Hill, J. O., (1997). Fat and energy balance. *Ann. N Y Acad. Sci., 827*, 431–448.

Pasman, W. J., Heimerikx, J., & Rubingh, C. M., (2008). The effect of Korean pine nut oil on *in vitro* CCK release, on appetite sensations and on gut hormones in post-menopausal overweight women. *Lipids in Health and Disease, 7*(10), 7–10.

Patil, S. G., Patil, M. P., Maheshwari, V. L., & Patil, R. H., (2015). In vitro lipase inhibitory effect and kinetic properties of di-terpenoid fraction from *Calotropis procera* (Aiton). *Biocatal. Agric. Biotechnol., 4*, 579–585.

Patra, S., Nithya, S., Srinithya, B., et al., (2015). Review of medicinal plants for anti-obesity activity. *Transl. Biomed., 6*(3), 1–22.

Peng, C. H., Chyau, C. C., Chan, K. C., Chan, T. H., Wang, C. J., & Huang, C. N., (2011). *Hibiscus sabdariffa* polyphenolic extract inhibits hyperglycemia, hyperlipidemia, and glycation- oxidative stress while improving insulin resistance. *J Agric Food Chem., 59*, 9901–9909.

Plantenga, M. W., Diepvens, K., Joosen, A. M. C. P., Parent, S. B., & Tremblay, A., (2006). Metabolic effects of spices, teas, and caffeine. *Physiology and Behavior, 89*, 85–91.

Poudyal, H., Campbell, F., & Brown, L., (2010). Olive leaf extract attenuates cardiac, hepatic, and metabolic changes in high carbohydrate-, high fat-fed rats. *J Nutr., 140*, 946–953.

Poulain-Godefroy, O., Lecoeur, C., Pattou, F., Frühbeck, G., & Froguel, P., (2008). Inflammation is associated with a decrease of lipogenic factors in omental fat in women. *Am. J. Physiol., 295*,R1–7.

Rains, T. M., Agarwal, S., & Maki, K. C., (2011). Anti-obesity effects of green tea catechins: A mechanistic review. *J. Nutr. Biochem., 22*.

Ramgopal, M., Attitalla, I. H., Avinash, P., & Balaji, M., (2010). Evaluation of antilipidemic and anti-obesity efficacy of *Bauhinia purpurea* bark extract on rats fed with high fat diet. *J. Plant Sci., 3*(3), 104–107.

Rani, N., Sharma, S. K., & Vasudeva, N., (2012). Assessment of anti-obesity potential of achyranthes aspera Linn. seed. *Evidence-Based Complement Altern. Med., 2012*, 715912.

Roberts, A. T., Martin, C. K., & Liu, Z., (2007). The safety and efficacy of a dietary herbal supplement and gallic acid for weight loss. *J. Med. Food, 10*(1), 184–188.

Rosen, E. D., Walkey, C. J., Puigserver, P., & Spiegelman, B. M., (2000). Transcriptional regulation of adipogenesis. *Genes Dev., 14*, 1293–1307.

Rucker, D., Padwal, R., Li, S. K., Curioni, C., & Lau, D. C. W., (2007). Long term pharmacotherapy for obesity and overweight: Updated meta-analysis. *BMJ: Br. Med. J., 335*(7631), 1194–1199.

Saminathan, M., (2013). Systematic review on anticancer potential and other health beneficial pharmacological activities of novel medicinal plant *Morinda citrifolia* (Noni). *Int J Pharmacol., 9*, 462–492.

Scharbert, S., & Hofmann, T., (2005). Molecular definition of black tea taste by means of quantitative studies, taste reconstitution, and omission experiments. *J. Agric. Food Chem., 53*, 5377–5384.

Sengupta, K., Mishra, A. T., Rao, M. K., Sarma, K. V. S., Krishnaraju, A. V., & Trimurtulu, G., (2012). Efficacy of an herbal formulation LI10903F Containing *Dolichos biflorus* and *Piper betle* extracts on weight management. *Lipids in Health and Disease, 11*(176), 1–9.

Seo, C. R., Yi, B., Oh, S., Kwon, S. M., Kim, S., Song, N. J., Cho, J. Y., et al., (2015b). Aqueous extracts of hulled barley containing coumaric acid and ferulic acid inhibit adipogenesis in vitro and obesity in vivo. *J. Funct. Foods, 12*, 208–218.

Sethi, A., (2011). Review on garcinia Cambogia - a weight controlling agent. International *Journal of Pharmaceutical Research and Development, 3*(10), 13–24.

Shidfar, F., Rajab, A., Rahideh, T., Khandouzi, N., Hosseini, S., & Shidfar, S., (2015). The effect of ginger (*Zingiber officinale*) on glycemic markers in patients with type 2 diabetes. *J. Complement Integr. Med., 12*, 165–170.

Shirin Hasani-Ranjbar, Neda Nayebi, Bagher Larijani, & Mohammad Abdollahi (2009). A systematic review of the efficacy and safety of herbal medicines used in the treatment of obesity, *World Journal of Gastroenterology, 15*(25), 3073–3085.

Shivaprasad, H. N., (2014). Ethnopharmacological and phytomedical knowledge of *Coleus forskohlii*: An approach towards its safety and therapeutic value. *Oriental Pharmacy and Experimental Medicine, 14*, 301–312.

Sidhu, S., Parikh, T., & Burman, K. D., (2017). Endocrine changes in obesity. In: Feingold, K. R., Anawalt, B., Boyce, A., et al., (eds), *Endo text* [*Internet*]. South Dartmouth (MA): MDText.com,Inc.

Smyth, S., & Heron, A., (2006). Diabetes and obesity: The twin epidemics. *Nature Medicine, 12*(1), 75–80.

Sun, N. N., Wu, T. Y., & Chau, C. F., (2016). Natural Dietary and Herbal Products in Anti-Obesity Treatment. Molecules. *Molecules, 21*, 1351.

Sung, J., Lee, J., & Capsicoside, G., (2016). A furostanolsaponin from pepper (*Capsicum annuum* L.) seeds, suppresses adipogenesis through activation of AMP-activated protein kinase in 3T3-L1 cells. *J. Funct. Foods, 20*, 148–158.

Suryawanshi, J. A. S., (2011). An overview of *Citrus aurantium* used in treatment of various diseases. *Afr. J. Plant Sci., 5*(7), 390–395.

Suzuki, R., Tanaka, M., Takanashi, M., Hussain, A., Yuan, B., Toyoda, H., & Kuroda, M., (2011). Anthocyanidins-enriched bilberry extracts inhibit 3T3-L1 adipocyte differentiation via the insulin pathway. *Nutr. Metab., 8*(1), 14.

Tembhurne, S. V., & Sakarkar, D. M., (2012). Anti-obesity and hypoglycemic effect of ethanolic extract of *Murraya koenigii* (L) leaves in high fatty diet rats. *Asian Pac. J. Trop. Dis.*, S166–S168.

Thaker, V. V., (2017). Genetic and epigenetic causes of obesity. *Adolesce Med State Art Rev., 28*(2), 379–405.

Trigueros, L., Pena, S., Ugidos, A. V., Sayas-Barbera, E., Perez-Alvarez, J. A., & Sendra, E., (2013). Food ingredients as anti-obesity agents: A review. *Crit. Rev. Food Sci. Nutr., 53*(9), 929–942.

Tsujita, T., Takaichi, H., Takaku, T., Aoyama, S., & Hiraki, J., (2006). Anti-obesity action of _ polylysine, a potent inhibitor of pancreatic lipase. *J. Lipid Res., 47*, 1852–1858.

Udani, J., Hardy, M., & Madsen, D. C., (2004). Blocking carbohydrate absorption and weight loss: A clinical trial using phase 2™ brand proprietary fractionated white bean extract. *Alternative Medicine Review, 9*(1), 63–69.

Uto-Kondo, H., Ohmori, R., Kiyose, C., Kishimoto, Y., Saito, H., Igarashi, O., & Kondo, K., (2009). Tocotrienol suppresses adipocyte differentiation and Akt phosphorylation in 3T3-L1 pre-adipocytes. *The Journal of Nutrition, 139*(1), 51–57.

Van, H. F. R., Vleggaar, R., Horak, R. M., Learmonth, R. A. V., Maharaj, V., & Whittal, R. D., (2002). *Pharmaceutical Compositions Having Appetite-Suppressant Activity*. US Patent 6376657 B1.

Van, H. F., (2008). Hoodia gordonii: A natural appetite suppressant. *Journal of Ethnopharmacology, 119*(3), 434–437.

Van, R. J., Esterhuyse, A. J., Engelbrecht, A. M., & Du Toit, E. F., (2008). Health benefits of a natural carotenoid rich oil: A proposed mechanism of protection against ischaemia/reperfusion injury. *Asia Pacific J. Clinical Nutri., 17*, 316–319.

Vaquero, M. R., Yanez-Gascon, M. J., Villalba, R. G., Larrosa, M., Fromentin, E., Ibarra, A., Roller, M., et al., (2012). Inhibition of gastric lipase as a mechanism for body weight and plasma lipids reduction in Zucker rats fed a rosemary extract rich in carnosic acid. *PLoS One, 7*e39773.

Verhaegen, A. A., & Van, G. L. F., (2019). Drugs that affect body weight, body fat distribution, and metabolism. In: Feingold, K. R., Anawalt, B., Boyce, A., et al., (eds.), *Endotext* [*Internet*]. South Dartmouth (MA): MDText.com,Inc.

Vermaak, I., Hamman, J. H., & Viljoen, A. V., (2011). Hoodia gordonii: An up-to-date review of a commercially important anti-obesity plant. *Planta Med., 77*, 1149–1160.

Walsh, D. E., Yaghoubian, V., & Behforooz, A., (1984). Effect of glucomannan on obese patients: A clinical study. *Int. J. Obes., 8*(4), 289–293.

Wang, L., Yamasaki, M., Katsube, T., Sun, X., Yamasaki, Y., et al., (2011). Anti-obesity effect of polyphenolic compounds from molokheiya (*Corchorus olitorius* L.) leaves in LDL receptor-deficient mice. *Eur. J. Nutr., 50*, 127–133.

World Health Organization (WHO), (2020). *Obesity and Overweight*. https://www.who.int/news-room/fact-sheets/detail/obesity-and-overweight (accessed on 01 November 2021).

Xu, Y., Zhang, M., Wu, T., Dai, S., Xu, J., & Zhou, Z., (2015). The anti-obesity effect of green tea polysaccharides, polyphenols and caffeine in rats fed with a high-fat diet. *Food Funct., 6*, 296–303.

Yamasaki, M., Ogawa, T., Wang, L., Katsube, T., Yamasaki, Y., Sun, X., & Shiwaku, K., (2013). Anti-obesity effects of hot water extract from Wasabi (*Wasabia japonica* Matsum.) leaves in mice fed high-fat diets. *Nutr. Res. Pract., 7*, 267–272.

Yao, Y., Li, X. B., Zhao, W., Zeng, Y. Y., Shen, H., Xiang, H., & Xiao, H., (2010). Anti-obesity effect of an isoflavone fatty acid ester on obese mice induced by high fat diet and its potential mechanism. *Lipids Health Dis., 9*.

Yasir, M., Das, S., & Kharya, M. D., (2010). The phytochemical and pharmacological profile of *Persea americana*. Mill. *Pharmacog Rev., 4*, 77.

Yudkin, J. S., (1999). C-reactive protein in healthy subjects: Associations with obesity, insulin resistance, and endothelial dysfunction: A potential role for cytokines originating from adipose tissue? *Arterioscler Thromb. Vasc. Biol., 19*, 972–978.

Zhao, Y. X., Liang, W. J., Fan, H. J., Ma, Q. Y., Tian, W. X., et al., (2011). Fatty acid synthase inhibitors from the hulls of *Nephelium lappaceum* L. *Carbohydr Res., 346*, 1302–1306.

Zhu, T., Wang, L., Wang, W., Hu, Z., Yu, M., Wang, K., & Cui, Z., (2014). Enhanced production of lipstatin from *Streptomyces toxytricini* by optimizing fermentation conditions and medium. *J. Gen. Appl. Microbiol., 60*, 106–111.

CHAPTER 19

ETHNOMEDICINAL PLANTS OF NORTH EASTERN HIMALAYAN REGION OF INDIA TO COMBAT HYPERTENSION

PINTUBALA KSHETRI, K. TAMREIHAO, SUBHRA SAIKAT ROY, THANGJAM SURCHANDRA SINGH, SUSHEEL KUMAR SHARMA, and MERAJ ALAM ANSARI

ICAR Research Complex for NEH Region, Manipur Center, Imphal – 795004, Manipur, India, E-mail: subhrasaikat@gmail.com (S. S. Roy)

ABSTRACT

Hypertension or high blood pressure (BP) is one of the major risk factors for many non-communicable diseases (NCD) such as strokes, heart failure, and coronary heart disease. Previously hypertension is considered to be prevalent in developed countries, but now its prevalence is also prominent in developing countries. Generally, for treatment of hypertension, patients have to undergo long-term medication, so conventional antihypertensive drugs are usually associated with many unwanted side effects in prolonged use. Hence, people are searching for alternative option such as complementary and alternative medicine (CAM) which has lesser side effect and cost-effective. In this regard, traditional folk medicine-based medication practiced by ethnic people of North Eastern Himalayan (NEH) Region of India is worth mentioning. From time immemorial they have been using more than 50 medicinal plants and their formulations for the treatment of hypertension. Some of the most common plants used by these people are *Clerodendrum colebrookianum, Clerodendrum viscosum, Rauwolfia serpentina, Solanum torvum*, etc. Among the plants reported for treatment of hypertension, only 25 plant species have scientific evidence based on the available scientific literature.

Most of the potential antihypertensive traditional medicinal plants lack the systematic studies on their mode of action, pharmacokinetics, toxicity, and safety. Hence, a comprehensive scientific study is required to validate the traditional medications as alternative and complementary drugs for the treatment of hypertension. Moreover, overexploitation, and correct identification of the plants is another challenge in traditional based medicines. Hence, it becomes mandatory to give proper awareness regarding GACP (guidelines on good agricultural and collection practices) for medicinal plants developed by WHO.

19.1   INTRODUCTION

Hypertension is regarded as one of the key risk factors for chronic disease burden worldwide and is estimated to cause 7.5 million deaths, about 12.8% of the total of all deaths (De Boer et al., 2017). It is the major leading causes of non-communicable disease (NCD) related mortality. The latest guidelines of the European heart association define the hypertension as the level of blood pressure (BP) >140/90 mmHg whereas, American heart association guidelines lowered the threshold to <130/80 mm Hg. While persons with a systolic BP of 120 to 139 mm Hg or a diastolic BP of 80 to 89 mm Hg, have been considered as prehypertensive (Chopra and Ram, 2019). Hypertension can be primary or secondary type. Primary hypertension is the most common type of hypertension found in the majority of the population. The cause of primary hypertension is not clear and is supposed to be linked to genetics, poor diet, lack of exercise and obesity. Secondary hypertension is triggered by other medical conditions such as pregnancy, chronic kidney disease, thyroid, and adrenal gland dysfunction, etc. The studies conducted by many researchers reveal a high occurrence of hypertension among the Indian population, across all age groups with almost in the ratio of 1:3 (Gupta et al., 2019; Ramakrishnan et al., 2019). Overall prevalence of the disease was found to be 30.7%, and the prevalence among men and women were 34.2% and 23.7% respectively (Ramakrishnan et al., 2019). Hypertension is a silent killer because in most of the cases it is asymptomatic and the patients are unaware of it. Uncontrolled high BP leads to heart attack, heart failure, dementia, aneurysm, kidney failure and many other health complications. Hence, control of BP at a normal level is becoming an important approach for preventing lethal lifestyle related NCD like strokes, heart failure and coronary heart disease. For combating the rise in BP, a holistic approach of treatment is required, which includes lifestyle changes, drugs, and other natural remedies. In the developing country like India, traditional folk medicine-based remedy is very common especially in area inhabited by tribals. Since, from the time immemorial to combat any aliments or disorder the native people have been practicing traditional knowledge using natural herbs.

In this regard, the traditional healing remedies practiced by indigenous people of the North-Eastern Himalayan (NEH) region of India which are mostly populated by tribal communities are also worth mentioning. The traditional healers of these regions have extensive knowledge on the use of plants and herbs for medicinal and nutritional purposes through experience gained from trial and error. The knowledge was passed from one generation to other by oral traditions. Moreover, these regions have also been conferred with rich diversity of flora and fauna. Most of the people inhabited in rural or hilly areas of these regions have relied on medicinal plants for mitigation of hypertension and other related diseases (Shankar et al., 2012). However, majority of these medicinal plants are not well documented in terms of the presence of bioactive compounds and scientific evidence of their medicinal/ healing properties. This chapter will give the summarization on ethnomedicinal plants and scientific mechanisms of action that are used by different ethnic groups of NEH region India for treating hypertension which is regarded as one of the key important risk factors for chronic disease worldwide.

19.2 STRATEGIES USED FOR TREATMENT OF HYPERTENSION

Hypertension is a chronic disease that can be controlled with medication, but it cannot be totally cured. Hence, patients need to continue with the treatment and lifestyle modifications. Lifestyle modifications such as dietary changes (consumption of diets low in sodium, high in potassium, rich in vegetables, fruits, and low-fat dairy products), increase physical activity, weight loss and stress reduction can manage BP effectively. However, lifestyle changes may not be adequate to mitigate the elevated BP; antihypertensive medication is also important in controlling BP. In general, the first target to control hypertension is to reduce the BP below 140/90 mm Hg. While it is recommended to lower BP to less than 130/80 in people older than age 65 and in patients with diabetes and high cholesterol (Gupta and Guptha, 2010). Generally, patients having primary hypertension are treated by administering medicines that function in reduction of blood volume; systemic vascular resistance and stroke volume. For patients with secondary hypertension, the best treatment is to control or eradicate the underlying disease condition with concomitant medication with antihypertensive drug. The main classes of drugs available for treatment of hypertension are (i) diuretics (ii) vasodilators (iii) enzyme inhibitors such as angiotensin-converting enzyme (ACE) and renin inhibitors (iv) receptor blockers such as Angiotensin II receptor blockers, beta-blockers, calcium channel blockers, alpha-blockers (Disi et al., 2016). These medications may be taken either alone or in combination with two or more drugs (Sinha and Agrawal 2019; Laurent 2017). The mechanism of action and target organs of antihypertensive drugs is illustrated in Figure 19.1. As the antihypertensive drugs have to be administered prolonged patients may face unwanted results due to high cost and undesired side effects. In this context herbal medicine is an important alternative option in combating hypertension as herbal medicine is cheaper with lesser undesired side effects. As people are more conscious of the adverse effects of taking conventional medicines, they are more inclined towards the use of herbal extract having antihypertensive activity to combat the disease (Malik et al., 2018). Herbal plant-based formulations or medicines are essential to traditional Chinese practices; traditional Indian medicine (Ayurvedic), Siddha, and Unani medicine which are well known traditional medicine (TM) practice worldwide (Disi et al., 2016).

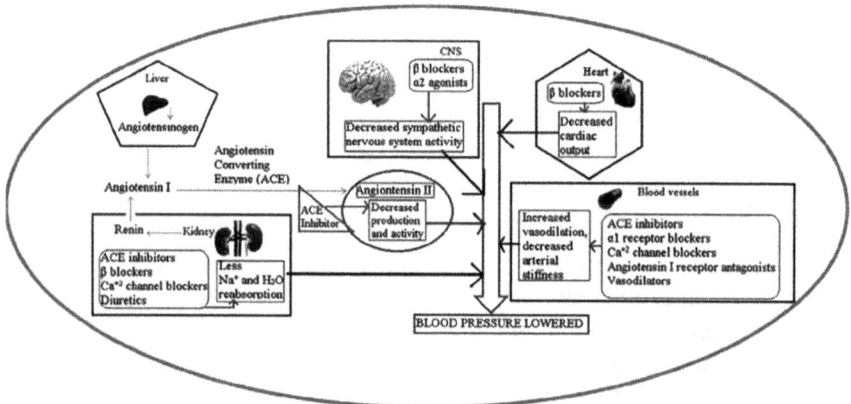

FIGURE 19.1 Mechanism of action of the antihypertensive drugs at different organs of the human body.

Source: Reprinted from: Yahaya, Rahman, and Abdullah (2014). © 2014 with permission from Elsevier.

Previously, the TM, often termed as complementary and alternative medicine (CAM), was widespread in underdeveloped and developing countries. But in recent years, CAM is also rapidly increasing in developed countries. The traditional knowledge on the use of ethnomedicinal plants in combating various diseases or ailments is more pronounced in the regions where accessibility to modern medication is limited. Generally, these regions are distributed in remote areas and inhabited by indigenous or tribal people. For example, in Africa, up to 80% of the population uses TM to help meet their health care needs (WHO, 2002). NEH region of India is also one of such places which are inhabited by diverse ethnic people and have rich traditional medicinal knowledge.

19.3   HYPERTENSION AND ITS CHALLENGES IN NEH REGION OF INDIA

Northeast (NE) India is located at the easternmost part of India. It comprises eight states viz. Assam, Arunachal Pradesh, Manipur, Meghalaya, Mizoram, Nagaland, Sikkim, and Tripura. Of the total 450 tribes inhabited in India about 225 tribes are found in these regions (Chatterjee et al., 2006). Hypertension is becoming a major cardiovascular disease among the population of NE India. The main factors for increasing hypertension in this region are due to change in the lifestyle, food habits, epidemiological, and demographic transition. Higher prevalence was reported in the NE states, namely Sikkim (20.2%), Nagaland (17.6%), Assam (17.6%), Arunachal Pradesh (16.6%) and Tripura (15.4%) as compared to other states of India (Ghosh and Kumar, 2019). Hypertension is distributed in people of all ages of this region. However, the prevalence differs depending on ethnic group, age, sex, and location (urban or rural), etc. For example, in a study conducted by Hazarika et al. (2000), the prevalence of hypertension was higher among the garden tea workers of Assam (30.1%) as compared to the Mizo community (2.04%). However, significance difference in prevalence among male and woman subjects was not observed. A pilot study conducted by Prasanta et al. (2018) showed that prevalence of hypertension was significantly higher in urban than rural population among the Mizo. The occurrence of hypertension among the children of age group between 5–14 years is also noteworthy (Borah et al., 2015; Thangjam et al., 2017). Thangjam et al. (2017) reported the total prevalence of pre-hypertension (17.5%) and hypertension (15.3%) among the children of 5–15 years from Manipur.

Considering the high incidence of hypertension in this region, regular examination and control of rise in BP in all the age groups is the need of the hour to avoid mortality and morbidity caused by hypertension. The major drawback that often delays treatment of hypertension is due to the lack of awareness, high costs, their availability and accessibility, and undesired side effects of antihypertensive drugs. Hence, indigenous people inhabited in these regions relied on TMs for treating hypertension and other health ailments. Many medicinal plants belonging to different families and genera have been reported from this region. And the use of TMs is deeply rooted in cultural and religious beliefs of all ethnic groups. Ethnomedicinal plants used by the indigenous people of this region in mitigation of hypertension are described in further sections.

19.4   ETHNOMEDICINAL PLANTS USED TO COMBAT HYPERTENSION BY THE PEOPLE OF NORTH EASTERN INDIA

The diverse indigenous people of NER of India have conserved much of their original cultural and ethnopharmacological practices as a means of strengthening the ethnic identity. Thus, many ailments including hypertension are often treated with traditional or folk medicines. And it is used alone or in combination with allopathic drugs. More than 50 ethnomedicinal plants used in the mitigation of hypertension have been reported from different states of NEH region. The medicinal plants used for treatment for hypertension by different communities of this region are summarized in Table 19.1. They belong to 29 different families; of which majority belongs to Asteraceae with 7 species, Lamiaceace with 5 species whereas Zingiberaceae and Solanaceae with 4 species each. Among these reported ethnomedicinal plants, *Clerodendrum colebrookianum* is widely used in mitigating the rise in BP by a large cross-section of people belonging to different communities. Decoction is the most common mode of application for traditional plant-based treatment. Sometimes extraction using ethanol is also used by traditional medical practitioners.

TABLE 19.1   Antihypertensive Medicinal Plants Used by Ethnic Groups of North Eastern India

SL. No.	Scientific Name	Family	Habitat	Parts Used	States	References
1.	*Ageratina adenophora*	Asteraceae	Shrub	Leaves	Manipur	Panmei et al. (2019)
2.	*Allium hookeri*	Alliaceae	Herb	Whole part	Manipur	Devi et al. (2011)

TABLE 19.1 *(Continued)*

SL. No.	Scientific Name	Family	Habitat	Parts Used	States	References
3.	*Alpinia galanga*	Zingiberaceae	Herb	Leaves and inflorescence	Manipur	Devi and Devi (2017)
4.	*Amomum dealbatum*	Zingiberaceae	Herb	Rhizome	Manipur	Devi et al. (2014)
5.	*Anaphalis contorta*	Asteraceae	Herb	Leaves and tender shoot	Manipur	Devi et al. (2014)
6.	*Andrographis paniculata*	Acanthaceae	Herb	Leaves	Manipur	Devi et al. (2011)
7.	*Antidesma acidum Retz.*	Phyllanthaceae	Tree	Leaves	Meghalaya	Sharma et al. (2014)
8.	*Artocarpus chaplasha Roxb.*	Moraceae	Tree	Leaves	Meghalaya	Hazarika et al. (2016)
9.	*Azadirachta indica*	Meliaceae	Tree	Leave	Nagaland	Jamir et al. (1999)
10.	*Basella alba Linn*	Basellaceae	Vine	Leaves	Manipur	Imotomba and Devi (2011)
11.	*Bauhinia variegata*	Fabaceae	Tree	Leaves	Meghalaya, Nagaland	Sharma et al. (2014); Sumi and Shohe (2018)
12.	*Bidens pilosa Linn*	Asteraceae	Herb	Leave	Manipur	Lokho (2012)
13.	*Blumea balsamifera Linn.*	Asteraceae	Herb	Leaves	Manipur	Nahakpam (2012)
14.	*Brugmansia suaveolens*	Solanaceae	Shrub	Leaves	Nagaland	Sumi and Shohe (2018)
15.	*Centella asiatica*	Apiaceae	Herb	whole plants	Arunachal Pradesh	Sen et al. (2008)
16.	*Chenopodium ambrosioides*	Amaranthaceae	Herb	Leaves	Manipur	Lokho (2012)
17.	*Clerodendrum colebrookianum* Walp	Lamiaceae	Shrub	Leaves	Arunachal Pradesh, Assam, Manipur, Nagaland, Sikkim	Lokho (2012); Lokesh and Amitsankar (2012); Devi et al. (2011); Kayang et al. (2005)
18.	*Clerodendrum serratum*	Lamiaceae	Shrub	Whole plant	Arunachal Pradesh	Perme et al. (2015)

TABLE 19.1 *(Continued)*

SL. No.	Scientific Name	Family	Habitat	Parts Used	States	References
19.	*Clerodendrum viscosum* Vent	Lamiaceae	Shrub	Leaves	Arunachal Pradesh, Manipur, Tripura	Khongsai et al. (2011); Devi et al. (2014)
20.	*Coptisteeta* Wall.	Ranunculaceae	Herb	Root	Arunachal Pradesh	Shankar and Rawat (2010); Payum (2017)
21.	*Crassocephalum crepidioides*	Asteraceae	Herb	Leaves	Manipur	Devi et al. (2011)
22.	*Croton caudatus*	Euphorbiaceae		Leaves	Manipur	Imotomba and Devi (2011)
23.	*Cuscuta reflexa* Roxb.	Convolvulaceae	Herb	Whole plant	Nagaland	Changkija (1999)
24.	*Dicentra scandens* (D. Don)	Fumariaceae	Herb	Tuber	Nagaland	Temsutola et al. (2019)
25.	*Dioscorea alata* Linn	Dioscoreaceae	Herb	Leaves	Manipur	Meetei and Singh (2007)
26.	*Elsholtzia blanda* Bentham	Lamiaceae	Herb	Leaves	Manipur	Meetei and Singh (2007)
27.	*Eryngium foetidum*	Apiaceae	Herb	Leaves	Manipur, Mizoram	Lokho (2012); Singh et al. (2014)
28.	*Fagopyrum esculentum*	Polygonaceae	Herb	Whole plant	Manipur	Devi and Devi (2017)
29.	*Gynura cusimbua*	Asteraceae	Herb	Whole plant	Manipur	Imotomba and Devi (2011)
30.	*Hydrocotyle Asiatica* Linn	Apiaceae	Herb	Whole plant	Sikkim	Meetei and Singh (2007)
31.	*Jatropha curcas* Linn.	Euphorbiaceae	Shrub	Leaves	Tripura	Das (2012)
32.	*Juglans regia* L.	Juglandaceae	Tree	Leaves, bark, Fruits	Nagaland	Temsutola et al. (2019)
33.	*Kaempferia rotunda*	Zingiberaceae	Herb	whole plant	Manipur	Devi et al. (2014)
34.	*Lygodium flexuosum*	Lygodiaceae	Herb	Leaves	Manipur	Nahakpam (2012)
35.	*Melia azedarach*	Meliaceae	Tree	Leaves	Manipur, Mizoram	Lokho (2012); Rai and Lalramnghinglova (2010)

TABLE 19.1   *(Continued)*

SL. No.	Scientific Name	Family	Habitat	Parts Used	States	References
36.	*Meriandra bengalensis* Benth	Lamiaceae	Herb	Leaves	Manipur	Meetei and Singh (2007)
37.	*Mikania micrantha*	Asteraceae	Vine	Leaves	Nagaland	Changkija (1999)
38.	*Momordica charantia* Linn	Cucurbitaceae	Vine	Leaves, fruits	Manipur, Arunachal Pradesh	Lokho (2012); Murtem and Chaudhry (2016)
39.	*Moringa oleifera*	Moringaceae	Tree	Leaves	Assam	Ghosh and Parida (2015)
40.	*Nardostachys grandiflora* DC	Valerianaceae	Herb	Whole plant	Sikkim	Tamang et al. (2017)
41.	*Oroxylum indicum*	Bignoniaceae	Shrub	Bark and root	Manipur, Sikkim	Lokho (2012); Panmei et al. (2019); Singh et al. (2002)
42.	*Passiflora eduli*s	Passifloraceae	shrub	Leaves	Nagaland	Jamir et al. (1999); Kichu et al. (2015)
43.	*Phlogacanthus thyrsiflorus*	Acanthaceae	Shrub	Leaves	Manipur	Panmei et al. (2019)
44.	*Physalis minima*	Solanaceae	Herb	Whole plant	Arunachal Pradesh	Perme et al. (2015)
45.	*Polygonum posumbu*	Polygonaceae.	Herb	Leaves	Manipur	Meetei and Singh (2007)
46.	*Rauwolfia serpentina*	Apocynaceae	Shrub	Roots and leave	Mizoram, Assam	Rai and Lalramngh-inglova (2010); Sharma and Das (2018)
47.	*Solanum indicum*	Solanaceae	Shrub	Fruit	Arunachal Pradesh	Kamum (2018)
48.	*Solanum nigrum*	Solanaceae	Shrub	Leaves and fruit	Nagaland	Changkija (1999)
49.	*Solanum torvum*	Solanaceae	Shrub	Fruit	Manipur, Arunachal Pradesh	Lokho (2012); Murtem and Chaudhry (2016)
50.	*Terminalia arjuna*	Combretaceae	Tree	Bark	Manipur	Devi and Devi (2017)

TABLE 19.1   *(Continued)*

SL. No.	Scientific Name	Family	Habitat	Parts Used	States	References
51.	*Thevetia peruviana* (pers.) Merill.	Apocynaceae	Shrub	Seed	–	Shankar et al. (2017)
52.	*Urtica parviflora* Roxb.	Urticaceae.	Herb	Roots and leaves	Sikkim	Panda (2012)
53.	*Valeriana jatamansi* Wall.	Caprifoliaceae	Herb	Root	–	Shankar et al. (2017)
54.	*Zingiber zerumbet*	Zingiberaceae	Herb	Flower	Arunachal Pradesh	Kamum (2018)

19.5   SCIENTIFIC EVIDENCE OF ANTIHYPERTENSIVE ACTIVITY OF ETHNOMEDICINAL PLANTS OF NEH INDIA

Of 54 plant species used in combating hypertension, 25 species have scientific evidence based on the available scientific literature. Of these, 10 of the selected important species are described below.

19.5.1   ALLIUM HOOKERI

Allium hookeri is a perennial herb widely cultivated and commonly used for culinary purposes in the South and Southeast Asia including NER of India. The ethanolic extract of leaves showed antihypertensive activity in vitro and in vivo conditions. Assay of angiotensin-converting enzyme (ACE) inhibition in vitro, the ethanolic leaves extract of *Allium hookeri* exhibited 82.67% inhibition which is comparable with standard drug captopril which showed 86.72% inhibition. Similarly, in vivo assay also showed a significant decrease in systolic BP and diastolic BP at a dose of 400 mg/kg in rats.

It also exhibits a reduction in blood cholesterol levels, triglycerides, low density lipoprotein (LDL) but significant increase in high density lipoprotein (HDL) level (Swarnalata, 2017).

19.5.2   ANDROGRAPHIS PANICULATA

Andrographis paniculata, commonly known as green chireta, is an annual herbaceous plant in the family Acanthaceae, native to Taiwan, China, India, and Sri Lanka (Verma et al., 2019). Ethanolic extract of *Andrographis paniculata* exert significant reduction in systolic (120%) and diastolic (150%) BPs in hypertensive Wistar rats induced by phenylephrine (Trilestari, 2015).

Andrographolide is the bioactive phytoconstituent isolated from various parts of *Andrographis paniculata*. It exhibits anti-HIV, anti-inflammatory, and antineoplastic properties (Chen et al., 2014; Jayakumar, 2013). Yoopan et al. (2007) studied the effects of three active diterpenoids viz., andrographolide (AP1), 14-deoxy-11, 12-didehydroandrographolide (AP3) and neoandrographolide on BP, vascular, and chronotropic responses by using conscious rats and their isolated Arotas as test model. They found that AP3 was most effective for inducing vasorelaxation and retarding heart rate and had a greater hypotensive effect in conscious rats than the AP1. Their result suggests that vascular muscle is the major site of hypotensive effect of AP3. Similarly, Mali et al. (2017) also showed that application of andrographolide loaded scleroglucan based formulation inhaler in rat increased lung deposition of andrographolide powder in lung and pulmonary antihypertensive activity.

19.5.3 *AZADIRACHTA INDICA*

Azadirachta indica belong to the Meliaceae family and commonly known as Neem or Indian lilac. It is native to the Indian subcontinent. It is well known medicinal plant used as ingredients folk/traditional and modern medicine for treating several infectious, metabolic or cancer diseases (Alzohairy, 2016). Some researchers have demonstrated the anti-hypertension activity of *Azadirachta indica* extract. Polyphenol rich fraction of *A. indica* could reduce the BP and cardiac and renal dysfunction induced by L-NAME in rats. Administration of L-NAME not only induced hypertension but also cause oxidative stress. *A. indica* extract could effectively restore BP to near normal and its effect is comparable to anti-hypertensive drug captopril. The extract also showed antioxidant, anti-inflammatory, and cardioprotective effects which are evidenced by the enhancement and upregulated activities of the non-enzymatic and enzymic antioxidants and erythroid 2-related factor 2 expressions. These two are the basic components of the first line of protection against oxidative stress associated with hypertension (Omóbòwálé et al., 2018). The protective effects of *A. indica* extract on Sodium fluoride (NaF) induced hypertension and genotoxicity in rats have also been reported. Treatment of NaF causes a decrease in production of nitric oxide (NO), a signaling molecule playing a key role in vasodilatation. Decrease in NO production in the body is closely related to hypertension. Co-administration of *A. indica* extract with NaF restored the NO concentration equal to control group (Omóbòwálé et al., 2018). In another study, Obiefuna and Youn (2005) observed that daily consumption of 20 mg/kg neem-leaf extract for 5 weeks in DOCA-salt-treated hypertensive rats, prevents the establishment of hypertension and the accompanying alterations in the ECG patterns.

19.5.4   *BIDENS PILOSA*

Bidens pilosa is a perennial herb widely distributed all over the globe and is well-known in African folk medicinal practices, especially in the western region of Cameroon and parts of Central America, as a potent hypotensive agent (Bartolome et al., 2013; Tom et al., 2017). There are several reports on the hypotensive activity of this plant. Dimo et al. (2001) studied the effects of the anti-hypertensive activity of the leaf extracts of *Bidens pilosa* on hypertensive rats induced by fructose. Chronic fructose treatment not only induces BP elevation but also causes metabolic abnormalities such as hyperinsulinemia, insulin resistance and hypertriglyceridemia. Administration of *B. pilosa* extract in their diet could reverse the elevation of BP and hypertriglyceridemia. But the extracts could not reduce the plasma insulin levels and insulin resistance (Dimo et al., 2001). They also studied the effect of the health beneficial compound present in the extract of the plant on acute and chronic hypertension and some related abnormalities induced by a high fructose diet in normal rats. During the study they observed that the methanolic extract of *B. pilosa* was able to subside the establishment of hypertension. The extract also reduced the highly elevated plasma insulin levels caused by the high fructose diet. Their results showed that crude leaf extract of *B. pilosa* can reduce BP and blood insulin level (Dimo et al., 2002). They further studied the effects of the intravenous administration of neutral extract obtained from the leaves of *B. pilosa* in spontaneously hypertensive and salt-loaded hypertensive rats. The antihypertensive activity of the neutral extract of *B. spilosa* has two consecutive phases. At the first phase, the plant extract acts on the cardiac pump efficiency, while a the second phase the extract may cause stimulation of gamma-receptor and vasodilation (Dimo et al., 2003). Furthermore, Bilanda et al. (2017) reported the hypotensive property of ethyl acetate extract of *B. pilosa* in L-NAME-induced hypertension rats.

19.5.5 CLERODENDRUM COLEBROOKIANUM WALP

Clerodendrum colebrookianum Walp generally grows in the south and south-east Asia. In India it is mostly grown in the NER up to an altitude of 1,700 m (Rajlakshmi et al., 2003). Its hypotensive activity was demonstrated by a study conducted by Lokesh and Amitsankar (2012) where they observed that the ethyl acetate fraction of *C. colebrookianum* Walp leaves exhibits Rho kinase (ROCK II) and phosphodiesterase-5 (PDE-5) inhibition. ROCK II and PDE-5 are the two important enzymes playing a key role in vasoconstriction. Around 21 compounds have been reported from *C. colebrookianum* Walp. And from the molecular docking studies, it was revealed that the three compounds (acteoside, martinoside, and osmanthuside b6) could interact with ROCK, ACE, and PDE5 which are well-known anti-hypertensive drug targets. The acteoside and osmanthuside b6 make stable interactions with the anti-hypertensive targets ROCK I/ROCK II and PDE5 (Arya et al., 2018).

19.5.6 CUSCUTA REFLEXA

Cuscuta reflexa commonly known as dodder or Devil's hair, is a rootless, leafless, perennial parasitic twining herb. A study conducted by Gilani and Aftab (1992) showed that the crude extract of *Cuscuta reflexa* subside the arterial BP and heart rate is dose-dependent in pentothal anesthetized rats. Pretreatment of the tissue with atropine (0.1 µM) did not change the negative inotropic and negative chronotropic activity of the plant extract. However, it could block the vasodilation activity of the acetylcholine. On contrary, *Cuscuta reflexa* extract could not reduce the increase in BP triggered by norepinephrine. These findings indicate that the antihypertensive and brady-cardiac activities of *Cuscuta reflexa* extract are independent of cholinergic receptor stimulation or adrenergic receptor blockade.

19.5.7 NARDOSTACHYS GRANDIFLORA DC.

Nardostachys grandiflora DC (syn *N. jatamansi*) commonly known as 'Spikenard' or 'Jatamansi,' is a small, perennial herb and its distribution is restricted on alpine Himalayas at an altitude of 3,000 to 5,200 m. This plant has been reported to use in various ailments including hypertension. A clinical study on management of essential hypertension using *N. jatamansi* was evaluated by Venkatachalapathy and his co-worker (2012) in 50 patients of both sexes in the age group of 30 to 70 years. The patients were given finely powdered dried rhizome of *N. jatamansi* at the dose of 1 gm thrice a day with honey for 30 to 60 days. Administration with dried rhizome for 3 weeks produced significant improvement of systolic BP and Diastolic BP. The study results reveal a substantial reduction in BP of the majority patient. Moreover, none of the patients showed any adverse side effects. In another study conducted by Rajyalakshmi et al. (2017), 10 patients suffering from diabetes and hypertension were given commercial 10 ml of Jatamansi extract twice a day for 15 days.

A significant reduction in BP, improvement of NO availability and improvement of endothelial function were observed among the patients. Methanolic root extract of both wild and in vitro derived of plants showed very promising ACE inhibitory activity with IC50 of 46.25 and 42.5 μg/ml, respectively. These values are comparable to a potent anti-hypertensive molecule, captopril which has an IC50 value of 32.36 μg/ml (Bose, 2019).

19.5.8   PASSIFLORA EDULIS

Oral application of the crude extract of *Passiflora edulis* rind (10 or 50 mg/kg) significantly reduce BP in spontaneously hypertensive rats (SHRs). Luteolin, a phenolic compound extracted from *Passiflora edulis* leaves also lowered BP for 1 to 7 h when orally administered in SHRs at a concentration of 50 mg/kg (Ichimura et al., 2006). Zibadi et al. (2007) also observed that diet supplemented with purple passion fruit extract (PFP extract) at a concentration of 50 mg/kg significantly lower systolic BP by 12.3 mm Hg in female SHRs. They further extended their study to hypertensive human subjects by administering with PFP extract or pill at a dose of 400 mg/day for 4-weeks. BP of the PFP extract-treated group was found to significantly decrease by 30.9 (systolic) and 24.6 (diastolic) mm Hg, as compared to the placebo group. Interestingly no adverse effects were reported by the patients. Similarly, in a study conducted by Konta et al. (2014) observed a significant reduction in systolic BP in male Wistar rats when a high dose of purple passion fruit pulp (8 g/kg) is orally given. Moreover, *Passiflora edulis* have also been reported to contain gamma-aminobutyric acid (GABA), a neurotransmitter involved in the reduction of BP (Inoue et al., 2003; Appel et al., 2011).

19.5.9   RAUWOLFIA SERPENTINA

R. serpentina is an evergreen shrub commonly known as Indian snakeroot widely distributed in the Indian subcontinent. It is a well-known folk medicine in India and is used in treating several important diseases. Clinical studies conducted by various researchers reveals that an active molecule "reserpine" extracted from the root is responsible for controlling the hypertensive activity of this plant (Wilkins and Judson, 1953). Reserpine, an alkaloid, is a drug used in treatment of hypertension. Sheldon and Kotte (1957) conducted 2-year double-blind study on the effect of reserpine on hypertensive patients, where they observed a significant reduction in BP of the patients. The mechanism of hypotensive activity is by inhibiting vesicular monoamine transporter (VMAT) 1 and 2 located at the neuroendocrine cells of the peripheral nervous system. The inhibition of VMAT's blocked the L-type voltage-gated calcium channels and catecholamine secretion thereby lowering BP (Loby 2015; Mahata et al., 1996).

19.5.10   SOLANUM TORVUM

Solanum torvum belong to the Solanaceae family and is commonly known as Turkey berry. It was native to West Indies but now spread to tropical areas of various countries. Intravenous injection of aqueous and methanol extract of fruit significantly reduces the arterial BP in Wistar rats. Aqueous extract significantly and dose-dependently inhabited the blood aggregation induced by thrombin and adenosine diphosphate. The hypotensive activity of *S. torvum* extract is due to their bradycardic effect (Nguelefack et al., 2008). Similarly, Mohan et al. (2009) also demonstrated that the ethanolic extract of *S. torvum* fruit could prevent the development of high BP in fructose induced hypertensive rats.

19.6   CHALLENGES AND FUTURE PROSPECTIVE OF USING ETHNOMEDICINAL PLANTS IN COMBATING HYPERTENSION

Generally, hypertensive patients need to be under medications for long-lasting and sometimes lifetime; hence, the use of modern drugs for long duration is associated with several adverse side effects to human health. For combating such type of chronic diseases, people are exploring for

CAM which have lesser side effects. Hence, plants can be used as the alternative source for production of new drug or compound to mitigate the chronic disease especially hypertension which is considered as the leading cause of NCD related mortality. Some of the important antihypertensive compounds have been extracted from plants such as deserpidine from *Rauwolfia canescens*, tetrandrine from *Stephania tetrandra,* and reserpine and rescinnamine from *Rauwolfia serpentina*. The advantages of using TM are due to its low cost, less side effects and easy accessibility or availability.

However, the main challenges for using the TM are the lack of scientific knowledge underlying the molecular mechanisms for mitigation of the disease, dosage, presence of active phytochemical compound(s), quality control, etc. In some cases, plants of close species are so similar that is difficult to differentiate morphologically which may to lead to application of wrong species. Hence, proper scientific identification of the plant is required in order to combat hypertension. Another important challenge is that plants are slow-growing species and most of these ethnomedicinal plants are confined in a specific region or habitat. So, overexploitation will lead to the extinction of indigenous, rare, ethnomedicinal plants disturbing the biodiversity as well as increasing the environmental damage. For example, in India, *Clerodendrum colebrookianum* having many medicinal properties including hypotensive activity is confined in the NER and is now placed under vulnerable category.

Hence, it becomes mandatory to give proper awareness regarding GACP (guidelines on good agricultural and collection practices) for medicinal plants developed by WHO. This guideline gives general technical guidance on procurement of good quality medicinal plant materials for sustainable production of herbal products and contributes to the quality assurance, safety, and efficacy of finished herbal products. It also encourages and supports the sustainable cultivation and prudent exploration of medicinal plants of good quality in ways that respect, protect, and conserve medicinal plants and environment (WHO, 2003).

North East India is endowed with rich flora and fauna as it falls under the Eastern Himalayan and the Indo-Burma mega-biodiversity hotspots that have diverse ecosystems ranging from wetland, tropical, and temperate (Myers et al., 2000). There is a great potential for further exploration and discovery of novel compound that helps in combating the chronic disease especially 'silent killer' hypertension. Moreover, exploration of endophytes such as bacteria and fungi associated with the antihypertensive ethnomedicinal plants that can also produce the same or novel compound is the need of the hour to protect the susceptible medicinal plants endemic to a particular region from overexploitation.

This is due to the fact that long association of endophytes with the host plants may lead to participation of the endophytes in metabolic pathways, or some genetic information may be transferred from the host to produce the same important bioactive compounds as their host plants (Golinska et al., 2015). Also, there is the possibility that the compound(s) produced by endophytes may possess less adverse effect as the compound(s) may not affect the human cell since the endophyte have a symbiotic relationship with the host plants. This will save the indigenous rare medicinal plants from extinction and also save the time to harvest slow-growing plants as the exploration of microbial source are easier, faster, production of bulk in short duration, cost-effective and, safer to human health and environment (Tamreihao et al., 2019).

19.7   CONCLUSION

Considering the predominance of chronic disease across the globe, it is becoming mandatory to search for a novel compound which is cost-effective, less adverse side effects and readily accessible or available for controlling hypertension. One such alternative option is CAM which main backbone is the traditional or folk medicine practiced by many local healers from time immemorial. For controlling hypertension, single-use of drug is not effective sometimes multiple drugs have been recommended. Plant based herbal medicine is generally composed of many metabolites which work together to control the BP by two or more mechanisms, and it also have lesser side effects. In addition, utilization of some of the edible antihypertensive herbs considered to be safe for thousands of years can be used as supplements in preparation of herbal tea for consumption to control BP. Nevertheless, it is worth mentioning that their safety must be supported by sound scientific evidence based on clinical trials with large population. These plants have huge potential as a natural remedy for hypertension as well as for ensuring a healthy living.

KEYWORDS

- **angiotensin-converting enzyme**
- **hypertension**
- **medicinal plants**
- **noncommunicable disease**
- **North Eastern Himalayan Region**

REFERENCES

Alzohairy, M. A., (2016). Therapeutics role of *Azadirachta indica* (Neem) and their active constituents in diseases prevention and treatment. *Evid. Based Complement Alternat. Med.,* 1–11. Article ID 7382506.

Appel, K., Rose, T., Fiebich, B., Kammler, T., Hoffmann, C., & Weiss, G., (2011). Modulation of the γ-aminobutyric acid (GABA) system by *Passiflora incarnata* L. *Phyther. Res., 25*(6), 838–843.

Arya, H., Syed, S. B., Singh, S. S., Ampasala, D. R., & Coumar, M. S., (2018). In silico investigations of chemical constituents of *Clerodendrum colebrookianum* in the anti-hypertensive drug targets: ROCK, ACE, and PDE5. *Interdiscip. Sci. Comput. Life Sci., 10*(4), 792–804.

Bartolome, A. P., Villaseñor, I. M., & Yang, W. C., (2013). *Bidens pilosa* L. (Asteraceae): Botanical properties, traditional uses, phytochemistry, and pharmacology. *Evid. Based Complement Alternat. Med.*

Bilanda, D. C., Dzeufiet, P. D. D., Kouakep, L., Aboubakar, B. F. O., Tedong, L., Kamtchouing, P., & Dimo, T., (2017). *Bidens pilosa* ethylene acetate Extract can protect against L-NAME-induced hypertension on rats. *BMC Complement. Altern. Med., 17*(1), 1–7.

Borah, P. K., Devi, U., Biswas, D., Kalita, H. C., Sharma, M., & Mahanta, J., (2015). Distribution of BP & correlates of hypertension in school children Aged 5–14 years from North East India. *Indian J. Med. Res., 142*, 293–300.

Changkija, S., (1999). Folk Medicinal Plants of the Nagas in India. *Asian Folkl. Stud., 58*(1), 205.

Chatterjee, S., Saikia, A., Dutta, P., Ghosh, D., Pangging, G., & Goswami, A. K., (2006). *Background Paper on Biodiversity Significance of North East India.* Forests Conservation Program. WWF-India, New Delhi.

Chen, Y. Y., Hsu, M. J., Hsieh, C. Y., Lee, L. W., Chen, Z. C., & Sheu, J. R., (2014). Andrographolide inhibits nuclear factor-κB activation through JNK-Akt-p65 signaling cascade in tumor necrosis factor-α-stimulated vascular smooth muscle cells. *Sci. World J.,* 10. Article ID 130381.

Chopra, H. K., & Ram, C. V. S., (2019). Recent guidelines for hypertension: A clarion call for BP control in India. *Circ. Res., 124*(7), 984–986.

Das, S., (2012). Ethnomedicinal uses of some traditional medicinal plants found in Tripura, India. *J. Med. Plants Res., 6*(36).

De Boer, I. H., Bangalore, S., Benetos, A., Davis, A. M., Michos, E. D., Muntner, P., Rossing, P., ET AL., (2017). Diabetes and hypertension: A position statement by the American Diabetes Association. *Diabetes Care, 40*(9), 1273–1284.

Devi, K. Y., & Devi, M. H., (2017). Survey of medicinal plants in Bishnupur District, Manipur, North-Eastern India. *Int. J. Appl. Res., 3*(4), 462–471.

Devi, M. R., Singh, P. K., & Dutta, B. K., (2011). Ethnomedicinal plants of Kabui Naga tribe of Manipur, India. *Pleione, 5*(1), 115–128.

Devi, R., Boruah, D. C., Sharma, D. K., & Kotoky, J. (2011). Leaf extract of *Clerodendron Colebrookianum* inhibits intrinsic hypercholesterolemia and extrinsic lipid peroxidation. *Int. J. Pharmtech Res, 3*(2), 960–967.

Devi, T. I., Devi, K. U., & Singh, E. J., (2014). Wild medicinal plants in the hill of Manipur, India: A traditional therapeutic potential. *Int. J. Sci. Res. Publ., 5*(6), 1–9.

Dimo, T., Azay, J., Tan, P. V., Pellecuer, J., Cros, G., Bopelet, M., & Serrano, J. J., (2001). Effects of the aqueous and methylene chloride extracts of *Bidens pilosa* leaf on fructose-hypertensive rats. *J. Ethnopharmacol., 76*(3), 215–221.

Dimo, T., Nguelefack, T. B., Tan, P. V., Yewah, M. P., Dongo, E., Rakotonirina, S. V., Kamanyi, A., & Bopelet, M., (2003). Possible mechanisms of action of the neutral extract from *Bidens pilosa* L. leaves on the cardiovascular system of anesthetized rats. *Phytother. Res., 17*(10), 1135–1139.

Dimo, T., Rakotonirina, S. V., Tan, P. V., Azay, J., Dongo, E., & Cros, G., (2002). Leaf methanol extract of *Bidens pilosa* prevents and attenuates the hypertension induced by a high-fructose diet in Wistar rats. *J. Ethnopharmacol., 83*(3), 183–191.

Disi, A., Sara, S., M., Anwar, A., & Eid, A. H. (2016). Anti-hypertensive herbs and their mechanisms of action: Part I. *Front. Pharmacol., 6*, 1–24.

Ghosh, D., & Parida, P., (2015). Medicinal plants of Assam, India: A mini-review medicinal plants of Assam, India: A mini-review. *Int. J. Pharmacol. Pharma. Sci., 2*(6), 5–10.

Ghosh, S., & Kumar, M., (2019). Prevalence and associated risk factors of hypertension among persons aged 15–49 in India: A cross-sectional study. *BMJ Open, 9*(12), e029714.

Gilani, A.H. Aftab, K., (1992). Pharmacological actions of Cuscuta reflexa. Int. J. Pharmacog., 30(4), 296-302.

Golinska, P., Wypij, M., Agarkar, G., Rathod, D., Dahm, H., & Rai, M., (2015). Endophytic actinobacteria of medicinal plants: Diversity and bioactivity. *Antonie Van Leeuwenhoek., 108*(2), 267–289.

Gupta, R., & Guptha, S., (2010). Strategies for initial management of hypertension. *Indian J. Med. Res., 132*(5), 531–542.

Gupta, R., Gaur, K. & Ram, C. V. S., (2019). Emerging trends in hypertension epidemiology in India. *J. Hum. Hypertens., 33*(8), 575–587.

Hazarika, N. C., Biswas, D., Narain, K., Phukan, R. K., Kalita, H. C., & Mahanta, J., (2000). Differences in BP level and hypertension in three ethnic groups of Northeastern India. *Asia-Pacific J. Public Heal., 12*(2), 71–78.

Hazarika, T. K., Marak, S., Mandal, D., Upadhyaya, K., Nautiyal, B. P., & Shukla, A. C., (*2016*). Underutilized and unexploited fruits of Indo-Burma hot spot, Meghalaya, North-East India: Ethno-medicinal evaluation, socio-economic importance and conservation strategies. *Genet. Resour. Crop Ev., 63*(2):289–304.

Ichimura, T., Yamanaka, A., Ichiba, T., Toyokawa, T., Kamada, Y., Tamamura, T., & Maruyama, S., (2006). Antihypertensive effect of an extract of *Passiflora edulis* rind in spontaneously hypertensive RATS. *Biosci. Biotechnol. Biochem., 70*(3), 718–721.

Imotomba, R. K., & Devi, L. S., (2011). Creation of geo-spatial data base of medicinal plants of Senapati district, Manipur. *National J. Chem. Biosis., 2*(2), 17–36.

Inoue, K., Shirai, T., Ochiai, H., Kasao, M., Hayakawa, K., Kimura, M., & Sansawa, H., (2003). Blood-pressure-lowering effect of a novel fermented milk containing γ-aminobutyric acid (GABA) in mild hypertensives. *Eur. J. Clin. Nutr., 57*(3), 490–495.

Jamir, T. T., Sharma, H. K., & Dolui, A. K., (1999). Folklore medicinal plants of Nagaland, India. *Fitoterapia, 70*(4), 395–401.

Jayakumar, T., Hsieh, C. Y., Lee, J. J., & Sheu, J. R., (2013). Experimental and clinical pharmacology of *Andrographis paniculata* and its major bioactive phytoconstituent andrographolide. *Evid Based Complement Alternat. Med.,*16. ArticleID846740.

Kamum, G., (2018). Ethnomedicinal plants used by Galo community of West Siang District, Arunachal Pradesh. *Int. J. Res. Appl. Sci. Eng. Technol., 6*(1), 438–444.

Kayang, H., Kharbuli, B., Myrboh, B., & Syiem, D., (2005). Medicinal plants of Khasi hills of Meghalaya, India. *Acta Hortic., 675*, 75–80.

Khongsai, M., Saikia, S. P., & Kayang, H., (2011). Ethnomedicinal plants used by different tribes of Arunachal Pradesh. *Indian J. Tradit. Knowl., 10*(3), 541–546.

Kichu, M., Malewska, T., Akter, K., Imchen, I., Harrington, D., Kohen, J., Vemulpad, S. R., & Jamie, J. F., (2015). An ethnobotanical study of medicinal plants of Chungtia Village, Nagaland, India. *J. Ethnopharmacol., 166*, 5–17.

Konta, E. M., Almeida, M. R., & Lira, C., (2014). Evaluation of the antihypertensive properties of yellow passion fruit pulp (*Passiflora edulis* Sims) in spontaneously hypertensive rats. *Phytother. Res., 28*(1), 28–32.

Laurent, S., (2017). Antihypertensive drugs. *Pharmacological Res., 124*, 116–125.

Lobay, D., (2015). Rauwolfia in the treatment of hypertension. *Integrative Medicine, 14*(3), 40–46.

Lokesh, D., & Amitsankar, D., (2012). Evaluation of mechanism for antihypertensive action of *Clerodendrum colebrookianum* walp.; used by folklore healers in North-East India. *J. Ethnopharmacol., 143*(1), 207–212.

Lokho, A., (2012). The folk medicinal plants of the Mao Naga in Manipur. *Int.J. Sci. Res. Pub., 2*(6), 1–8.

Mahata, M., Mahata, S. K., Parmer, R. J., & O'Connor, D. T. (1996). Vesicular monoamine transport inhibitors novel action at calcium channels to prevent catecholamine secretion. *Hypertension, 28*(3), 414–420.

Mali, A. J., Bothiraja, C., Purohit, R. N., & Pawar, A. P., (2017). *In Vitro* and *In Vivo* performance of novel spray-dried andrographolide loaded scleroglucan based formulation for dry powder inhaler.*Curr. Drug. Deliv., 14*(7), 968–980.

Malik, K., Ahmad, M., Bussmann, R. W., Tariq, A., Ullah, R., Alqahtani, A. S., Shahat, A. A., ET AL., (2018). Ethnobotany of anti-hypertensive plants used in Northern Pakistan. *Front. Pharmacol., 9*, 1–18.

Meetei, S. Y., & Singh, P. K., (2007). Survey for medicinal plants of Thoubal district, Manipur. *Flora and Fauna, 13*(2), 355–358.

Mohan, M., Jaiswal, B. S., & Kasture, S., (2009). Effect of *Solanum torvum* on BP and metabolic alterations in fructose hypertensive rats. *J. Ethnopharmacol., 126*(1), 86–89.

Murtem, G., & Chaudhry, P., (2016). An ethnobotanical study of medicinal plants used by the tribes in upper Subansiri district of Arunachal Pradesh, India. *Am. J. Ethnomedicine, 3*(3), 35–49.

Myers, N., Mittermeier, R. A., Mittermeier, C. G., Da Fonseca, G. A. B., & Kent, J., (2000). Biodiversity hotspots for conservation priorities. *Nature, 403*, 853–858.

Nahakpam, L., (2012). Ethno-medicinal plants of Manipur used in the treatment of BP. *NeBIO, 3*(1), 39–41.

Nguelefack, T. B., Mekhfi, H., Dimo, T., Afkir, S., Nguelefack-Mbuyo, E. P., Legssyer, A., & Ziyyat, A., (2008). Cardiovascular and anti-platelet aggregation activities of extracts from *Solanum torvum* (Solanaceae) fruits in rat. *J. Complement. Integr. Med., 5*(1).

Obiefuna, I., & Young, R., (2005). Concurrent administration of aqueous *Azadirachta indica* (Neem) leaf extract with DOCA-salt prevents the development of hypertension and accompanying electrocardiogram changes in the rat. *Phytotherapy Res., 19*(9), 792–795.

Omóbòwálé, T. O., Oyagbemi, A. A., Alaba, B. A., Ola-Davies, O. E., Adejumobi, O. A., Asenuga, E. R., Ajibade, T. O., et al., (2018). Ameliorative effect of *Azadirachta indica* on sodium fluoride-induced hypertension through improvement of antioxidant defense system and upregulation of extracellular signal-regulated kinase 1/2 signaling. *J. Basic Clin. Physiol. Pharmacol., 29*(2), 155–164.

Omóbòwálé, T. O., Oyagbemi, A. A., Ogunpolu, B. S., Ola-Davies, O. E., Olukunle, J. O., Asenuga, E. R., Ajibade, T. O., Adejumobi, O. A., Afolabi, J. M., Falayi, O. O., et al., (2018). Correction: Antihypertensive effect of polyphenol-rich fraction of *Azadirachta indica* on Nω-Nitro-L-arginine methyl ester-induced hypertension and cardiorenal dysfunction. *Drug Res. (Stuttg).*

Panda, D., (2012). Medicinal plants use and primary health care in Sikkim. *Int. J. Ayurvedic Herb. Med., 2*(2), 253–259.

Panmei, R., Gajurel, P. R., & Singh, B., (2019). Ethnobotany of medicinal plants used by the zeliangrong ethnic group of Manipur, Northeast India. *J. Ethnopharmacol., 235*, 164–182.

Payum, T., (2017). Distribution, ethnobotany, pharmacognosy and phytoconstituents of *Coptis teeta* wall.: A highly valued and threatened medicinal plant of Eastern Himalayas. *Pharmacogn. J., 9*(6), 28–34.

Perme, N., Choudhury, S. N., Choudhury, R., Natung, T., & De, B., (2015). Medicinal plants in traditional use at Arunachal Pradesh, India. *IJPP, 5*(5), 86–98.

Rai, P. K., & Lalramnghinglova, H., (2010). Ethnomedicinal plant resources of Mizoram, India: Implication of traditional knowledge in health care system. *Ethnobot. Leafl., 14*, 274–305.

Rajlakshmi, D., Banerjee, S. K., Sood, S., & Maulik, S. K., (2003). *In-vitro* and *in-vivo* antioxidant activity of different extracts of the leaves of *Clerodendron colebrookianum* walp in the rat. *J. Pharm. Pharmacol., 55*(12), 1681–1686.

Rajyalakshmi, I., Rao, A. V., Potti, R. B., & Murty, K. V. G. S., (2017). Effect of *Nardostachys jatamansi* extract on vascular endothelial dysfunction in hypertensive, hyperglycemic patients: An open-label, prospective study. *J. Pharmacy Res., 11*(9), 1180–1183.

Ramakrishnan, S., Zachariah, G., Gupta, K., Shivkumar, R. J., Mohanan, P. P., Venugopal, K., Sateesh, S., Sethi, R., Jain, D., Bardolei, N., et al., (2019). Prevalence of hypertension among Indian Adults: Results from the great India BP Survey. *Indian Heart J., 71.*

Sen, P., Dollo, M., Choudhury, M. D., & Choudhury, D., (2008). Documentation of traditional herbal knowledge of Khamptis of Arunachal Pradesh. *Indian J. Tradit. Knowl., 7*(3), 438–442.

Shankar, R., & Rawat, M. S., (2010). Biodiversity of medicinal plants in North East India: Their systematic utilization. *Natl. Conf. Biodivers. Med. Aromat. Plants Collect. Charact. Util., 1*(2), 584–591.

Shankar, R., Kumar, T. A., Anku, G., Neyaz, S., & Rawat, M. S., (2017). Indigenous medicinal plants of Northeast India in human health: Literary Note. *J. Drug Res. Ayurvedic Sci., 2*(2), 104–117.

Shankar, R., Lavekar, G. S., & Sharma, B. K., (2012). Traditional healing practice and folk medicines used by Mishing community of North East India. *J. Ayurveda Integr. Med., 3*(3), 124–129.

Sharma, M., & Das, B., (2018). Medicinal plants of North-East Region of India: A small review. *Int. J. Curr. Pharm. Res., 10*(4), 11.

Sharma, M., Sharma, C. L., & Marak, P. N., (2014). Indigenous uses of medicinal plants in North Garo Hills, Meghalaya, NE India. *Res. J. Recent Sci., 3*, 137–146.

Singh, B. K., Ramakrishna, Y., & Ngachan, S. V., (2014). Spiny Coriander (*Eryngium foetidum* L.): A commonly used, neglected spicing-culinary herb of Mizoram, India. *Genet. Resour. Crop Evol., 61*(6).

Singh, H. B., Prasad, P., & Raj, L. K., (2002). Folk medicinal plants in the Sikkim Himalayas of India. *Asian Folkl. Stud., 61*(2).

Sinha, A., & Agrawal, R., (2019). Clinical pharmacology of antihypertensive therapy for the treatment of hypertension in CKD. *CJASN., 14*(5), 757–764.

Sumi, A., & Shohe, K., (*2018*). Ethnomedicinal plants of Sumi Nagas in Zunheboto district, Nagaland, Northeast India. *Acta Sci. Pharma. Sci., 2*(8), 15–21.

Swarnalata, N., (2017). To study antihypertensive potential of ethanolic extract of *Allium Hookeri* thaw Enum leaves (maroi napakpi). *Int. J. Eng. Tech. Management Appl. Sci, 5*(3), 407–416.

Tamang, M., Pal, K., Kumar, R. S., Kalam, A., & Ahmed, S. R., (2017). Ethnobotanical survey of threatened medicinal plants of West Sikkim. *Bot. Stud., 2*(6), 116–125.

Tamreihao, K., Mukherjee, S., Ningthoujam, D. S., & Roy, S. S., (2019). Prospects of Actinobacteria from underexplored ecosystems as anti-infective agents against *Mycobacterium Tuberculosis*. In: Tamreihao, K., Mukherjee, S., Ningthoujam, & Debananda, S., (ed.), *Frontiers in Anti-infective Agents: Current Perspective on Anti-infective Agents* (Vol. 1, pp. 1–13). Bentham Science: U.A.E.

Temsutola, Ngullie, O. L., & Vepu., (2019). Ethnomedicinal study of plants used by Chang Naga tribe of Tuensang, Nagaland, India. *Int. J. Botany Stud., 4*(2), 107–109.

Thangjam, R. S., Singh, A. I., Rothangpui, Cindy, L., & Rameshchandra, T., (2017). The Profile of BP (BP) and the prevalence of hypertension in school going children Aged 5–15 Years of Manipur, a North-Eastern Hilly Indian State. *Int. J. Contemp. Pediatr., 4*(6), 2151.

Trilestari, Nurrochmad, A., Ismiyati, Wijayanti, A., & Nugroh, A. E., (2015). Antihypertensive activity of ethanolic extract of *Andrographis paniculata* herbs in Wistar rats with a non-invasive method. *Int. J. Toxicol. Pharmacol. Res., 7*(5), 247–255.

Venkatachalapathy, V., Balakrishnan, S., Musthafa, M., & Natarajan, A., (2012). A clinical evaluation of *Nardostachys jatamansi* in the management of essential hypertension. *Int. J. Pharm. Phytopharmacol. Res., 2*(2), 96–100.

Verma, H., Negi, M. S., Mahapatra, B. S., Shukla, A., & Paul, J., (2019). Evaluation of an emerging medicinal crop Kalmegh [*Andrographispaniculata* (Burm. F.) Wall. Ex. Nees] for commercial cultivation and pharmaceutical & industrial uses: A review. *J. Pharmacogn. Phytochem., 8*(4), 835–848.

WHO, (2002). *WHO Traditional Medicine Strategy 2002–2005* (pp. 1–74). World Health Organization: Geneva.

WHO, (2003). *WHO Guidelines on Good Agricultural and Collection Practices (GACP) for Medicinal Plants* (p. 45). World Health Organization: Geneva.

Wilkins, R. W., & Judson, W. E., (1953). The use of *Rauwolfia serpentina* in hypertensive patients. *New Engl. J. Med., 248*(2), 48–53.

Yoopan, N., Thisoda, P., Rangkadilok, N., Sahasitiwat, S., Pholphana, N., Ruchirawat, S., Satayavivad,J.(2007).Cardiovascular effects of 14-deoxy-11,12-didehydroandrographolide and Andrographis paniculata extracts. *Planta Med, 73*(6), 503–11.

Zibadi, S., Farid, R., Moriguchi, S., Lu, Y., Foo, L. Y., Tehrani, P. M., Ulreich, J. B., & Watson, R. R., (2007). Oral administration of purple passion fruit peel extract attenuates BP in female spontaneously hypertensive rats and humans. *Nutr. Res., 27*(7), 408–416.

CHAPTER 20

MEDICINAL PLANTS: CONSUMPTION, SUPPLY CHAIN, MARKETING, AND TRADE IN INDIA

DEBASHIS MANDAL

Department of Horticulture, Aromatic, and Medicinal Plants,
Mizoram University, Aizawl – 796004, Mizoram, India,
E-mail: debashismandal1982@gmail.com

ABSTRACT

India, the land is having enormous indigenous knowledge of ethnomedicine and herbal formulation since time immemorial for remedies to health ailments of its tribes. This masterpiece geographical area is blessed with a bounty of natural diversity, which is storehouse of several elite therapeutic herbs across its higher hills, valleys, and river basin. Starting from wild forest to cultivated land, it is having diverse sources of medicinal plants either in wild habitat or under cultivation. Indian Himalaya-possesses the well-respected repute of magical mysterious herbs to strengthen immune and to prolong the beauty and youthfulness. However, though the country has its star presence in the galaxy of medicinal plants producers of globe, yet having a very unexposed supply chain management system which people perhaps had little understanding or knowledge of it. But Indian's medicinal plants export are increasing with a growth rate over 14% for the past 10 years and had exported around 330.18 million USD of crude herbs and 465.12 million USD of processed herbs in 2017–2018. This chapter will therefore enumerate the existing consumption and supply chain of medicinal plants in India along with glimpses of its marketing and trade under global context.

20.1 INTRODUCTION

With the advancement of the society and the developmental process across the nation, it was expected that the traditional medicinal practices, majority based of different type of botanical plant species will be substituted by the modern chemical-based medicines. However, it is worth noted, that the present generation is more conscious about health and aware of the side effects for the use of chemical medicinal preparations. Thus, we can notice a resurgence of herbal medicine, not only for health care but also for general well-being. Herbal medicine was defined as "crude drug of the vegetable origin utilized for the treatment of diseased state often of a chronic nature or to attain or maintain a condition of improved health" by Tyler (Tyler, 1994). But herbs or herbal preparation are not only being used for health care or chronic diseases any more. We can get an ample number of beauty products, cosmetic formulations and even functional food preparations based on herbal constitutes. However, the folklore uses by folk healers and house hold consumption for traditional uses remain unchanged in the core of the Indian villages, in particular to those areas which are geographically more isolated. Thus, medicinal plants, which holds a major proportion of flora, supply raw materials for pharmaceutical, drug, and cosmetic industries with a high demand within and outside of the country (Nagaraju et al., 2018; Rathore and Mathur, 2019). Furthermore, a transformation of choice by the end users is taking place globally for using traditional medicine (TM), is that to depend much on ready herbal products available at market which are being prepared by pharmaceutical industries rather than own preparations of the practitioners. It is the era of "herbs for wellness." Now-a-days there are large number of ready to use commercial herbal formulation for reducing stress problem, increasing nutritional power, skin health, vitality, increasing body energy level as well as anti-aging, which broadly for general well-being of human. Therefore, there is a high demand for medicinal plants, both cultivated and of wild origin, into herbal health care and wellness sector. As per the report of Global Wellness Institute, the estimated value of the global wellness industry in 2013 was US$ 3.4 trillion (Bodekar, 2015). Goraya and Ved (2017) reported that total commercial demand of raw herbal drug in India, is 5,12,000 MT in 2014–2015, where, 1.95 lakhs MT is for domestic herbal industry, 1.345 lakhs MT to meet the export demand and 1.675 lakhs MT for household consumption apart from an estimated wastage of 14.91000 MT. After study by the EXIM Bank through the Foundation for Revitalization of Local Health Tradition (FRHLT) in 2003, found that there are 880 medicinal plant species in trade which includes 42 species in foreign trade. Moreover, it was reported that the total consumption of raw herbal drug was around 1.28 Lakhs MT worth Rs. 847 Crore with a projected annual growth of 10%. National Medicinal Plant Board (NMPB), Government of India, in 2002, through Center for Research, Planning, and Action (CERPA) estimated annual demand of 2.34 lakhs MT including export trade value of Rs. 1275.68 Crores (CERPA, 2002). Previous reports suggested that around 2,500 (Chauhan, 1999) to 7,500 (Pushpangadan, 1995) medicinal plants species are in use; however, at 2006–2007 survey of NMPB resulted with the information of using 960 plant species into herbal trade. More recently, Goraya and Ved (2017) opined that the Indian classical and folk health care system depends on about 6,500 medicinal species, which are being used by 1 million folk healers and around 138 million rural households. Kesari and Pradeep (2018) reported 90% of the traded medicinal plants of India are of wild collection and caused around 1,000 species into threat to loss. Further threat assessment resulted that around 344 native medicinal plant species of India are already marked as red-listed (Tables 20.1 and 20.2) at regional, national or international level (Goraya and Ved, 2017; Holley and Cherla, 1998).

TABLE 20.1   Red Listed Medicinal Plants of South India

Status	Medicinal Plant Species
Critically endangered	*Adhatoda beddomei, Cayratia pedata var. glabra, Coscinium fenestratum, Cycas circinalis, Janakia arayalpatra, Kaempferia galanga, Paphiopedilium druyi, Piper barberi, Syzygium travancoricum, Utleria salicifolia, Vateria macrocarpa*
Endangered	*Ampelocissus indica, Cyclea fissicalyx, Heliotropium keralense, Kingiodendron pinnatum, Lamprachaenium microcephalum, Madhuca diplostemon, Myristica malabarica, Nervilla aragoana, Nilgirianthus ciliatus, Pterocarpus, santalinus, Rauwolfia serpentina, Saraca asoca*
Extinct	*Aerva wightii, Asparagus rottleri, Madhuca insignis*
Extinct in wild	*Plectranthus vettiveroides*
Vulnerable	*Acorus calamus, Adenia hondala, Aegle marmelos, Amorphophallus paeonifolius, Ampelocissus araneosa, Aristolochia tagala, Commiphora, mukul, Drosera peltata, Garcinia indica, Garcinia morella, Holostemma annulare, Hydnocarpus macrocarpa, Michellia champaca, Moringa concanensis, Ochreinauclea missionis, Oroxylum indicum, Piper mullesua, Piper nigrum, Schrebera sweitenodes, Symplocus cochinchinsis subsp. laurina, Tinospora sinensis, Tragia bicolor, Trichopus zeylanicus subsp. travancoricus*

TABLE 20.1   *(Continued)*

Status	Medicinal Plant Species
Low risk	*Andrographis paniculata, Aristolochia bracteolata, Artemisia nilagirica, Balanites aegyptica, Buchanania lanzan, Drosera indica, Elaeagnus conferta, Embelia ribes, Gardenia gummifera, Gloriosa superba, Glycosmis macrocarpa, Hedychium coronarium, Operculina turpethum, Phoenix pusilla, Piper longrum, Pseudarthria viscida, Puereria tuberosa, Symplocos racemosa, Vateria indica, Vernonia anthelmintica, Woodfordia fruticosa*

TABLE 20.2   Highly Traded Red Listed Medicinal Plants Species of India

Aconitum ferox, Aconitum heterophyllum, Aquilaria malaccensis, Berberis aristata, Bergenia ciliata, Boswellia serrata, Buchanania lanzan, Celastrus paniculatus, Chlorophytum tuberosum, Cinnamomum sulphuratum, Cinnamomum tamala, Commiphora wightii, Coscinium fenestratum, Decalepis hamiltonii, Embelia ribes, Embelia tsjeriam-cottam, Ephedra gerardiana, Garcinia indica, Gloriosa superba, Gymnema sylvestre, Holostemma ada-kodien, Jurinea dolomiaea, Litsea glutinosa, Mesua ferra, Nardostachys grandiflora, Nilgirianthus ciliatus, Operculina turpethum, Oroxylum indicum, Picrorhiza kurrooa, Pseudarthria viscida, Pterocarpus marsupium, Pterocarpus santalinus, Rauvolfia serpentina, Rheum emodi, Rheum moorcroftianum, Rhododendron antopogon, Rubia cordifloia, Santalum album, Saraca asoca, Saussurea costus, Schrebera sweietenioides, Smilax glabra, Sterculia urens, Swertia chirayita, Symlocos racemosa, Taxus wallichiana, Valeriana hardwickii, Valeriana jatamansi, Vateria indica

Therefore, cultivation, and conservation of commercially important medicinal plants is very much needed. Chowti et al. (2018) reported that medicinal plants were cultivated in 2.62 lakh hectares area with an annual production of 2.02 lakh tons in 2005–2006 which got increased and in 2015–2016 the area under cultivation is 6.34 lakhs hectares with a production of 10.23 lakh tons in India with a growth rate of 2.76%. It was further reported that currently Rajasthan (56%) holds the largest area share under medicinal plants cultivation followed by Uttar Pradesh (25%) whereas, production share in Madhya Pradesh (44%) followed by Rajasthan (19%). Important medicinal plant species under cultivation in India (Table 20.3).

TABLE 20.3   Important Medicinal Plants Species Under Cultivation in India

Medicinal Plant Species	Area (1,000 Hectare)	Production (1,000 MT)
Acorus calamus	0.4	3.5
Aloe vera	1.0	15.0
Artemisia annua	0.4	2.0

TABLE 20.3   *(Continued)*

Medicinal Plant Species	Area (1,000 Hectare)	Production (1,000 MT)
Cymbopogon vetiveroides	1.5	0.5
Lawsonia inermis	40.0	25.0
Mentha arvensis	40.0	8.0 lakhs liter oil
Ocimum tenuiflorum	5.0	5.0
Piper longum	5.5	4.0
Plantago ovata	80.0	45.0
Saussurea costus	0.25	0.12
Senna alexandrina	22.0	20.0
Withania somnifera	6.0	5.0

Sources: Goraya and Ved (2017).

There are 528 wild life sanctuaries, 108 national parks and 65 conservation reserves in India for protection and conservation of red listed medicinal plants. Further, Government of India, through its different projects has developed 108 medicinal plants conservation areas (MPCA) in different states of the country. Out of 108 MPCAs, Tamil Nadu (12), Kerala (9), Karnataka (13), Andhra Pradesh (8), Maharashtra (13), Madhya Pradesh (13), Rajasthan (7), Chhattisgarh (7), Odisha (5), Arunachal Pradesh (7), Uttarakhand (7) and West Bengal is having 7 nos. of MPCA. Further, through NMPB initiatives, there are 76 medicinal plants conservation and development areas (MPCDA) (Table 20.4) in addition to MPCAs for *in situ* conservation of medicinal plants in different states viz. Haryana (1), West Bengal (7), Nagaland (4), Gujarat (6), Mizoram (4), Manipur (3), Karnataka (13), Himachal Pradesh (5), Sikkim (4), Maharashtra, and Tamil Nadu (14), each.

TABLE 20.4   MPCDAs and MPCAs of North East India

Name of the State	Name of MPCDA/MPCAs
Arunachal Pradesh	Tezu-Parsuramkund
	Roing-Mayodia
	Kanubari-Wannu
	Bomdila
	Hake-Tari
Manipur	Khangkhuikulle
	Kailam Churachanpur
	Langol Imphal

TABLE 20.4   *(Continued)*

Name of the State	Name of MPCDA/MPCAs
Mizoram	Bilkhawthlir Kolasib Division
	Vairangte Kolasib Division
	Hmunpui Reik Division
	Sialsuk Thenzawl Division
Nagaland	Jalukie Village Peren District
	Changtonya Mokochung District
	Chipvu Luhro Park
	Intaki National Park
Sikkim	Lashar Valley Lachen
	Latui RF East Sikkim
	Mangrhing RF South Sikkim
	Bhudang, West Sikkim

20.2   DOMESTIC CONSUMPTION OF MEDICINAL PLANTS AND ASSOCIATED INDUSTRIES

There are 8,610 licensed herbal units that constitute the Indian herbal industry of contemporary time, which consume an estimated 1.95 lakhs MT of herbal raw drugs with a total turnover of 20,000 crores and on an annual growth rate of about 9–10% (Goraya and Ved, 2017). Annual turnover of herbal industries were reported as 8.80,000 crores in 2005–2006 (Ved and Goraya, 2008). Currently, among the states, Uttar Pradesh has the highest share (26.09%) of licensed herbal units followed by Kerala (10.51%) and Maharashtra (8.18%). Only five states of India viz. Uttar Pradesh, Kerala, Maharashtra, Madhya Pradesh and Andhra Pradesh hold the 59.21% share of the total licensed herbal units of India.

20.2.1   CLASSIFICATION OF HERBAL UNITS

The herbal industries can be broadly classified into three viz. based on registrations under different traditional health system (Ayurved, Unani, Siddha, and Homeopathy), based on annual turnover and based on annual consumption. There are approximately 7,494 numbers of licensed units in India registered under Ayurveda (Goraya and Ved, 2017). Among the different states, the maximum numbers of such units are there in Uttar Pradesh (1,974 units) followed by Kerala (880 units) and Maharashtra (660 units). Madhya Pradesh (625 units), Gujarat (480 units), Andhra Pradesh (473 units) and Tamil Nadu (323 units) are the other important states in the map of licensed herbal units registered for Ayurveda. Under Unani System, there are 421 licensed herbal units and state Uttar Pradesh has the maximum number of such units (237 units). Andhra Pradesh (106 units) and Bihar (27 units) are the other important states having good number of registered herbal units for Unani. Out of the total 367 units for Homeopathy system, West Bengal possess the maximum units (105) followed by Bihar (40 units) and Maharashtra (39 units). Only two states viz. Tamil Nadu (324 units) and Kerala (4 units) constitute the licensed herbal unit registered under Siddha in India.

Herbal units can further be classified into Large (annual turnover above 50 crores), Medium (annual turnover above 5 to 50 crores), Small (annual turnover above 1 to 5 crores) and Very Small (less than 1 crore) (Anon., 2002). There are 20 numbers of large units, 50 numbers of medium units, 2,000 numbers of small and 6,540 numbers of very small units in the country.

Herbal units are classified into Large (annual consumption above 500 MT), Medium (annual consumption above 50 to 500 MT), Small (annual consumption above 10 to 50 MT) and Very Small (annual consumption below 10 MT) based on the annual consumption (Goraya and Ved, 2017). There are about 50 licensed large herbal units, 200 medium units, 2,000 small and 6,360 very small units in terms of annual consumption of raw herbal drugs. Based on the annual consumption, it is evident that 75% of the total volume of raw drugs been consumed by merely <3% of total licensed herbal units falls under Large and Medium category whereas, 97% of the total licensed herbal units constitute the small and very category have access to only 25% of the total volume of raw herbal drugs.

20.2.2   MAJOR INDIAN INDUSTRIES IN HERBAL SECTOR

There are ample numbers of industrial units consuming raw herbal drugs or extracts, mostly being used in patented and proprietary preparations for treating joint pains, gastric problems, diabetes, kidney, and urinary stones, obesity, skin, and hair problems and sexual disorders, etc. (Goraya and Ved, 2017). Around 500 medicinal plant species being used for medicinal extracts by Pharma Industries. Further, information is there of using extracts for cereals, vegetables, pulses, fruits along with herbs in herbal products by these industries. De Silva (1997) reported that the majority of the medicinal plants used in industries for phytopharmaceuticals, galenicals, TM, inter-mediate drugs, TM, herbal teas and pharmaceutical or industrial ancillary products. The major Indian industries into the herbal sector are Dabur India Ltd., Ghaziabad; Zandu Pharmaceutical Works Ltd., Bombay; The Himalaya Drug Co., Banglore; Patanjali Ayurved Limited, Haridwar; Shree Baidyanath Ayurveda Bhavan, Jhansi; Arya Vaidya Sala, Kerala; Emami Ltd., Kolkata; Vicco Laboratories, Mumbai; Charak Pharmaceuticals, Mumbai; Hamdard (Wakf) Laboratories, Delhi; Indian Herb and Research Supply Co., Saha-ranpur; Allen Laboratories, Kolkata; J&J Dechane Laboratories Pvt. Ltd., Hyderabad; Dattatraya Krishan Sandu Bros., Mumbai; Kruzer Herbals, New Delhi; Ansar Drug Laboratories, Surat; Herbals Pvt. Ltd., Patna; Acis Laboratories, Kanpur; Madona Pharmaceutical Research Pvt. Ltd., Kolkata; Shilpachem, Indore; Herbo-med (P) Ltd., Kolkata; ALRASIN Marketing, Mumbai; Bharti Rasanagar, Kolkata; Amil Pharmaceutical, New Delhi, etc. (Nirmal et al., 2013; Sharma et al., 2008 and Rathore and Mathur, 2019).

20.2.3 CONSUMPTION OF RAW HERBAL DRUGS IN INDIAN INDUSTRIES

There are many medicinal plants species being used by the Indian Pharma industries for developing herbal products, out of those 198 species of medic-inal plants, almost occupies 95% of the total demand of raw herbal drugs in the country. The top 10 lists of such plants species has been described below (Table 20.5).

TABLE 20.5 Top 10 Medicinal Plants Species Used for Industries for Raw Herbal Drug

SL. No.	Name of the Medicinal Plant Species	Amount Consumed (Dry Weight, 1,000 MT)
1.	*Aloe vera*	15.68
2.	*Phyllanthus Emblica*	14.18
3.	*Plantago ovata*	13.71
4.	*Mentha arvensis*	6.29
5.	*Terminalia chebula*	6.07
6.	*Withania somnifera*	4.20
7.	*Mentha piperita*	3.86
8.	*Tinospora cordifolia*	3.78
9.	*Gaultheria procumbens*	3.13
10.	*Cinnamomum camphora*	2.95

Sources: Goraya and Ved (2017).

These plants are collected from wild or from the cultivated sources apart from imported species. The main species which dominates the large and medium scale industries are Aloe, Aonla, Mentha, and Gaultheria oil, whereas, species like *Tecomella undulate, Pendulum murex, Chlorophytum tuberosum, Mucuna pruriens* and *Amorphophallus paeonifolius* mostly used in small and very small industries in larger quantities. Further, medicinal plants species like *Gaultheria procumbens, Glycyrrhiza glabra, Bambusa arundinacea, Gaultheria fragrantissima, Commiphora wightii, Atropa belladonna, Salix caprea, Piper Chaba, Anacyclus pyrethrum, Onosoma bracteata, Tamarix gallica, Smilax china, Melaleuca leucadendra* and *Quercus infectoria* are imported to cater the need of the industries. More than 53% of these identified 198 important species being collected from wild and around 40% come from cultivated source along with 7% imported species to cater the major need of the Indian herbal industries. Apart from these licensed industries, there are cottage scale manufacturing units also where raw herbal drugs are being used and sold as formulations or 'churans' at roadside temporary outlets, near parks and village market, and at fairs or even in front of religious places.

20.2.4   RURAL HOUSEHOLD AND FOLK HEALERS CONSUMPTION OF RAW HERBAL DRUGS

NMPB, Government of India; has classified the country into six zones for identifying area wise or zone wise consumption pattern for raw herbal drugs. These zones are Northern, North Eastern, North Western, Central Western and Southern zones. It was reported around 677 raw herbal drugs from 479 medicinal plant species are in use by rural people (Goraya and Ved, 2017). Tulsi, Amla, Neem, Bael, Sajina, Bahera, Asthissamhrta, Karnasphota, Harar, Harshingar, and Ghritakuamri are consumed more than 3,000 MT per annum by rural communities. Most commonly used plant species in almost all the identified zones are *Phyllanthus Emblica, Ocimum tenuiflorum, Azadirachta indica, Terminalia bellirica, Moringa oleifera, Aloe vera and Asparagus racemosus*. Whereas, species like *Terminalia chebula, Catharanthus roseus, Calotropis procera, Justicia adhatoda, Syzygium cumini, Phyllanthus amarus, Mentha arvensis, Ficus religiosa* being used in five zones out of six. Moreover, there are ample numbers of medicinal plant species like *Zanthoxylum armatum, Adhatoda zeylanica, Azadirachta indica, Acacia nilotica, Juglans regia, Salvadora oleides, Prunus cerasoides,*

Murraya koenigi and *Salix tetrasperma*, etc., are being used for dental care, oral hygiene and as chewing sticks. Leaves, roots, tubers, rhizomes are the important plant part mostly used in rural household along with other parts like fruits, bark, stem, flower, seed, gum/latex, exudates or whole plants for managing issues like flu and common cold, cough, body injuries and wounds, skin problems, snake bite, digestive disorders, abdominal problems and post-delivery nourishment, etc. Goraya and Ved (2017) after interacting with 89 randomly selected folk healers under NMPB survey found that annually around 9.82 MT of 340 types of medicinal plants are used by them for their folk medicinal preparation and practice. Top 10 medicinal plant species frequently used by the folk healers are listed in Table 20.6.

TABLE 20.6   Top 10 Medicinal Plants Species Used by the Folk Healers

SL. No.	Medicinal Plant Species	Plant Parts Used
1.	*Withania somnifera*	Root
2.	*Aloe vera*	Leaf
3.	*Terminalia bellirica*	Fruit
4.	*Terminalia chebula*	Fruit and seed
5.	*Piper longrum*	Flower, fruit, and seed
6.	*Phyllanthus Emblica*	Fruit
7.	*Tinospora cordifolia*	Stem, root, and leaf
8.	*Aegle marmelos*	Bark, leaf, and fruit
9.	*Alpinia galangal*	Root and rhizome
10.	*Asparagus racemosus*	Rhizome/root, leaf, and stem

20.3   MARKETING, TRADE, TRADE CHANNEL AND SUPPLY CHAIN OF MEDICINAL PLANTS WITHIN INDIA

Herbal trade in domestic markets are performed through different categories on mandis which had been described by Ved and Goraya (2008) as large mandis, regional mandis, roadside, and intermediate *mandis* based on annual transaction capacity whereas, to organized *Agri-mandis* and traditional *jari-buti mandis* based of transaction types. However, in more recent NMPB survey report, it was stated that current trading of medicinal plants in India is happening through conventional raw herbal mandis, krishi upaj mandis, specialized herbal mandis, trading through corporations/federations or cooperatives and buy-back system of trade (Goraya and Ved, 2017).

20.3.1 CONVENTIONAL RAW HERBAL MANDIS

Major conventional raw herbal mandis are located at Delhi, Tamil Nadu, Madhya Pradesh, Uttarakhand, Chhattisgarh, Uttar Pradesh, Maharashtra, Odisha, Bihar, West Bengal and Jammu and Kashmir:

1. **Khari Baoli, Delhi:** It is Asia's largest spice market and also the largest conventional raw herbal mandi in India with an estimated annual marketing volume of 1.47 Lakhs MT with more than 300 raw herbal entities. The major herbal raw drugs traded here are *Glycyrrhiza glabra, Lawsonia inermis, Ocimum tenuiflorum, Berberis sp., Picrorhiza kurroa, Terminalia chebula, Phyllanthus emblica, Rubia cordifloia, Sapindus mukorossi* and *Plantago ovata.*

2. **Tamil Nadu Herbal Raw Drug Mandi:** Chennai, Dindigul, and Virudhnagar are the main location of conventional raw herbal mandi in Tamil Nadu with a cumulative trade volume of approx. 20,000 MT. The main medicinal plants entities here are *Azadirachta indica, Abutilon indicum, Cissus quadrangularis, Cyperus rotundus, Curculigo orchioides, Eclipta prostrate, Sida acuta, Phyllanthus maderaspatensis,* and *Tephrosia purpurea,* etc.

3. **Conventional Herbal Raw Drug Mandi of Madhya Pradesh:** Shivpuri, Indore, Jabalpur, Betul, Chhindwara, Bhopal, Shahdol, and Balaghat are the prime locations of the herbal raw drug mandi at Madhya Pradesh and deal with major medicinal plant species like *Terminalia bellirica, Terminalia chebula, Madhuca indica, Phyllanthus Emblica, Andrographis paniculata, Chlorophytum tuberosum, Asparagus racemosa, Tinospora cordifolia, Mucuna pruriens, Aegle marmelos,* etc.

4. **Raw Herbal Drug Mandi of Uttarakhand:** Ramnagar and Tanakpur are the two main conventional raw herbal mandi of Uttarakhand having an annual herbal trade volume of 13,000 MT and mainly deal with Chirayta and Tejpatta supply to Khari Baoli market at Delhi.

5. **Raw Herbal Drug Mandi of Chhattisgarh:** Raipur, Kankar, Bilaspur, Katni, Dhamatari, and Jagdalpur are the major such mandis at Chhattisgarh which mainly reroute raw herbs like *Woodfordia fruticosa, Emblica tjeriumcottam, Aegle marmelos, Andrographis paniculata, Cassia tora,* and *Semecarpus Anacardium* to herbal mandis of Delhi, Kanpur or Mumbai.

6. **Raw Herbal Drug Mandi of Odisha:** Cuttak and Koraput are the prime locations of Odisha's raw herbal drug mandi and mainly deal with *Phyllanthus Emblica, Terminalia chebula* and *Terminalia bellirica* and reroute produce to Khari Baoli market of Delhi.

There are conventional raw herbal mandis at Amritsar (Punjab); Saharanpur, Lucknow, Banaras, Kanpur, Kannauj (Uttar Pradesh); Mumbai, Amravati, Nagpur, and Chandrapur (Maharashtra), Patna (Bihar), Kolkata (West Bengal), Ranchi (Jharkhand) and at Jammu and Srinagar (Jammu and Kashmir).

20.3.2 KRISHI UPAJ AND SPECIALIZED HERBAL MANDIS

Main locations of krishi upaj mandis are at Sojat (Rajasthan), Unjha mandi (Gujrat) and Neemuch mandi (Madhya Pradesh). Neem, Isabgol, kalonji, ashwagandha, kalmegh, amla, tulsi, and Mehendi are the mainly traded medicinal plants at Neemuch mandi, whereas, senna, castor, Mehendi, and isabgol are the important traded produce at Sojat mandi and saunf, jeera, fennel, isabgol, fenugreek, mustard, coriander, castor, and dill are in Unjha mandi.

The important specialized herbal mandis are located at Tanakpur Depot (Tanakpur), Bibiwala (Rishikesh) and Amanda (Ramnagar) of Uttarakhand and mainly deal with three medicinal plant species viz. *Parmelia sp., Cinnamomum tamala* and *Chondrus sp.* There are specialized herbal mandis at Himachal Pradesh (Shamshi, Kullu) and Rajasthan (Udaipur).

20.3.3 TRADING THROUGH CORPORATIONS/FEDERATIONS OR COOPERATIVES AND BUY-BACK SYSTEM OF TRADE

In the state of Gujarat, medicinal plant trade is also done by Gujarat State Forest Development Corporation Ltd. and the main herbal entities are different kinds of gums, tendu leaf and mahua flowers. There are Co-operative federations at Madhya Pradesh [Madhya Pradesh State Minor Forest Produce (Trading and Development) Co-operative Federation Ltd.] and Chhattisgarh [Chhattisgarh State Minor Forest Produce (Trading and Development) Co-operative Federation Ltd.] involved in trade of herbal produce like kullu gum, sal seed, dhawada gum, tendu leaf, babool, and khair gum, etc. Andhra Pradesh Girijan Co-operative Corporation Ltd. and Telangana

Girijan Co-operative Corporation Ltd. are trading important herbal entities like myrobalan, soapnut, marking, and cleaning nuts, mohwa, litsea, nux-vomica, karaya gum, decalepsis, and tamarind, etc.

There are only few Indian Pharma giants like Dabur India Ltd., Himalaya Drug Company, Natural Remedies and Sami Labs, etc., are involved in buy-back system of trade for medicinal plants like *Picrorhiza kurroa, Phyllanthus amarus, Aconitum heterophyllum, Ocimum tenuiflorum, Swertia chirayata* and *Uraria picta*, etc.

Goraya and Ved (2017) reported that there are around 65 important medicinal plant species traded in India across line of control to the mandis of Srinagar and Jammu and the mostly traded medicinal plant species are *Valeriana jatamansii, Glycyrrhiza glabra, Peganum hermala, Terminalia chebula, Santalam album, Phoenix dactylifera, Trillium govanianum* and *Quercus infectoria*, etc.

20.3.4 HIGHLY TRADED HERBAL PRODUCE ACROSS THE COUNTRY IN DOMESTIC TRADE

From the NMPB survey data of 2014–2015, it was found that around 700 herbal entities are involved in herbal trade of India, out of which 139 plant species are highly traded (>100 MT) for contributing around 165 raw drug entities. Details of the medicinal plant species are listed below according to the plant parts traded (Table 20.7).

TABLE 20.7   List of Highly Traded Medicinal Plant Species According to the Plant Parts Traded

Plant Parts Traded	Medicinal Plant Species
Seed	*Abrus precatorius, Abutilon indicum, Althaea officinalis, Apium graveolens, Azadirachta indica, Buchanania cochinchinensis, Centratherum anthelminticum, Chamaecrista absus, Cichorium intybus, Datura metel, Holarrhena pubescens, Hyoscyamus niger, Juniperus macropods, Lactuca sativa, Lepidium sativum, Linum usitatissimum, Madhuca longifolia var. latifolia, Moringa oleifera, Mucuna pruriens, Nigella sativa, Ocimum basilicum, Peganum harmala, Plantago ovata, Ricinus communis, Semecarpus anacardium, Senna tora, Solanum americanum, Strychnos nux-vomica, Syzygium jambos, Trigonella foenum-graecum, Withania somnifera, Wrightia tinctoria, Zanthoxylum armatum*
Rhizome	*Alpinia galanga, Zingiber officinale*
Tuber	*Curculigo orchioides*

TABLE 20.7   *(Continued)*

Plant Parts Traded	Medicinal Plant Species
Thallus	*Parmelia spp.*
Leaf	*Abrus precatorius, Abutilon indicum, Aegle marmelos, Aloe barbadensis, Azadirachta indica, Bergenia ciliata, Catharanthus roseus, Cinnamomum tamala, Datura metel, Gymnema sylvestre, Justicia adhatoda, Lawsonia inermis, Moringa oleifera, Murraya koenigii, Ocimum tenuiflorum, Senna alexandrina, Senna auriculata, Chrysopogon zizanioides, Withania somnifera*
Flower	*Althaea officinalis, Butea monosperma, Calendula officinalis, Carthamus tinctorius, Hibiscus rosa-sinensis, Jasminum sambac, Madhuca longifolia var. latifolia, Onosma bracteata, Rosa damascena, Rosa cymosa, Senna auriculata, Woodfordia fruticosa*
Fruit	*Acacia concina, Aegle marmelos, Citrullus colocynthis, Embelia ribes, Phyllanthus emblica, Momordica charantia, Morinda coreia, Papaver somniferum, Piper longum, Sapindus mukorossi, Semecarpus anacardium, Tamarindus indica, Terminalia arjuna, Terminalia bellirica, Terminalia chebula, Trapa natans, Tribulus lanuginosus, Tribulus terrestris, Vitis vinifera, Ziziphus jujuba*
Root	*Acorus calamus, Asparagus racemosus, Berberis spp., Bergenia ciliata, Boerhavia diffusa, Bombax ceiba, Chlorophytum borivilianum, Chrysopogon zizanioides, Curcuma zedoaria, Cyperus rotundus, Cyperus scariosus, Glycyrrhiza glabra, Hedychium spicatum, Helicteres isora, Homalomena aromatica, Inula racemosa, Nardostachys grandiflora, Onosoma hispidum, Operculina turpethum, Picrorhiza kurroa, Piper longum, Plumbago zeylanica, Rauvolfia serpentina, Rheum australe, Ricinus communis, Rubia cordifolia, Saussurea costus, Trillium govanianum, Valeriana jatamansi, Withania somnifera, Zaleya decandra*
Bark	*Azadirachta indica, Betula utilis, Butea monosperma, Cinnamomum cassia, Cinnamomum Verum, Ficus benghalensis, Ficus religiosa, Litsea glutinosa, Moringa oleifera, Symplocos racemosa, Terminalia arjuna*
Stem	*Berberis spp., Cissus quadrangularis, Symplocos racemosa, Tinospora cordifolia*
Wood	*Pterocarpus santalinus, Santalum album*
Aerial part	*Centratherum anthelminticum*
Whole plant	*Achyranthes aspera, Andrographis paniculata, Bacopa monnieri, Boerhavia diffusa, Centella asiatica, Chondrus spp., Eclipta prostrata, Holostemma ada-kodien, Mollugo cerviana, Ocimum tenuiflorum, Phyllanthus amarus, Phyllanthus maderaspatensis, Sida acuta, Sida cordifolia, Solanum americanum, Solanum virginianum, Swertia chirayita, Tephrosia purpurea, Viola odorata*
Gum and exudates	*Boswellia serrata, Commiphora wightii, Sterculia urens, Asphaltum punjabianum*

20.3.5 TRADE CHANNELS AND SUPPLY CHAIN

The traditional trade channel of wild herbs involves primary collectors, local aggregators and large traders (Goraya and Ved, 2017). Depending upon the demand they make collection of raw drugs and do the primary operations like cleaning and drying and send it to the local aggregator or sometimes sell into weekly market of the village. Village level local aggregators are the local shopkeeper who used to collect the material from primary collector or directly purchase it from the weekly village market and store in their warehouse or godown. They also do the primary processing like cleaning, grading, drying, and then packing for transport to the herbal mandis. Large traders are generally located at herbal mandis of the big cities in the state, where they received the graded, dried, and properly packed material that they use for domestic or foreign trade. Rathore and Mathur (2019) after their exclusive study on the supply chain of the two mostly traded medicinal plants viz. Isabgol and *Aloe vera* has reported that for cultivated medicinal plant species, there are broadly three chains in working, i.e., from farmer or producer to local trader to processing unit; farmer/ producer to local trader to wholesaler to processing unit and farmer/producer to wholesaler to consumer. From the previous study on supply chain by Belt et al. (2003); and Van De Kop et al. (2006) it can be summarized that there are five layers in existing supply chain or trade channel of medicinal plant. These are collector, trader/intermediate, processors, retailers, and consumers. There are contractors, cooperative, intermediate companies, or informal traders as trader/ intermediates, whereas pharmaceutical companies, ayurvedic companies, small scale processers, and local or traditional healers as processors. Local and traditional healers, national retail shops and pharmacies largely act as retailers. Besides, consumers at the national level or international market is being the base of consumers. Collectors are directly linked with either traders/ intermediates or with informal traders for handing the material or to feed the local level folk healers for selling the produce. From traders or intermediates, it use to reach pharmaceutical /ayurvedic companies, whereas, informal traders dispense to the intermediate trading companies or to the small-scale processors. The finished products of the processors reach consumers through national retail shops or pharmacies or directly to the consumer, for example, through folk healers. Small scale processing units are further linked to the international market for foreign trading, sometimes. In general, there is 5–8% wastage involved in this traditional supply chain. Therefore, processing within the supply chain is very crucial to reduce the wastage and to increase the value of the produce through the chain and even in case of the finished product and thus required to strengthen the supply chain into value chain (Alam and Belt, 2009; Chhabra, 2018; Rathore and Mathur, 2019).

20.4 EXPORT AND IMPORT OF MEDICINAL PLANTS IN INDIA

India has exported 330.18 million worth of crude herbs and 456.12 million of processed and value-added herbal products during 2017–2018 (Anon., 2019). Export largely depends on the production level of the medicinal plants under cultivation or status of conservation of the wild medicinal plant resources along with availability of the raw herbs to the herbal industries within the country. In the year 2014–2015 India has exported raw botanical drug of about 134.44000 MT worth around 321.13 million and imported 64.54000 MT worth 107.57 million (Goraya and Ved, 2017). It was found that additionally India had exported 4.50000 MT of Gum worth 11.75 million, botanical extracts of 11.64000 MT worth 151.73 million, and Ayurved, Siddha, Unani, and Homeopathy medicaments of 15.74000 MT worth 70.84 million in 2014–2015. Major exported raw herbal produce are psyllium seeds and husk, senna leaves and pods, long pepper, *cassia tora* seeds, pyrethrum, galangal rhizome and roots, sandalwood chips and dust, *Vinca*, tukmaria, zedovary roots, henna leaves and powder, etc., whereas, gymnema, camboge, belladonna, neem, nux-vomica, and agar are the major medicinal extracts which are exported besides, important gums like karaya gum, gum Arabic, guggal, and Asian gum, etc. (Table 20.8). India's major export destination for the herbal raw drugs are USA, Vietnam, China, Pakistan, Germany, Taiwan, Japan, Bangladesh, United Kingdom, France, UAE, Mexico, Korea Republic, Spain, Belgium, Italy, Malaysia, Australia, and Sri Lanka, etc.

TABLE 20.8 Top 15 Herbal Produce (in Quantity) Exported from India

SL. No.	Exported Herbal Produce	Quantity (1,000 MT)	Value (1,000 Lakhs)
1.	Psyllium husk	32.33	92.41
2.	*Cassia tora* seed	28.19	12.34
3.	Senna leaves and pods	13.24	8.82
4.	Camboge extracts	5.05	12.96
5.	Basil, hyasop, rosemary sage, savory	1.29	2.44

TABLE 20.8   *(Continued)*

SL. No.	Exported Herbal Produce	Quantity (1,000 MT)	Value (1,000 Lakhs)
6.	Pepper long	1.21	1.27
7.	Zedovary roots	1.12	1.38
8.	Psyllium seed	1.00	1.17
9.	Asafetida	0.89	4.10
10.	Galangal rhizomes	0.71	0.79
11.	*Vinca rosea*	0.57	0.57
12.	Tukmaria	0.43	0.81
13.	Asian gum	0.41	1.78
14.	Gum Arabic	0.40	1.10
15.	Sweet flag rhizome	0.23	0.11

Source: Goraya and Ved (2017).

Psyllium husk, Tribulus fruit, neem leaf, etc., are high valued exported produce having high unit price also (Table 20.9).

TABLE 20.9   Indian Medicinal Produce with Unit Export Price

SL. No.	Medicinal Plant Produce	Unit Export Price (US$ per Kg)
1.	Aniseed	1.06–1.80
2.	Cassia bark	1.19
3.	Cinnamon bark	1.25
4.	Coriander fruit	0.62
5.	Fennel fruit	1.06
6.	Fenugreek seed	0.36
7.	Garlic bulb	0.41
8.	Ginger rhizome	1.2
9.	Gymnema leaf	0.85
10.	Neem leaf	3.9
11.	Psyllium husk	3.7–4.1
12.	Senna leaf	0.85
13.	Senna pods	0.68
14.	Tribulus fruit	5.90
15.	Turmeric rhizome	1.05–1.20

Source: FAO (2004).

India use to import raw herbal drugs from countries like Nigeria, Sudan, Nepal, Pakistan, Congo, Vietnam, Indonesia, Afghanistan, Sri Lanka, Chad, Ghana, China, Cameroon, Tanzania, Iran, Netherland, Australia, and Morocco, etc. Gum Arabic, *Garcinia* fruit, pepper long, liquorice root, ginseng root-extract and powder, sandalwood, basil, rosemary, savory, cubeb powder, chirayta, pyrethrum, and agarwood, etc., are the major produce that India use to import.

20.5   GLOBAL HERBAL MARKET AND INDIAN STAKE

India is considered to be one of the main raw herbal drug producers of South Asia. Moreover, it was projected that Indian Pharmaceutical industries will grow to 150 billion US dollars compared with the current 15–20 billion US dollars (Ramawat and Goyal, 2008). In India, around 3,000 medicinal plant species are in use, next to China (4,941 plant species) and followed by USA (2,564 plant species) (Table 20.10).

TABLE 20.10   Top 10 Global Consumers of Medicinal Plant Species

SL. No.	Name of the Country	Number of Medicinal Plant Species in Use
1.	China	4,941
2.	India	3,000
3.	United States of America	2,564
4.	Thailand	1,800
5.	Malaysia	1,200
6.	Indonesia	1,000
7.	Philippines	850
8.	Nepal	700
9.	Sri Lanka	550
10.	Pakistan	300

Source: Ramawat and Goyal (2008).

It was reported that main global market for medicinal plants are at Europe, North America and Asia, where, Europe has sole share of about 50% and China, India, and Germany leads as individual countries (CUTS, 2004). Wakdikar (2004) estimated the global market of herbal supplement of about 15 billion US dollar and reported Europe, North America and Asia have contribution of about 7 billion, 3 billion and 2.7 billion US dollar in it. From

FAO published medicinal plants trade report it was found that Hongkong, USA, Japan, Germany, Korea Republic, France, China, Malaysia, Italy, Pakistan, Spain, United Kingdom and Singapore were the major importing countries whereas, China, India, Germany, USA, Chile, Egypt, Bulgaria, Singapore, Morocco, Mexico, Bulgaria, Pakistan, and Albania were the major exporters (FAO, 2004; Ramawat and Gopal, 2008). Five most important countries in global import and export of medicinal plant produce are listed in Table 20.11.

TABLE 20.11   Top Five Importers and Exporters of Medicinal Plant Produce in the Globe

SL. No.	Importing Country	Import Volume (Tons)	Import Value (US$ 1000)
1.	Hong Kong	73,650	314,000
2.	Japan	56,750	146,650
3.	USA	56,000	133,350
4.	Germany	45,850	113,900
5.	Republic of Korea	31,400	52,550
SL. No.	**Exporting Country**	**Export Volume (Tons)**	**Export Value (US$ 1000)**
1.	China	139,750	298,650
2.	India	36,750	57,400
3.	Germany	15,050	72,400
4.	USA	11,950	114,450
5.	Chile	11,850	29,100

Source: Ramawat and Goyal (2008).

20.6   CONCLUSION

India is bestowed with such a large agro-climatic variation suitable for cultivation of so many plant species which are potent herbal drug value. Top of that wild areas of Himalayas, Nilgiris along with other tropical or subtropical deciduous and evergreen forests are storehouse of variety of medicinal plant species. But indiscriminate consumption of wild resources will certain made more and more species to enter into red list. Community harvesting, *in situ* conservation and strengthening the other biodiversity conservation programs of national or by local government and agencies or NGO's and Cooperative(s) are crucial. Area under location specific medicinal crop production has to be increased to meet the consistent increasing demand both of domestic and foreign trade. Identification and standardization of active principles and bio-prospection of indigenous medicinal plants are of immense importance. Mass production of commercially cultivable medicinal species through tissue culture should be emphasized to cater the need of quality planting material in area expansion programs and also *in situ* cultivation of wild medicinal plants through indigenous farmers' or self-help group is worth need of time. We should understand that with the present volume of production and export, India holds only around 2% global market shares (Kumar and Janagram, 2011; Aneesh et al., 2009) which fall below the potentiality. Improper assessment of crude drug for carcinogen or mutagenic contamination or of arsenic/lead and mercury traces, mycotoxin hazard of stored drug samples and even adulteration of raw herbal drugs has to be stringently controlled and overcome (Dubey et al., 2004). Strategic and practical intervention is crucially needed for large scale organic production, processing, product standardization and R&D, regulatory market framework, etc. To strengthen our foreign exchange foot print, a consistent supply of botanically well identified, contaminants free, unadulterated quality raw herbal drugs meeting regulatory requirements are essentially needed.

KEYWORDS

- Ayurveda
- consumption
- export
- Himalaya
- India
- market
- medicinal plants
- supply chain

REFERENCES

Alam, G., & Belt, J., (2009). *Developing a Medicinal Plant Value Chain: Lessons from an Initiative to Cultivate kutki Picrorhiza Kurrooa) in Northern India.* KIT Working Papers Series C5. Amsterdam: KIT.

Aneesh, T. P., Hisham, M., Sonal, S. M., Manjushree, M., & Deepa, T. V., (2009). International market scenario of traditional Indian herbal drugs – India declining. *International Journal of Green Pharmacy.* doi: 10.4103/0973-8258.56271.

Anonymous, (2002). *National Policy on ISM & H.* Government of India.

Anonymous, (2019). *Export of Herbs and Herbal Products.* Press Information Bureau, Ministry of Commerce & Industry, Government of India.

Belt, J., Lengkeek, A., & Van, D. Z. J., (2003). *Cultivating a Healthy Enterprise: Developing a Sustainable Medicinal Plant Chain in Uttaranchal-India.* KIT Publishers, Amsterdam. KIT Bulletin no. 350.

Bodekar, G., (2015). *Herbs for Wellness: Key Drivers in the New US$ 3.4 Trillion Global Wellness Industry.* NWFP Update. Issue 6: Health & Well-being, FAO.

CERPA Demand Study for Selected Medicinal Plants, (2002). *A Report Prepared for the Ministry of Health and Family Welfare, Government of India, Department of Indian Systems of Medicine and Homoeopathy and World Health Organization* (Vol. I).

Chauhan, N. S., (1999). *Medicinal and Aromatic Plants of Himachal Pradesh.* Indus Publishing Company, New Delhi.

Chhabra, T., (2018). Value chain analysis for medicinal plant based products in India: Case study of Uttarakhand. *An archive of Organic and Inorganic Chemical Sciences, 4*(1), 449–457.

Chowti, S. P., Rudrapur, S., & Naik, B. K., (2018). Production scenario of medicinal and aromatic crops in India. *Journal of Pharmacognosy and Phytochemistry, SP3,* 274–277.

CUTS Database on medicinal plants, (2004). CUTS Center for International Trade, Economics & Environment, Consumer Unity & Trust Society CUTS, Calcutta, India.

De Silva, T., (1997). Industrial utilization of medicinal plants in developing countries. In: *FAO, 1997. Medicinal Plants for Forest Conservation and Healthcare* (p. 34). Non-Wood Forest Products 11, Food and Agriculture Organization of the United Nations, Rome.

Dubey, N. K., (2004). Global promotion of herbal medicine: India's opportunity. *Current Sci., 8,* 61, 37–41.

FAO, (2004). *Trade-in Medicinal Plants.* Raw Materials, Tropical and Horticultural Products Service Commodities and Trade Division, Economic and Social Department, Food and Agriculture Organization of the United Nations, Rome.

Goraya, G. S., & Ved, D. K., (2017). *Medicinal Plants in India: An Assessment of their Demand and Supply.* National Medicinal Plants Board, Ministry of AYUSH, Government of India, New Delhi and Indian Council of Forestry Research & Education, Dehradun.

Holley, J., & Cherla, K., (1998). *The Medicinal Plants Sector in India: A Review.* Medicinal & Aromatic Plants Program in Asia, IDRC-SARO, New Delhi.

Keshari, P., & Pradeep, (2018). A review of conservation and sustainable use of medicinal plant with special reference of *Tecomella undulata* (Sm.) Seem. *Journal of Pharmacognosy and Phytochemistry, SP3,* 09–13.

Kumar, M. R., & Janagram, D., (2011). Export and import pattern of medicinal plants in India. *Indian Journal of Science and Technology, 4*(3), 245–248.

Nagaraju, K., Vishwanath, M., & Aruna, K., (2018). Seed quality enhancement techniques in medicinal and aromatic crops. *Journal of Pharmacognosy and Phytochemistry, SP3,* 104–109.

Nirmal, S. A., Pal, S. C., Otimenyin, S. O., Aye, T., Elachouri, M., Kundu, S. K., Thandavarayan, R. A., & Mandal, S. C., (2013). Contribution of herbal products in global market. *The Pharma Rev.,* 95–104.

Pushpangadan, P., (1995). *Ethnobiology in India: A Status Report.* All India Coordinated Research project on Ethnobiology. Ministry of Environment & Forests, Government of India, New Delhi.

Ramawat, K. G., & Goyal, S., (2008). The Indian herbal drug scenario in global perspectives. In: Ramawat, K. G., & Merillon, J. M., (eds.), *Bioactive Molecules and Medicinal Plants* (pp. 325–347.). Springers, Netherlands.

Rathore, R., & Mathur, A., (2019). Scope of cultivation and value chain perspectives of medicinal herbs in India: A case study on aloe Vera and Isabgol. *Journal of Pharmacognosy and Phytochemistry, 8*(2), 243–246.

Sharma, A., Shanker, C., Tyagi, L. K., Singh, M., & Rao, C. V., (2008). Herbal Medicine for Market Potential in India: An Overview. *Academic Journal of Plant Science, 1*(2), 26–36.

Tyler, V. E., (1994). *Herbs of Choice: The Therapeutic Use of Phytomedicals, Pharmaceutical, Products.* Binghampton, New York.

Van De Kop, P., Alam, G., & Piter, B. D. S., (2006). Developing a sustainable medicinal -plant chain in India, linking people, markets and value. In: Ruben, R., Slingerland, M., & Nijhoff, H., (eds.), *Agro-food Chains and Netwroks for Development* (pp. 191–202). Springer, Netherlands.

Ved, D. K., & Goraya, G. S., (2008). *Demand and Supply of Medicinal Plants in India.* Bishen Singh Mahendra Pal Singh, Dehradun & FRLHT, Bangalore.

Wakdikar, S., (2004). Global health care challenge: Indian experiences and new prescriptions. *Electronic Journal of Biotechnology, 7*(3), 214–220.

CHAPTER 21

POTENTIAL OF SPICES AS MEDICINES AND IMMUNITY BOOSTERS

MINOO DIVAKARAN,[1] K. NIRMAL BABU,[2] and K. V. PETER[3]

[1]*Associate Professor, Providence Women's College, Calicut – 673009, Kerala, India, E-mail: minoodivakaran@gmail.com*

[2]*Director, ICAR Indian Institute of Spices Research, Calicut – 673012, Kerala, India*

[3]*Former Vice-Chancellor, Kerala Agricultural University and Former Director, ICAR Indian Institute of Spices Research, Calicut; Mullakkara, P O Mannuthy – 680651, Thrissur, Kerala, India*

ABSTRACT

'Let food be thy medicine and medicine be thy food,' as said by Hippocrates. In times of global pandemics and search for safer medicines, remembering the potential of spices and inclusion in daily cuisine can be a savior, to protect humanity from myriad pathogens and viruses, by their immunoprotective properties, and this seems to be need of the hour. Demand for golden milk (inclusion of turmeric in milk) and Indian rasam (spices' concoction) grows as people from diverse expertise, be it scientists, medical practitioners, or traditional healers, all advocate use of spices in enhancing immunity while lowering the risks of viral attacks. The most commonly used herbs and spices that are medicinal and have proven to act against diseases are Black pepper-the king of spices, cardamom-known as the queen of spices, black cumin (kala jeera), caraway, chili, cinnamon, cloves, coriander, dill, fenugreek, nigella, ginger, sage, turmeric, and vanilla-prince of spices, etc. One of the most commonly used spices in Ayurveda, Unani, and Siddha, systems of medicine, is Black pepper. Cardamom has antimicrobial properties. Cumin seeds aid digestion and are incorporated to flavor by the bakers'

industry. Caraway is stomachic, carminative, and antihelminitic. Cloves and Chilies are used in relieving pain, flatulence and against rheumatic ailments. Cinnamon is a neuro-stimulant, helping in the contraction of cells and tissues. Coriander, dill, fenugreek, and sage are used in Indian cooking systems to promote appetite and assist digestion. Ginger is known to be a diuretic, also lowers cholesterol levels, while turmeric is used against microbial infections. Vanilla, popular for its flavor, also exhibits antiseptic activity against various pathogens.

21.1   INTRODUCTION

Since times immemorial, priests used the 'technique' of Phytotherapy to keep the sick alive and if possible, cure them, but from the times of Hippocrates onwards, the herbalist-physicians, practiced 'Medicine,' as the art of knowing how to administer precise herbal extracts, chosen, and proportioned according to the illnesses diagnosed. The oldest evidence of plant cure comes from the Egyptians, Chinese, Tibetans, and Indians. The Chinese text from 3000 BC (Pen Tsao), compiles many natural cure methods for diseases including cancer.

Chronic conditions, and diseases like Alzheimer's, arthritis, cancer, cardiovascular (CVD), diabetes and Parkinson's, remain the primary death and disability causes, worldwide. The major factors associated with these conditions are unhealthy practices in daily life, coupled with reduced physical activities, lack of balanced diet, stress, and anxiety, unwanted addictions, atmospheric radiations and prone to pathogenic infections. Such agents induce inflammation and disrupt their pathways, leading to chronic ailments (Prasad et al., 2012). Since ancient times, phytochemicals, both in their natural and in synthetic forms, are being used for the treatment of chronic conditions. Spices have been used for different culinary purposes, and the plant parts used are also diverse, like buds, seeds, bark, stem, roots, leaves, fruits (berry or pods), floral stigma, etc., in addition to rendering flavor, fortify the food with tremendous health advantages (Nilius and Appendino 2013). Congregate evidences suggest that a diet rich in plant-based items, including spices, has the ability to keep most of the chronic diseases at bay. Humans have been using spices since 5000 B.C., and extensive studies, on their biological activities, made by Sung et al. (2012), showed that nutraceuticals derived from spices like clove, coriander, garlic (Judith et al., 1990), ginger, onion, pepper, and turmeric are preventive and curative in action to various chronic diseases primarily by addressing the inflammatory pathways.

Inflammation is a body's natural response against harmful pathogens and stimuli which occur in two stages, namely, acute, and chronic. Modifying inflammatory pathways has a high probability in protecting against deadly diseases. Most of the drugs developed by pharmaceutical companies till today for these chronic diseases are costly and also known to produce adverse side effects. Hence the urgency to develop an efficient, safer and affordable, remedy for the management of these diseases (Aggarwal et al., 2009), is a priority. In countries like India, where spices are included daily in cooking, studies on disease incidence indicate, low occurrence of cancer (94/100,000) than in countries, where spices are not regularly consumed (318/100,000), clearly indicative of the likelihood of spices as a medicine and especially in cancer prevention.

The efficiency of active principles in spices help to prevent various diseases like arthritis, asthma, cancer, cardiovascular diseases (CVD), diabetes, etc., was proven by preclinical and clinical studies (Opara and Chohan, 2014). Black pepper, cardamom, cinnamon, clove, cumin, fenugreek, fennel, garlic, ginger, onion, rosemary, and turmeric, possessing desirable biological activities are some of the most commonly used spices for culinary purposes. History of Indian Spices is more than 7,000 years old, and it was the lure for these spices that brought many seafarers to the shores of India. History of world trade in the 1400s, was destined by spice missions that were led with the support of European rulers.

These navigations were later to become the world's first steps in globalization, in the search of more flavorful food. Due to different climatic conditions across the country, India grows 53 of the 109 spices as per the list of the International Organization for Standardization (ISO). Indian spices have thus shaped the history as well as played an important role in strengthening the economic conditions since the ancient ages. Thus, the pursuit of spices triggered the global explorations which formed the world history and also helped to create a global economy.

Herbs and spices have occupied a pivotal role throughout history. Most of the spices were noted for their medicinal properties, as much as culinary uses. Present day science has revealed that most of them do deliver remarkable health benefits. "Spices assure supply of antioxidants," says Diane Vizthum, research nutritionist for the Johns Hopkins University School of Medicine. The triangular relationship of a host, a pathogen and a conducive environment, for creating a pathos condition, is irrevocable, hence usage of spices in one's daily life, can modify the environment component to a 'non-conducive' one. Many spices which have indicated proven results in healing many diseases are compiled below;

21.2   MEDICINAL VALUES OF SELECTED HERBS AND SPICES

21.2.1   ANETHUM GRAVEOLENS (DILL)

Dill, botanically belongs to the genus *Anethum* is derived from Greek word aneeson or aneeton, indicating its strong odor. Dill is commonly used in Ayurvedic medicine to relieve abdominal pain and discomfort, and aiding for digestion. It also cures ulcers, eye diseases and uterine pains. A paste of linseed, castor seeds and dill, in milk for external applications in rheumatic disorders, was prescribed by Charaka. *Kashyapa samhitaa*, one of the earliest treatises on Indian systems of medicine, endorsed stimulant, revitalizing, and brainpower promoting properties to the herb (*A. graveolens*). Used in Unani medicine for gripes, digestive problems (Jana and Shekhawat, 2010), it is also effective against reducing fevers.

21.2.2   CAPSICUM FRUTESCENS, C. ANNUM (CAYENNE PEPPER, PAPRIKA)

Capsaicinoids (mainly capsaicin) are active ingredients used in pharmaceutical industry to prepare certain drugs (sprays), which are applied externally to stop the pain of arthritis (rheumatoid arthritis, osteoarthritis), acyl derivatives of capsanthin and acyl derivatives of cansorubin inhibit LDL oxidation *in vitro* (Kumar et al., 2006). Maoka et al., 2001, reported that capsanthin and capsorubin can improve the cytotoxic action of chemotherapy used in treating cancer and has the potential of carotenoids as possible resistance modifiers. The concept of 'bio-chemoprevention' by incorporation of lutein, zeaxanthin, capsanthin, crocetin, and phytoene have been proven to be potent anticarcinogenic in activity than β-carotene (Nishino et al., 2002). It is a source of capsasin, capsorubin, and vitamins C, A, and E and is used both as a flavorant and food colorant.

Capsaicin based creams and lotions have been prescribed for application to reduce post-operative pain of mastectomy patients, and the insect-repellent property of capsaicinoids has also been proved. Stringed mature fruits are stringed when mature, are hung at the entrance to homes, traditionally, in New Mexico, as a symbol of hospitality (Bosland, 1992).

21.2.3   CARUM CARVI (CARAWAY)

Caraway, a plant similar in appearance to members of the carrot family, is recommended as a remedy for digestive problems like flatulence bloating, stomach aches, constipation, lack of appetite and nausea. In small children, caraway is used to treat the accumulation of gases in the alimentary canal and accompanying pains. Fruits of caraway ingested orally produce an effect on the digestive tract, liver, and kidneys. They have smooth muscle relaxing properties, whereby bile ducts and the sphincter normalize the flow of bile and pancreatic secretions to the duodenum and thus enhance gastric juices' secretion, resulting in better appetite. Enhanced production of milk by use of caraway fruits in women and bovines was observed, which also had an indirect beneficial effect on the baby's digestive system, because of the muscle-relaxing properties. The component promoting milk secretion in caraway seed has not been known, however limonene and carvone, which is most abundantly found in caraway, contribute to the antigripping qualities and used in alternative medicine (Malhotra, 2006).

21.2.4   CINNAMOMUM VERUM (CINNAMON)

Cinnamon of commerce is obtained from the dried inner bark of the trees of the *Cinnamomum verum*, of family Lauraceae, has played an important role in human cuisine. R&D efforts were initiated in Sri Lanka and India, and a comprehensive volume is compiled providing on all aspects of cinnamon by Ravindran et al. (2003).

Effect of cinnamon, in Type 2 diabetes, to improve glucose, triglyceride, total cholesterol, HDL cholesterol, and LDL cholesterol levels in the blood, as reported by Anderson (2003). In the study, comprising of a population segregated into six groups, of men and women (30 each in number), aged 52.2 ± 6.32 years. The first 3 groups were given cinnamon at 1, 3, or 6 g, respectively, and the last 3 groups were administered placebo capsules dosage similar to that of cinnamon consumed. Cinnamon was administered for 40 days continuously followed by a break of 20-days period, and it was observed that at the end of the two months, the three levels of cinnamon led to lowering of average values of serum glucose during fasting (18–29%), triglyceride (23–30%), LDL cholesterol (7–27%), and total cholesterol (from 12–26%) levels; whereas remarkable differences were not noted in the groups fed with placebo. However, no significant differences were observed in HDL cholesterol. Thus, these observations revealed significant protection by, inclusion of cinnamon in the diet of people with type 2 diabetes which could modify the risk factors of diabetes and CVD substantially (Crawford 2009). The cinnamon bark is anti-asthmatic, enhances renal functions, stops bleeding, astringent, stomachic, and germicide. Producers of pain relievers have been including cinnamon in their commercial preparations, which is also antimicrobial and an anti-oxidant (Peter and Nirmal Babu, 2012).

21.2.5   CORIANDRUM SATIVUM (CORIANDER)

Coriander, is a plant, with both leaves and seeds having an aroma, and was one of the earliest spices to be used as a flavoring agent. The tender whole plant is ground into chutneys, and the leaves are used for garnishing various dishes like curries, sauces, and soups. Dry seeds are powdered and stored for preparations of curry powder, pickles, spices and seasoning and also to cure fevers, vomiting, and stomach disorders (Sharma and Sharma 2006). Fruits are stimulants and are known to counteract hepatological disorders. The entire plant is administered against colic, giddiness, renal stones, indigestion, and sore throat (Peter and Nirmal Babu, 2012).

21.2.6   CROCUS SATIVUS (SAFFRON)

Saffron, the world's most expensive spice, is valued both for its traditional value, as a food additive, and therapeutic properties. Used as an anti-depressant in Persian traditional medicine (TM), a comparative study has been made on the effect of combining hydro-alcoholic extract of *Crocus sativus* (stigma) with fluoxetine, for the management of depression. A population, which was administered saffron 30 mg/day two times a day and another which was given fluoxetine capsules alone, in the dosage of 20 mg/day (twice) for 6-weeks, showed at the end of the study period, that saffron was similar to fluoxetine in the treatment of depression, without any significant differences in terms of observed side effects (Noorbala et al., 2005). When saffron (50 mg) dissolved in 100 ml of milk was fed, to 20 people, a major decrease in lipoprotein oxidation susceptibility (LOS), was observed in 10 of them, who suffered from Coronary Artery Disease (CAD). This indicated the potential of Saffron as an antioxidant (Verma and Bordia, 1998). Similar studies have indicated its action as a tonic, stomachic, and protectant against carcinogenesis (Peter and Shylaja, 2012).

21.2.7   CURCUMA LONGA (TURMERIC)

Turmeric (has been the most commonly used spice and medicine around the world. Curcumin, the active principle of turmeric (2–5%), was first isolated by Vogel and Pelletier (1818), renders the golden color to turmeric. The earliest reference about turmeric can be seen in Atharva Veda (Ca. 6000 yr B.P.), in which *C. longa* is quoted as to lure away jaundice and was prescribed in leprosy treatment. Turmeric was listed as a plant used in coloring, in an Assyrian herbal epic, dating about Ca 2600 yr B.P. Marco Polo (1280) has mentioned the presence of turmeric in the Fokien region, China. Sharma (1976) studied the anti-oxidative properties of curcumin and its derivatives and demonstrated how it provides a protection for hemoglobin from oxidation (Ravindran et al., 2007). As an ingredient of curry powders, improves flavor and functions as an antiseptic, antipoison factor, while functioning as an anti-oxidant, anti-carcinogenic, and anti-AIDS and anti-inflammatory properties.

21.2.8   ELETTARIA CARDAMOMUM (CARDAMOM)

Cardamom of commerce is the dried seed capsule of a group of plants belonging to the family Zingiberaceae. Small cardamom (*Elettaria cardamomum* Maton), native to India, is known as the 'Queen of spices' is cultivated commonly in the southern states of Kerala, Karnataka, and Tamil Nadu. Kazemi et al. (2017) have investigated supplementation effects of cardamom in obese pre-diabetic women (population size of 80), with high lipid levels in blood, with regards to their inflammation and oxidative stress, thus reducing complications associated with it. Cardamom is added as an enhancer of immune responses, in the pharmaceutical industry, to drugs which are carminative, stomachic. It is a common home remedy for indigestion, morning sickness, oral odor, bronchial infections, skin diseases, inflammations, itching, and poisons.

21.2.9   NIGELLA SATIVA (BLACK CUMIN)

The seeds of *Nigella* have melanthin, a chemical similar to helleborin and, have diuretic, anthelmintic, and emmenagogue properties, like saponin, therefore used as a corrective of laxatives. Possessing actions as a galactagogue, they are given to lactating mothers, along with other medicines. Seeds mixed with powdered camphor, are used to protect wardrobes from insect damage all over India. The seeds possess antibilious property administered internally to arrest vomiting. Relief from cold and inflammation of mucous membranes in the airways of the nose are obtained by inhaling fried seeds tied in a muslin bag. A concoction with Nigella seeds, cumin seeds, black pepper, raisins, tamarind pulp, pomegranate juice and sonchal salt with molasses syrup and honey is used to overcome loss of appetite and distaste for food. Application of seed powder in vinegar for skin infestations and baldness has been indicated by Weiss (2002). However, usage of Nigella seeds is to be done with caution, as its volatile oil yields melanthin, nigelline, damascene, and tannin, of which melanthin is toxic, when consumed in large dosages and nigelline is paralytic. The traditional use of Nigella seeds in curing dyslipidemia, hyperglycemia, and related abnormities, indicated a relative toxicity of this plant (Malhotra 2006). Nigella is also used in preservation as its alcoholic extract shows antibacterial activity.

21.2.10   SYZYGIUM AROMATICUM (CLOVES)

Extracts from clove (both ethanolic extract and essential oils (EOs)) are able to reduce the multiplication of human cancer cells and led to cell death in cancer cells of the colon, and human breast cancer cells. Hence cloves might play a positive role in the future of cancer treatment by lowering the cancerous cells' multiplication rate. Cloves are aromatic, stimulant, and used in gastric irritation and dyspepsia. When administered in powdered form they help alleviate feelings of nausea and vomiting, and oil serves as a local analgesic to correct flatulence and hypersensitive dentine and carious cavities, as it has antiseptic and pain-relieving qualities (Peter and Nirmal Babu, 2012).

21.2.11   PIPER NIGRUM (BLACK PEPPER)

Piper species is medicinal owing to the presence of piperine. Black pepper is used as a spice and adjuvant in various traditional systems of medicine and piperine is used as a bioavailability-enhancer. The effect of piperine was studied by Pattanaik et al. (2009), in epilepsy patients who were sustained on carbamazepine monotherapy, and it was revealed that when piperine was administered along with carbamazepine, piperine made a remarkable increase in the bioavailability of carbamazepine, either by reducing the elimination or by enhancing its absorption.

Pattanaik et al. (2006) had also showed how piperine, the active principle in P. *longum*, *P. nigrum* and *Zingiber officinalis*, increased the oral bioavailability of phenytoin in patients with uncontrolled epilepsy. Black pepper is used as an aromatic stimulant in cholera, vertigo, and coma and as a stomachic in dyspepsia and flatulence, and also as protection against filariasis.

21.2.12 SALVIA OFFICINALIS (SAGE)

Sage gets its name from the Latin word *Salvere,* which means "to save." It had a strong reputation for its healing properties, and was even used to prevent the plague. Studies have indicated that sage may be able to improve brain power and memory, beneficial for people with Alzheimer's disease (AD), which is accompanied by an acetylcholine (a molecular messenger) drop, in the brain. Sage blocks the disintegration of acetylcholine and can enhance memory in healthy people, both young and old (Perry et al., 2003). Sage is administered in cases of excessive sweating, fever, and nervous disorders too.

21.2.13 ZINGIBER OFFICINALE (GINGER)

Ginger is the underground rhizome of herbaceous perennial *Zingiber officinale* Rosc. Ginger, finds use in fresh and dry forms, and is the third most important spice prized for its flavor and medicinal properties. It is useful as a spice and condiment, to alleviate liver complaints, state of anemia, arthritic pain, piles, and jaundice in both Indian and Chinese medicine. The genus *Zingiber* consisting of about 150 species, is widely distributed in tropical and subtropical Asia. Traditional usage reports effectiveness in gastrointestinal complaints and also as a viable adjuvant against nausea and vomiting in the cancer treatment, especially chemotherapy. Marx et al. (2017) revealed that gingerol and shojail, the bioactive compounds in ginger, interfere with the biochemical pathways linked to chemotherapy induced nausea and vomiting (CINV) pathways, by modulation of cellular redox signaling process.

These studies were followed by different workers incorporating crude ginger powder for preventing CINV, and it was found that those patients who were on gingerol supplementation, were less tired, and had an improved appetite and quality of life when compared to other cancer patients who were on chemotherapy treatments (Konmun et al., 2017).

The study that was inclusive of healthy individuals, coronary artery disease (CAD) affected, and non-insulin-dependent diabetic patients, with/ without CAD, indicated that in CAD patients, powdered ginger when given in a dose of 4 g/day for 90 day-period, did not result in platelet aggregation, whereas a dose of 10 g /day ginger powder, showed a decreased platelet aggregation, however, no effect on blood profile *viz.*, lipids, and sugar, was observed. Ginger Tea brewing is common in households for curing and providing relief from coughs and colds. Ginger Compresses are known to relieve sinus congestions of the nasal and respiratory pathways, urological problems, menstrual cramps, etc.

21.2.14   *TRIGONELLA FOENUM-GRAECUM (FENUGREEK)*

Fenugreek known for reducing cholesterol levels, when 2.5 g was given twice daily for 3 months to healthy individuals, could not modify the blood profile, but, when administered in the same daily dose for the same period to CAD patients with NIDDM, led to reduced values in lipids profiles, with no effect on the HDL-c. However, the same dose, when administered to NIDDM (non-CAD) patients (mild cases), did lead to a reduction in blood sugar levels. Bordia et al. (1997) concluded that administration of fenugreek did not affect platelet aggregation, fibrinolytic activity and fibrinogen. Fenugreek seeds are widely used against arthritis and galactogog. Fenugreek extract (aqueous) revealed antibiotic activity, and also used to cure chronic bronchitis, hepato-and splenomegaly, diabetes (Peter and Nirmal Babu, 2012).

21.2.15   *VANILLA PLANIFOLIA (VANILLA OF COMMERCE)*

Vanilla, the only orchid spice, is one of the most sought-after flavor, and the second-costliest spice, only to saffron. Vanilla produces vanillin which is a proven antioxidant, antidepressant, and exhibits anti-tumor properties.

Vanilla contains about 500 compounds that render its unique flavor and fragrance, and vanillin is the most prominent and studied compound. Though the world seeks vanilla as a flavoring agent, benefits of its consumption, have indicated its effects which are promising on human health too. The pleasant aroma of vanilla, calms stresses, refreshes the mind and revitalizes energy, and has a direct impact on the nervous system, and can help with anxiety, calm, and relieve stress, hence also popular as part of aromatherapy treatment.

The diverse health benefits of vanilla include antibacterial properties, and application of its essential oil to medical devices, inhibited the proliferation of specific bacterial cells (Bilcu et al., 2014). Results of the study by Gokce et al. (2011) have shown that vanillin, ethyl vanillin, and vanillic acid play an inhibitory role in control of *Cronobacter* spp. in food preparation and storage industries. Vanillin exhibited antidepressant activity in mice which is comparable with fluoxetine, which could be due to the antioxidant property (Ahsan et al., 2013).

Shifting our life styles would be the best alternative to get healed of the pathological conditions, which seem to lead the world towards pandemics. Man has the right to define and defend his health, and the knowledge of medicinal potential of these spices can be utilized to live a longer and healthier life, in good mental and physical health condition.

Curcumin in turmeric is an antiviral compound with a potent fighting potential against most viruses that cause strong common colds and flues. As cumin seeds are rich in iron, its intake ensures availability of an integral component of hemoglobin that transports oxygen from the lungs to the entire body, keeping the immune system healthy. Loaded with antibacterial and antioxidant properties, black pepper boosts the immunity while working as an excellent antibiotic. Clove helps to break up phlegm and prevent respiratory tract infections, being an organic expectorant. Carom seeds have been traditionally used in dealing with respiratory ailments associated with myriad flues.

21.3 FUTURE OF RESEARCH ON EXPLOITING SPICES AS MEDICINES

All the 109 herbs and spices listed by ISO have medicinal and therapeutical uses and values. Cultivated organically, spice, and herbs based Neutra-pharmaceuticals would become the ideal targets for internal and external medicines. The recent occurrence of COVID-19 due to Coronavirus necessitates anticipatory research on spices and herbs for developing curative and preventive medicines. Being part of food, herbs, and spices are taken and absorbed as synthetic and chemical molecules without side effects. The document Vision-2050 of ICAR-IISR, Kozhikode (www.spices.res.in) envisages Improvement, Production, Protection, Natural Resource Management, Value Addition and Product Development, as its mission. Being exported to more than 100 countries, emphasis is on 'clean rather not cleaned' herbs and spices. Indian Council of Medical Research (ICMR), Council for Scientific and Industrial Research (CSIR), Indian Council of Agricultural Research (ICAR) and Ministry of AYUSH (www.ayush.gov.in) are mandated with plant-based drug discovery. Ministry of AYUSH guides and supports Ayurveda, Yoga, and Naturopathy, Unani, Siddha, Homoeopathy, and SOWA-RIGPA, where herbs and spices are base materials for new drug development and pharmaceutical uses.

KEYWORDS

- antioxidant
- bioactive compounds
- flavor
- immunity
- medicine
- spices

REFERENCES

Aggarwal, B. B., Van, K. M. E., Iyer, L. H., Harikumar, K. B., & Sung, B., (2009). Molecular targets of nutraceuticals derived from dietary spices: potential role in suppression of inflammation and tumorigenesis. *Exp. Biol. Med. (Maywood), 234*(8), 825–849.

Ahsan, S., Mukta, C., Gokul, P., Amritha, R., & Ashish, S., (2013). Evaluation of antidepressant activity of vanillin in mice *Indian J. Pharmacol., 45*(2), 141–144.

Anderson, R. A., (2003). Cinnamon improves glucose and lipids of people with type 2 diabetes. *Diabetes Care., 26*(12), 3215–3218.

Bilcu, M., Grumezescu, A. M., Oprea, A. E., Popescu, R. C., Mogoșanu, G. D., Hristu, R., Stanciu, G. A., et al., (2014). Efficiency of vanilla, patchouli and Ylang Ylang essential oils stabilized by iron oxide@C14 nanostructures against bacterial adherence and bio-films formed by *Staphylococcus aureus* and *Klebsiella pneumonia* clinical strains. *Molecules, 19*(11), 17943–17956.

Bordia, A., Verma, S. K., & Srivastava, K. C., (1997). Effect of ginger (*Zingiber officinale*) and fenugreek (*Trigonella foenum-graecum*) on blood lipids, blood sugar and platelet aggregation in patients with coronary artery disease. *Prostaglandins Leukot Essent Fatty Acids, 56*(5), 379–384.

Bosland, P. W., (1992). Chillies: A diverse crop. *Hort. Tech., 2*, 6–10.

Crawford, P., (2009). Effectiveness of cinnamon for lowering hemoglobin A1C in patients with type 2 diabetes: A randomized, controlled trial. *J. Amer. Board. Fam. Med., 22*, 507–512.

Gokce, P., Yemiş, F. P., Susan, B., & Pascal, D., (2011). Effect of vanillin, ethyl vanillin, and vanillic acid on the growth and heat resistance of *Cronobacter* species. *Journal of Food Protection, 74*(12), 2062–2069.

Jana, S., & Shekhawat, G. S., (2010). *Anethum graveolens:* An Indian traditional medicinal herb and spice. *Pharmacognosy Reviews, 4*(8), 179–184.

Judith, G., Dausch, D., & Nixon, W., (1990). Garlic: A review of its relationship to malignant disease. *Preventive Medicine, 19*, 346–361.

Kazemi, S., Yaghooblou, F., Siassi, F., Rahimi, F. A., Ghavipour, M., Koohdani, F., & Sotoudeh, G., (2017). Cardamom supplementation improves inflammatory and oxidative stress biomarkers in hyperlipidemic, overweight, and obese pre-diabetic women: A randomized double-blind clinical trial. *J. Sci. Food Agric., 97*(15), 5296–5301.

Konmun, J., Danwilai, K., Ngamphaiboon, N., Sripanidkulchai, B., Sookprasert, A., & Subongkot, S., (2017). A phase II randomized double-blind placebo-controlled study of 6-gingerol as an anti-emetic in solid tumor patients receiving moderate to highly emetogenic chemotherapy. *Med. Oncol., 34*(4), 69.

Kumar, S., Kumar, R., & Singh, J., (2006). Cayenne / American pepper. In: Peter, K. V., (ed.), *Handbook of Herbs and Spices* (Vol. 3, pp. 299–312). CRC Press, Woodhead Publishing Limited England.

Malhotra, S. K., (2006). Caraway. In: Peter, K. V., (ed.), *Handbook of Herbs and Spices* (Vol. 3, pp. 270–298). CRC Press, Woodhead Publishing Limited, England.

Malhotra, S. K., (2006). Nigella. In: Peter, K. V., (ed.), *Handbook of Herbs and Spices* (Vol. 2, pp. 206–214). CRC Press, Woodhead Publishing Limited, England.

Maoka, T., Mochida, K., Kozuka, M., Ito, Y., Fujiwara, Y., Hashimoto, K., Eno, F., et al., (2001). Cancer chemopreventive activity of carotenoids in the fruits of red paprika *Capsicum annuum* L. *Cancer Letter, 172*, 103–109.

Marx, W., Ried, K., McCarthy, A. L., Vitetta, L., Sali, A., McKavanagh, D., & Isenring, L., (2017). Ginger-Mechanism of action in chemotherapy-induced nausea and vomiting. *Crit. Rev. Food Sci Nutr., 57*(1), 141–146.

Nilius, B., & Appendino, G., (2013). Spices: The savory and beneficial science of pungency. *Rev. Physiol. Biochem. Pharmacol., 164*, 1–76.

Nishino, H., Murakosh, M., Il, T., Takemura, M., Kuchide, M., Kanazawa, M., Mou, X. Y., et al., (2002). Carotenoids in cancer chemoprevention. *Cancer Metastasis Rev., 21*, 257–264.

Noorbala, A. A., Akhondzadeh, S., Tahmacebi-Pour, N., & Jamshidi, A. H., (2005). Hydro-alcoholic extract of *Crocus sativus* L. versus fluoxetine in the treatment of mild to moderate depression: A double-blind, randomized pilot trial. *J. Ethnopharmacol., 97*(2), 281–284.

Opara, E. I., & Chohan, M., (2014). Culinary herbs and spices: Their bioactive properties, the contribution of polyphenols and the challenges in deducing their true health benefits. *Int. J. Mol. Sci., 15*(10), 19183–19202.

Pattanaik, S., Hota, D., Prabhakar, S., Kharbanda, P., & Pandhi, P., (2006). Effect of piperine on the steady-state pharmacokinetics of phenytoin in patients with epilepsy. *Phytother Res., 20*(8), 683–686.

Pattanaik, S., Hota, D., Prabhakar, S., Kharbanda, P., & Pandhi, P., (2009). Pharmacokinetic interaction of single dose of piperine with steady-state carbamazepine in epilepsy patients. *Phytother. Res., 23*(9), 1281–1286.

Perry, N. S., Bollen, C., Perry, E. K., & Ballard, C., (2003). *Salvia* for dementia therapy: Review of pharmacological activity and pilot tolerability clinical trial. *Pharmacol. Biochem. Behav., 75*(3), 651–659.

Peter, K. V., & Nirmal, B. K., (2012). Introduction to herbs and spices and sustainable production. In: Peter, K. V., (ed.), *Handbook of Herbs and Spices* (Vol. II, pp. 1–15). CRC Press.

Peter, K. V., & Shylaja, M. R., (2012). Introduction to herbs and spices: Definitions, trade and application. In: Peter, K. V., (ed.), *Handbook of Herbs and Spices* (Vol. I, pp. 1–24). CRC Press.

Prasad, S., Sung, B., & Aggarwal, B. B., (2012). Age-associated chronic diseases require age-old medicine: Role of chronic inflammation. *Prev. Med., 54*(Suppl), S29–37.

Ravindran, P. N., Nirmal, B. K., & Shylaja, M., (2003). *Cinnamon and Cassia: The Genus Cinnamomum, Medicinal and Aromatic Plants - Industrial Profiles*. CRC Press.

Ravindran, P. N., Nirmal, B. K., & Sivaraman, K., (2007). *Turmeric: The genus Curcuma, Medicinal and Aromatic Plants - Industrial Profiles*. CRC Press.

Sharma, M. M., & Sharma, R. K., (2006). Coriander. In: Peter, K. V., (ed.), *Handbook of Herbs and Spices* (Vol. 2, pp. 145–161). CRC Press, Woodhead Publishing Limited, England.

Sung, B., Prasad, S., Yadav, V. R., & Aggarwal, B. B., (2012). Cancer cell signaling pathways targeted by spice-derived nutraceuticals. *Nutr Cancer, 64*(2), 173–1797.

Verma, S. K., & Bordia, A., (1998). Antioxidant property of Saffron in man. *Indian J. Med. Sci., 52*(5), 205–207.

Weiss, E. A., (2002). *Spice Crops* (pp. 356–360). CABI Publishing, Wallingford.

CHAPTER 22

MEDICINAL PLANTS: FUTURE THRUST AREAS AND RESEARCH DIRECTIONS

K. V. PETER[1] and A. B. SHARANGI[2]

[1]*Former Vice-Chancellor, Kerala Agricultural University and Director, ICAR Indian Institute of Spices Research, Calicut; Mullakkara, P. O. Mannuthy – 680651, Thrissur, Kerala, India*

[2]*Department of Plantation, Spices, Medicinal, and Aromatic Crops, Bidhan Chandra Krishi Viswavidyalaya (Agricultural University), Mohanpur, Nadia, West Bengal – 741235, India, E-mail: absharangi@gmail.com*

ABSTRACT

"Let the earth bring forth grass, the herb that yields seed, and the fruit tree that yields fruit according to its kind, whose seed is in itself, on the earth" and it was so.   *–Genesis 1.11*

Therapeutic uses of plants-herbs, spices, fruits, vegetables, tubers, medicinal, and aromatics, bamboos, and mushrooms- are well established against diseases-viral, viroidal, fungal, bacterial-, and disorders-deficiency and allergic. Role of plants in health and wellness finds mention in ancient books, archives, and folk songs. Civilizations like Chinese, Greek, Aryan, Dravidian, Persian and Buddhist mention plants as neutra-pharmaceuticals and cleansers of human body and habitats. Psychosomatic influences of plants on the human mind to drive away depression are well known. Herbs like tulsi (*Ocimum sanctum*), brahmi (*Bacopa monnieri*) and spices like ginger (*Zingiber officinale*), turmeric (*Curcuma longa*), cardamom (*Elettaria cardamomum*) and black pepper (*Piper nigrum*) are used to make home remedies against ailments. "Health for All" is the global goal of WHO. Organic cultivation of medicinal and aromatic plants (MAPs) following GAP is being encouraged. The MAP sector faces several challenges-loss of MAP ecotypes and ecology and non-availability of novel varieties with high yield, quality, and tolerance to biotic and abiotic stresses. The estimated global herbal industry is valued at US$ 60 billion mainly in the form of pharmaceuticals (US$ 40 billion), spices, and herbs (US$ 5.9 billion), natural cosmetics (US$ 7 billion) and essential oil (US$ 4 billion)-growing at 7% per year. Essential oils (EOs) from MAP used in food and flavoring industry, beverages, toiletries, pharmaceuticals, and pesticide industry are in growing demand. Viral diseases like Corona-16 are threatening the very existence of human and animal race. In the fight against dreaded diseases, MAP has a vital role. Systems of medicine like Chinese, Ayurveda, Siddha, Unani, Amchi (Tibetan), Greek, African, and Tribal make use of MAP in alleviating agony of diseases and disorders through drug discovery and uses. Preference for plant based drugs over conventional medicines is growing with the rising global population from present 6.8 billion to 9.1 billion by 2050 (ICAR-DMAPR, 2015).

22.1 INTRODUCTION

Nature is sustaining a considerable number of medicinal and aromatic plants (MAPs) which contain active Neutra-pharmaceuticals and complex phytomolecules, a few of which are to be scientifically recognized and analyzed. These plants are used for health and wellness of both body and mind since millennia. Out of anticipated 2,50,000 to 3,50,000 plant species recognized so far, about 35,000 are used globally for health, wellness, preventive, and curative purposes. The World Health Organization (WHO) reports that plants and herbs based drugs provide the health requirements of approximately 80% of the world's population and more than ever so for millions of people in the vast rural areas of developing countries. For the moment, increased frustration of the consumers in developed countries with existing healthcare practices led to a further search for suitable alternatives. Several factors, viz., the efficacy of pro-nature phytomedicines, the harmful downbeat side effects of most modern drugs and the development of science and technology are responsible for the current resurgence of remedies with natural plant-based drugs.

22.2 CONSERVATION AND IMPROVEMENT OF EXISTING GENETIC RESOURCES

More than one-tenth of plant species (50,000) are used in the manufacture of drugs leading to health and wellness products. Medicinal plants are not distributed consistently across the world (Huang, 2011; Rafieian-Kopaei, 2013). China and India uphold the uppermost spots in the usage of medicinal plants, with 11, 146, and 7,500 species, respectively, followed by Colombia, South Africa, the United States of America, and 16 other countries with sizeable percentages of medicinal plants (Rafieian-Kopaei, 2013; Hamilton, 2003; Marcy et al., 2005; Srujana et al., 2012). Enhanced number of MAPs in certain species of several plant families is often associated with a higher magnitude of vulnerability compared to others (Huang, 2011). A few of them which undergo genetic erosion and resource obliteration are scheduled to be listed as threatened (Schippmann, 2005; Deeb et al., 2013).

Infrequency index of species is used to appraise the extinction risk of medicinal plants, and to identify the one with a huge risk of extinction before conservation initiatives (Figueiredo and Grelle, 2009). It is necessary to determine how uncommon and sporadic each species is and in which ways extraordinary species differ from the rest individually. Harvesting pressure-based destruction is not similar to all medicinal plants (Wagh and Jain, 2013; Andel and Havinga, 2008). Overexploitation, random collection, uninhibited deforestation, and habitat destruction all influence species rarity, but are inadequate to elucidate individual species vulnerability or resilience to harvest pressure. Multiple biological characters show a relationship with extinction risk, such as habitat specificity, allocation range, population size, species diversity, intensification rate and reproductive system.

Wealth of MAP is being harvested in increasing volumes; mainly from wild populations in recent decades. In Europe, North America, and Asia the demand for natural resources is augmented to the extent of 8–15% annually. There is a threshold below which reproductive competence of plant species becomes irrevocably reduced (Soule et al., 2005; Semwal et al., 2007). A good number of recommendations involving *in situ* and *ex situ* conservation of medicinal plants are formulated (Huang, 2011; Liu et al., 2011). Natural reserves and wild nurseries are classic examples to keep hold of the medicinal effectiveness of plants in their usual habitats, whereas botanic gardens and seed banks are imperative for *ex situ* conservation and potential replanting (Sheikh et al., 2002; Coley et al., 2003). A knowledge of the geographic distribution and biological characteristics of MAPs is essential to steer conservation initiatives with a view to compare species conservation between nature or in a protected nursery. Studying the conservation status of all species in trade is also obligatory. This clearly opens up a big challenge for conservationists, policymakers, researchers, industry, and farmers to manage MAPs wisely and economically (Figure 22.1).

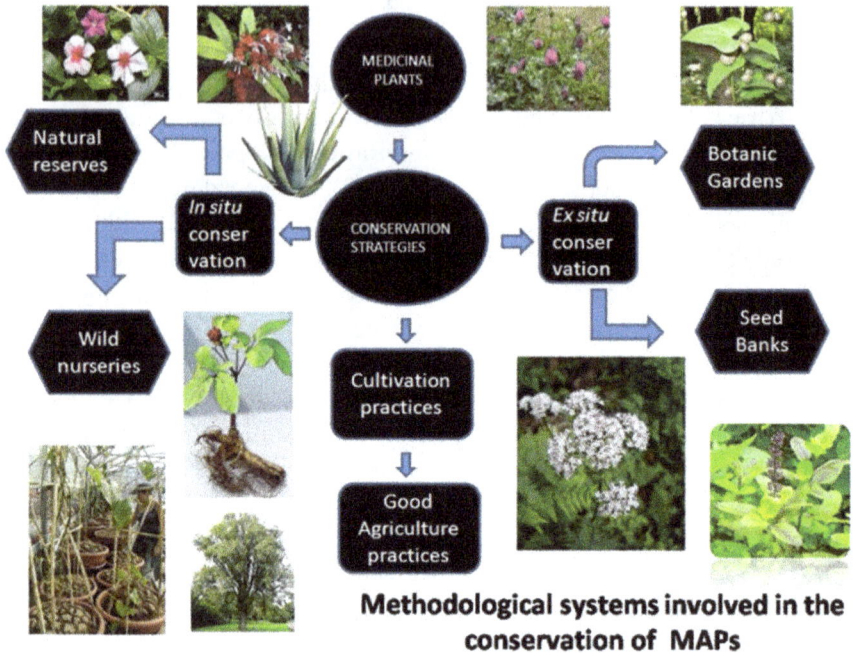

FIGURE 22.1 Methodological systems involved in the conservation of medicinal and aromatic plants.

Source: Adapted after: Chen et al. (2016).

22.3 SUSTAINING STRATEGIES FOR DEVELOPMENT OF HERBAL PLANTS

The of scope bringing cultivable lands under MAPs is limited as the demand for food grains, sugar cane, pulses, oilseeds, fruits, vegetables, and tubers are increasing. Medicinal plants can very well be accommodated as intercrops in plantations and field crops to derive maximum benefit of limited space, soil moisture, nutrients, and other inputs. Intercropping of one medicinal plant with other or with cereals, vegetables, and fruits, will give extra income without affecting the growth and yield of the target crop. Chickpea was more successful than safflower, linseed, mustard, and wheat intercropped with Senna (*Cassia angustifolia*) in obtaining better senna herb yield and maximum net return. Growing *patchouli (Pogostemon cablin)* with French bean is much remunerative over growing p*atchouli* alone when *patchouli* essential oil equivalent and gross returns are considered. Radish gave more returns with the highest mint oil equivalent yield among various intercrops tried with menthol mint. Growing lentil, a legume as intercrop is highly favorable as this combination over-yields the sole citronella even in terms of yield of citronella oil. Palms, being widely spaced perennial crops, provide excellent scope for intercropping with MAPs. Lemongrass adopts well under coconut shade and yields more than the sole crop. Yield of most of the intercrops kalmegh (*Andrographis paniculata*), makoi (*Shorea assamica*), medicinal coleus (*Coleus forskolin*), garden rue (*Ruta graveolens*), Lepidium (*Lepidium spp.*), tulsi (*Ocimum sanctum*), arrowroot (*Curcuma aromaticum*), kacholam (*Kaempferia galanga*), cowhage (*Mucuna pruriens*), roselle (*Hibiscus sabdariffa*), ambrette (*Abelmoschus moschatus*), citronella (*Cymbopogon nardus*) and vetiver (*Chrysopogon zizanioides*) are reduced due to shade effect. Inter-spaces of black pepper gardens can be effectively utilized for growing MAPs. The rice-wheat rotation with mint has been successfully accomplished over large area growing MAPs. Forests in alpine, sub-alpine, Northwest Himalayas, Afro-mountain areas, humid tropics or temperate regions of Asia offer cultivation scope of highly cherished MAPs. Aromatic grasses like vetiver (*Chrysopogon zizanoides*), lemongrass (*Cymbopogon flexuosus*) and citronella (*Cymbopogon nardus*) can be grown on-field and soil conservation bunds in croplands in contour strips or as a live hedge barrier. Medicinal trees like amla and bael endure saline and alkaline conditions and are recommended for salt-affected soils. Protected cultivation of MAPs is standardized to save space, moisture, and energy. Vertical farming, hydroponics, and aeroponics of MAPs are practiced in urban and peri-urban areas. *In vitro* production of active principles of MAPs is successfully achieved and phytochemistry of *in vitro* metabolites-primary and secondary-is elucidated. There are significant increased harvestable products from MAPs under protected cultivation.

The most crucial stage in any drug development program, using plants as the starting material is the collection and analysis of information on the use(s) of plant(s) by various native habitats. Ethnobotany, ethnomedicine, folk medicine and tribal and traditional medicine (TM) provide information useful as a 'pre-screen' to decide on plants for pharmacological studies. The following scheme represents a summary of the stages involved in the development of pure drug from a plant source.

- Collection and conservation;
- Ancient and current literature survey;

- Extraction with solvent(s) and preparation of non-polar and polar extracts for initial biological testing;
- Evaluation of plant extract(s) by receptor binding, enzyme inhibition and /or cytotoxicity assays;
- Activity guided fractionation on the extract by monitoring each chromatographic fraction with bioassay;
- Structure and elucidation of pure active isolate(s) using spectroscopic techniques and chemical methods;
- *In vitro* and *in vivo* biological tests of each active compound to determine strength and selectivity of the drug;
- Molecular modeling studies and preparation of derivatives of active compounds;
- clinical trials (Phases I–III).

22.4   GENETIC IMPROVEMENT AND BREEDING STRATEGIES

In general, a very few medicinal plant species are only sexually sterile, but the majority have some sexual fertility. Based on the breeding objectives, any breeding program involves three important steps, i.e., induction of variability, selection of desired traits and propagation and multiplication of new varieties. For meeting the above goal, either of the conventional breeding methods like introduction, selection, hybridization-intra, and interspecific, polyploidy, and mutation, alone or in combination are effective. Additional tools like tissue culture techniques (micropropagation, selection, embryo culture, anther culture, cell suspension culture, and protoplast fusion) and recombination techniques (marker-assisted selection (MAS) and genetic transformation) are also being utilized. At each step, different techniques can be applied which have an impact at plant/population level, cell/tissue level and DNA level.

Under conventional breeding, the general selection methods available for medicinal plant improvement are mass and progeny selection, pure line selection, pedigree method, bulk breeding, backcross method, population improvement, recurrent selection, clonal selection, mutation breeding, polyploidy, and distant hybridization which improve the yield and quality of secondary metabolites. These methods do not always bestow the desirable level of improvement for several reasons, viz., sterility, elongated generation time, perenniallity, and complex biosynthetic pathway, etc. Even though the breeding objectives may be different for each species, the following objectives may be common for most of the medicinal plants:

- to increase the content and chemical profile of active compounds above and beyond higher yield;
- to have the basic agronomic characters related to uniformity, stability, growth, and development and resistance/tolerance to biotic and abiotic stresses.

The organic systems approach requires varieties which match a different crop ideotype in which it is more important to adapt the variety to the (given) organic environment rather than the environment to the variety. This includes (i) organic soil fertility management, (ii) a better root system and ability to interact with beneficial soil micro-organisms), (iii) ability to suppress weeds, (iv) contributing to soil and crop health, (v) good product quality, (vii) elevated yield level and high yield stability, and (viii) ability to produce healthy propagules under organic conditions.

22.5 BIOTECHNOLOGY: EMERGING AREAS OF INTERVENTION

Agro-biotechnology aids to increase the biosynthetic ability of neutra-pharmaceutical crops and to produce commercial biopharmaceuticals, functional proteins and edible vaccines in the plant body. Research targets are focused on identifying the genes involved in the biosynthesis of secondary metabolites for treatments of diseases and disorders. Metabolic control through genetic manipulation of plants is key to regulate biosynthetic pathways. Unlike cereals and other economic crops, the progress in the field of biotechnology of MAPs is slow.

Different types of markers like restriction fragment length polymorphism (RFLP), random amplified polymorphic DNA (RAPD), inter simple sequence repeats (ISSR), simple sequence repeats (SSR) and amplified fragment length polymorphism (AFLP) markers are used for validation purpose in MAPs. DNA barcodes using second internal transcribed spacer (ITS2) region are used for discriminating medicinal plant species (Pang and Chen, 2014). RAPD analysis was used for evaluation of genetic relationships in several medicinal plant species. ISSR markers were used to evaluate the genetic diversity in many of the medicinal plants. Molecular markers can be employed to characterize any phenotypic trait, biochemical, and/or physiological mechanisms. The direct measurement of such traits can be simultaneously mapped. The number of loci controlling genetic variation of any important agronomic trait(s) in segregating population can be estimated, and the map positions of these loci in the genome be determined by means of molecular linkage genetic maps and QTL mapping technology.

In setting up priorities for conserving and researching MAPs, wild plants with small populations have greater precedence over plants already in cultivation. For wild plants, priority precedence is to be given to perennials over annuals as priority. Furthermore, MAPs grown for their roots and barks should receive special attention. Meanwhile, the future of MAPs harvested for leaves, flowers, and fruits are to a certain extent quite safe, and they may be exposed in danger of extinction if they are sensitive to habitat disturbances and grow only in virgin forests.

The science of genetic engineering has led to large-scale biosynthesis of natural products, and advancements in tissue and cell culture and fermentation of medicinal plants. As a consequence, newer avenues for large-scale and highly efficient production of desirable bioactive compounds and secondary metabolites have opened up. Micro plant culture (including plant, tissue, cell, and transgenic hairy root culture) is a potential substitute for the production of rare and high-value secondary metabolites of medicinal importance (Rao and Ravishankar, 2002). Micropropagation via tissue encapsulation of propagules facilitates storage and transportation and promotes higher regeneration rates as well (Baker et al., 2007). Synthetic seed technology (artificially encapsulated somatic embryos) could be used for cultivation *in vitro* or *ex vitro* and is a feasible alternative in times of inadequate availability of normal seeds (Zych et al., 2005; Lata et al., 2008). Harnessing the genetic potential of MAPs through application of biotechnology is still at infancy. With the availability of genome sequencing of model plants and the availability of high output sequencing technology and understanding of genetic control, MAPs can be tailored to human needs.

22.6   ENHANCING QUALITY AND VALUE ADDITION

To achieve uniform standards of herbal medicines worldwide, the harvesting process and period, incidents of adulteration, presence of microorganisms and pesticides/residues, have high impact. Quality of herbal medicines is contingent upon good agricultural practices (GAPs), good manufacturing practices (GMPs), packaging of finished herbal products, and in post-marketing quality assurance surveillance (Fong, 2002). Broad-based screening of plant materials, specific activity evaluation, chemical evaluation, pharmacological, and clinical evaluation; drug designing, pharmacogenomics, drug safety and efficacy evaluation along with clinical studies of herbal medicines are principle requirements towards drug development and quality control as reported by Kurian and Sanker (2007). GAPs and GMPs are also given due emphasis in this regard (Kurian and Sanker, 2007). GMPs ensure raw materials used in the manufacture of drugs are authentic, of prescribed quality and free from contamination-physical, microbiological. Adequate quality control measures are prescribed and guidelines followed till the drugs reach the consumers. Some of the technologies for metabolite characterization and quality control include NMR-based metabolic fingerprinting, HPLC, GC, HPLC-PDA-ESI/MS, HPLC-DAD-ESI/MS, GC/MS, GCxGC-qMS, TOF/MS, GCxGC-TOF/MS, MALDI-TOF/MS, HPLC/UV, TLC, UPLC, UPLC-Q/TOF-MS, IT-TOF-MS, CEC, TFC, HPLC/ESI/MS, etc.

22.7   ADULTERATION ISSUES

Proper use of herbal medicinal products of 'assured quality' ensures beneficial therapeutic effects on users and decreases the risks associated with allopathic medicines. It should also be noted that, similar to allopathic drugs, herbs and herbal products are not free from side effects. Regulations and registration of herbal drugs are often neglected, ill-planned, poorly developed in most of the countries, and the quality of herbal products sold is, therefore, not guaranteed. Till date, taxonomists could identify and name only about a third of the million or so species of higher plants. Of those named, only a minuscule fraction is studied. Furthermore, the use of impure herbal ingredients and wrong formulations have definite consequences in the production of low-quality and harmful or even unsafe herbal medicines.

The herbal medicines hold good future prospects and they may come out as good substitutes or superior alternatives for synthetic chemicals-based allopathic drugs or may even substitute them. At the present time, a new approach provides the linking of the indigenous knowledge of medicinal plants to contemporary research activities turning the rate of discovery of drugs much more efficient than with unsystematic collection. Herbal medicines should be brought under officially authorized legal control across countries, and efforts should be made to elevate public awareness level on the risks and benefits of using herbal medicines.

22.8 OMICS AND OTHER TECHNOLOGIES

The post-genomic period witnessed the emergence of "omic" studies in biological research. System science and omics-biotechnology-driven strategies can be used potentially to unravel the yet to be untapped potential for novel molecular target discovery. An array of technology platforms, viz., System biology, Bioinformatics, Genomics, Proteomics, Transcriptomics, Metabolomics, Automated separation techniques, Computer-aided drug design, Transgenic, and RNAi technology, Biochip, and Automated separation techniques are there in course of herbal drug development through system biology. The understanding of the mechanism of action of herbal bioactive principles has introduced vistas of scientific methods for the modernization and standardization of several herbal medicines including those of Chinese (Buriani et al., 2012). Epigenomics, metagenomics, toxicogenomics, pharmacogenomics, herbogenomics, metallomics, etc., are a few "omic" approaches at the genetic level. Newer approaches and insights into herbal medicine through Research and Development (R&D) led to development of abundant traditional remedies and ground-breaking drug discovery systems (Pang et al., 2011), which will make an immense impact on the typical biomedical science (Trusheim et al., 2007; Parekh et al., 2009).

22.9 DEVELOPMENT OF HERBAL DRUGS AND ITS CHALLENGES

For developing newer drugs, medicinal plants are the fundamental natural inputs (Heinrich, 2000; Shakya et al., 2012). More than 80% of drugs are either straightway derivatives of natural products or developed from a natural compound (Maridass and John de Britto, 2008). Around 50% of pharmaceuticals are derivatives of compounds first identified or isolated from herbs/plants, including micro-organisms, animals, and insects, as active ingredients (Krief et al., 2004). The development of plant based drugs started in the prehistoric period and flourished gradually with concurrent developments in analytical chemistry, isolation techniques, purification, characterization of active plant compounds, application in synthesis of new molecules and introduction of robotics, artificial intelligence and big data. Herbal medicine is effective in particular, having lesser side effects, and reasonably priced than the allopathic and/or synthetic medicines. It is well documented that herbal plants and their derivatives play crucial roles in contemporary drug development.

Chinese herbal medicine (CHM) and Indian Herbal Medicine (IHM), developed in ancient China, Japan, Korea, and India, are still having immense influence on the current healthcare (Samy et al., 2008). Herbal drug discovery may be on three stages, namely, pre-drug stage, quasi-drug stage, and full-drug stage. The "quasi drug" stage in drug discovery from herbal medicine starts with the preparation of extracts from herbs, phytochemical grouping and identification of lead compounds by using modern and conventional research tools. When potential drug candidates undergoing clinical trials succeed to prove their efficacy fully, they reach to their full-drug stage. The distinctive herbal drug development process includes a number of aspects including isolation of bioactive ingredient(s), evaluation of safety and efficacy by conventional pharmacological methods and regulatory approval of the therapeutic agents to be used in the market and post-market monitoring.

Quality of an herbal product is often questioned and challenged. Standardization of raw material, therefore, emerges as the foremost issue for herbal industry (Yadav et al., 2014; Patwardhan et al., 2004). Two major problems reported in herbal medicines are adulteration and heavy metal contamination demanding immediate attention. Ecological ethics and resource-dependent sustainable development are also to be addressed. A strategy of drug discovery from nature resources-forests, gardens, and wild growths-differs to a great extent from their synthetic counterparts. Accumulated knowledge, traditional wisdom and technical skill in TM, therefore, plays a pivotal role in enhancing the accomplishment of drug discovery from MAPs.

22.10 FUTURE PROSPECTS AND CONSTRAINTS

22.10.1 PROSPECTS

1. MAPs and their derivatives play a major role in health and wellness therapy in spite of advances in chemical technology. The reaction involved is either difficult or expensive to replicate by common chemical methods. In plants-derived diosgenin and solasodine, where stearic forms are possible, chemical synthesis yields a blend of the isomers which may be somewhat difficult to separate. The synthetic products may, therefore, be noxious or having a divergent curative consequence than the natural ones.

2. The demand for phytopharmaceuticals from MAPs and Vegetables of Indian origin are remarkably high in Western nations. The scenario

is almost similar in the domestic market for raw materials used for perfumeries, pharmacies, and bio-pesticides. The harmful effects of synthetic chemical drugs, lesser side effects of natural drugs, increased number of pharmaceutical companies manufacturing natural drug formulations, ever-increasing health consciousness and reliance on naturopathy all contributed to the enhanced demand for traditional herbal drugs.

3. Cost of drug development out of MAPs is less than synthetic drug production. Reserpine is an excellent example. Cost of synthesis of reserpine is approximately twice compared to one extracted from the plant.

4. Readiness of many countries to absorb and adopt technological changes according to available skill and manpower is another perspective dimension.

5. MAPs have a couple of intrinsic merits like drought hardiness and capability to grow on marginal lands and are relatively free from wild and domesticated animal damage. The MAPs are better earners than many of the field crops.

6. Since they are new crops, there is scope for further improvement in their productivity and adaptability for enhanced returns.

22.10.2 CONSTRAINTS

1. Rate of growth of MAPs in relation to their economic prospects is not always satisfactory in spite of separate Ministry of AYUSH in India and major growing countries.

2. In spite of the positive policy support by the Government of India through institutions like the CSIR-Center for Medicinal and Aromatic Plants (CIMAP): CSIR-Regional Research Laboratories (RRL), at Jammu, Bhubaneshwar, and Jorhat; ICAR-directorate of medicinal and aromatic plants (DMAPR) and ICAR-All India Co-ordinated Research Project on MAPs, Boravi, Anand, Gujarat, National Botanical Gardens, State Botanical Gardens, Indian Forest Research Institute, Dehradun, Uttarakhand, State Forest Research Institutes, State Cinchona Directorates in Tamil Nadu and West Bengal, the replenishments of renewable inputs like quality planting materials of improved varieties, good extension literature, training, and quality testing are extremely inadequate.

3. The other major constraints are climate change, biotic, and abiotic stresses, lack of testing facilities at the procurement and trading centers, unscientific market handling, wide fluctuations in prices and speculative trade practices.

4. Cultivation of a few MAPs is a discouraging enterprise, mainly because of their commercially unviable proposition. There is need for minimum support price (MSP) based on cost of cultivation and marginal income to growers.

5. Although most of them are industry oriented crops, the land-holding model does not provide for commercial cultivation on a wide scale. In a few perennial MAPs, viz., Aonla (*Emblica officinalis*), Asoka (*Saraca asoca*), Arjun (*Terminalia arjuna*), bael (*Aegle marmelos*), nutmeg (*Myristica fragrans*), neem (*Azardicta indica*), the land is occupied for a longer period.

22.11   FUTURISTICS OF RESEARCH

In the face of escalating usage pattern coupled with fast-growing market of herbal medicines and related herbal healthcare products, in both developing and developed countries, policy-makers, health professionals and the general public are gradually more concerned about the safety, efficacy, quality, accessibility, safeguarding, and further development problems of these herbal products. To alleviate these concerns and to congregate community demands, wide-ranging research on herbal medicines is a must, not only for their nature-friendly healthcare values but also for the huge commercial benefits. Fortunately, phytochemical and pharmacological researches on MAPs and their herbal medicines are already quite advanced all through the world, and efforts are being made to segregate and categorize their active chemical constituents to validate the claims of their efficiency and safety. Scientific evidences from randomized clinical trials are reasonably relevant options for the reliance and sustainability of herbal medicines over the time.

The future R&D of MAPs need to address following challenges:

- Production of quality planting materials;
- Conservation, management, and enhancement of MAP germplasm with novel traits;
- Development of good agricultural and collection practices for MAPs;
- Cultivation of MAPs in different cropping and land-use systems;
- Enhancement of input use efficiencies (nutrients, light, and water);

- Elucidation and engineering of biosynthetic pathways of various active compounds;
- Post-harvest operations including value addition;
- Certification of MAP based products and quality assurance of raw drugs;
- Management of pests and diseases in MAPs;
- Identification of promising bio-pesticide molecules from MAPs;
- Ensuring linkages among different MAP stakeholders;
- Creation of the highest level of communications, documentation, and management of databases and indigenous traditional knowledge and use of apps.

KEYWORDS

- **bioprospecting**
- **climate change**
- **future research**
- **ICT**
- **improvement**
- ***in vitro* conservation**
- **indigenous and modern system of healthcare**
- **medicinal and aromatic plants**
- **protection**
- **quality**

REFERENCES

Andel, T. V., & Havinga, R. M., (2008). *Sustainability Aspects of Commercial Medicinal Plants Harvesting in Surinam, 256*,1540–1545.

Buriani, A., Garcia-Bermejo, M. L., Bosisio, E., Xu, Q., Li, H., Dong, X., Simmonds, M. S. J., et al., (2012). Omic techniques in systems biology approaches to traditional Chinese medicine research: Present and future. *J. Ethnopharmacol., 140*, 535–544.

Coley, P. D., Heller, M. V., Aizprua, R., Arauz, B., Flores, N., Correa, M., Gupta, M., et al., (2003). Using ecological criteria to design plant collection strategies for drug discovery. *Front Ecol. Environ., 1*, 421–428.

Deeb, T., Knio, K., Shinwari, Z. K., Kreydiyyeh, S., & Baydoun, E., (2013). Survey of medicinal plants currently used by herbalists in Lebanon. *Pak. J. Bot., 45*, 543–555.

Figueiredo, M. S. L., & Grelle, C. E. V., (2009). Predicting global abundance of a threatened species from its occurrence: Implications for conservation planning. *Divers. Distrib., 15*, 117–121.

Fong, H. H. I., (2002). Integration of herbal medicine into modern medical practices: Issues and prospects. *Integr. Cancer Ther., 1*, 287–293.

Hamilton, A., (2003). *Medicinal Plant and Conservation: Issues and Approaches*. UK: WWF.

Heinrich, M., (2000). Ethnobotany and its role in drug development, *Phytotherapy Res., 14*(7), 479–488.

Huang, H., (2011). Plant diversity and conservation in China: Planning a strategic bioresource for a sustainable future. *Bot. J. Linn. Soc., 166*, 282–300.

ICAR DMAPR, (2015). *Directorate of Medicinal and Aromatic Plants Research* (p. 27). Vision 2050.

Krief, S., Martin, M. T., Grellier, P., Kasenene, J., & S´evenet, T., (2004). Novel antimalarial compounds isolated in a survey of self-medicative behavior of wild chimpanzees in Uganda, *Antimicrobial Agents and Chemotherapy, 48*(8), 3196–3199.

Kurian, A., & Shanker, A., (2007). In: Peter, K. V., (ed.), Medicinal Plants. (p. 351). NewIndia Publishing Agency, New Delhi.

Lata, H., Chandra, S., Khan, I. A., & Elsohly, M. A., (2008). Propagation of *Cannabis sativa* L. using synthetic seed technology. *Plant Med., 74*, 328.

Liu, C., Yu, H., & Chen, S. L., (2011). Framework for sustainable use of medicinal plants in China. *Zhi Wu Fen Lei Yu Zi Yuan Xue Bao., 33*, 65–68.

Marcy, J., Balunasa, A., & Kinghornb, D., (2005). Drug discovery from medicinal plants. *Life Sci., 78*, 431–441.

Maridass, M., & John De, B. A., (2008). Origins of plant derived medicines. *Ethnobotanical Leaflets, 12*, 373–387.

Pan, S. Y., Chen, S. B., Dong, H. G., Yu, Z. L., Dong, J. C., et al., (2011). New perspectives on Chinese herbal medicine (Zhong-yao) research and development. *Evid. Based Complement. Alternat. Med.*, 403–709.

Pang, X., & Chen, S., (2014). Identification of medicinal plants using DNA barcoding technique. *Encyclopedia of Analytical Chemistry* (doi: 10.1002/9780470027318.a9935).

Parekh, H. S., Liu, G., & Wei, M. Q., (2009). A new dawn for the use of traditional Chinese medicine in cancer therapy. *Mol. Cancer, 8*, 21.

Patwardhan, B., Vaidya, A. D. B., & Chorghade, M., (2004). Ayurveda and natural products drugs discovery. *Current Science., 86*(6), 789–799.

Rafieian-Kopaei, M., (2013). Medicinal plants and the human needs. *J. Herb. Med. Pharm., 1*, 1–2.

Samy, R. P., Pushparaj, P. N., & Gopalakrishnakone, P., (2008). A compilation of bioactive compounds from Ayurveda. *Bioinformation, 3*(3), 100–110.

Schippmann, U., Leaman, D. J., Cunningham, A. B., & Walter, S., (*2005*). Impact of cultivation and collection on the conservation of medicinal plants: Global trends and issues. *III WOCMAP Congress on Medicinal and Aromatic Plants: Conservation, Cultivation and Sustainable Use of Medicinal and Aromatic Plants, Chiang Mai.*

Semwal, D. P., Saradhi, P. P., Nautiyal, B. P., & Bhatt, A. B., (2007). Current status, distribution and conservation of rare and endangered medicinal plants of Kedarnath Wildlife Sanctuary, Central Himalayas, India. *Curr. Sci. India, 92*, 1733–1738.

Shakya, A. K., Sharma, N., Saxena, M., Shrivastava, S., & Shukla, S., (2012). Evaluation of the antioxidant and hepatoprotective effect of Majoon-e-Dabeed-ul-ward against carbon tetrachloride induced liver injury. *Experimental Toxicology and Pathology.*, *64*(7, 8), 767–773.

Sheikh, K., Ahmad, T., & Khan, M. A., (2002). Use, exploitation and prospects for conservation: People and plant biodiversity of Naltar Valley, northwestern Karakorum, Pakistan. *Biodivers. Conserv., 11*, 715–742.

Soule, M. E., Estes, J. A., Miller, B., & Honnold, D. L., (2005). Strongly interacting species: Conservation policy, management, and ethics. *Bioscience, 55*, 168–176.

Srujana, S. T., Babu, K. R., & Rao, B. S. S., (2012). Phytochemical investigation and biological activity of leaves extract of plant Boswellia serrata. *Pharm Innov., 1*, 22–46.

Trusheim, M. R., Berndt, E. R., & Douglas, F. L., (2007). Stratified medicine: Strategic and economic implications of combining drugs and clinical biomarkers. *Nat. Rev. Drug Discov, 6*, 287–293.

Wagh, V. V., & Jain, A. K., (2013). Status of threatened medicinal plants of Jhabua district, Madhya Pradesh, India. *Ann Plant Sci., 2*, 395–400.

Yadav, M., Chatterji, S., Gupta, S. K., & Watal, G., (2014). Preliminary phytochemical screening of six medicinal plants used in traditional medicine. *International Journal of Pharmacy and Pharmaceutical Sciences, 6*(5), 539–542.

Zych, M., Furmanowa, M., Krajewska, P. A., Lowicka, A., Dreger, M., & Mendlewska, S., (2005). Micropropagation of *Rhodiola kirilowii* plants using encapsulated axillary buds and callus. *Acta Biol. Cracov. Bot., 47*, 83–87.

INDEX